The Essentials of Respiratory Care

The Essentials of Respiratory Care

Fourth Edition

Robert M. Kacmarek, PhD, RRT, FAARC
Professor
Department of Anesthesia
Harvard Medical School
Director, Respiratory Care
Massachusetts General Hospital
Boston, Massachusetts

Steven Dimas, RRT
Retired President, STAT Home Care
Elmhurst, Illinois

Craig W. Mack, MM, RRT
Director of Professional Services
Gottlieb Memorial Hospital
Melrose Park, Illinois

with over 400 illustations

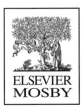

ELSEVIER
MOSBY

ELSEVIER
MOSBY

11830 Westline Industrial Drive
St. Louis, Missouri 63146

The Essentials of Respiratory Care, Fourth Edition

ISBN 0-323-02700-8

NOTICE

Pharmacology is an ever-changing field. Standard safety precautions must be followed, but as new research and clinical experience broaden our knowledge, changes in treatment and drug therapy may become necessary or appropriate. Readers are advised to check the most current product information provided by the manufacturer of each drug to be administered to verify the recommended dose, the method and duration of administration, and contraindications. It is the responsibility of the licensed prescriber, relying on experience and knowledge of the patient, to determine dosages and the best treatment for each individual patient. Neither the Publisher nor the author assumes any liability for any injury and/or damage to persons or property arising from this publication.

The Publisher

Previous editions copyrighted 1990, 1985, 1979.

International Standard Book Number 0-323-02700-8

Managing Editor: Mindy Hutchinson
Senior Developmental Editor: Melissa K. Boyle
Publishing Services Manager: Pat Joiner
Project Manager: David Stein
Senior Designer: Amy Buxton

Printed in the United States of America

Last digit is the print number: 9 8 7 6 5 4 3 2 1

Neila Altobelli, AS, RRT
Staff Respiratory Therapist
Respiratory Care Services
Massachusetts General Hospital
Boston, Massachusetts
CHAPTER 35, *Aerosol and Humidity Therapy*
CHAPTER 38, *Airway Care*

Peter Betit, BS, RRT
Assistant Director
Respiratory Care Services
Boston Children's Hospital
Boston, Massachusetts
CHAPTER 30, *Assisted Ventilation for Pediatric Patients*

Edward Burns, BA, RRT
Quality Assurance Coordinator
Respiratory Care Services
Massachusetts General Hospital
Boston, Massachusetts
CHAPTER 37, *Analyzers*

Daniel W. Chipman, BA, RRT
Assistant Director
Respiratory Care Services
Massachusetts General Hospital
Boston, Massachusetts
CHAPTER 20, *Obstructive Pulmonary Disease and General Management Principles*
CHAPTER 22, *Restrictive Lung Diseases: General and Ventilatory Management*

Gary W. Collymore, BSM, RRT
Senior Respiratory Therapist
Respiratory Care Services
Massachusetts General Hospital
Boston, Massachusetts
CHAPTER 33, *Gas Therapy*

Patricia English, MS, RRT
Senior Respiratory Therapist
Respiratory Care Services
Massachusetts General Hospital
Boston, Massachusetts
CHAPTER 28, *Mechanical Ventilation of the Newborn*

Daniel F. Fisher, BS, RRT
Senior Respiratory Therapist
Respiratory Care Services
Massachusetts General Hospital
Boston, Massachusetts
CHAPTER 24, *Nutrition*

Robert Goulet, MS, RRT
Senior Respiratory Therapist
Respiratory Care Services
Massachusetts General Hospital
Boston, Massachusetts
CHAPTER 17, *Pharmacology*

Joseph Kratohvil, LPN, RRT
Clinical Support Coordinator
Respiratory Care Services
Massachusetts General Hospital
Boston, Massachusetts
CHAPTER 34, *Oxygen, Helium, and Nitric Oxide Therapy*

Steven C. Mason, RRT/NPS
Staff Respiratory Therapist
Respiratory Care Services
Massachusetts General Hospital
Boston, Massachusetts
CHAPTER 26, *Assessment and Management of the Newborn*
CHAPTER 29, *Respiratory Disorders of the Pediatric Patient*

Christopher M. Piccuito, AS, RRT, NPS
Senior Respiratory Therapist
Respiratory Care Services
Massachusetts General Hospital
Boston, Massachusetts
CHAPTER 36, *Airway Clearance Techniques*

John Thompson, RRT
Director
Respiratory Care Services
Boston Children's Hospital
Boston, Massachusetts
CHAPTER 30, *Assisted Ventilation for Pediatric Patients*

Purris F. Williams, BS, RRT
Senior Respiratory Therapist
Respiratory Care Services
Massachusetts General Hospital
Boston, Massachusetts
CHAPTER 19, *Pulmonary Function Testing*
CHAPTER 27, *Respiratory Disorders of the Newborn*

With love to Jan, Robert, Julia, Katie, and Callie
Carol, Eric, Cassandra, James, and Max
Karen, Brian, and Justin

The profession of respiratory care has matured. Over the 15 years since the last edition of this book, the knowledge required for a respiratory care practitioner has increased and markedly developed into a more uniform and consistent body of information. We hope we have captured the essentials of this in our new edition. This edition is completely revised and expanded about 25%. We have removed the detailed technical information on mechanical ventilation and other technology. This information changes so rapidly that it is impossible for a book detailing it to be current. In addition, the current textbooks addressing these issues are excellent. All other areas of the book have been expanded.

The organization of the book has been revised to more logically group the chapters on various topics. All anatomy and physiology and basic science chapters have been updated. The chapters covering mechanical ventilation and neonatal/pediatric respiratory care have been completely rewritten and expanded. A number of chapters have been added detailing newer adjunctive therapies in critical care. The chapters on pharmacology, pulmonary rehabilitation, home care, modes of mechanical ventilation, PEEP, and initiation, maintenance, and weaning from ventilatory support in particular have been completely rewritten.

As in previous editions, the stated goal of this text is to present what we believe is the knowledge base required of respiratory care practitioners in a logical and concise manner. The entire text is in outline form and as a result is probably best used as a secondary text, since a certain level of overall understanding is assumed. We have found that this text is best used for review and quick reference. Following each chapter is a bibliography of both primary texts and periodicals to guide the practitioner to original presentations of material.

We believe one of the primary uses of this text is in the preparation for certification, registration, and licensure examination.

Robert M. Kacmarek, PhD, RRT, FAARC
Steven Dimas, RRT

A very sincere and special thank you to Julia Kacmarek and Katie Kacmarek for their assistance with artwork.

In addition, a sincere thank you to all of our students and associates, past and present, who have provided the enthusiasm and dedication to inspire us to grow, develop, and continually question.

Finally we are eternally indebted to Jane Donohue and Debra Duffy for their understanding, skill, and everlasting patience in the preparation of this manuscript.

3 Microbiology, Sterilization, and Infection Control, *42*

SECTION II:
Cardiopulmonary and Related Anatomy and Physiology

4 Anatomy of the Respiratory System, *69*

5 Mechanics of Ventilation, *96*

SECTION III:
The Nervous System and Pharmacology

SECTION IV:
Cardiopulmonary Assessment and Diseases and Their Management

18 Clinical Assessment of the Cardiopulmonary System, *325*

19 Pulmonary Function Testing, *344*

BY PURRIS F. WILLIAMS

20 Obstructive Pulmonary Disease and General Management Principles, *365*

BY DANIEL W. CHIPMAN

24 Nutrition, *428*

SECTION V:
Neonatal and Pediatric Respiratory Care

25 Intrauterine Development and Comparative Respiratory Anatomy, *445*

29 Respiratory Disorders of the Pediatric Patient, *522*

By *STEVEN C. MASON*

30 Assisted Ventilation for Pediatric Patients, *542*

By *PETER BETIT AND JOHN THOMPSON*

SECTION VIII:
Advanced Respiratory Care

Chapter 1

Basic Chemistry

I. **Atomic Structure**
  A. **Atom:** The smallest subdivision of a substance that still maintains the properties of that substance, frequently referred to as the building blocks of the universe. An atom is composed of the following (Figure 1-1):
  1. **Nucleus:** Central portion of an atom, which contains protons and neutrons.
    a. **Proton:** Positively charged particle with a mass of one atomic mass unit.
    b. **Neutron:** Neutral particle with a mass of one atomic mass unit.
  2. **Electron:** Negatively charged particle that revolves around the nucleus of the atom with a mass of approximately 1/1000 of an atomic mass unit. Electrons exist in well-defined orbitals that establish the chemical reactivity of an atom.
  3. Normally, in its nonreactive state, an atom contains the same number of protons and electrons. The number of neutrons in the nucleus of a substance varies among atoms (isotopes).
  B. **Element:** General term applied to each of the 109 specifically named different types of atoms.
  C. **Isotope:** Atom of a substance with the same number of protons but with a varying number of neutrons. All elements have at least two isotopes. The following are the three primary isotopes of oxygen:

  0–16, 8 neutrons (99.76% of all oxygen)
  0–17, 9 neutrons (0.04% of all oxygen)
  0–18, 10 neutrons (0.20% of all oxygen)

  D. **Atomic weight:** Average weight of an atom of a particular substance based on its comparison with the atomic weight of the carbon 12 isotope. The atomic weight is approximately equal to the sum of the number of protons and neutrons in the nucleus of an atom but is not a whole number because of the presence of isotopes (Table 1-1).
  E. **Gram atomic weight:** Mass in grams of an element equal to its atomic weight (see Table 1-1).
  F. **Atomic number:** Equal to the number of protons in the nucleus of an atom (see Table 1-1).
  G. **Ion:** Charged species of a particular atom; occurs as a result of the loss or gain of electrons from an atom.

II. **Molecular Structure**
  A. **Molecule:** Particle that results from the chemical combination of two or more atoms normally having a neutral charge but may be positively or negatively charged.
  B. **Compound:** Molecule formed from two or more elements.
  C. **Free radical:** A charged compound, reacting as any other ion reacts.

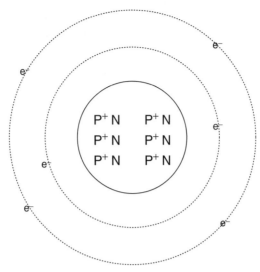

FIG. 1-1 Atomic structure of a carbon atom. P, Protons. N, neutrons. e, electrons.

D. Molecular formula: Chemical expression indicating the types and number of atoms in a molecule. The particle that is positively charged is usually listed first.
    Examples:

    NaCl = 1 sodium atom and 1 chloride atom contained in the molecule.
    H_2SO_4 = 2 hydrogen atoms, 1 sulfur atom, and 4 oxygen atoms contained in the molecule.

E. Molecular weight (MW): Sum total of all individual atomic weights of atoms that make up a molecule.
    Example (H_2SO_4):

Atom	No. of Atoms		Atomic Weight	Total Contributing Weight
H	2	×	1	2
S	1	×	32	32
O	4	×	16	64
				MW 98

Example (CO_2):

Atom	No. of Atoms		Atomic Weight	Total Contributing Weight
C	1	×	12	12
O	2	×	16	32
				MW 44

F. Gram molecular weight (GMW): Mass in grams of a molecule equal to its MW.
G. One mole of a substance is equal to one GMW of the substance.

III. Valence
    A. Valence: Number given to an atom that indicates its tendency to gain or lose electrons in a chemical reaction.
        Examples (see Table 1-1):
            Na^{+1} (sodium): Valence of +1 indicates that in a chemical reaction it will react by losing one electron.

TABLE **1-1**

Symbol, Atomic Number, Atomic Weight, and Valence of the 26 Elements Commonly Found in the Human Body and Other Elements Commonly Seen in Medicine

Element	Symbol	Atomic No.	Atomic Weight	Valence
Elements Commonly Seen in the Body				
Aluminum	Al	13	26.98	+3
Boron	B	5	10.83	+3
Calcium	Ca	20	40.08	+2
Carbon	C	6	12.0	+ or −4
Chlorine	Cl	17	35.5	−1
Chromium	Cr	24	51.99	−1 or −2
Cobalt	Co	27	58.93	+2
Copper	Cu	29	63.55	+1 or +2
Fluorine	F	9	18.99	−1
Hydrogen	H	1	1.00	+1
Iodine	I	53	126.9	−1
Iron	Fe	26	55.84	+1 or +2
Magnesium	Mg	12	24.31	+2
Manganese	Mn	25	54.94	−2 or −3
Molybdenum	Mo	42	95.94	−1 or −2
Nitrogen	N	7	14.01	−3
Oxygen	O	8	15.99	−2
Phosphorus	P	15	30.97	−3
Potassium	K	19	39.09	+1
Selenium	Se	34	78.96	−2
Silicone	Si	14	28.09	+ or −4
Sodium	Na	11	22.98	+1
Sulfur	S	16	32.06	−2
Tin	Sn	50	118.7	+ or −4
Vanadium	V	23	50.94	−2 or −3
Zinc	Zn	40	91.22	+1 or +2
Other Elements Commonly Seen in Medicine				
Barium	Ba	56	137.34	+2
Gallium	Ga	31	69.72	+3
Helium	He	2	4.00	+ or −2
Lead	Pb	82	207.19	+1 or +2
Lithium	Li	3	6.94	+1
Mercury	Hg	80	200.59	+1 or +2

Ca^{+2} (calcium):   Valence of +2 indicates that in a chemical reaction it will react by losing two electrons.

F^{-1} (fluorine):   Valence of −1 indicates that in a chemical reaction it will react by gaining one electron.

    B. Generally, valences of elements allow predictions of their chemical reactivity with each other.

    C. Inert gases (noble gases) have an electron distribution that has full outer orbitals. These elements (e.g., helium, neon, argon, krypton, and xenon) do not react with other elements under normal atmospheric conditions.

IV. Types of Chemical Compounds

    A. Ionic compound: A compound formed by atoms in the compound transferring electrons, one atom gaining and the other losing electrons. Ionic compounds form ions when dissolved in solution.

Examples:

NaCl: Na^{+1} has a valence of +1, and Cl^{-1} has a valence of −1. The Na^{+1} atom has lost an electron, and the Cl^{-1} atom has gained an electron during the formation of NaCl.

CaF_2: Ca^{+2} has a valence of +2, and each F^{-1} atom has a valence of −1. The Ca^{+2} atom has lost two electrons, and each F^{-1} atom has gained one electron during the formation of CaF_2.

1. Properties of ionic compounds:
   a. High boiling points.
   b. High melting points.
   c. Dissolve readily in polar solvents (solvents formed by hydrogen bonding).
   d. Strong electrolytes: dissociate readily in polar solvents:

$$NaCl + H_2O \rightarrow Na^{+1} + Cl^{-1} + H_2O$$
$$CaF_2 + H_2O \rightarrow Ca^{+2} + 2\ F^{-1} + H_2O$$

B. Covalent compound: A compound formed by the sharing of electrons between the various atoms in the compound. In solution the molecule does not disassociate into its component parts.

$$O^{-2} + O^{-2} \rightarrow O_2$$
$$N^{-3} + N^{-3} \rightarrow N_2$$
$$Cl^{-1} + Cl^{-1} \rightarrow Cl_2$$

1. Properties of covalent compounds:
   a. Exist only between atoms of the same element.
   b. Low melting points.
   c. Low boiling points.
   d. Dissolve poorly in polar solvents.

C. Hydrogen bonding (polar covalent compound): An intermediate compound between a pure covalent compound and an ionic compound characterized by an incomplete (partial) sharing of electrons. In solution the molecule only partially disassociates into its component parts.

Examples:

$$H^{+1} + OH^{-1} \rightarrow H_2O$$
$$H_2O + CO_2 \rightarrow H_2CO_3$$

1. Properties of hydrogen bond compounds:
   a. Vary according to the particular compound.
   b. These compounds normally are weak electrolytes. Only a small percentage of ionization takes place when hydrogen bond compounds are added to a polar solution.
   c. May have high or low boiling points.
   d. May have high or low melting points.
   e. Dissolve in polar or nonpolar solutions.

V. **Types of Chemical Reactions**
   A. Synthesis reactions: Two substances react to form a third releasing energy

$$H^{+1} + OH^{-1} \ energy \ H_2O$$

   B. Decomposition reaction: A substance breaks up into its component parts with the release of energy, normally in the form of heat.

$$Carbohydrate \rightarrow sugar\ molecules + energy$$

C. Exchange reaction: Two substances exchange parts to form two new substances, such as the reaction of an acid and base to form a salt and water.

$$HCl + NaOH \rightarrow NaCl + H_2O$$

VI. **Volume Percent and Gram Percent**
   A. Volume percent (vol%): Method of indicating the number of milliliters of a substance in 100 ml of solution.
      1. 10 vol% = 10 ml/100 ml of solution
      2. 3.5 vol% = 3.5 ml/100 ml of solution
   B. Gram percent (g%): Method of indicating the number of grams of a substance in 100 ml of solution.
      1. 5.2 g% = 5.2 g/100 ml of solution
      2. 14.2 g% = 14.2 g/100 ml of solution

VII. **Chemical Solutions**
   A. Solution: Homogeneous mixture of two substances.
   B. Solute: Substance dissolved in a solution.
   C. Solvent: Substance that is the dissolving agent.
   D. Effects of a solute on the physical characteristics of water:
      1. Solutes cause the boiling point of water to increase.
      2. Solutes cause the freezing point of water to decrease.
      3. The osmotic pressure of a solution containing a solute is higher than that of pure water.
   E. As the temperature of the solvent increases, the volume of solute that can be dissolved in the solvent also increases.
   F. Dilute solution: A solution with a small amount of solute dissolved in each unit of solvent at a particular temperature.
   G. Saturated solution: A solution with the maximum amount of solute dissolved in each unit of solvent at a particular temperature. In a saturated solution a precipitate is seen at the bottom of the solution.
   H. Supersaturated solution: A solution with a greater amount of solute than the solvent would normally hold, dissolved at a particular temperature. However, any physical disturbance of this solution causes the excess solute to precipitate.
   I. Precipitate: A crystallized solid formed at the bottom of a saturated solution.

VIII. **Solution Concentrations**
   A. Ratio solution: Solution concentration represented as a ratio (1:100) between solute and solvent in number of grams to number of milliliters.
      Examples:
         2:500 means 2 g to 500 ml: 2 indicates the number of grams of solute, and 500 indicates the number of milliliters of solvent.
         1:1000 means 1 g to 1000 ml: 1 indicates the number of grams of solute, and 1000 indicates the number of milliliters of solvent.
      Problems:
      1. How many milligrams of solute are there in 1 ml of a 1:200 solution?

         1:200 means 1 g to 200 ml, 1 g = 1000 mg, thus

         $$\frac{1000\,mg}{200\,ml} = \frac{x}{1\,ml}$$
         $$x = 5\ mg$$

      2. How many milligrams are there in 5 ml of a 1:500 solution?

         1:500 means 1 g to 500 ml, 1 g = 1000 mg, thus

$$\frac{1000\,mg}{500\,ml} = \frac{x}{5\,ml}$$
$$x = 10 \text{ mg}$$

B. Percent weight/volume (w/v): Solution concentration in which the actual percentage indicates the number of grams of solute per 100 ml of solution.
    Example:
       1% w/v solution means 1 g of solute is contained in 100 ml of solution.
    Problems:
    1. How many milligrams are there in 10 ml of a 3% w/v solution?

    3% w/v means 3 g per 100 ml, 1 g = 1000 mg, thus
    3 g = 3000 mg

$$\frac{3000\,mg}{100\,ml} = \frac{x}{10\,ml}$$
$$x = 300 \text{ mg}$$

    2. How many milligrams are there in 3 ml of a 0.5% w/v solution?

    0.5% w/v means 0.5 g per 100 ml, 1 g = 1000 mg, thus
    0.5 g = 500 mg

$$\frac{500\,mg}{100\,ml} = \frac{x}{3\,ml}$$
$$x = 15 \text{ mg}$$

C. True percent solution: Solution concentration in which solute and solvent are expressed in either weight (% w/w) or volume (%v/v). The solute is expressed as a true percentage of the solution.
    Examples:
       10% w/w solution, where the total solution volume is 100 g, there is 10 g of solute and 90 g of solvent.
       3% v/v solution, where the total solution volume is 500 ml, there is 15 ml of solute and 485 ml of solvent.
    Problems:
    1. How many grams of solute are there in 250 g of a 5% w/w solution.

    (250)(0.05) = 12.5 g
    solution   solute

    (250 − 12.5) = 237.5 g
                        solvent

    2. How many milliliters of solute are there in 500 ml of a 10%v/v solution.

    (500)(0.10) = 50 ml
    solution   solute

    (500 − 50) = 450 ml
                      solvent

D. Molal solution: Solution concentration in which the solute is expressed in moles, and the solvent is expressed in kilograms, or millimoles per gram (mmol/g).
    Example:
       2.5 molal solution contains 2.5 moles of solute in 1 kg of solvent.
       1.5 molal solution of KCl contains 1.5 moles, or 111.9 g of KCl (1.5 × MW of KCl) in 1 kg of solvent.

Problems:

1. What is the molality of a solution with 117 g of NaCl in 1000 g of water?

$$1 \text{ molal solution of NaCl} = \frac{58.5 \text{ g}}{1000 \text{ g}} \text{ of water}$$

$$\frac{117 \text{ g}}{58.5 \text{ g}} = 2 \text{ moles}$$

2 moles of NaCl/1000 g of water = 2 molal solution

2. How much H_2SO_4 must be dissolved in 500 g of H_2O to make a 0.5 molal solution?

$$1 \text{ mole of } H_2SO_4 = 98 \text{ g}$$
$$1 \text{ molal solution} = 98 \text{ g}/1000 \text{ g of water}$$
$$0.5 \text{ molal solution} = \frac{98}{2} \text{ or } \frac{49 \text{ g}}{1000 \text{ g}} \text{ of water}$$

$$\frac{49 \text{ g of } H_2SO_4}{1000 \text{ g of water}} = \frac{x}{500 \text{ g of water}}$$
$$x = 24.5 \text{ g of } H_2SO_4 \text{ needed}$$

E. Molar solution (M): Solution containing 1 mole of solute per liter of solution (or mmol/ml).
   Examples:
   1.75 M solution contains 1.75 moles of solute per liter (L) of solution.
   2.0 M solution of NaOH contains 2 moles, or 80 g of NaOH/L of solution (2 × MW of NaOH).

Problems:

1. What is the molarity of 5.85 g of NaCl in 1 L of solution?

$$1 \text{ M solution} = 58.5 \text{ g of NaCl/L}$$
$$\frac{5.85}{58.5} = 0.1 \text{ mole of NaCl}$$
$$0.1 \text{ mole of NaCl/L} = 0.1 \text{ M solution}$$

2. In what volume of solution must 149.2 g of KCl be dissolved to make a 4 M solution?

$$1 \text{ M solution} = 74.6 \text{ g/L}$$
$$4 \text{ M solution} = 4 \times 74.6, \text{ or } 298.4 \text{ g/L}$$

$$\frac{298.4 \text{ g}}{1000 \text{ ml}} = \frac{149.2}{x}$$
$$x = 500 \text{ ml}$$

F. Normal solution (N): Solution concentration containing 1 g equivalent weight (GEW; see Section X, A, Gram Equivalent Weights) of solute/L of solution (or 1 mg equivalent weight/ml).
   Examples:
   1.25 N solution contains 1.25 GEW/L of solution.
   2.00 N solution of HCl contains 2 GEWs, or 73 g of HCl/L of solution (1 GEW of HCl = 36.5 g).

Problems:

1. What is the normality of a solution containing 42 g of $NaHCO_3$?

$$1 \text{ GEW of } NaHCO_3 = 84 \text{ g}$$
$$1 \text{ N solution} \qquad = 84 \text{ g/L}$$
$$42 \text{ g}/84 \text{ g} \qquad = 0.5 \text{ GEW}$$
$$42 \text{ g/L} \qquad = 0.5 \text{ N solution}$$

2. How many grams of NH_3Cl must be dissolved in 250 ml of solution to make a 2 N solution?

$$1 \text{ GEW of } NH_3Cl = 52.5 \text{ g}$$
$$2 \text{ N solution} = 2 \text{ GEWs } (105 \text{ g})/L$$
$$\frac{105 \text{ g}}{1000 \text{ ml}} = \frac{x}{250 \text{ ml}}$$
$$x = 26.25 \text{ g}$$

IX. **Dilution Calculations**
   A. The following formula is used to determine the concentration that will result when a solution is diluted:

$$V_1 \times C_1 = V_2 \times C_2 \tag{1}$$

   where
   V_1 is the volume before dilution
   C_1 is the concentration before dilution
   V_2 is the volume after dilution
   C_2 is the concentration after dilution

   B. Before equation 1 can be used, three of the four variables must be known.
   Problems:
   1. What volume of water should be added to 50 ml of a 40% v/v solution of alcohol to dilute it to a 20% v/v solution?

$$V_1 \times C_1 = V_2 \times C_2$$
$$(50)(40) = (x)(20)$$
$$x = 100 \text{ ml}$$
$$100 \text{ ml} = V_2$$
$$V_2 - V_1 = \text{added volume}$$
$$100 \text{ ml} - 50 \text{ ml} = 50 \text{ ml of water to be added}$$

   2. If 4 ml is added to 0.5 ml of a 15% v/v solution, what is the solution's final concentration?

$$V_1 \times C_1 = V_2 \times C_2$$
$$(0.5)(15\%) = (4.5)(x)$$
$$x = 1.67\% \text{ v/v}$$

X. **Gram Equivalent Weights**
   A. GEW: Amount of a substance that will react completely with 1 mole of H^{+1} or OH^{-1} or 1 mole of any monovalent substance.
   B. The GEW of an element is determined by dividing the gram atomic weight of the substance by its valence. The charge of the valence is disregarded.
   Examples:

$$Na^{+1} \text{ atomic weight, 23 g}$$
$$\frac{23 \text{ g}}{1} = 23 \text{ g/GEW}$$

$$Al^{+3} \text{ atomic weight, 27 g}$$
$$\frac{27 \text{ g}}{3} = 9 \text{ g/GEW}$$

$$S^{-2} \text{ atomic weight, 32 g}$$
$$\frac{32 \text{ g}}{2} = 16 \text{ g/GEW}$$

   C. The GEW of an acid is determined by dividing its GMW by the number of replaceable hydrogen ions in the molecular formula. Normally all H^{+1} are replaceable. However, H_2CO_3 is an exception: only 1 H^{+1} is replaceable.

Examples:

$$H_2SO_4 \text{ GMW} = 98 \text{ g, 2 replaceable } H^{+1}$$
$$\frac{98 \text{ g}}{2} = 49 \text{ g/GEW}$$

$$H_3PO_4 \text{ GMW} = 98 \text{ g, 3 replaceable } H^{+1}$$
$$\frac{98 \text{ g}}{3} = 32.66 \text{ g/GEW}$$

$$H_2CO_3 \text{ GMW} = 62 \text{ g, 1 replaceable } H^{+1}$$
$$\frac{62 \text{ g}}{1} = 62 \text{ g/GEW}$$

D. The GEW of a base is determined by dividing its GMW by the number of replaceable hydroxyl ions (OH^{-1}) in the molecular formula. Normally all OH^{-1} are replaceable.
Example:

$$NaOH \text{ GMW} = 40 \text{ g, 1 replaceable } OH^{-1}$$
$$\frac{40 \text{ g}}{1} = 40 \text{ g/GEW}$$

$$Ca(OH)_2 \text{ GMW} = 74 \text{ g, 2 replaceable } OH^{-1}$$
$$\frac{74 \text{ g}}{2} = 37 \text{ g/GEW}$$

$$Al(OH)_3 \text{ GMW} = 78 \text{ g, 3 replaceable } OH^{-1}$$
$$\frac{78 \text{ g}}{3} = 26 \text{ g/GEW}$$

E. The GEW of a salt is determined by dividing its GMW by the total valence of the positive ions or free radicals in the molecule.
Examples:

$$NaCl \text{ GMW} = 58.5 \text{ g, 1 } Na^{+1} \text{ with a total valence of } +1$$
$$\frac{58.5 \text{ g}}{1} = 58.5 \text{ g/GEW}$$

$$CaF_2 \text{ GMW} = 78 \text{ g, 1 } Ca^{+2} \text{ with a total valence of } +2$$
$$\frac{78 \text{ g}}{2} = 39 \text{ g/GEW}$$

$$Al_2(CO_3)_3 \text{ GMW} = 234 \text{ g, 2 } Al^{+3} \text{ with a total valence of } +6$$
$$\frac{234 \text{ g}}{6} = 39 \text{ g/GEW}$$

F. The GEW of a free radical is determined by dividing its GMW by its valence, disregarding the charge of the valence.
Examples:

$$HCO_3^{-1} \text{ GMW} = 61 \text{ g, valence 1}$$
$$\frac{61 \text{ g}}{1} = 61 \text{ g/GEW}$$

$$PO_4^{-3} \text{ GMW} = 95 \text{ g, valence 3}$$
$$\frac{95 \text{ g}}{3} = 31.67 \text{ g/GEW}$$

$$CO_3^{-2} \text{ GMW} = 60 \text{ g, valence 2}$$
$$\frac{60 \text{ g}}{2} = 30 \text{ g/GEW}$$

G. Milliequivalent weight (mEq): Weight of a substance that will react with 1 mmole of H^{+1}, OH^{-1}, or any monovalent substance. Numerically, the mEq of a substance is equal to its GEW.

Examples:

NaCl 58.5 g/GEW, 58.5 mg/mEq
H_2CO_3 62 g/GEW, 62 mg/mEq
Na 23 g/GEW, 23 mg/mEq

H.   Equivalent weights are used to determine the precise quantity of a substance that reacts completely with a given quantity of another substance.

XI.   **Other Types of Liquid Mixtures**
   A.   Suspension: A mixture formed by placing a solid unable to dissolve (dissociate into its component parts) into a liquid. Particles suspended are large (>100 μm). A suspension is characterized by:
      1.   An insoluble substance dispersed in a liquid
      2.   The dispersion is heterogenous
      3.   The solid settles out over time
      4.   The solid does not pass through filter paper or membranes
   B.   Colloid: A mixture formed the same way as a suspension except the particles are between 1 and 100 μm in size. A colloid is characterized by:
      1.   The solid in the mixture does not settle over time
      2.   Colloids can pass through filters
      3.   Colloids do not pass through membranes
      4.   Colloids possess an electrical charge
      5.   Colloids exhibit the *Tyndall effect* or the ability to disperse or scatter a beam of light passing through the mixture
      6.   Colloids exhibit *Brownian movement*, the constant movement of the colloid particles by bombardment from the liquid medium
      7.   Colloid dispersions (mixtures) can be either *hydrophilic* (attracting water) or *hydrophobic* (repelling water)
      8.   Gels: Systems in which there is a strong attraction between the colloid particles and water
      9.   Sols: Systems in which there is little attraction between the colloid particles and water

XII.   **Inorganic Molecules and Compounds**
   A.   Compounds generally formed by ionic or hydrogen bonds that do not contain C-C or C-H covalent bonds
   B.   Acids, bases, and salts are inorganic compounds or molecules

XIII.   **Organic Compounds or Molecules**
   A.   Compounds generally formed by covalent bonds containing a high proportion of C-C and C-H bonds
   B.   Biologically important organic molecules include:
      1.   Carbohydrates
      2.   Lipids
      3.   Proteins
      4.   Nucleic acids
      5.   Vitamins
      6.   Hormones
      7.   Enzymes

XIV.   **Temperature Scales**
   A.   Temperature scales (in degrees) in general use:
      1.   Fahrenheit (F)
      2.   Celsius or centigrade (C)
      3.   Rankine (R)
      4.   Kelvin (K)

B. The Rankine and Kelvin scales are absolute zero scales (i.e., zero on their scales represents the point where all molecular activity stops).
C. Conversion formulas for temperature scales:
  1. C = 5/9 (F − 32)
  2. F = (9/5 C) + 32
  3. K = C + 273
  4. R = F + 460

Problems:
  1. Convert 55° F to degrees K:

$$C = 5/9 \ (F - 32)$$
$$C = 5/9 \ (55 - 32)$$
$$C = 12.80$$
$$K = C + 273$$
$$K = 12.8° \ C + 273$$
$$K = 285.8$$

  2. Convert 30° C to degrees R:

$$F = 9/5 \ (C) + 32$$
$$F = 9/5 \ (30) + 32$$
$$F = 86$$
$$R = F + 460$$
$$R = 86° \ F + 460$$
$$R = 546$$

XV. **Diffusion**
  A. The movement of water and the dissolved solute from an area of high concentration of each to an area of low concentration of each across a membrane permeable to both (Figure 1-2).

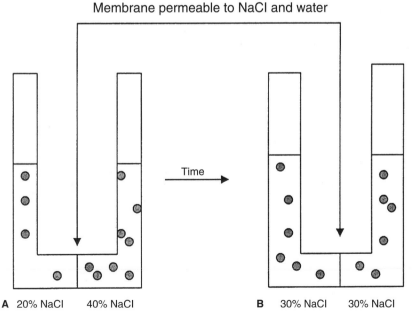

FIG. 1-2 Simple diffusion **(A)** of water and NaCl across a permeable membrane. Note that the original and final volume of water is unchanged, but the concentration of NaCl equilibrated across the membrane **(B)**.

B. When complete, the concentration of water and the solute is equal on each side of the membrane.

C. Refer to Chapter 2 for details on diffusion of gases.

XVI. **Osmosis**

A. Osmosis is the movement of water from an area of high concentration of water to an area of low concentration of water.

B. Osmosis occurs when a membrane that is selectively permeable only to water separates two compartments of fluid (Figure 1-3).

C. Osmosis will proceed in a system until the concentration of water in the involved compartments is equal. When concentrations are equal, no net movement of fluid occurs; however, molecules of water still move back and forth across the membrane.

D. Osmosis occurs between two solutions as a result of osmotic pressure differences in the solutions.

1. The potential pressure of the molecules of pure H_2O is approximately 1,073,000 mm Hg.

2. When a solute is dissolved in H_2O, the potential pressure of the H_2O is decreased.

3. The osmotic pressure of a solution is equal to the potential pressure of pure water minus the potential pressure of the solution.
Example:

$$
\begin{array}{rl}
\text{Pure } H_2O & 1{,}073{,}000 \text{ mm Hg} \\
\text{Solution} & \underline{1{,}000{,}000 \text{ mm Hg}} \\
\text{Osmotic pressure} & 73{,}000 \text{ mm Hg}
\end{array}
$$

4. Osmotic pressure is a force drawing water into the solution.

5. Osmosis can be stopped by exerting a force on a solution equal to the osmotic pressure of the solution (Figures 1-4 and 1-5).

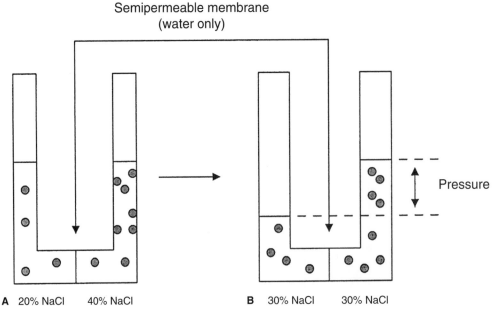

Semipermeable membrane (water only)

A   20% NaCl   40% NaCl   B   30% NaCl   30% NaCl

Pressure

FIG. 1-3 Osmosis of water across a semipermeable membrane **(A)**. Here the membrane is permeable only to water. Sodium chloride concentrations are equilibrated but purely as a result of the movement of water. The final volume of water on each side of the membrane has markedly changed **(B)**.

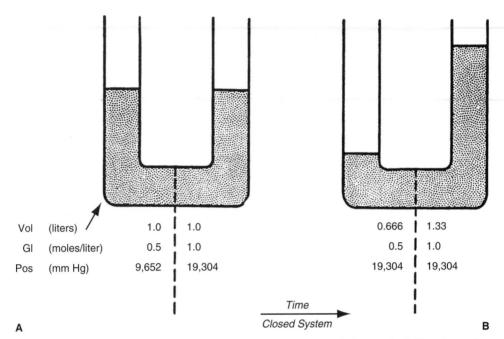

Vol	(liters)	1.0	1.0	0.666	1.33
Gl	(moles/liter)	0.5	1.0	0.5	1.0
Pos	(mm Hg)	9,652	19,304	19,304	19,304

Time

A   *Closed System*   **B**

FIG. 1-4 Two solutions separated by a membrane permeable only to water. **A,** As a result of different osmotic pressure, a total potential pressure gradient favoring water movement from the left to right. Any 1 mol/L solution creates an osmotic pressure (Pos) of 19,304 mm Hg within the solution. The osmotic pressure gradient causing movement is 9,652 mm Hg (19,304 – 9,652 mm Hg). **B,** At equilibrium the concentration of glucose (Gl) and the osmotic pressure are equal on both sides of the membrane. However, the volume on the left increased 0.33 L and on the right decreased 0.33 L.

XVII. **Starling's Law of Fluid Exchange**
   A. Fluid movement across capillaries is controlled by the interaction of hydrostatic and osmotic pressures (colloid osmotic pressure caused as a result of protein being the only nondiffusible substance).
   B. As a result of this interaction there is a net movement of a small amount of fluid from capillaries into the interstitial space.
   C. An imbalance in the forces controlling fluid exchange can result in edema.
   D. Edema can occur either in the lungs (pulmonary edema) or in the legs (systemic edema).
   E. Starling's law is:

$$Q = K\,[(Pcap - Pis) - \sigma\,(\pi cap - \pi is)] \tag{2}$$

   where Q is net fluid movement across a capillary, K is the capillary filtration coefficient, Pcap is the capillary hydrostatic pressure, Pis is the interstitial hydrostatic pressure, πcap is the capillary (plasma) colloid osmotic pressure, $\pi$is is the interstitial colloid osmotic pressure, and σ is refection coefficient (the membrane's ability to prevent the passage of protein).

XVIII. **Hydrostatic Pressure**
   A. Hydrostatic pressure is the amount of force exerted by the weight of a column of water (cm H_2O).

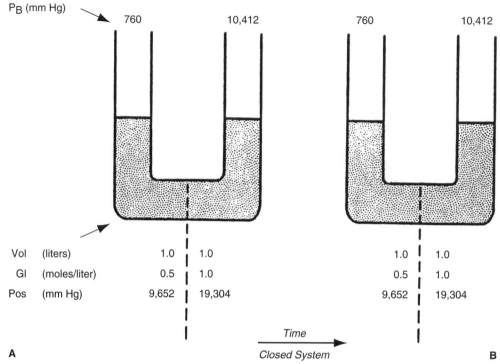

FIG. 1-5 Two solutions separated by a membrane permeable only to water. **A,** An osmotic pressure (Pos) gradient exists between the two glucose solutions (Gl), which is equal to 9,652 mm Hg (19,304 mm Hg – 9,652 mm Hg). However, a barometric pressure (Pb) difference also equal to 9,652 mm Hg (10,412–760 mm Hg) exists. Thus, the Pb gradient on the right side counteracts the effects of the Pos gradient. **B,** At equilibrium no movement has occurred because no total pressure gradient exists between the two sides of the system.

XIX. **Expressions of H^+ Ion Concentration**
   A. pH: Negative log of the H^+ concentration per liter of solution; [ ] is used to symbolize molar concentration.
      1. $pH = -\log_{10}[H^+]$ or $\log_{10}\frac{1}{[H^+]}$
      2. pH of 7.0: Neutral
      3. pH >7.0: Basic or alkalotic
      4. pH <7.0: Acidic or acidotic
      5. pH scale: 1 to 14, equivalent to an $[H^+]$ of 10^{-1} to 10^{-14} mol/L
   B. Nanomoles per liter (nmol/L): H^+ concentration in number of billionths of moles of H^+ per liter.
      1. The $[H^+]$ is expressed as a number multiplied by 10^{-9}.
      2. A pH of 7.0 = 3.98×10^{-8} mol/L, or 39.8×10^{-9} mol/L, or 39.8 nmol/L.
      3. Nanomole expressions normally are used for $[H^+]$ in the physiologic range.
         a. pH of 6.90 = 126 nmol/L
         b. pH of 7.70 = 20.1 nmol/L

XX. **Acids and Bases**
   A. Acid: A compound that donates H^+ when placed into solution.
      1. The active compound responsible for the properties of acids is the hydronium ion (H_3O^{+1}).
      2. In solution the liberated H^+ reacts with H_2O to form the H_3O^{+1} ion:

$$H^+ + H_2O \rightarrow H_3O^{+1}$$

B. Base: A compound that accepts H^+ when placed into solution. The active compound responsible for the properties of most bases is the OH^{-1} (hydroxyl ion).

C. Neutralization reaction: The reaction between an acid and a base where the results are a salt plus water:

$$NaOH + HCl \rightarrow NaCl + H_2O$$

XXI. Oxidation and Reduction
  A. Oxidation: Process in a chemical reaction whereby a substance loses electrons.
  B. Reduction: Process in a chemical reaction whereby a substance gains electrons.

XXII. Metric System
  A. Length
    1. The basic unit of length is the meter (m). One meter is equal to 39.37 inches (in.).
    2. One meter is equal to all of the following, and they are thus equal to each other:
       a. 100 centimeters (10^2 cm)
       b. 1000 millimeters (10^3 mm)
       c. 1,000,000 micrometers (10^6 μm)
       d. 10,000,000,000 angstroms (10^{10} Å)
    3. Basic factors used to convert the metric to the British system or the British to the metric system:
       a. 1 m = 39.37 in.
       b. 1 in. = 2.54 cm
    Problems:
    1. How many angstroms are equal to 2.2×10^2 cm?

$$1 \text{ m} = 10^2 \text{ cm}$$
$$\frac{1 \text{ m}}{10^2 \text{ cm}} = \frac{x}{2.2 \times 10^2 \text{ cm}}$$
$$x = 2.2 \text{ m}$$
$$1 \text{ m} = 10^{10} \text{ Å}$$
$$\frac{1 \text{ m}}{10^{10} \text{ Å}} = \frac{2.2 \text{ m}}{x}$$
$$x = 2.2 \times 10^{10} \text{ Å}$$

    2. How many inches are equal to 5.3×10^6 mm?

$$1 \text{ cm} = 2.54 \text{ cm}$$
$$10^3 \text{ mm} = 10^2 \text{ cm}$$
$$\frac{10^3 \text{ mm}}{10^2 \text{ cm}} = \frac{5.3 \times 10^6 \text{ mm}}{x}$$
$$x = 5.3 \times 10^5 \text{ cm}$$
$$\frac{1 \text{ in.}}{2.54 \text{ cm}} = \frac{x}{5.3 \times 10^5 \text{ cm}}$$
$$x = 2.09 \times 10^5 \text{ in.}$$

  B. Weight
    1. The basic unit of weight in the metric system is the kilogram (kg). One kilogram is equal to 2.2 pounds (lb).
    2. One kilogram is equal to all of the following, and they are thus equal to each other:
       a. 1000 g (10^3 g)
       b. 1,000,000 mg (10^6 mg)
    3. Basic factors used to convert from metric to British system or from British to metric system:
       a. 1 kg = 2.2 lb
       b. 1 lb = 454 g

Problems:
1. How many milligrams are there in 1.5×10^2 kg?

$$1 \text{ kg} = 10^6 \text{ mg}$$
$$\frac{10^6 \text{ mg}}{1 \text{ kg}} = \frac{x}{1.5 \times 10^2 \text{ kg}}$$
$$x = 1.5 \times 10^8 \text{ mg}$$

2. How many grams are equal to 0.6 lb?

$$1 \text{ kg} = 2.2 \text{ lb}$$
$$1 \text{ kg} = 10^3 \text{ g, therefore}$$
$$10^3 \text{ g} = 2.2 \text{ lb}$$
$$\frac{10^3 \text{ g}}{2.2 \text{ lb}} = \frac{x}{0.6 \text{ lb}}$$
$$x = 277.2 \text{ g}$$

C. Volume
1. The basic unit of volume in the metric system is the liter, which is equal to 1.057 quarts (qt).
2. One liter is equal to 1000 ml (10^3 ml) and also to 1000 cc (cubic centimeters) (10^3 cc).
   a. The volume of 1 cc is 1 ml.
   b. 1 ml of water weighs 1 g.
3. One cubic meter contains 10^3 L.
4. Basic factors used to convert from the metric to British system or from British to metric system:
   a. 1 L = 1.057 qt
   b. 1 cubic ft = 28.3 L

Problems:
1. How many liters are equal to 2.5×10^9 m?

$$1 \text{ L} = 10^3 \text{ ml}$$
$$\frac{1 \text{ L}}{10^3 \text{ ml}} = \frac{x}{2.5 \times 10^9 \text{ ml}}$$
$$x = 2.5 \times 10^6 \text{ ml}$$

2. How many cubic feet are equal to 3.5×10^6 L?

$$1 \text{ cubic ft} = 28.3 \text{ L}$$
$$\frac{1 \text{cubic ft}}{28.3 \text{ L}} = \frac{x}{3.5 \times 10^6 \text{ L}}$$
$$x = 1.3 \times 10^5 \text{ cubic ft}$$

BIBLIOGRAPHY

Brooks SM: *Integrated Basic Sciences,* ed 4, St. Louis, Mosby, 1979.

Burton GG, Hodgkin JE, Ward JJ: *Respiratory Care: A Guide to Clinical Practice,* ed 4, Philadelphia, Lippincott, 1997.

Ebbing DD: *General Chemistry,* ed 4, Boston, Houghton Mifflin Publishers, 1993.

Epstein LI, Kuzava BA: *Basic Physics in Anesthesiology: A Programmed Approach,* Chicago, Year Book Medical Publishers, 1976.

Hess D, MacIntyre N, Mishoe S, et al: *Respiratory Care: Principles and Practice,* St. Louis, Mosby, 2002.

Sachheim GI, Lehamn DD: *Chemistry for the Health Sciences,* ed 5, New York, Macmillan, 1985.

Shapiro BA, Harrison RA, Cane R, et al: *Clinical Application of Blood Gases,* ed 4, Chicago, Year Book Medical Publishers, 1989.

Thomas G: *Chemistry for Pharmacy and the Life Sciences,* Hereforshire, UK, Prentice Hall, 1996.

Wilkins R, Stoller J, Scanlan CL: *Egan's Fundamentals of Respiratory Therapy,* ed 8, St. Louis, Mosby, 2003.

Wojciechowski WV: *Respiratory Care Sciences: An Integrated Approach,* Albany, NY, Delmar, 1996.

Chapter 2

General Principles of Gas Physics

I. **Basic Units and Relationships**
   A. Mass: The ability of matter to occupy space, and if in motion to remain in motion, and if at rest to remain at rest.
   B. Weight: The quantification of the mass of an object; the effect of gravitational attraction on an object.
   C. Velocity: The speed that an object moves between two points; expressed in miles per hour or centimeters per second.
   D. Acceleration: The rate at which the velocity of an object increases. The units of acceleration are cm/sec^2 or $miles/hour^2$.
   E. Work: The force needed to move an object multiplied by the specific distance the object is moved.

$$\text{Work} = \text{Force} \times \text{Distance} \tag{1}$$

   1. Force is defined as mass × acceleration. The units of force are:
      a. Dyne = gm × cm/sec
      b. Newton = kg × m/sec
   2. Work is not performed unless the applied force causes movement; if no movement, no work.
   3. The units of work are:
      a. ERG = dyne-centimeter
      b. Joule = Newton-meter
   4. When relating work to the respiratory system:
      a. Pressure replaces force
      b. Volume replaces distance
      c. Thus work can be expressed as (see Chapter 5):

$$\text{Work} = \text{Pressure} \times \text{Volume} \tag{2}$$

      d. Respiratory work is normally expressed as (m = meter):
         (1) kg × m/L
         (2) joules/L (1 kg × m/L = 10 joules/L)
      e. Work performed over time is power expressed as:
         (1) kg × m/min
         (2) joules/min
   F. Energy is defined as the ability to do work.
   1. Potential and kinetic energy are the two types of mechanical energy.
   2. Potential energy (PE) is the energy of position.
   3. PE is equal to:

$$\text{PE} = \text{M} \times g \times \text{h} \tag{3}$$

where M = mass, g = gravitational attraction of the earth, and h = height.

4. Mass times gravitational attraction is frequently represented as weight (W):

$$PE = W \times h \tag{4}$$

5. Kinetic energy (KE) is the energy of motion.
6. KE is equal to:

$$KE = 0.5 \, MV^2 \tag{5}$$

where M = mass and V = velocity.

7. KE of gases is normally expressed as:

$$KE = 0.5 \, DV^2 \tag{6}$$

where D = density of the gas.

G. Pressure is the force applied per unit area. The units of pressure are:
1. Pounds per square inch (lb/in.^{2} or psi)
2. Grams per square centimeter (g/cm^2)

II. **States of Matter**
A. All matter exists in one of three basic states (Figure 2-1):
1. Solid: High degree of order, little random molecular motion, and strong intermolecular attraction
2. Liquid: Limited degree of order, some freedom of movement, and moderate intermolecular attraction
3. Gas: No order, complete freedom of motion, and weak intermolecular attraction
B. The state of a substance is determined by the relationship of two forces.
1. KE of the molecules.
2. Intermolecular attractive forces among the molecules.
C. The KE of a substance is directly related to temperature.
1. The greater the KE of a substance, the greater its tendency to exist as a liquid or gas.
2. Molecules of every substance are in constant motion as a result of KE.
3. At absolute zero, the KE of a substance is theoretically zero.
D. Intermolecular attractive forces oppose the KE of molecules and tend to force them to exist in less free (solid or liquid) states. Basically there are three types of intermolecular attractive forces: dipole, hydrogen bonding, and dispersion.

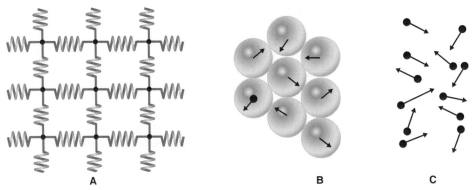

FIG. 2-1 Simplified models of three states of matter. **A,** Solid, strong intermolecular attraction. **B,** Liquid, moderate intermolecular attraction. **C,** Gas, weak intermolecular attraction.

1. Dipole forces: Forces that exist between molecules that have electrostatic polarity; the negative aspect of one molecule is lined up and attracted to the positive aspect of another molecule, as seen with NaCl. These substances frequently form crystals.
2. Hydrogen bonding: A force that exists between molecules formed by hydrogen reacting with fluorine, oxygen, or nitrogen.
   a. As a result of the electronegative difference between hydrogen and fluorine, oxygen, or nitrogen, the hydrogen atom in the molecule exists essentially as a pure proton.
   b. The hydrogen end of one molecule is thus attracted to the negative aspect of another molecule of the same substance.
   c. Hydrogen bonding occurs only with compounds of fluorine, oxygen, and nitrogen because of these atoms':
      (1) Strong electronegativity
      (2) Small atomic diameter
3. Dispersion forces (London or van der Waals forces): Forces between molecules of relatively nonpolar substances.
   a. In nonpolar substances the electron cloud normally is distributed equally among all of the atoms in the molecule.
   b. However, at some point in time the electron cloud may be instantaneously concentrated at one end of the molecule. When this occurs, a polarity is set up on the molecule.
   c. This instantaneous polarity allows weak attraction between adjacent molecules.
   d. Dispersion forces are the weakest of all intermolecular forces.

E. Heat
1. The first law of thermodynamics states that energy (heat) is neither created nor lost but simply transformed from one form to another.
2. That is, any energy a substance gains must be lost by its surrounding environment.
3. Heat (energy) always moves from the hotter object to the cooler object until there is thermal equilibrium between the two objects.
4. Heat transfer occurs in four ways:
   a. Conduction: Transfer of heat by direct contact between objects. Thermal conductivity is a measure of a substance's ability to absorb heat.
      (1) Metals have high thermal conductivity; they tend to feel cool because they readily absorb heat from the body.
      (2) Liquids have low thermal conductivity.
      (3) Gases have the lowest thermal conductivity.
   b. Convection: Heating by the mixing of two fluids (liquids or gases). Heat is allowed to freely transfer in the mixture. Fluid currents carrying heat energy are called convection currents.
   c. Radiation: Heating without direct contact, heat energy in the visible and infrared light ranges transferred to the objects they encounter—heating by the sun.
   d. Vaporization/condensation: Heating by the transfer of energy as water changes from one state to another.
5. Heat and moisture exchangers function by the process of vaporization and condensation. Water is condensed, and heat is transferred to the device during exhalation. During inspiration the inhaled gas picks up water vapor by vaporization, and heat as a result is transferred to the inhaled gas (see Chapter 35).
6. Calorie: Unit of heat in the metric system. Essentially it is the amount of heat necessary to cause a 1° C increase in the temperature of 1 g of water.
7. British thermal unit (BTU): Unit of heat in the British system. Essentially it is the amount of heat necessary to cause a 1° F increase in the temperature of 1 lb of water.
8. One BTU is equal to 252 calories of heat.
9. Heat capacity: Number of calories needed to raise the temperature of 1 g of a substance 1° C.

10. Specific heat: Ratio of the heat capacity of a substance compared with the heat capacity of water.

F. Change of state
1. A specific defined amount of heat is needed to cause the molecules of a substance to change their state of matter without a change in temperature.
2. Latent heat of fusion is the amount of heat necessary to change 1 g of a substance at its melting point from a solid to a liquid without causing a change in temperature.
   a. The melting point is the temperature (at 1 atm of pressure) at which a substance changes from a solid to a liquid.
   b. The total volume of a substance must change from a solid to a liquid before its temperature can change.
   c. Generally, a large amount of heat gain is required to change from a solid to a liquid.
   d. Changing from a liquid to a solid requires the same amount of heat loss.
   e. Latent heats of fusion and melting points for various substances:

Substance	Heat of fusion (calories/g)	Melting point (° C)
Water	80	0
Hydrogen	13.8	−259.25
Carbon dioxide	43.2	−57.6
Nitrogen	6.15	−210
Oxygen	3.3	−218.8

3. The latent heat of vaporization is the amount of heat necessary to change 1 g of a substance at its boiling point from a liquid to a gas without causing a change in temperature.
   a. Boiling point is the temperature at 1 atm of pressure at which a substance changes from a liquid to a gas.
   b. The total volume of a substance must change from a liquid to a gas before its temperature changes.
      (1) For a substance to boil, its vapor pressure must equal the pressure of the atmosphere above it.
      (2) Evaporation is a surface phenomenon whereby individual molecules of a substance gain enough heat to change their state. Boiling, on the other hand, occurs throughout the entire volume of the substance.
   c. Latent heats of vaporization are generally much greater than latent heats of fusion.
   d. Latent heats of vaporization and boiling points for various substances:

Substance	Heat of vaporization (calories/g)	Boiling point (° C)
Water	540	100
Hydrogen	40	−252.5
Carbon dioxide	83	−78.5
Nitrogen	. . .	−196
Oxygen	50	−183

G. Effects of pressure on melting and boiling points
1. In general, the greater the pressure over a substance, the higher the temperature necessary to cause the substance to change its state. However, pressure has a greater effect on the boiling point of a substance than on its melting point.
2. Critical temperature: The highest temperature at which a substance can exist as a liquid, regardless of the amount of pressure applied to it ($O_2 = -118.8°$ C).
3. Critical pressure: The lowest pressure necessary at the critical temperature of a substance to maintain it in its liquid state ($O_2 = 49.7$ atm pressure).

4. Critical point: The combination of the critical temperature and the critical pressure of a substance.
   H. Triple point: Specific combination of temperature and pressure in which a substance can exist in all three states of matter in dynamic equilibrium.
   I. Sublimation: Transition of a substance from a solid directly to a gas without existence in a liquid state. The heat of sublimation equals the heat of fusion plus the heat of vaporization.

III. **Properties of Liquids**
   A. Liquids flow and assume the shape of their containers.
   B. Liquids exert pressure that varies with the depth of the liquid and its density.
   C. According to Pascal's principle the shape or volume of a container does not affect the pressure of a liquid; pressure is only affected by the liquid's height and density.
   D. Variations in liquid pressure in a column produce an upward force referred to as buoyancy.
   E. As a result of buoyancy, objects in water appear to weigh less in water than in air.
   F. Liquids exert a buoyancy force because the pressure below a submerged object always exceeds the pressure above the object.
   G. According to Archimedes principle, the buoyancy force must equal the weight of the fluid displaced by the object.
   H. If the weight of the object exceeds the weight of the displaced water, it sinks, but if it weighs less than the displaced water, it floats.
   I. Archimedes principle is used to determine the specific gravity of liquids such as urine.

IV. **Kinetic Theory of Gases**
   A. The kinetic theory of gases normally is applied to relatively dilute gas volumes.
   B. Principles of the kinetic theory of gases are:
      1. Gases are composed of molecules that are in rapid continuous random motion.
      2. The molecules undergo near collisions with each other and collide with the walls of their container.
      3. All molecular collisions are elastic, and as long as the container is properly insulated, the temperature of the gas remains constant.
      4. The KE of molecules of a gas is directly proportional to the absolute temperature.
         a. An increase in temperature causes an increase in KE of the gas.
         b. The increased KE causes an increase in the velocity of the gas molecules.
         c. The increased velocity causes an increase in the frequency of collisions.
         d. The increased frequency of collisions causes an increase in the pressure in the system.
         e. With an increase in temperature, the degree of increase in the velocity of gas molecules is indirectly related to their molecular weight (MW).

V. **Avogadro's Law**
   A. One gram molecular weight (GMW), 1 g atomic weight, 1 g ionic weight, and so on, of a substance contains $6.02 = 10^{23}$ particles of that substance.
   B. The above mass of any substance is referred to as a mole.
   C. One mole of a gas at $0°$ C and 760 mm Hg (standard temperature and pressure; STP) occupies a volume of approximately 22.4 L. (There is a small percent variation in this number for individual gases; e.g., CO_2 = 22.3 L.)
   D. An equal number or fractions of moles of different gases at a specific temperature and pressure occupy the same volume and contain the same number of particles.

VI. **Density**
   A. Density (D) is the mass of an object per unit volume (V) and usually is expressed as g/L:

$$D = \frac{M}{V}$$

(7)

B. On the surface of the earth, mass in equation 7 may be replaced by weight.

C. Calculation of densities of solids and liquids is straightforward because their volumes are relatively stable at various temperatures and pressures.

D. The volumes of gases, on the other hand, are severely affected by temperature and pressure.

E. For this reason, the standard density of all gases is determined at STP (0° C and 760 mm Hg pressure) conditions where the volume used is 22.4 L and the weight used is the GMW of the particular gas:

$$\text{Density of gas} = \frac{\text{GMW}}{22.4 \text{ L}} = x \text{ g/L} \tag{8}$$

$$\text{Density of oxygen} = \frac{32 \text{ g (GMW)}}{22.4 \text{ L}} = 1.43 \text{ g/L}$$

F. Standard densities of various substances:
1. Oxygen: 1.43 g/L
2. Nitrogen: 1.25 g/L
3. Carbon dioxide: 1.965 g/L
4. Helium: 0.179 g/L

G. The density of a mixture of gases is determined by the following equation:

$$D = \frac{(\%_A)(\text{GMW}_A) + (\%_B)(\text{GMW}_B) + (\%_C)(\text{GMW}_C)}{22.4 \text{ L}} \tag{9}$$

Example: The density of a gas containing 40% oxygen, 55% nitrogen, and 5% carbon dioxide would be computed as follows:

$$D = \frac{(0.4)(32) + (0.55)(28) + (0.05)(44) \text{ g}}{22.4 \text{ L}}$$

$$D = \frac{(12.8) + (15.4) + (2.2) \text{ g}}{22.4 \text{ L}}$$

$$D = \frac{30.4 \text{ g}}{22.4 \text{ L}}$$

$$D = 1.36 \text{ g/L}$$

H. Specific gravity: Ratio of the density of a substance to the density of a standard. The specific gravity of solids and liquids is determined using water as the (density, 1 kg/L) standard; for gases, oxygen is used as the standard. When it is stated that the specific gravity of urine is 1.10, it means the urine is 1.10 times heavier than H_2O because of the dissolved substances in the urine.

VII. Gas Pressure

A. Pressure (P) in any sense is equal to force per unit area:

$$P = \frac{\text{g}}{\text{cm}^2}; \quad P = \frac{\text{lb}}{\text{in.}^2} \tag{10}$$

B. The pressure of a gas is directly related to the KE of the gas (see Section II, States of Matter) and to the gravitational attraction of the earth.

C. With an increase in altitude, the gravitational attraction of the earth on the molecules of gas in the atmosphere decreases.
1. This causes a decrease in density of the atmospheric gases.
2. Decreased density results in fewer molecular collisions.
3. Thus, with increasing altitude there is a nonlinear decrease in the pressure of the total atmosphere and of individual gases.
4. Even though there is a steady decrease in the pressure of the atmosphere with altitude, the concentration of gases in the atmosphere remains stable to an elevation of approximately 50 miles.

5. Concentration of atmospheric gases:
   a. Oxygen: 20.95%
   b. Nitrogen: 78.08%
   c. Argon: 0.93%
   d. Carbon dioxide: 0.03%
   e. Trace elements: 0.01%
D. The barometric pressure (PB) of the atmosphere is equal to the height of a column of fluid times the fluid's density (Figure 2-2):

$$P_B = (\text{height of column of fluid})(\text{fluid's density}) \tag{11}$$

If the fluid used is mercury, normal atmospheric pressure is equal to psi:

$$14.7 \text{ psi} = (29.9 \text{ in. Hg})(0.491 \text{ lb/in.}^3)$$

E. Mercury's density in the metric system is 13.6 g/ml; in the British system it is 0.491 lb/in.^{3}.
F. Gas pressure is frequently expressed as the height of a substance (i.e., mm Hg, cm H_2O). These are not true pressure expressions, but they may be easily converted to the proper pressure notation by use of equation 11 if necessary.
G. Atmospheric pressure can be determined by a number of pressure-measuring devices (Figure 2-3).
   1. Fluid manometer
      (a) Simple mercury type
      (b) U-tube
      (c) Slanted tube
   2. Pressure gauges (aneroid barometer)

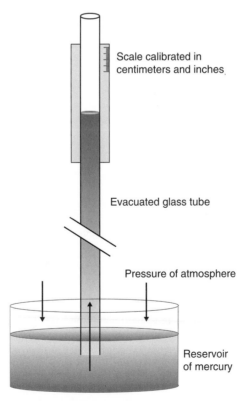

Scale calibrated in centimeters and inches

Evacuated glass tube

Pressure of atmosphere

Reservoir of mercury

FIG. 2-2 The major components of a mercury barometer.

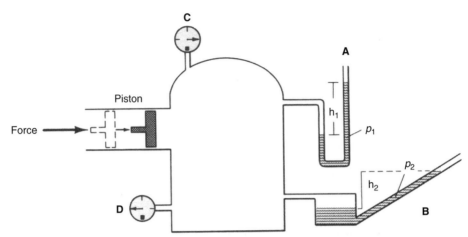

FIG. 2-3 Types of manometers. **A,** U-tube manometers determine the pressure as a difference in the height between the two limbs of the U-tube. The more dense the fluid in the manometer (P_1), the smaller the height difference (h_1). **B,** Slanted tubes can magnify small pressure changes (P_2 density of fluid, h_2 height of the fluid). **C,** Gauges measure a pressure change by converting the pressure to the displacement of a diaphragm. A gear mechanism converts displacement into motion of a needle on a scale. The measurement of "absolute pressure" adds the change in pressure within the chamber to atmospheric pressure. **D,** This gauge only measures pressure change within the chamber similar to A and B, referred to as "gauge pressure."

    H. Equivalent expressions of normal atmospheric pressure:
        1. 14.7 psi
        2. 760 mm Hg
        3. 1034 g/cm^2
        4. 33 ft of salt H_2O
        5. 33.9 ft of fresh H_2O
        6. 29.9 in. Hg
        7. 76 cm Hg
        8. 1034 cm H_2O

VIII. Humidity
    A. Water vapor content of the air under atmospheric conditions is variable. Temperature is the factor that most significantly affects water vapor content in the atmosphere.
        1. The process of a liquid changing into a gas at a temperature lower than its boiling point is referred to as evaporation.
        2. The process of a gas changing into liquid at a temperature lower than its boiling point is called condensation.
    B. At a particular temperature, there is a maximum amount of water that a gas can hold, capacity for water vapor.
    C. Because the boiling point of water (100° C) is considerably higher than the normal temperature of the atmosphere, the maximum water vapor content of the atmosphere varies with temperature.
        1. As the temperature increases, the rate of evaporation of water accelerates, and the capacity of the atmosphere to hold water increases.
        2. All other standard gases in the atmosphere have boiling points much lower than atmospheric temperature. This causes stability in their concentrations.
        3. Water is the only standard atmospheric gas that responds to temperature changes in this manner.

D. Expressions of water vapor content
1. Absolute humidity is defined as the actual weight of water vapor contained in a given volume of gas.
    a. Absolute humidity may be expressed as grams per cubic meter or milligrams per liter.
    b. The maximum absolute humidity at 37° C is 43.8 g/m^3, or 43.8 mg/L.
2. Partial pressure (PP) of water vapor (PH$_2$O), maximum PH$_2$O at 37° C, is equal to 47 mm Hg.
3. Maximum weight of water and water vapor pressure at different temperatures:

Temperature (° C)	Weight (mg/L)	PH$_2$O (mm Hg)	Temperature (° C)	Weight (mg/L)	PH$_2$O (mm Hg)
20	17.30	17.5	29	28.75	30.0
21	18.35	18.7	30	30.35	31.8
22	19.42	19.8	31	32.07	33.7
23	20.58	21.1	32	33.76	35.7
24	21.78	22.4	33	35.61	37.7
25	23.04	23.8	34	37.57	39.9
26	24.36	25.2	35	39.60	42.2
27	25.75	26.7	36	41.70	44.6
28	27.22	28.3	37	43.80	47.0

4. Relative humidity (RH) is defined as a relationship between the actual weight or pressure (content) of water in air at a specific temperature and the maximum weight or pressure (capacity) of water that air can hold at that specific temperature. RH is expressed as a percentage.
    a. Expressions of actual and maximum amounts of water:
        (1) mm Hg
        (2) g/m^3
        (3) mg/L
    b. Formula for calculating RH:

$$RH = \frac{Content}{Capacity} \times 100 \qquad (12)$$

Example: At 37° C, if the actual water vapor pressure is 20 mm Hg, what is the RH?

$$RH = \frac{20 \text{ mm Hg}}{47 \text{ mm Hg}} \times 100 = 43\%$$

    c. If water content is kept constant and temperature is increased, RH decreases because capacity of air for water increases. As temperature decreases, the opposite effect is seen (Figure 2-4).
5. Gases in the lungs exist under body temperature and pressure saturated conditions: 37° C, RH 100%, pressure is equal to atmospheric pressure.
6. A humidity deficit exists when the actual content of water in a gas entering the lungs is less than the capacity of the gas at 37° C.

IX. **Dalton's Law of Partial Pressure**
A. Dalton's law states that the sum of the individual PPs of the gases in a mixture is equal to the total PB of the system.
1. PO$_2$ is the PP of oxygen in a mixture.
2. PCO$_2$ is the PP of carbon dioxide in a mixture.
B. The PP of a gas is equal to the PB times the concentration of the gas in the mixture:

$$(PP) = (PB)(Concentration) \qquad (13)$$

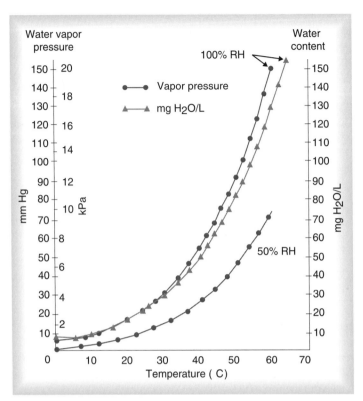

FIG. 2-4 Water vapor pressure (P_{H_2O}) and absolute humidity (mg H_2O/L) curves for gas that is fully saturated (relative humidity 100%) at various temperatures, and water vapor pressures at 50% relative humidity at various temperatures.

Example: If the P_B is 760 mm Hg and the concentration of O_2 is 21%, what is the P_{O_2}?

$$P_{O_2} = (760)(0.21) = 159.6 \text{ mm Hg}$$

C. The concentration of a gas is equal to the P_P of the gas divided by the P_B times 100:

$$\text{Concentration} = P_P/P_B \times 100 \qquad (14)$$

Example: If the P_B is 750 mm Hg and the P_{O_2} is 200 mm Hg, what is the concentration of O_2?

$$O_2 \text{ concentration} = 200 \text{ mm Hg}/750 \text{ mm Hg} \times 100 = 26.7\%$$

X. **Effect of Humidity on Dalton's Law**
   A. Water vapor pressure does not follow Dalton's law because under normal atmospheric conditions, the P_{H_2O} is dependent primarily on temperature and available water for evaporation.
   B. When the P_P of a gas is calculated and water vapor is present, the total P_B of the system must be corrected for water vapor before the P_P of any other gas can be calculated.
   C. The following is a modification of Dalton's law to account for the presence of water vapor:

$$(P_P) = (P_B - P_{H_2O})(\text{Concentration}) \qquad (15)$$

Example: If P_B is 770 mm Hg, P_{H_2O} is 30 mm Hg, and the concentration of O_2 is 50%, what is the P_{O_2}?

$$P_{O_2} = (770 \text{ mm Hg} - 30 \text{ mm Hg})(0.50)$$
$$P_{O_2} = 370 \text{ mm Hg}$$

D. When the temperature is 37° C with P_B 760 mm Hg, the gas saturated with water vapor, and the oxygen concentration 21%, the P_{O_2} is 149.7 mm Hg:

$$P_{O_2} = (760 \text{ mm Hg} - 47 \text{ mm Hg})(0.21) = 149.7 \text{ mm Hg}$$

XI. Ideal Gas Laws
A. The ideal gas laws apply to dilute gases at temperatures above the gases' boiling point.
B. The closer the temperature to the boiling point of a gas, the greater the error involved in using the gas laws.
C. The *ideal gas law* demonstrates the interrelationships among volume, pressure, temperature, and amount of gas.
  1. According to the ideal gas law, multiplying the pressure of the system by the volume of the system and dividing this by the product of the absolute temperature and amount of gas in any gas system yields a constant. This is referred to as *Boltzmann's constant*, which can be applied to all gas systems.
  2. The ideal gas law is normally expressed as:

$$PV = nRT \tag{16}$$

or

$$R = PV/nT$$

  where P = pressure, V = volume, n = amount of gas (expressed normally in moles), R = Boltzmann's constant, and T = absolute temperature (expressed in ° K).
  3. Boltzmann's constant is equal to:
    a. 82.1 ml × atm/mole × ° K when pressure is expressed in atmospheres and volume is expressed in milliliters.
    b. 62.3 L × mm Hg/mole × ° K when pressure is expressed in millimeters of mercury and volume is expressed in liters.
D. *Boyle's law* states that pressure and volume of a gas system vary inversely if the temperature and amount of gas in the system are constant.
  1. Boyle's law mathematically is:

$$PV = nRT \tag{17}$$

where nRT is equal to a constant, thus

$$PV = K \tag{18}$$

  2. In a system where temperature and amount of gas are constant, the original pressure and volume equal the final pressure and volume:

$$P_1V_1 = P_2V_2 \tag{19}$$

Problem:
  If a patient's exhaled volume (dry) at a P_B of 760 mm Hg is 300 ml, what is the exhaled volume (dry) during air transport if the atmospheric pressure during transport is 500 mm Hg?

$$P_1 = 760 \text{ mm Hg} \qquad P_2 = 500 \text{ mm Hg}$$
$$V_1 = 300 \text{ ml} \qquad V_2 = x$$

$$P_1V_1 = P_2V_2$$
$$(760 \text{ mm Hg})(300 \text{ ml}) = (500 \text{ mm Hg})(x)$$
$$x = 456 \text{ ml}$$

E. *Charles' law* states that the temperature and volume of a gas system vary directly if the pressure and amount of gas in the system are constant.

1. Charles' law mathematically is:

$$\frac{V}{T} = \frac{nR}{P} \tag{20}$$

where nR/P is equal to a constant, thus

$$\frac{V}{T} = K \tag{21}$$

2. In a system where the pressure and amount of gas are constant, the original temperature and volume equal the final temperature and volume:

$$\frac{V_1}{T_1} = \frac{V_2}{T_2} \tag{22}$$

Problem:

A patient's exhaled vital capacity measured at 20° C is 2.5 L. What is the patient's actual exhaled volume at body temperature?

$$
\begin{array}{ll}
V_1 = 2.5\ \text{L} & V_2 = x \\
T_1 = 20°\ \text{C} + 273° & T_2 = 37°\ \text{C} + 273° \\
T_1 = 293°\ \text{K} & T_2 = 310°\ \text{K}
\end{array}
$$

$$\frac{V_1}{T_1} = \frac{V_2}{T_2}$$

$$\frac{2.5\ \text{L}}{293°\ \text{K}} = \frac{x}{310°\ \text{K}}$$

$$x = 2.65\ \text{L}$$

F. *Gay-Lussac's law* states that the pressure and temperature of a gas system vary directly if the volume and amount of gas in the system are constant.

1. Gay-Lussac's law mathematically is:

$$\frac{P}{T} = \frac{nR}{V} \tag{23}$$

where nR/V is equal to a constant, thus

$$\frac{P}{T} = K \tag{24}$$

2. In a system where the volume and amount of gas are constant, the original pressure and temperature equal the final pressure and temperature:

$$\frac{P_1}{T_1} = \frac{P_2}{T_2} \tag{25}$$

Problem:

An arterial blood gas analyzed at 37° C reveals a P_{O_2} of 100 mm Hg. What is the patient's actual P_{O_2} if body temperature is 34° C?

$$
\begin{array}{ll}
P_1 = 100\ \text{mm Hg} & P_2 = x \\
T_1 = 37°\ \text{C} + 273° & T_2 = 34°\ \text{C} + 273° \\
T_1 = 310°\ \text{K} & T_2 = 307°\ \text{K}
\end{array}
$$

$$\frac{P_1}{T_1} = \frac{P_2}{T_2}$$

$$\frac{100\ \text{mm Hg}}{310°\ \text{K}} = \frac{x}{307°\ \text{K}}$$

$$x = 99.03\ \text{mm Hg}$$

G. The *combined gas law* states that pressure, temperature, and volume of gas are specifically related if the amount of gas remains constant.
   1. The combined gas law mathematically is:

$$\frac{PV}{T} = nR \qquad (26)$$

where nR is equal to a constant, thus

$$\frac{PV}{T} = K \qquad (27)$$

   2. In a system where the amount of gas in a system is constant, the original pressure, temperature, and volume are equal to the final pressure, temperature, and volume:

$$\frac{P_1 V_1}{T_1} = \frac{P_2 V_2}{T_2} \qquad (28)$$

   Problem:
   If the original pressure of a system is 700 mm Hg, temperature 30° C, and volume 100 L, what will the final volume be if the pressure is increased to 750 mm Hg and temperature to 37° C?

$$
\begin{array}{ll}
P_1 = 700 \text{ mm Hg} & P_2 = 750 \text{ mm Hg} \\
V_1 = 100 \text{ L} & V_2 = x \\
T_1 = 30° \text{ C} + 273 & T_2 = 37° \text{ C} + 273 \\
T_1 = 303° \text{ K} & T_2 = 310° \text{ K}
\end{array}
$$

$$\frac{P_1 V_1}{T_1} = \frac{P_2 V_2}{T_2}$$

$$(700 \text{ mm Hg})(100 \text{ L})/303° \text{ K} = (750 \text{ mm Hg})(x)/310° \text{ K}$$
$$x = 95 \text{ L}$$

H. All gas law calculations must use temperature on the Kelvin scale for accurate results.
I. Water vapor does not react as an ideal gas; therefore, in a system where water vapor is present, water vapor pressure must be subtracted from the total system pressure before calculations are made.
   Problem:
   If the original pressure of a system is 760 mm Hg, the temperature 37° C saturated with water vapor, and volume 1000 ml, what will the final volume be if the pressure is decreased to 500 mm Hg?

$$
\begin{array}{ll}
P_1 = 760 \text{ mm Hg} & P_2 = 500 \text{ mm Hg} \\
P_{H_2O} = 47 \text{ mm Hg} & P_{H_2O} = 47 \text{ mm Hg} \\
P_{1C} = 713 \text{ mm Hg} & P_{2C} = 453 \text{ mm Hg} \\
T_1 = 37 + 273° & T_2 = 37 + 273° \\
T_1 = 310° \text{ K} & T_2 = 310° \text{ K} \\
V_1 = 1000 \text{ ml} & V_2 = x
\end{array}
$$

$$P_{1C} V_1 = P_{2C} V_2$$
$$(713 \text{ mm Hg})(1000 \text{ ml}) = (453 \text{ mm Hg})x$$
$$x = 1573.95 \text{ ml}$$

J. When precision is needed, the P_B reading should be corrected for the expansion of mercury as affected by temperature.

XII. **Diffusion**
   A. Diffusion is movement of gas from an area of high concentration of a gas to an area of low concentration of that gas (Figure 2-5).

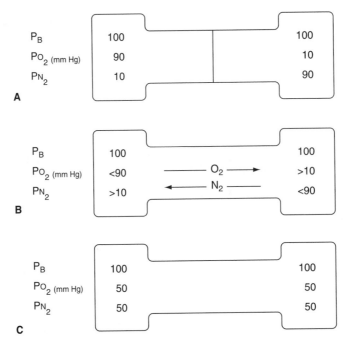

FIG. 2-5 Diffusion of two gases in a closed system. **A,** The system is separated into two parts in which the barometer pressure (P_B) is equal but the P_{O_2} and P_{N_2} differ. **B,** When the two systems are allowed to communicate, O_2 and N_2 diffuse as a result of partial pressure gradients. **C,** Diffusion continues until the partial pressure of O_2 and N_2 is equal throughout the system; however, P_B remains constant.

    B. As diffusion occurs, gases occupy the total container volume as if they were the only gas present; in other words, a gas in a container distributes itself with time equally throughout the whole container volume.

    C. The rate of diffusion of a gas through another gas is affected by the following factors:

        1. The concentration gradient, which is directly related to the rate of diffusion.

        2. The temperature, which is directly related to the rate of diffusion.

        3. The cross-sectional area available for diffusion, which is directly related to the rate of diffusion.

        4. The MW, which is indirectly related to the rate of diffusion.

        5. The distance the gas has to diffuse, which is indirectly related to the rate of diffusion:

$$\text{Rate of diffusion of a gas through a gas} = \frac{\text{(pressure) (temperature) (cross-sectional area)}}{\text{(MW) (distance)}} \qquad (29)$$

    D. *Henry's law* states that the amount of a gas that can dissolve in a liquid is directly related to the P_P of the gas over the liquid and indirectly related to the temperature of the system.

        1. Henry's law establishes the solubility coefficients of gases in liquids.

        2. Solubility coefficients of oxygen and carbon dioxide in plasma at 37° C:

            a. 0.023 ml of O_2/ml of blood/760 mm Hg P_{O_2}

            b. 0.510 ml of CO_2/ml of blood/760 mm Hg P_{CO_2}

    E. *Graham's law* states that the rate of diffusion of a gas through a liquid is indirectly related to the square root of the GMW of the gas.

F. If Henry's law and Graham's law are combined, the rates of diffusion of carbon dioxide to oxygen can be compared under conditions of equal pressure gradients, distances, cross-sectional areas, and temperatures.
  1. When the aforementioned variables are equal, the only factors affecting the comparison would be the GMWs of the gases and their solubility coefficients.
  2. The comparison may be mathematically represented as follows:
  Rate of diffusion of

$$\frac{CO_2}{O_2} = \frac{(\text{sol. coef. } CO_2)(\sqrt{\text{GMW } O_2})}{(\text{sol. coef. } O_2)(\sqrt{\text{GMW } CO_2})}$$

$$\frac{CO_2}{O_2} = \frac{(0.510)(5.66)}{(0.023)(6.66)} \tag{30}$$

$$\frac{CO_2}{O_2} = \frac{19}{1}$$

  3. Thus, under the previously mentioned conditions, carbon dioxide would diffuse approximately 19 times faster than oxygen.
  4. However, at the alveolar capillary membrane, pressure gradients for oxygen and carbon dioxide are not equal.
    a. Diffusion gradient for oxygen is 60 mm Hg.
    b. Diffusion gradient for carbon dioxide is 6 mm Hg.
    c. As a result of these pressure gradients, oxygen equilibrates across the alveolar-capillary membrane slightly faster than carbon dioxide.
    d. Oxygen equilibrates in approximately 0.23 second, whereas carbon dioxide equilibrates in approximately 0.25 second.

XIII. **Elastance and Compliance**
  A. Elastance (E) is the ability of a distorted object to return to its original shape.
  B. Compliance (C) is the ease with which an object can be distorted.
  C. Compliance and elastance are inversely related:

$$C = \frac{1}{E} \tag{31}$$

  D. If the compliance of a system increases, the elastance of the system decreases.
  E. If the compliance of a system decreases, the elastance of the system increases.
  F. *Hook's law* defines the response of elastic bodies to distorting forces (Figure 2-6).
    1. It states that an elastic body stretches equal units of length or volume for each unit of weight or force applied to it.
    2. This relationship holds until the elastic limit of the system is reached.
    3. Beyond the elastic limit, each unit of weight or force produces smaller and smaller changes in length or volume.
    4. With a true spring, exceeding the elastic limit results in permanent distortion of the spring.
    5. This principle can be applied to the lung. Overstretching with large tidal volumes results in disruption to the alveolar-capillary membrane and the development of ventilator-induced lung injury (see Chapter 23).
  G. Elastance can be mathematically defined as:

$$E = \frac{\Delta P}{\Delta V} \tag{32}$$

  where ΔP = change in pressure and ΔV = change in volume.
  H. Compliance can be mathematically defined as:

$$C = \frac{\Delta V}{\Delta P} \tag{33}$$

  I. See Chapter 5 for more details related to respiratory physiology.

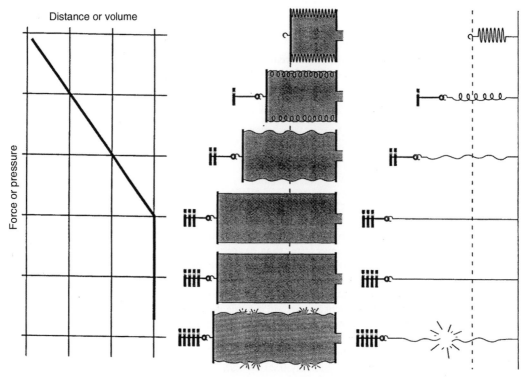

FIG. 2-6 Hooke's law applied to a spring. For an elastic structure, the increase in length (or volume) varies directly with the increase in force (or pressure) until the elastic limit is reached. Further stretching results in destruction of the system.

XIV.   **Surface Tension**
   A.   Surface tension (ST) is a force that exists at the interface between a liquid and a gas or between two liquids.
   B.   The ST of a liquid is the result of like molecules being attracted to each other and thus moving away from the interface. This causes the liquid to occupy the smallest volume possible (Figure 2-7).
   C.   As a result of ST, a force is necessary to cause a tear in the surface of the liquid.
   D.   The ST of a liquid is expressed in dynes per linear centimeter.
   E.   ST is indirectly related to temperature.

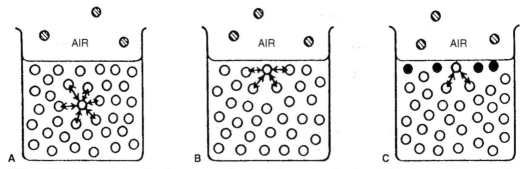

FIG. 2-7 A, Intermolecular attraction among molecules in the center of a given liquid volume. **B,** Intermolecular attraction among molecules at the surface of a liquid. **C,** Surface-active particles (black circles) interfere with the molecular attraction among molecules at the surface of the liquid.

F. *LaPlace's law* is used to determine the amount of pressure generated inside a system as a result of ST.
1. The law states that the P in dynes per square centimeter as a result of ST in dynes per centimeter is equal to the ST of the liquid multiplied by 1 over the radii (r) of curvature in centimeters:

$$P = ST \left(\frac{1}{r_1} + \frac{1}{r_2} + \frac{1}{r_3} + \ldots \frac{1}{r_n} \right) \tag{34}$$

2. LaPlace's law as applied to a drop is:

$$P = \frac{2\,ST}{r} \tag{35}$$

Here reference is made to a perfect sphere that has only two equal radii of curvature, one in the vertical plane and one in the horizontal plane.
3. LaPlace's law as applied to a bubble is:

$$P = \frac{4\,ST}{r} \tag{36}$$

There are two interfaces in a bubble, one on the inside of the bubble and one on the outside; thus, there are four radii. All radii are considered equal because the film of the bubble is only angstroms in diameter.
4. LaPlace's law as applied to a blood vessel is:

$$P = \frac{ST}{r} \tag{37}$$

When the radii of curvature of a blood vessel are considered, the only radius used in the calculation is that of the vessel's width because the radius of length is so great. When the inverse of the radii of length is calculated, the number essentially goes to infinity and is meaningless in calculating the pressure as a result of ST.
5. It is important to remember that the pressure as a result of ST is indirectly related to the radius. The smaller the sphere, the greater the pressure as a result of ST (Figure 2-8).
6. See Chapter 5 for details on the effect of ST on lung mechanics.
G. *Critical volume* is a volume below which the effects of ST are so great that the structure collapses. Once the critical volume is reached, collapse is always imminent.
H. The force necessary to inflate a deflated object increases markedly as the critical volume is reached but rapidly decreases once the critical volume is exceeded.

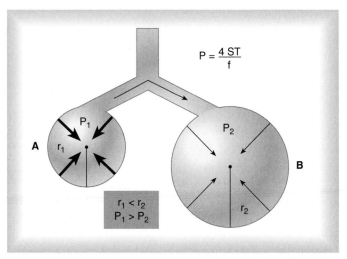

FIG. 2-8. When two bubbles of different sizes (**A** and **B**) but with the same surface tension are allowed to communicate, the greater pressure as a result of surface tension in the smaller bubble causes it to empty into the larger.

I. It is difficult to reinflate a collapsed lung. It requires high pressure to reopen, but once reopened the pressure needed to keep the lung open rapidly decreases.

J. Chemicals referred to as surfactants reduce the ST of a fluid. Surfactants are surface-active agents that interfere with the molecules of the fluid at the surface, causing a reduction in the force (ST) that draws the fluid centrally. Soaps and detergents are common surfactants (see Figure 2-7).

XV. **Fluid Dynamics**
   A. Law of continuity
      1. The product of the cross-sectional area of a system and the velocity for a given flow rate is constant (Figure 2-9).
      2. Thus, if the flow of gas is constant, the cross-sectional area and gas velocity are inversely related.
      3. In any system with varying radii, the velocity of gas movement must change inversely as the radius changes.
   B. Velocity versus flow
      1. Velocity is the speed with which movement between two points occurs (e.g., miles/hour, cm/sec).
      2. Flow is the volume passing a single point per unit of time (L/min).
      3. The two are related and may change directly or indirectly with each other, depending on the specific changes that occur in the structure of the system.
   C. Resistance to gas flow
      1. In general, resistance is defined as the force (pressure) necessary to maintain a specific flow in a particular system (Figure 2-10).
      2. For gas movement to occur, there must be a pressure gradient. The overall resistance of the system determines the magnitude of the pressure gradient. Resistance to flow is defined by Ohm's law. It states that resistance is equal to the change in pressure divided by flow:

$$R = \frac{\Delta P}{\dot{V}} \qquad\qquad (38)$$

where R = airway resistance, ΔP = change in pressure, and $\dot{V}$ = flow.
      3. Resistance is a physical property of the system.
      4. The change in pressure reflects the amount of pressure necessary to maintain a *specific flow* in the system.
      5. The resistance of a system is increased under the following situations:
         a. Decreased lumen of the system.
         b. Directional changes in the system.
         c. Branching of the system.
      6. If the resistance of a system is constant, an increase in pressure gradient results in an increase in system flow.
      7. An increase in resistance with a constant pressure gradient results in a decrease in flow.

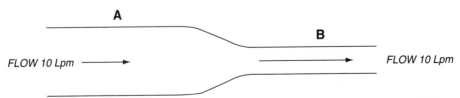

FIG. 2-9 Representation of the law of continuity. Because the cross-sectional area A is greater than B and the flow is constant, the velocity at B must be greater than the velocity of A. However, the product of velocity and cross-sectional area is equal at A and B.

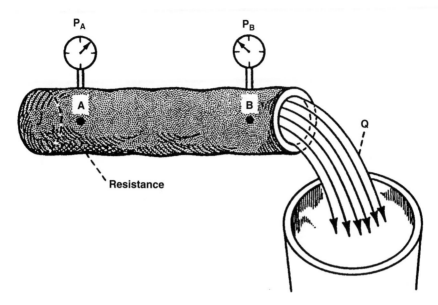

FIG. 2-10 Fluid flowing past two points, A and B, in a channel or pipe produces a pressure decrease that is related to the bulk flow of the fluid (Q) and the resistance of the channel or pipe. P_A = pressure at point A, P_B = pressure at point B, and resistance = the walls or structure of the channel.

8. In general, if resistance is constant, pressure gradient and system flow are directly related.

D. Series and parallel resistances (Figure 2-11)
  1. Series resistances are resistance elements arranged sequentially in the direction of flow (e.g., heat and moisture exchanges attached to an endotracheal tube). The exchanger and the tube are series resistors.
    (a) When resistors are placed in series their individual resistances are additive.
    (b) The pressure necessary to maintain flow is equal to flow times the sum of the individual resistance.

$$P = \dot{V}\,(R_1 + R_2 + R_3) \qquad (39)$$

  where R_1, R_2, and R_3 represent three resistances in series.
  2. Parallel resistances are resistance elements arranged next to each other where flow is divided between resistive elements. The mouth and nose are arranged in parallel.
    (a) When resistors are placed in parallel the pressure gradient across them is equal, but flow through each is related to the resistance of each resistor.
    (b) The pressure necessary to maintain flow across a parallel system is equal to the sum of the flow times resistance of each resistor.

$$P = (\dot{V}_1)\,(R_1) + (\dot{V}_2)\,(R_2) + (\dot{V}_3)\,(R_3) \qquad (40)$$

  where $\dot{V}_1$, $\dot{V}_2$, $\dot{V}_3$ represent the flow through each resistor, and R_1, R_2, and R_3 represent the resistance of each resistor.

E. Conductance
  1. Conductance is the capability of a system to maintain flow.
  2. Conductance is the inverse of resistance.

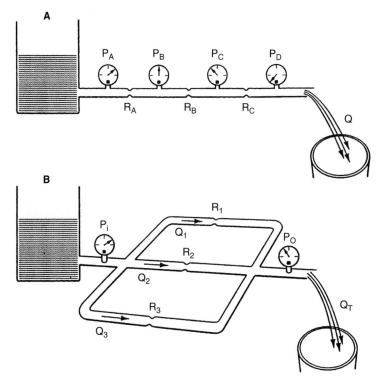

FIG. 2-11 Series and parallel resistors. **A,** Resistances connected in series have a common flow (Q), but the pressure before each resistor decreases based on the magnitude of the resistance across each resistor. **B,** Resistances connected in parallel divide flow among all resistors based on the actual resistance of each resistor.

3. Mathematically:

$$\text{Conductance} = \frac{\Delta \dot{V}}{\Delta P} \qquad (41)$$

F. Types of flow
   1. *Laminar flow* is a smooth, even, nontumbling flow.
      a. Laminar flow proceeds with a cone front. The molecules of gas in the center of the system encounter the least frictional resistance and move at a greater velocity than those at the sides of the system (Figure 2-12).
      b. In all laminar flow situations, the pressure necessary to overcome airway resistance is directly related to flow:

$$R = \frac{\Delta P}{\dot{V}} \qquad (42)$$

   2. *Turbulent flow* is a rough, tumbling, uneven flow pattern.
      a. Turbulent flow proceeds with a blunt front. Because of a tumbling effect, all of the molecules in the system encounter the walls of the vessel (see Figure 2-12).
      b. In a turbulent flow system, the pressure necessary to overcome airway resistance is directly related to the *square* of the flow:

$$R = \frac{\Delta P}{\dot{V}^2} \qquad (43)$$

      c. *The pressure gradient necessary to maintain turbulent flow is much higher than that necessary to maintain laminar flow.*
      d. A marker substance (smoke) is rapidly mixed with the primary gas in a turbulent system but not in a laminar system (Figure 2-13).

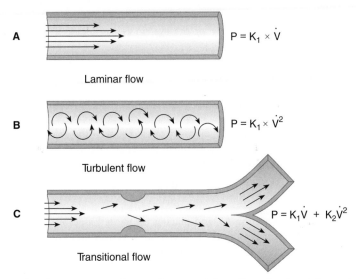

FIG. 2-12 A, In laminar flow, movement is smooth, no tumbling with molecules at the center of the flow proceeding more rapidly than those at the walls of the system. **B,** In turbulent flow, movement is rough and tumbling with no direct path followed by any molecules. **C,** In transitional (tracheobronchial) flow, a combination of laminar and turbulent flow occurs. Flow becomes turbulent at bifurcations or points where direction changes.

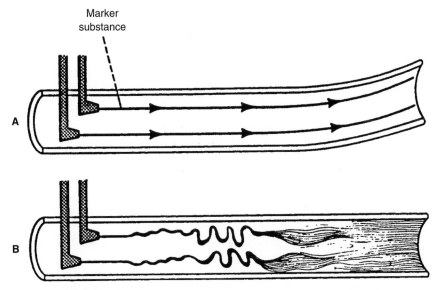

FIG. 2-13 A, During laminar flow, a marker substance (smoke) added to a flowing fluid remains stationary and follows gradual changes in the direction of flow. **B,** During turbulent flow, the paths of the marker become unsteady and rapidly mix with the primary fluid.

3. *Tracheobronchial flow* is a combination of areas of laminar and turbulent flow. Tracheobronchial flow is believed to be the type of flow maintained throughout the respiratory system (see Figure 2-12).
G. *Reynold's number*
   1. Reynold's number (RN) is a dimensionless number that indicates whether flow through a system is laminar or turbulent.
   2. RN is calculated as follows:

$$RN = \frac{(Diameter)(Velocity)(Density)}{(Viscosity)} \qquad (44)$$

where the diameter refers to the diameter of the system, and velocity, density, and viscosity refer to the gas that is flowing in the system.

3. If RN is ≥2000, the flow in the system is turbulent. If it is < 2000, the flow is laminar.

H. *Poiseuille's law*
   1. Poiseuille's law was originally used to determine the viscosity of a fluid.
   2. It also defines the factors that effect the pressure required to maintain laminar flow.
   3. Viscosity is defined as a fluid's resistance to deformity and for gases increases with increased temperature.
   4. Poiseuille's law states that viscosity (n) is equal to the change in pressure (ΔP) times pi (π) times the radius to the fourth power (r^4) divided by eight times the length of the system ($8l$) times flow ($\dot{V}$):

$$n = \frac{\Delta P \pi r^4}{8l\dot{V}} \tag{45}$$

   5. Rearranging equation 45 and placing on the left side of the equation those factors that would be constant when ventilating a patient and on the right side of the equation those factors that would vary, the result is:

$$\frac{n8l}{\pi} = \frac{\Delta P r^4}{\dot{V}} \tag{46}$$

   6. The right side of equation 46 indicates the relationship between pressure, flow, and radius of a laminar gas flow system.
   7. If the radius were to decrease by one half, there would be a 16-fold change in the right side of the equation.
   8. To maintain the left side of the equation constant, a 16-fold change in pressure or flow or a combination of both would be necessary to minimize the effects of the decrease in radius.
   9. Thus, to minimize the effects of an airway diameter decrease, it would be necessary to increase the pressure gradient and/or decrease the flow in the system. As gas enters deeper into the respiratory tract, flow through individual segments decreases.
   10. Theoretically, Poiseuille's law can be applied only to homogeneous fluid systems that are nonpulsatile and laminar through a single cylinder.
   11. Thus, Poiseuille's law cannot be directly applied to the respiratory and cardiovascular systems, but it does provide insights into the interrelationships between pressure, flow, and system radius in physiologic systems.

I. *Bernoulli effect*
   1. Bernoulli effect: As a gas moves through a free-flowing system, transmural pressure is inversely related to velocity of the gas (i.e., as the velocity of the gas increases, the transmural pressure decreases; Figure 2-14).
   2. Statement 1 holds true because the total energy in a free-flowing system is equal at all points (conservation of energy).
   3. In a free-flowing system of limited size functioning essentially as a non–gravity-dependent system, the total energy is equal to the sum of the KE and the transmural pressure energy.
   4. Transmural pressure energy is purely a measure of the force that the gas flow exerts on the walls of the system (Figure 2-15).
   5. KE in this sense is equal to 0.5 times the gas density times the gas velocity squared:

$$\text{KE} = 0.5 \ (\text{D})(\text{V}^2) \tag{47}$$

   6. Thus, in a free-flowing system:

$$\text{Total energy} = 0.5 \ (\text{D})(\text{V}^2) + \text{P}_{\text{transmural}} \tag{48}$$

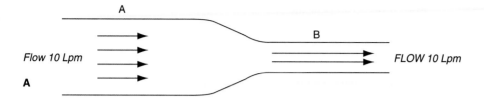

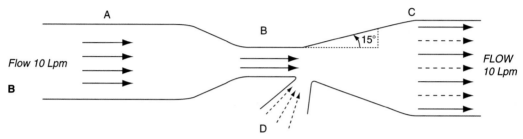

FIG. 2-14 A, (top) The Bernoulli effect. The velocity at B is greater than at A. The transmural pressure is greater at A than at B as a result of the law of conservation of energy. **B,** (bottom) The Venturi effect. At B the transmural pressure is subatmospheric because of the increased kinetic energy. A second gas is entrained at D. If the angle of divergence distal to the stenosis (point B) is not greater than 15°, the transmural pressure at C and A is equal.

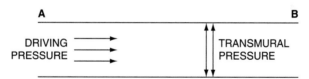

FIG. 2-15 Driving pressure, the force necessary to maintain flow, is the difference in pressure across a system: pressure at A – pressure at B. Transmural pressure is the force exerted on the lateral wall of a system. In a given system actual transmural pressure may vary depending on the structure of the system, even though the driving pressure is constant.

This illustrates the fact that velocity and transmural pressure are inversely related.

7. As the radius of the system decreases and velocity of the gas moving through the system increases, transmural pressure decreases, per equation 48.

8. The lower the density of a gas, the smaller the decrease in transmural pressure as the gas moves through a stenosis. This relationship demonstrates the effect of density on maintaining a more laminar flow (see Chapter 34).

9. *Venturi principle*
   a. The Venturi principle is an extension of the Bernoulli effect (see Figure 2-14).
   b. It states that distal to a stenosis in a free-flowing system, prestenotic pressure can be restored if the angle of divergence of the system from the midline does not exceed 15°.

    c. Also, if the stenosis in the system is small enough, subatmospheric transmural pressure can be developed and used to entrain a second gas or liquid.

    d. Venturi systems can be designed to deliver specific oxygen concentrations.

    e. The concentration of oxygen delivered by a Venturi system can be varied by:

       (1) Altering the size of the Venturi's stenosis.

       (2) Altering the size of the entrainment ports.

    f. Backpressure on a Venturi system decreases the volume of fluid or gas entrained. This causes the oxygen concentration delivered by such a system to increase.

J. Jet mixing

    1. The use of a constant flow of gas (jet) to entrain a second gas (Figure 2-16).

    2. No pressure gradient exists between the jet flow and the ambient environment.

    3. Air entrainment is a result of the viscous shearing force between a dynamic fluid and a stationary fluid resulting in a change in velocities.

      a. The dynamic fluid's velocity decreases.

      b. The stationary fluid's velocity increases.

    4. Provided free access is allowed for the entrained gas, mixing at specific ratios can be maintained.

    5. Altering the *flow* of the gas from the jet alters the total volume exiting the system but does not alter entrainment ratios or resulting gas concentration.

    6. Changing the size of the jet orifice or the size of the entrainment port alters entrainment ratios.

    7. Entrainment ratios are the same as those commonly listed for Venturi systems (see Chapter 34).

    8. Backpressure on the system decreases entrainment and increases $F_I O_2$.

    9. Jet mixing is responsible for the function of air entrainment masks and most other systems in respiratory care commonly attributed to the Venturi effect.

K. Driving pressure as illustrated in Figure 2-15 is the pressure necessary to maintain flow between point A and B in a gas flow system.

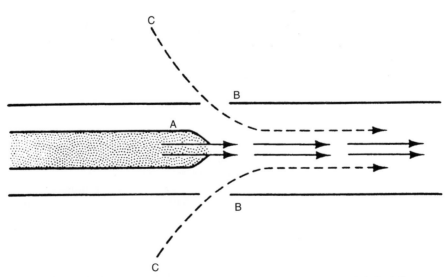

FIG. 2-16 Jet mixing results from the shearing force of a rapid flow of gas A on a relatively stationary gas C. The velocity of the stationary gas is thus increased, resulting in entrainment at point B.

BIBLIOGRAPHY

Comroe JH: *The Lung,* ed 2. Chicago, Year Book Publishers, 1962.

Comroe JH: *Physiology of Respiration,* ed 2. Chicago, Year Book Medical Publishers, 1974.

Guyton AC, Hall JE: *Textbook of Medical Physiology,* ed 10. Philadelphia, WB Saunders, 2000.

Hess DR, MacIntyre NR, Mishoe SC, Galvin WF, Adams AB, Saposnick AB: *Respiratory Care Principles and Practices.* Philadelphia, WB Saunders, 2002.

Kacmarek RM, Hess DR, Stoller JK: *Monitoring in Respiratory Care,* St. Louis, Mosby–Year Book, Inc., 1993.

Murray JF: *The Normal Lung,* ed 2. Philadelphia, WB Saunders, 1987.

Nunn JF: *Applied Respiratory Physiology With Special Reference to Anesthesia,* ed 2. Stoneham, MA, Butterworth, 1977.

Pierson DJ, Kacmarek RM: *Foundations of Respiratory Care,* New York, Churchill Livingstone, 1992.

Scacci R: Air entrainment masks: Jet mixing is how they work; the Bernoulli and Venturi principles is how they don't. *Respir Care* 24:928-934, 1979.

Shapiro BA, Harrison RA, Kacmarek RM, et al: *Clinical Application of Respiratory Care,* ed 3. Chicago, Year Book Medical Publishers, 1985.

Shapiro BA, Harrison RA, Cane R, et al: *Clinical Application of Blood Gases,* ed 4. Chicago, Year Book Medical Publishers, 1989.

Wojciechowski WV: *Respiratory Care Sciences: An Integrated Approach,* Clifton Park, NY, Delmar, 1996.

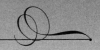

Chapter 3

Microbiology, Sterilization, and Infection Control

I. **Classification of Microorganisms by Cell Type**
   A. Eukaryotic (Protista)
      1. Algae (except blue-green)
      2. Protozoa
      3. Fungi
      4. Slime molds
   B. Prokaryotic (lower Protista)
      1. Blue-green algae
      2. Bacteria
      3. Rickettsiae
      4. Mycoplasmas
   C. Viruses
      1. Simple nucleic acid chain (DNA or RNA)
      2. Protein coat

II. **Eukaryotic Cell Structure (Figure 3-1)**
   A. Surface layers
      1. Cell membrane: Complex lipoprotein structure.
      2. Cell wall: Rigid to moderately rigid polysaccharide structure.
   B. Nucleus
      1. Well-defined nucleus surrounded by nuclear membrane.
      2. Control center for cell growth and development.
         a. Contains chromosomes
         b. Contains RNA
         c. Nuclear membrane continuous with endoplasmic reticulum (ER)
   C. Cytoplasmic structures
      1. Endoplasmic reticulum: System of large sacs and smaller tubules responsible for macromolecular transport.
         a. Smooth ER (without attached ribosomes): Involved in lipid and steroid synthesis.
         b. Rough ER (with attached ribosomes): Involved in protein synthesis.
      2. Mitochondria: Responsible for production of adenosine triphosphate and aerobic metabolism (Krebs' cycle and electron transport chain); seen in animal cells.
      3. Chloroplasts: Contain pigments, starches, and enzymes used in photosynthesis; seen in plant cells.
      4. Ribosomes: Free or attached to ER; responsible for protein synthesis.
      5. Lysosomes: Contain proteolytic enzymes for metabolism of ingested organic material.

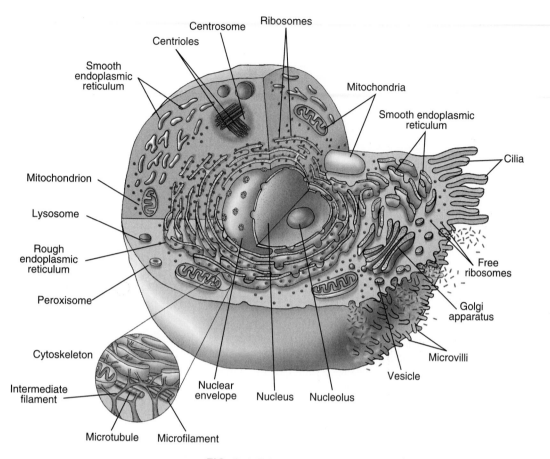

FIG. 3-1 Eukaryotic cell.

D. Motility organelles
   1. Cilia
      a. Numerous on cell exterior
      b. Move in coordinated waves
   2. Flagella
      a. Singular or present in small numbers
      b. Move in undulating motion
      c. Longer than cilia

III. **Prokaryotic Cell Structure (Figure 3-2)**
   A. Surface layers
      1. Cell membrane or plasma membrane
         a. A lipoprotein structure.
         b. The inner layer beneath the cell wall.
         c. Acts as osmotic barrier and is the site of some enzyme activity.
      2. Cell wall: Moderately rigid to very rigid structure
         a. Protects cell from bursting in low osmotic pressure conditions.
         b. Maintains cell shape.
      3. Cell wall in gram-positive bacteria
         a. High lipid content
         b. Murein network: Peptide chains attached to larger polysaccharide chains
         c. Stains violet on Gram stain because of peptidoglycan in the cell wall

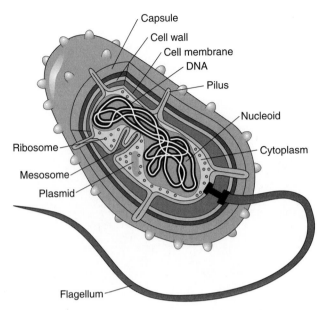

FIG. 3-2 A typical bacterial prokaryotic cell.

4. Cell wall in gram-negative bacteria: three layers
   a. The inner layer is a mucopeptide.
   b. The middle layer is lipopolysaccharide.
   c. The outer layer is a lipoprotein.
   d. Stains pink on Gram stain with counter-safranin stain because of lack of peptidoglycan.
5. Capsule
   a. Layer surrounding outside of cell produced by the cell itself; common in pathogenic organisms.
   b. Functions
      (1) Prevents phagocytosis.
      (2) Prevents virus attachment.
      (3) Functions as external nutrient storage.
   c. Causative factors
      (1) High sugar concentration
      (2) Presence of blood or serum in culture
      (3) Microorganism living in a host organism
   d. Composition: Mucilaginous
      (1) Polypeptides
      (2) Dextran
      (3) Polysaccharides
      (4) Cellulose
B. Nucleus
   1. No distinct nucleus; no separation from the cytoplasm.
   2. The cell may contain one or more regions of nuclear material called *nucleoids*.
   3. No mitotic apparatus.
   4. Chromosomes exist freely in cytoplasm; may be circular or attached to the cell membrane.
C. Cytoplasmic structures
   1. The ER is absent.
   2. Mitochondria are absent. Aerobic metabolic enzymes are present in the form of multienzyme complexes; they are attached to the cell membrane or other internal membranes.

3. Chloroplasts are absent. Photosynthetic enzymes and pigments are present in special arrangements; these are not separated from the cytoplasm by a membrane.
4. Ribosomes: Slightly smaller than eukaryotic ribosomes; exist freely in cytoplasm.
5. Mesosome: They are found in the cell membrane and allow for attachment of DNA in cell division. They are found chiefly in gram-positive forms.
6. Lysosomes are absent.
7. Cytoplasmic granules store cell nutrients.

D. Motility organelles
   1. Flagella
      a. They are different from eukaryotic flagella.
      b. One or many are on each cell.
   2. Pili
      a. They are short, fine filaments.
      b. Their function is not known; may function in specialized bacterial sexual reproduction.

E. Bacterial spores
   1. They are the intermediate form of the organism that develops in response to adverse environmental conditions.
   2. They will regenerate to a vegetative cell when conditions improve.
   3. They are notably produced by the aerobic genus *Bacillus* and the anaerobic genus *Clostridium*, and *Sporosarcina*.
   4. They resist adverse environmental conditions of dryness, heat, and poor nutrition.
   5. A true spore is a highly refractile body formed within the vegetative bacterial cell.
   6. They function as a protective coat around nucleic material that may remain inside the cell (endospore) or extend beyond the width of the cell (exospore).
   7. They are metabolically active and contain essential enzymes of Krebs' cycle.

IV. Bacterial Growth Requirements

A. Growth medium: Needs vary with specific bacteria.
   1. Simple nutrients: Water, carbon, hydrogen, nitrogen, oxygen, sulfur, phosphorus, calcium, potassium, and magnesium
   2. Complex nutrients: Sugar, amino acids, and blood products

B. Atmospheric gas requirements
   1. *Obligate anaerobes* reproduce only in an oxygen-free environment. Oxygen is toxic to these organisms.
   2. *Aerotolerant anaerobes* are organisms unaffected by exposure to oxygen.
   3. *Facultative anaerobes* reproduce under aerobic or anaerobic conditions.
   4. *Microaerophilic anaerobes* reproduce best at low oxygen tensions. High oxygen tensions are inhibitory.
   5. *Obligate aerobes* require oxygen for reproduction.
   6. *Chemolithotrophic* and *photolithotrophic bacteria* use carbon dioxide as their principal source of carbon.

C. Temperature requirements, optimal growth ranges:
   1. Psychrophilic: −5° C to 30° C (optimum 10° C to 20° C)
   2. Mesophilic (pathogenic): 10° C to 45° C (optimum 20° C to 40° C)
   3. Thermophilic: 25° C to 80° C (optimum 50° C to 60° C)

D. The osmotic pressure requirement varies with each bacterial species. Most require a 0.9% saline environment.

E. Hydrogen ion (pH variations)
   1. Pathogens: 7.2 to 7.6 (optimum range)
   2. Acidophiles: 6.5 to 7.0
   3. Neutrophiles: 7.5 to 8.0
   4. Alkalophiles: 8.4 to 9.0

F. Moisture: Water is essential for all bacterial growth.

G. Light
1. Most bacteria prefer darkness.
2. Ultraviolet (UV) and blue light are destructive to bacteria.

V. **Microbial Reproduction**
A. Asexual (binary fission)
1. This is the most common form of reproduction.
2. Two identical daughter cells result from a single parent cell.
3. Chromosome replication is normal.
B. Sexual (conjugation)
1. This is present in a few bacterial species.
2. DNA is transferred from one bacterium to another.

VI. **Growth Pattern: A new culture of bacteria will develop similar to the growth curve seen in Figure 3-3.**
A. Lag phase: Adaptation to new environment; little reproduction.
B. Exponential phase: Stage of rapid cell growth.
C. Stationary phase: Equal death and growth rates.
D. Death phase: Depletion of culture nutrients and buildup of toxic waste; death rate exceeds growth rate.

VII. **Measurement of Growth**
A. Cell concentration: Expressed as the number of viable cells.
B. Cell density: Expressed as dry weights.

VIII. **Microbial Relationships**
A. Autotroph: An organism capable of using simple inorganic matter as nutrients (nonpathogenic).
B. Heterotroph: An organism that requires organic matter for growth and survival (pathogenic).
C. Symbiosis: Two dissimilar organisms existing together.
1. Amensalism: One organism is inhibited, and the other is not affected.
2. Commensalism: One organism benefits, and the other is not affected.
3. Mutualism: Each organism benefits and is unable to survive without the other.
4. Parasitism: One organism benefits, and the other is harmed.
5. Synnecrosis: Both organisms are harmed by the relationship.

IX. **Microbial Shapes (Figure 3-4)**
A. Spherical: Coccus
B. Rod: Bacillus
C. Spiral: Spirillum, spirochete
D. Comma-shaped: Vibrios
E. Spindle-shaped: Fusiform

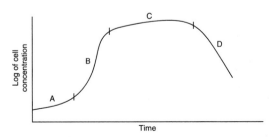

FIG. 3-3 Growth pattern of a new closed culture. **A,** Lag phase. **B,** Exponential phase. **C,** Stationary phase. **D,** Death phase.

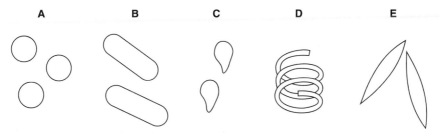

FIG. 3-4 Bacterial shapes. **A,** Cocci. **B,** Bacilli. **C,** Vibrios. **D,** Spirillum, spirochete. **E,** Fusiform.

X. **Staining**
  A. Purpose: Used to identify and categorize bacteria based on cell components.
  B. Gram staining
    1. Bacteria can be separated into two general categories by virtue of their staining properties: gram-positive or gram-negative.
    2. Variation in staining is determined by cell wall construction.
    3. Staining sequence
      a. Basic dye is crystal violet (all organisms take up this dye).
      b. The specimen is then covered with Gram's iodine.
      c. A water rinse is then performed.
      d. The specimen is then decolorized with acetone.
      e. A water wash is then performed.
      f. The specimen is counterstained with red dye (usually safranin).
      g. A final water rinse is done.
    4. Gram-positive organisms stain blue or violet.
    5. Gram-negative organisms stain red or pink.
  C. Acid-fast (Ziehl-Neelsen) stain
    1. Used to identify bacteria of the genus *Mycobacterium.*
    2. Acid-fast bacteria appear red against a blue background.
    3. Staining sequence
      a. Carbolfuchsin (red)
      b. Water rinse
      c. Destain with hydrochloric acid alcohol
      d. Counterstain with methylene blue

XI. **Definitions Related to Microorganisms**
  A. Contamination: Presence of a microorganism in an otherwise sterile environment.
  B. Pathogen: Any disease-producing microorganism.
  C. Virulence: Heightened ability of an organism to produce infection in its host.
  D. Aerobic: Growth only in the presence of oxygen.
  E. Anaerobic: Growth in the absence of oxygen.
  F. Toxins: Poisonous substances produced by bacteria.
    1. Exotoxin
      a. Produced primarily by gram-positive bacteria.
      b. Composed of protein and normally excreted by bacteria into surrounding media.
      c. Some are extremely lethal.
    2. Endotoxin
      a. Produced primarily by gram-negative bacteria.
      b. A lipopolysaccharide normally released when the bacterial cell is destroyed.
  G. Vegetative cell: Metabolically active form of a bacterium in which reproduction can occur.
  H. Vector: An insect, animal, or other carrier that transfers an infecting agent or pathogen from one host to another.

I. Host: An organism that harbors or furnishes nutrition to a dissimilar organism.
J. Bacteremia: The presence of bacteria in the blood.
K. Septicemia: A condition in which pathogens and their associated toxins are present in the blood.
L. Toxemia: The presence of bacterial toxins in the blood.
M. Pyogenic: Pus producing.
N. Pyemia: Condition in which pus-forming bacteria have entered the bloodstream.
O. Pyrogenic: Fever producing.

XII. **Definitions Related to Immunologic Response**
A. Infection: An inflammatory process resulting from the presence and growth of a pathogenic organism.
B. Inflammation: A tissue response to injury or stress that can cause local vascular dilation, fluid exudation, and/or leukocyte accumulation at the site caused by a microorganism or some other stress.
C. Superinfection: Infection developed primarily in the debilitated or immunosuppressed patient previously treated with antibiotics.
D. Nosocomial infection: Hospital-acquired infection.
E. Immunity: The ability of the body to resist or overcome infection or disease.
F. Plasma cell: Cells that specialize in the production of antibodies.
G. Eosinophils: White blood cells with two- or three-lobed nucleus and large cytoplasmic granules.
    1. They are able to phagocytize antigen-antibody complexes.
    2. Increase in number occurs with hypersensitivity and parasitic infections.
H. Lymphocyte: White blood cells formed in the lymphatic system and by the thymus gland.
    1. Have a single nucleus with no granules.
    2. Can become plasma cells that may form antibodies.
    3. Can attract and localize macrophages to an area of infection.
I. T lymphocytes: Specialized white blood cells formed by the thymus gland.
J. Macrophage: Large mononuclear phagocytic cell.
    1. Travels to sites of infection.
    2. Can phagocytize antigens or microbes.
K. Monocyte: White blood cell (leukocyte) with a single nucleus (mononuclear) that is capable of phagocytosis.
L. Polymorphonucleated leukocyte (neutrophil): White blood cell with a multilobed nucleus capable of phagocytosis.
    1. Can migrate into tissues.
    2. Acts as a defensive mechanism against bacteria.
M. Antibody: Developed in response to antigen.
    1. Produced by lymphoid tissue in response to an antigen.
    2. Antibodies can cause invading antigens or microbes to clump, rendering them easier for ingestion by macrophages and granulocytes.
    3. Can cause lysis of some microbial cells.
N. Antigen: A substance, often a protein, that gains access to the bloodstream or a body tissue.
    1. It stimulates or induces antibody formation.
    2. Certain antigens cause specific lymphocytes to gather at the site of an infection.
O. Immunoglobulins: Circulating antibodies.
    1. IgA: A surface immunoglobulin found on mucous membranes of the gastrointestinal tract and upper respiratory tract.
    2. IgE: Involved with allergic responses.
    3. IgG: Most abundant of the immunoglobulins; serves to activate the complement system.
    4. IgM: Helps agglutinate antigenic matter.

XIII. Development of Infection
  A. Infection occurs when a pathogen is able to overcome the barriers of a host.
  B. Three elements must be present for an infection to develop:
    1. A source of pathogens
    2. A susceptible host
    3. A route of transmission
  C. Factors that increase host susceptibility to infection include:
    1. Diabetes mellitus
    2. Lymphoma
    3. Leukemia
    4. Neoplasia
    5. Uremia
    6. Previous treatment with:
      a. Antimicrobials (some)
      b. Corticosteroids
      c. Irradiation
      d. Immunosuppressive agents
    7. Older age
    8. Chronic disease
    9. Shock
    10. Coma
    11. Traumatic injury
    12. Recent surgical procedure
  D. The high incidence of nosocomial gram-negative bacterial pneumonias is associated with factors that promote colonization of the pharynx (Box 3-1).
  E. Patients with artificial airways are at highest risk of nosocomial pneumonia.
  F. Pathogens can be transmitted to a host by five major routes (Table 3-1).
    1. Contact
      a. Direct: Body surface-to-body surface contact between host and colonized or infected person.
      b. Indirect: Contact between host and contaminated object.
    2. Droplet: Contact with large droplets produced by an infected or contaminated individual.
      a. Produced by coughing, sneezing, talking, and so on.
      b. Droplet only travels short distances (i.e., ≤3 feet).
    3. Airborne
      a. Contaminate is spread by dust particles or droplet nuclei.
      b. Normally ≤5 μm in size.
      c. Capable of remaining suspended in air for long periods.
    4. Common vehicle: Pathogen transmitted to host in contaminated food or water.
    5. Vectorborne: Transmission by an animal from infected individual to host, usually by insects.

BOX 3-1

Conditions Associated with Oropharyngeal Colonization by Gram-Negative Bacilli

• Acidosis	• Hypotension
• Azotemia	• Nasogastric tube
• Chronic alcohol abuse	• Neutralization of gastric secretions
• Coma	• Respiratory distress syndrome
• Diabetes mellitus	• Underlying respiratory disease
• Endotracheal intubation	

From Wilkins RL, et al: *Egan's Fundamentals of Respiratory Care,* ed 8. St. Louis, Mosby, 2003, p. 43.

TABLE **3-1**

Routes of Infectious Disease Transmission

Mode	Type	Examples
Contact	Direct	Hepatitis A
		Venereal disease
		HIV
		Staphylococcus
		Enteric bacteria
	Indirect	*Pseudomonas aeruginosa*
		Enteric bacteria
		Hepatitis B and C
		HIV
Droplet		*Haemophilus influenzae* (type B) pneumonia and epiglottitis
		Neisseria meningitidis pneumonia
		Diphtheria
		Pertussis
		Streptococcal pneumonia
		Influenza
		Mumps
		Rubella
		Adenovirus
Vehicle	Waterborne	Shigellosis
		Cholera
	Foodborne	Salmonellosis
		Hepatitis A
Airborne	Aerosols	Legionellosis
	Droplet nuclei	Tuberculosis
		Varicella
		Measles
	Dust	Histoplasmosis
Vectorborne	Ticks and mites	Rickettsia, Lyme disease
	Mosquitoes	Malaria
	Fleas	Bubonic plague

From Wilkins RL, et al: *Egan's Fundamentals of Respiratory Care,* ed 8. St. Louis, Mosby, 2003,

XIV. **Notable Gram-Positive Pathogenic Bacteria**
  A. *Bacillus anthracis*: Causes skin infections, septicemia, enteritis, meningitis, anthrax, and pneumonia (woolsorter's disease).
    1. Rod shaped, arranged in chains, spore forming.
    2. Secretes exotoxin.
  B. *Clostridium botulinum*
    1. Causes botulism: Toxic food poisoning (a flaccid paralysis).
    2. Rod shaped in pairs, spore forming.
  C. *Clostridium perfringens*
    1. Causes gas gangrene.
    2. Rod shaped in pairs, spore forming.
  D. *Clostridium tetani*
    1. Produces tetanus: Rigid descending paralysis.
    2. Rod shaped in pairs, spore forming.
  E. *Streptococcus pneumoniae* (*Diplococcus* pneumonia)
    1. Gram-positive aerobe.
    2. Coccus, arranged in chains.
    3. May produce capsules.

        4. Can cause empyema, septicemia, meningitis, and peritonitis.

        5. Causes lobar pneumonia (most common cause of community-acquired pneumonia).

  D. *Staphylococcus aureus*

        1. Gram-positive, aerobic, and facultative anaerobe.

        2. Coccus arranged in irregular (grapelike) clusters.

        3. Produces an exotoxin and enterotoxin.

        4. Causes pneumonia, empyema, and wound infections.

XV. Notable Gram-Negative Bacteria (see Box 3-1)

  A. *Pseudomonas aeruginosa*

        1. Gram-negative aerobe and facultative anaerobe.

        2. Rod shaped and found as a single organism.

        3. Causes up to 10% of all hospital-acquired infections.

        4. Causes pneumonia with characteristic green odoriferous sputum.

        5. Causes wound infection, urinary tract infection, empyema, meningitis, and septicemia.

  B. *Serratia marcescens*

        1. Gram-negative aerobe.

        2. Rod shaped.

        3. Causes empyema, septicemia, and wound infections and is responsible for some hospital epidemics.

  C. *Escherichia coli*

        1. Gram-negative aerobe and facultative anaerobe.

        2. Rod shaped and found as a single organism.

        3. Responsible for approximately 45% of all nosocomial infections.

        4. Causes necrotizing pneumonia, septicemia, endocarditis, meningitis, wound infections, and urinary tract infections.

  D. *Klebsiella pneumoniae*

        1. Gram-negative aerobe and facultative anaerobe.

        2. Short rod and found as a single organism.

        3. Produces capsules.

        4. Causes necrotizing pneumonia with characteristic "red currant jelly" sputum.

        5. Causes lung abscesses, endocarditis, and septicemia.

  E. *Haemophilus influenzae*

        1. Gram-negative aerobe and facultative anaerobe.

        2. Minute rod found as a single organism.

        3. Most common cause of epiglottitis in children.

        4. Causes meningitis, laryngitis, croup, and subacute bacterial endocarditis.

  F. *Salmonella typhi*

        1. Gram-negative aerobe and facultative anaerobe.

        2. Rod shaped and found as single organism.

        3. Produces exotoxin.

        4. Resistant to freezing.

        5. Transmitted through contaminated water and, less frequently, contaminated food.

  G. *Salmonella enteritidis*

        1. Found in animals, particularly shellfish, swine, and fowl.

        2. Causes enteritis that may progress to meningitis, encephalitis, or nephritis.

        3. Transmitted orally via contaminated milk, turtles, eggs, undercooked chicken, fish, clams, and pork.

  H. *Bordetella pertussis*

        1. Gram-negative.

        2. Minute, nonmotile coccobacilli.

        3. Hemolytic bacillus responsible for whooping cough.

  I. *Neisseria meningitidis*

        1. Gram-negative aerobe.

    2. Coccus is found as diplococci with their adjacent sides flattened.

    3. Causes meningococcal meningitis, bacteremia, and pneumonia.

  J. *Proteus mirabilis* and *Proteus vulgaris*

    1. Gram-negative aerobe and facultative anaerobe.

    2. Rod shaped and found as a single organism.

    3. Causes chronic urinary tract infections, pneumonia, gastroenteritis, and bacteremia.

  K. Normal human flora by body site (Table 3-2)

  L. Common causes of community, hospital, and nosocomial pneumonias are listed in Box 3-2.

XVI. *Mycobacterium*: **Genus Characteristics**

  A. Consists of acid-fast, gram-positive, aerobic rods.

  B. Inert forms are found singly; virulent strains are found in "cords"; two chains in a side-by-side parallel arrangement.

  C. Identified by acid-fast staining and immunofluorescence staining.

  D. *Mycobacterium tuberculosis*

    1. Very slow growing organisms, requiring 3 to 6 weeks for culturing.

    2. Reaction time in newly infected individuals 3 to 6 weeks for a positive skin test.

    3. Causes pulmonary tuberculosis, spinal tuberculosis, and miliary tuberculosis.

    4. Transmitted through inhalation of droplet nuclei.

    5. Causes a necrotizing lesion with caseating center.

    6. Treatment is long-term therapy (6 to 12 months) with a combination of various agents.

  E. *Mycobacterium leprae*

    1. Causes leprosy, a true parasite found in the host.

    2. Transmission is via intimate contact.

  F. *Mycobacterium avium* complex (MAC) and *Mycobacterium avium intracellulare* (MAI)

    1. Nontuberculous-forming mycobacterium.

    2. Does not require the level of precautions used with tuberculous mycobacterium.

    3. Cause chronic pulmonary infections.

TABLE **3-2**

Normal Human Flora by Body Site

Site	Normal Flora
Pharynx and upper gastrointestinal tract	*Moraxella catarrhalis*; *Staphylococcus epidermidis* and *Staphylococcus aureus*; α-hemolytic streptococci; viridans-group streptococci; *Streptococcus pneumoniae*; *Peptostreptococcus*, *Lactobacillus*, and *Fusobacterium* species; *Actinomyces israelii*; *Haemophilus influenzae* and *Haemophilus parainfluenzae*; *Corynebacterium* species; *Neisseria meningitidis*, *Bacteroides* species and other anaerobes; and *Candida* (yeast) species.
Colon	*Enterococcus* species; *Escherichia coli*; *Pseudomonas*, *Bacteroides*, and *Clostridium* species and other gram-negatives and anaerobes; also *Candida* (yeast) species; organisms known as coliforms or enteric bacteria because of their location in the colon.
Skin	*Staphylococcus epidermidis* and *Staphylococcus aureus*; streptococci; *Corynebacterium* species; *Clostridium perfringens*; *Propionibacterium acnes*; and *Candida* (yeast) species.
Lower respiratory tract	Essentially sterile; possibility of colonization when illness or structural lung disease compromises immune function.

From Hess D, et al: *Respiratory Care: Principles and Practice.* Philadelphia, WB Saunders, 2002.

BOX 3-2

Etiologies of CAP, VAP, and Nosocomial Pneumonia

The microorganisms associated with each type of pneumonia are listed in descending order of prevalence.

CAP, Age <60 Years
Streptococcus pneumoniae
Mycoplasma pneumoniae
Viruses
Chlamydia pneumoniae
Haemophilus influenzae
Legionella species
Staphylococcus aureus
Mycobacterium tuberculosis
Fungi (*Histoplasma, Coccidioides, Blastomyces* species)
Gram-negative bacilli, nonpseudomonal enteric species

CAP, Age >60 Years
Streptoccous pneumoniae
Viruses
Haemophilus influenzae
Gram-negative bacilli, nonpseudomonal species
Mycobacterium tuberculosis
Fungi (*Histoplasma, Coccidioides, Blastomyces* species)

Nosocomial (Non-VAP) Pneumonia
Polymicrobial organisms
Staphylococcus aureus
Streptococcus pneumoniae
Gram-negative bacilli, nonpseudomonal
Pseudomonas species

VAP
Polymicrobial organisms
Staphylococcus aureus
Pseudomonas species
Haemophilus influenzae
Streptococcus pneumoniae
Gram-negative bacilli, nonpseudomonal

CAP, Community-acquired infection; *VAP,* ventilator-associated infection.
From Hess D, et al: *Respiratory Care: Principles and Practice.* Philadelphia, WB Saunders, 2002.

XVII.   Legionellaceae
    A.   Family characteristics
        1.   Gram-negative motile rods (difficult to stain).
        2.   Can survive as long as 139 days at room temperature in distilled water.
        3.   Can survive >1 year in tap water.
        4.   Growth can occur in tap water.
        5.   Found in air-conditioning cooling towers and evaporative condensers.
        6.   *Legionella pneumophila*
            a.   Causes 10% to 30% of hospital-acquired pneumonias.
            b.   Causes epidemic pneumonia, sporadic pneumonia, and a mild upper respiratory illness called "Pontiac fever."
            c.   Legionnaire's disease varies from mild pneumonia to adult respiratory distress syndrome.
            d.   Incubation is 2 to 10 days.
            e.   There is rapid onset of high fever, nonproductive cough, chills, headache, myalgias, and diarrhea.
            f.   A productive cough follows in 3 to 4 days, with patchy or segmental alveolar infiltrates usually in one lobe.
            g.   May be accompanied by pleural effusion, empyema, pneumothorax, hyponatremia, and respiratory failure.

XVIII.   Mycoplasma
    A.   Structure: Smallest bacteria (0.3 μm)
        1.   Surface layer
            a.   Three-layer membrane.
            b.   No cell wall.
         2.   Nucleus
            a.   No distinct nucleus.
            b.   Circular DNA.

      3. Cytoplasmic structures
         a. Ribosomes: Randomly distributed; occasionally seen in helical formation.
         b. Granules: Contain various enzymes.
      4. Motility organelles: None present.
      5. Gram-negative, highly pleomorphic, aerobic, and present as singular organisms.
      6. *Mycoplasma pneumoniae*
         a. Most common cause of atypical pneumonias.
         b. Causes a self-limiting respiratory syndrome that may have generalized symptoms or be asymptomatic.

XIX. **Rickettsiae**
    A. A true bacterium but is an obligate intracellular organism.
      1. Contains DNA and RNA.
      2. Multiplies by binary fission.
      3. Has metabolic enzymes.
    B. Gram-positive but requires special staining techniques for identification.
    C. It is a pleomorphic rod or coccus.
    D. Occurs singly, paired, chained, or in filaments.
    E. Diseases have clinical findings of fever, headaches, malaise, and rash.
      1. Typhoid fever
      2. Rocky Mountain spotted fever
      3. Q fever
      4. Trench fever
    F. It is transmitted via a bite of an infected organism.

XX. **Chlamydia**
    A. Gram-negative bacteria.
    B. Nonmotile and coccoidal.
    C. An obligate intracellular parasite.
      1. Developmental cycle in cytoplasm.
      2. Metabolically limited.
    D. *Chlamydia pneumoniae* is responsible for some atypical pneumonias.

XXI. **Viruses**
    A. Structure
      1. Surface layers
         a. Simple virus: Protein coat.
         b. Complex virus: Protein coat with some polysaccharides and lipids present (lipoprotein membrane).
      2. Nucleus: No nucleus; single strand of DNA or RNA present.
      3. Cytoplasmic structure
         a. No organelles present.
         b. Contains no metabolic enzymes.
      4. Motility organelles: None present.
    B. Characteristics
      1. Do not stain by conventional means.
      2. Come in a variety of shapes and forms, all of which are small (maximum diameters, 0.02 to 0.3 µm).
      3. Obligate intracellular parasite.
      4. Replication by diverting host metabolism to produce new viruses.
    C. Table 3-3 lists viruses important in human respiratory disease.

XXII. **Fungi (Yeasts and Molds)**
    A. These are primarily decomposers of dead and decaying matter (saprophytes).
      1. Occasionally they result in a pulmonary infection or pneumonia.

TABLE **3-3**	

Viruses Important in Human Respiratory Disease

Virus	Resulting Disease
Rhinoviruses, adenoviruses, coronaviruses	URI; "common cold"
Herpesviruses	Diverse important diseases
Herpes simplex virus (HSV)	Herpetic skin lesions; infection of the lungs and brain, causing pneumonia and encephalitis
Varicella zoster virus (VZV)	Chickenpox and shingles, both of which may involve the lung and central nervous system
Cytomegalovirus (CMV)	Systemic infection, including pneumonia, usually in immunocompromised individuals
Epstein-Barr virus (EBV)	Infectious mononucleosis ("mono")
Retroviruses (include HIV)	Diverse respiratory manifestations resulting from HIV
Flaviviruses (include yellow fever and dengue viruses)	Yellow fever and dengue, diseases common in Central and South America
Orthomyxoviruses	Influenza
Paramyxoviruses	Measles, mumps, parainfluenza
Respiratory syncytial virus (RSV)	Bronchiolitis in infants; milder disease in children and adults
Togaviruses	Diverse illnesses, including rubella
Coronavirus	Severe acute respiratory syndrome (SARS)

From Hess D, et al: *Respiratory Care: Principles and Practice.* Philadelphia, WB Saunders, 2002.

2. Usually they are acquired through inhalation of the spore form.
3. Some parasitic fungi can derive their food directly from living plants or animals.
4. Diseases in humans are usually restricted to the skin or mucous membranes (e.g., lung, pneumonia).

B. Structure
 1. Single cells: Yeasts.
 2. Tubular strands of single cells: More complex forms; hyphae, or series of branching filaments, that form mycelium.
  a. Vegetative mycelium: Part of fungus feeding and growing in medium.
  b. Aerial mycelium: Part of fungus protruding from medium.
  c. Reproduction
   (1) Sexual or asexual sporulation
   (2) Asexual sporulation

C. Table 3-4 lists important fungal respiratory pathogens in normal hosts.

D. Table 3-5 lists opportunistic fungal respiratory pathogens.

E. *Pneumocystis carinii*
 1. Widely distributed in animals in nature but is normally not pathogenic.
 2. Rarely problematic in healthy people.
  a. In most individuals it may be dormant, with no host damage.
  b. Seventy percent of healthy subjects have humoral antibody to the organism.
  c. Subclinical infection may be widespread.
 3. An extracellular opportunist that can cause a diffuse pneumonia.
 4. Assumed mode of transmission is by inhalation.
 5. In an immunocompromised host, the organism occurs in massive numbers; a common infection in patients with HIV.
 6. Usually there is panlobular involvement in the lungs.
 7. Clinical onset is usually abrupt, with fever, tachypnea, hypoxia, cyanosis, and asphyxia in the acute stage.

TABLE 3-4

Important Fungal Respiratory Pathogens in Normal Hosts

Organism	Disease	Comments
Coccidioides immitis	Coccidioidomycosis	The organism is commonly found in the arid regions of the southwest United States (e.g., Arizona and central California), and the disease causes valley fever, with high fever and bilateral pneumonia and may later form thin-walled pulmonary cavities.
Histoplasma capsulatum	Histoplasmosis	The organism is commonly found along the Mississippi and Ohio river valleys, and inhaled *Histoplasma inoculum* may cause acute fever and pneumonia. Some patients develop disseminated infection, often causing skin lesions; in rare cases, fibrosis of the mediastinum may result. Most residents of endemic areas have had asymptomatic infection, causing elevated antibody titers, and often one or more calcified granulomas visible on chest x-ray film.
Blastomyces dermatitidis	Blastomycosis	The organism is common in the southern United States, and the disease varies from mild fever and pulmonary infiltrates to severe illness, nodular pulmonary infiltrates, and dissemination.
Paracoccidioides brasiliensis	Paracoccidioidomycosis	Occurring in Central America, this clinical disease is similar to mild coccidioidomycosis.

From Hess D, et al: *Respiratory Care: Principles and Practice*. Philadelphia, WB Saunders, 2002.

TABLE 3-5

Opportunistic Fungal Respiratory Pathogens

Organism	Disease	Comments
Candida albicans	Candidiasis (e.g., thrush, esophagitis, and intertrigo	Organism is commonly found in infants and the elderly and also in HIV-infected and critically ill patients. Thrush also may be precipitated by inhaled steroid deposition in the mouth. True candidal pneumonia is rare.
Aspergillus species	Aspergillosis	Disease causes otitis externa in normal hosts; may infect skin, sinuses, or lung of immunocompromised individuals; and can disseminate, with extremely high mortality. Preexisting lung cavities from tuberculosis or emphysema are particularly prone to infection, with formation of a "fungus ball" inside.
Cryptococcus neoformans	Cryptococcosis	Organism is found in kitten feces and causes pneumonia and meningitis, a feared complication of AIDS.
Mucor and *Rhizopus* species	Mucormycosis	Organism can infect the sinuses, lungs, or gut, forming a black eschar. Treatment is difficult, often requiring surgical debridement.

HIV, Human immunodeficiency virus; *AIDS,* acquired immunodeficiency syndrome.
From Hess D, et al: *Respiratory Care: Principles and Practice*. Philadelphia, WB Saunders, 2002.

XXIII. **Definitions Related to Disinfection and Sterilization**
- A. Suffixes
  1. *-cide*: When a killing action is applied to a microorganism.
  2. *-statis* or *-static*: When the organism is only inhibited in growth or prevented from reproducing.
- B. Bactericide (bactericidal): Kills or destroys bacteria.

   C. Fungicide (fungicidal): Kills or destroys fungi.

   D. Virucide (virucidal): Kills or destroys viruses.

   E. Tuberculocide (tuberculocidal): Kills or destroys *Mycobacterium tuberculosis* and related mycobacterium.

   F. Sporicidal: Killing of bacterial spores.

   G. Germicide: Chemical agent that kills vegetative cells of microorganisms.

   H. Bacteriostatic: Inhibits or retards growth of bacteria.

   I. Antiseptic: Opposes sepsis or putrefaction either by killing microorganisms or by preventing their growth; free from living organisms.

   J. Antisepsis: Preventing the growth of bacteria or stopping bacterial activity.

   K. Medical asepsis: Killing or inhibiting the growth of pathogenic microorganisms to prevent their transmission from one person to another.

   L. Surgical asepsis: Sterilization or decontamination of items used in the operating room.

   M. Antiseptic: Free from living microorganisms; also an agent that destroys or inhibits the growth of microorganisms.

   N. Cleaning: The removal of all foreign matter such as sputum, blood, dirt, or organic matter from an item that may provide a favorable environment for bacterial growth; precedes sterilization.

   O. Disinfectant: Germicidal agent used on inanimate objects.

   P. Sanitizer: An agent that reduces the number of bacteria to a safer level for handling of material.

   Q. Sterilization: Complete destruction or inactivation of all forms of microorganisms.
1. The implication of this term is absolute destruction.
2. Sterile: Free from all living microorganisms.

   R. Disinfection: A process that eliminates vegetative, pathogenic microorganisms on inanimate objects.

   S. High-level disinfectants: Germicidal agents capable of killing all microorganisms except their spores.

   T. Intermediate-level disinfectants: Germicidal agents capable of killing all gram-negative bacteria and fungi but have variable activity against spores and certain viruses.

   U. Low-level disinfectants: Germicidal agents capable of killing some, but not all, vegetative bacteria, fungi, and lipophilic viruses.

   V. Decontamination: The process of removing a contaminant by chemical or physical means.

   W. Sanitization: Any process that reduces total bacterial contamination to a level consistent with safety in handling.

   X. Semicritical items: Objects that come in contact with mucous membranes but that do not enter tissue or the vascular system.

   Y. Noncritical items: Objects that do not come in contact with mucous membranes or skin that is not intact.

   Z. Critical items: Devices introduced in the bloodstream or other parts of the body.

XXIV. Dynamics of Disinfection and Sterilization

   A. Selection of the procedure is determined by the situation.
1. Items used for surgery, intravascularly, or within tissues must be sterile.
2. Media and glassware for the microbiology laboratory must be sterile.
3. Items not in contact with mucous membranes or that touch only intact skin may only need to be disinfected.

   B. Death rate of microorganism
1. Criterion of death is the irreversible loss of the ability to reproduce.
2. Exposure of a bacterial population to a lethal agent results in a time interval in which there is a progressive reduction in the number of survivors.
    a. This reduction may be logarithmic with time when the sterilizing agent is strong.
    b. This reduction may be sigmoidal, the rate being slower at the beginning, if the agent is less potent.

3. The larger the initial number of cells to be killed, the longer and more intense the required treatment for sterilization.
4. The rate of disinfection is related to the concentration of the disinfecting agent.

C. Factors affecting the potency of disinfectants
1. Concentration and type of agent and organism involved.
2. Amount of exposure time.
3. Hydrogen ion concentration, which affects bactericidal action.
   a. pH change may affect the organism and the bacterial agent.
   b. The pH determines the degree of ionization of the agent, which can alter its level of activity and ability to penetrate the cell membrane.
   c. Generally, nonionized agents pass through cell membrane quickly.

D. Temperature
1. Killing action increases with temperature.
2. At low temperatures, a 10° C increase doubles the death rate.

E. Nature of the organism
1. Species and presence of special structures such as capsules or spores.
2. Growth phase of culture and previous history.
3. The number of organisms present.

F. Presence of extraneous material such as organic or foreign matter

XXV. Processing of Equipment for Disinfection or Sterilization

A. Cleaning the equipment: Removal of dirt and organic material is the first step in processing equipment.
1. Should take place in a designated facility.
2. Clean and dirty equipment should always be separated.
3. Before cleaning, all equipment should be dissembled and parts examined for function.
4. Detergents should be used to clean equipment.
5. Equipment that cannot be immersed in water should have its surface disinfected with 70% ethyl alcohol or equivalent solution.

B. After cleaning, equipment should be completely dried.
1. Water dilutes and alters the pH of chemical disinfectants.
2. Water combines with ethylene oxide to form ethylene glycol, which is toxic to tissue.

C. After drying, equipment should be reassembled and packed appropriately when indicated.

D. Cleaning should always be performed in an aseptic manner.
1. Disinfect surfaces
2. Sterile towels
3. Gloves
4. Gowns when indicated

XXVI. Sterilization and Disinfection by Temperature Change (Table 3-6)

A. Heat is the most reliable and universally applied method of sterilization.
1. The time required is inversely related to temperature.
2. Heat causes denaturation of proteins and coagulation.
3. The efficiency of heat sterilization is determined by the heat capacity of the gas involved in the sterilization process.
4. The heat capacity of water at any temperature significantly exceeds the heat capacity of air.
5. Steam has a heat capacity many times greater than that of water at the same temperature because of the latent heat of vaporization of water molecules.
6. The heat capacity of steam increases logarithmically with increasing pressure.
7. Order of efficiency of sterilization and disinfection by heat
   a. Steam under pressure (autoclave)

TABLE 3-7

Common Chemical Disinfectants

Disinfectant	CDC Level	Gram-positive Bacteria	Gram-negative Bacteria	Tubercle Bacillus	Spores	Viruses	Fungi
Acetic acid	Low	+	+	?	?	?	±
Quaternary ammoniums	Low	+	±	0	0	±	+
Alcohols	Intermediate	+	+	+	0	±	±
Iodophors	Intermediate	+	+	+	0	±	+
Phenolics	Intermediate	+	+	+	0	±	+
Glutaraldehyde	High	+	+	+	±	+	+
Hydrogen peroxide	High	+	+	+	±	+	+
Peracetic acid	High	+	+	+	+	+	+
Sodium hypochlorite	High	+	+	+	±	+	+

+, Highly effective against; ±, moderately effective against; 0, not effective against; ?, effectiveness not established.
From Wilkins RL, et al: *Egan's Fundamentals of Respiratory Care,* ed 8. St. Louis, Mosby, 2003.

4. It is only slightly irritating, leaves no residue, removes fats and lipids from skin surfaces, and is inexpensive.
5. Alcohols are *not* sporicidal or virucidal to all viruses.
   a. Ethanol has been shown to be effective against HIV.
   b. Neither ethanol nor isopropanol is effective against tubercle bacillus in sputum.
6. Alcohol is a volatile and a powerful organic solvent that may damage rubber and plastic materials.
7. Ethanol (ethyl alcohol) is used at 70% concentration.
8. Isopropyl alcohol is used at 90% concentration.
9. Toxic effects of isopropanol are greater and longer lasting than ethanol if ingested or inhaled in large quantities.
10. Sometimes alcohol is used as part of the composition of other disinfecting agents such as Lysol spray (ethanol).

B. Quaternary ammonium compounds
   1. These are surface-acting, cationic agents containing the ammonium ion that cause a loss of membrane semipermeability and leakage of nitrogen- and phosphorus-containing compounds from the cell.
      a. Lysis of the cell is followed by the action of the cell's own autolytic enzymes.
      b. The agent may then enter the cell and denature its proteins.
   2. Activity is greatest at an alkaline pH.
   3. These compounds are bactericidal for a wide range of organisms, but gram-positive species are more susceptible.
   4. Antibacterial activity is reduced by the presence of organic matter.
   5. They can be reused.
   6. Ineffective against tuberculosis bacillus spores, enteroviruses, hepatitis B, bacterial spores, or some fungi and notably are not very pseudomonocidal.

C. Acetic acid
   1. Acetic acid has long been known as a preservative.
   2. It inhibits the growth of many bacteria and fungi.
   3. Antimicrobial activity is related to its acidity.
      a. Acidotic pH prevents organisms from maintaining a normal pH balance as excessive hydrogen ions enter the cell and cannot be expelled rapidly enough.
      b. It can result in denaturation of cellular proteins.
      c. It has an indirect effect because of ionization of organic compounds in the medium that permits them to penetrate the cell more rapidly and disrupt cell metabolism.

4. A 1.25% acetic acid solution seems to be sufficiently effective to disinfect equipment; one part vinegar (5% acetic acid) and three parts water.
5. Used extensively in the cleaning of respiratory care equipment, such as hand-held nebulizers, in the home.
6. Effectiveness is significantly reduced if a solution is reused.

D. Phenols
1. They cause leakage of cell contents and irreversible inactivation of membrane-bound enzymes.
2. Cresols are simple alkyl phenols obtained industrially from the distillation of coal tar.
3. The three primary types are orthocresol, metacresol, and paracresol (usually used as a mixture of tricresol).
4. Examples are Lysol and Creolin, which are emulsified mixtures of cresols and green soap.
   a. Some have virucidal properties.
   b. They are not sporicidal.
   c. They are used for cleaning instruments and general housekeeping.

E. Chlorine and related compounds
1. Like iodine, they are strong oxidizing agents that inactivate enzymes.
2. In addition to chlorine compounds, the hypochlorites and the inorganic and organic chloramines are also oxidizing disinfectants.
3. They are effective against most bacteria, viruses, and fungi.
4. They are not sporicidal at room temperatures.
5. They have no effect in the presence of organic matter.
6. They are highly corrosive to metals and cannot be used with rubber.
7. Chlorine is used to purify the water supply and is widely used in swimming pools (0.6 to 1.0 ppm).
8. Hypochlorites are widely used in the food and dairy industries for sanitization.
   a. They are also used as sanitizers in hospitals, households, and public buildings.
   b. A 0.2% solution of sodium hypochlorite has been recommended by the Pasteur Institute for use on inanimate objects for inactivation of HIV with a 10-minute contact time.
9. Commercial household bleach is usually bottled as a 5.25% hypochloride solution (storage reduces percentage and effectiveness).
10. A 1:50 dilution of household bleach is able to kill gram-negative bacteria, bacterial spores, and *M. tuberculosis* in 10 minutes.
11. The Centers for Disease Control and Prevention recommends a 1:10 dilution of bleach to clean blood spills after the area is cleaned of gross organic matter.

F. Hydrogen peroxide
1. This is a strong oxidizing agent similar to iodine and chlorine in bacterial activity.
2. The reaction of peroxide with iron may produce additional free hydroxide radicals that may account for part of its germicidal activity.
3. A 3% solution is used as a mild antiseptic for wound cleaning.
4. At room temperature a 6% solution is bactericidal, fungicidal, and virucidal in 10 minutes.
5. A 6% solution is sporicidal in 6 hours.
6. Used increasingly in recent years as a disinfectant of medical-surgical devices and soft plastic contact lenses.
7. It is also used for cleaning tracheostomy tubes and the incision site.

XXXI. Precautions
A. To avoid contamination of yourself and cross-contamination of patients, the Centers for Disease Control and Prevention has outlined specific precautions that should be taken with *all* patient contact and specific precautions that should be exercised when certain infections are present.

B. Standard precautions: Should be used wherever there is a probability that a caregiver will be exposed to blood, body fluids, or other excretions from *any* patient or contaminated medical equipment.
   1. The most important aspect of disease transmission prevention is *handwashing*.
      a. Hands should be disinfected with an alcohol-based hand rinse.
         (1) Before entering a patient's room.
         (2) After interaction with a patient.
         (3) After removal of any protective equipment, gloves, gowns, or mask.
      b. If hands are visibly soiled they should be vigorously washed with soap and water before applying the alcohol-based disinfectant.
   2. Gloves
      a. Clean, nonsterile gloves must be worn when touching blood, body fluids, secretions, mucous membranes, and contaminated medical equipment.
      b. Remove gloves after use and before touching any noncontaminated object.
   3. Gowns
      a. Clean, nonsterile gowns must be worn to protect skin and to prevent soiling of clothing during activities that may generate splashes or spray of blood, body fluids, secretions, or excretions.
      b. Remove soiled gown immediately on completing activity.
   4. Mask and eye protection or face shield should be worn to protect mucous membranes of the eyes, nose, and mouth during activities that could result in splashes of blood, body fluids, secretions, or excretions.
C. Contact precautions
   1. Required in treatment of patients where transmission of pathogen occurs by body-to-body contact.
   2. See Box 3-3 for a listing of diseases requiring contact precautions.
   3. Gloves when entering room.
   4. Gowns for direct contact with patient, environmental surfaces, or equipment in room.
   5. Private room required or patients need to be cohorted by infection.
   6. Equipment should be dedicated to the single patient for length of stay.
   7. If equipment is removed from room it must be properly disinfected.
   8. Standard precaution procedures also apply.
D. Airborne precautions
   1. Required in treatment of patients where transmission of pathogen occurs by droplet nuclei or dust particles.
   2. Respiratory protection is critical; an N-95/HEPA-filtered mask must be worn when entering the room.
   3. See Box 3-4 for a list of diseases requiring airborne precautions.
   4. If immune to chickenpox and measles, an N-95 mask is unnecessary.
   5. Patient should be placed in a negative pressure isolation room. *Door must remain closed.*
   6. Standard precaution procedures also apply.
E. Droplet precautions
   1. Surgical mask when within 3 ft of patient.
   2. See Box 3-5 for a list of diseases requiring droplet precautions.
   3. Private room required or cohort patients by disease.
   4. Door to room may remain open.
   5. Standard precaution procedures also apply.

XXXII. **Equipment-Related Infection Control Issues (Table 3-8)**
   A. Ventilator circuits and humidifiers
      1. Ventilator circuits and their condensate have been implicated for decades in the development of ventilator-associated pneumonia (VAP).
      2. However, recent data clearly indicate that VAP is primarily associated with aspiration of oral secretions and gastric contents.

BOX 3-3

Diseases Requiring Contact Precautions

Abscess (draining, major, not contained)	Herpangina (infants)
Adenovirus (infants/children)[D]	Herpes simplex (severe or neonatal)
Adenovirus pneumonia (adult)[D]	Marburg virus (viral hemorrhagic fever)[A]
Bronchiolitis (in infants)	MRSA (methicillin-resistant *Staphylococcus*
Chickenpox (varicella)[A]	*aureus*)
Clostridium difficile (patients with diarrhea)	Multidrug-resistant organisms (as defined by
Congenital rubella	Infection Control)
Conjunctivitis (acute viral)	Parainfluenza virus (infants)
Coxsackievirus (diapered or incontinent)	Pediculosis (lice)[P]
Croup (infants)	Pleurodynia (enterovirus, infants)
Decubitus ulcer (infected, major)	Pneumococcus, penicillin-resistant
Diphtheria (cutaneous)	Pneumonia (adenovirus, infants/children)[D]
Ebola viral hemorrhagic fever[A]	Respiratory syncytial virus (RSV)
Echovirus (diapered or incontinent)	Rotavirus (diapered or incontinent)
Enterococcus, vancomycin-resistant (VRE)	Scabies[P]
Enterocolitis (*C. difficile*)	Staphylococcal infection (major)
Enterovirus (diapered or incontinent)	*Staphylococcus aureus* (glycopeptide- or
Erysipelas	vancomycin-resistant)
Furunculosis (infants)	*Staphylococcus aureus* (methicillin-resistant)
Gastroenteritis (diapered or incontinent)	Streptococcal infection (major)
E. coli (enteropathogenic)	Varicella (chickenpox)[A]
Shigella	Viral infection, if not covered elsewhere (infants)
VRSA/GISA/VISA (glycopeptide- or vancomycin-	VRE (vancomycin-resistant enterococci)
intermediate *Staphylococcus aureus*)	Wound infection, major, not contained
Hemorrhagic fevers (Ebola, Lassa, Marburg)[A]	Zoster, herpes (immunocompromised host or if
Hepatitis A (diapered or incontinent)	disseminated)

A, Airborne precautions also required; *D,* droplet precautions also required; *P,* private room *not* required.
From Infection Control Manual, Massachusetts General Hospital, Boston, MA, 2004.

    a. Steps should always be taken to ensure that cuffs on airways are properly inflated, but this cannot prevent the small silent aspiration that continually occurs via folds in inflated airway cuffs during mechanical ventilation.

    b. Ideally, the head of the bed should be elevated 30 degrees to prevent regurgitation of gastric fluid.

    c. Some also recommend the use of pharmacologic agents to decontaminate the upper digestive tract of gram-negative bacteria and *Candida* species, but this is still controversial.

    d. Good oral hygiene and the removal of secretions above the cuff assist in minimizing aspiration.

  3. American Association for Respiratory Care practice guidelines recommend that ventilator circuits be changed no more frequently than every 7 days.

  4. Good evidence indicates that circuits need not be changed at all provided they are functional.

  5. Ideally, the circuit should not be disconnected from the patient once attached.

  6. Inline suction catheters eliminate contamination of the circuit by repeated removal for suctioning.

  7. Properly maintained inline catheters need only be changed when ventilator circuits are changed.

 B. Ventilator circuit condensate

  1. Normally, within hours the condensate of ventilator circuits is contaminated.

BOX 3-4

Diseases Requiring Airborne Precautions

Chickenpox (varicella)^C
Hemorrhagic fevers (Ebola, Lassa, and
  Marburg)^C
Herpes zoster (immunocompromised patient or if
  disseminated)^C
Measles (rubeola)
	Tuberculosis (pulmonary in any patient,
	  pulmonary or extrapulmonary in HIV+
	  patient)^D
	Varicella (chickenpox)^C
	SARS (coronavirus)^C + eye protection
	Smallpox^C
	Avian influenza^C + eye protection

C, Contact precautions also required; D, droplet precautions also required.
From Infection Control Manual, Massachusetts General Hospital, Boston, MA, 2004.

BOX 3-5

Diseases Requiring Droplet Precautions

Adenovirus (infants/children)^C
Adenovirus pneumonia (adult)^C
Bacterial meningitis (meningococcal or
  H. influenzae)
Diphtheria
Epiglottitis (*Haemophilus influenzae*)
Fifth disease (erythema infectiosum, parvovirus
  B19)
Patients with immunocompromised/aplastic
  crisis*
Patients with transient aplastic and/or erythrocyte
  crisis*
	German measles (rubella)
	Influenza
	Meningococcal pneumonia
	Meningococcemia (meningococcal sepsis)
	Mumps
	Pertussis (whooping cough)
	Pneumonia: *H. influenzae* (children)
	        Group A Strep (children)
	Pneumonic plague
	Scarlet fever (infants and young children)
	Whooping cough (pertussis)

A, Airborne precautions also required; C, contact precautions also required; *no pregnant staff.
From Infection Control Manual, Massachusetts General Hospital, Boston, MA, 2004.

TABLE 3-8

Frequency of Respiratory Care Equipment Change for Infection Control Purposes

Equipment	Change Frequency
Ventilator circuits and humidifiers	Most frequent every 7 days
	Least frequent when equipment malfunctions
Inline suction catheter	When ventilator circuit changed
	When system malfunctions
Heat and moisture exchangers	Every 48-96 hours
Nebulizers	Every 24 hours
Oxygen therapy equipment	Between patients or if malfunctioning
Ventilator	Surface disinfection between patients
Pulmonary function equipment	Circuits, mouthpieces, etc. between patients
	External surfaces no recommended cleaning frequency
Manual ventilators (Ambu Bags)	Weekly

From Infection Control Manual, Massachusetts General Hospital, Boston, MA, 2004.

   2. However, this contaminate is from the patient's airway provided appropriate pre-
      cautions are taken while handling the circuit.
   3. Condensate is an infectious hazard to caregivers, but it should not be a hazard to
      the patient.
   4. Careful regular drainage of condensate away from the patient should occur.
   C. Heat and moisture exchanges
      1. Current data indicate that they can be changed as infrequently as every 48 to 96
         hours without an increased risk of nosocomial pneumonia.

    D. Nebulizers
        1. Because they produce aerosols that can carry bacteria, they must be changed every 24 hours.
    E. Oxygen therapy equipment
        1. Because no aerosol is produced during humidification of delivered oxygen if appropriate precautions are taken, equipment only needs to be changed between patients or if equipment fails.
    F. Ventilators
        1. The outside surface of the ventilator should be cleaned periodically while in use.
        2. Disinfection should always occur between patients.
        3. The use of a filter at the ventilator on the exhalation side can prevent internal contamination of the ventilator. No data indicate that the ventilator itself is a cause of nosocomial pneumonia.
    G. Pulmonary function equipment
        1. Change circuits and mouthpieces between patients.
        2. HEPA filters may be placed in circuits to avoid internal equipment contamination.
        3. Disinfect external surfaces between patients if taken into patient's rooms on precaution.
        4. No recommended disinfection frequency for nonmobile units.
    H. Manual ventilators (Ambu Bags)
        1. Always changed between patients.
        2. During use, weekly change is recommended because of environmental contamination of the patient connection port.
        3. When not in use, the patient connection port should be capped to avoid environmental contamination.

BIBLIOGRAPHY

AARC Clinical Practice Guidelines: Infection control, *Respiratory Care*, 48:773-790, 2003.

Block SS: *Disinfection, Sterilization and Preservation,* ed 2. Philadelphia, Lea & Febiger, 1977.

Boyd RF, Hoerl BG: *Basic Medical Microbiology,* ed 2. Boston, Little Brown & Co., 1981.

Centers for Disease Control and Prevention: Hospital Infection Control Practices Advisory Committee Members: Guideline for Prevention of Nosocomial Pneumonia. *Respir Care* 39:942-951, 1994.

Dreyfuss D, Djedaini K, Weber P, et al: Prospective study of nosocomial pneumonia and of patient and circuit colonization during mechanical ventilation with circuit changes every 48 hours vs. no change. *Am Res Respir Dis* 143:738-743, 1991.

Fink JB, Krause SA, Barrett L, et al: Extending ventilator circuit change interval beyond 2 days reduces the likelihood of ventilator-associated pneumonia, *Chest* 113:405-411, 1998.

Garner JS: Hospital control practices advisory committee. Guideline for isolation precautions in hospitals. *Infect Control Hosp Epidemiol* 17:53-80, 1996.

Hess D, Burns E, Romagnoli D, et al: Weekly ventilator circuit changes: a strategy to reduce costs without affecting pneumonia rates. *Anesthesiology* 82:903-911, 1995.

Hess DR, MacIntyre NR, Mishoe SC, Galvin WF, Adams AB, Saposnick AB: *Respiratory Care Principles and Practices.* Philadelphia, WB Saunders, 2002.

Huxley EJ, Viroslav J, Gray WR, et al: Pharyngeal aspiration in normal adults and patients with depressed consciousness. *Am J Med* 64:564-568, 1978.

Jawetz E, Melinick JL, Adelbert EA: *Review of Medical Microbiology,* ed 16. Los Altos, CA, Lange Medical Publications, 1996.

Joklik WK, Willett HP, Amos DB, et al, editors: *Zinsser Microbiology,* ed 21. Norwalk, CT, Appleton and Lange, 1998.

Kirton OC, DeHaven B, Morgan J, et al: A prospective, randomized comparison of an in-line heat moisture exchange filter and heated wire humidifiers: rates of ventilator-associated early onset (community-acquired) or late-onset (hospital-acquired) pneumonia and incidence of endotracheal tube occlusion. *Chest* 112:1055-1059, 1997.

Kollef MH, Shapiro SD, Fraser VJ, et al: Mechanical ventilation with or without 7-day circuit changes: a randomized controlled trial. *Ann Intern Med* 123:168-174, 1995.

Thompson RE: Incidence of ventilator-associated pneumonia (VAP) with 14-day circuit change in a subacute environment, *Respir Care* 41:601-606, 1996.

Wilkins RL, Stoller JK, Scanlan CL: *Egan's Fundamentals of Respiratory Care,* ed 8. St. Louis, Mosby, 2003.

Chapter **4**

Anatomy of the Respiratory System

I. **Boundaries and Functions of the Upper Airway**
   A. Boundaries: From the anterior nares to the true vocal cords.
   B. Functions:
      1. Heating or cooling inspired gases to body temperature (37° C).
      2. Filtering inspired gases.
      3. Humidifying inspired gases to a relative humidity of approximately 100% at body temperature.
      4. Olfaction: Act of smelling.
      5. Phonation: Production of sound.
      6. Conduction: Passageway for ventilating gases.
   C. The nose
      1. The nose is a rigid structure of cartilage and bone; the superior one third is made up of the nasal and maxilla bones, and the inferior two thirds is made up of five large pieces of cartilage (Figure 4-1).
      2. The two external openings are called the nostrils, external nares, or anterior nares. Their lateral borders are termed the alae.
      3. The nasal cavity is divided into two nasal fossae by the septal cartilage.
      4. Each nasal fossa is divided into three regions: vestibular, olfactory, and respiratory.
         a. Vestibular region: An area of slight dilation inside the nostril, bordered laterally by the alae and medially by the nasal septal cartilage.
            (1) The vestibular region is lined with stratified squamous epithelium (Table 4-1). Layers of relatively flat cells continuously are being produced, replacing those lost at the surface.
            (2) Coarse nasal hairs (vibrissae) project anteriorly and inferiorly.
            (3) Sebaceous glands secrete sebum, a greasy substance that keeps the nasal hairs soft and pliable.
            (4) The nasal hairs are the first line of defense for the upper airway, acting as very gross filters of inspired air.
         b. Olfactory region: An area in each nasal cavity defined by the superior concha laterally, nasal septal cartilage medially, and roof of the nasal cavity superiorly.
            (1) Contained is the olfactory epithelium responsible for the sense of smell.
            (2) The olfactory epithelium is yellowish brown and appears as pseudostratified columnar epithelial cells. These cells are interspersed with more deeply placed olfactory cells, whose sensory filament, the olfactory hairs, protrudes to the epithelial surface. Similar in structure to the ciliated cells lining the respiratory region but without the cilia (Figure 4-2).

69

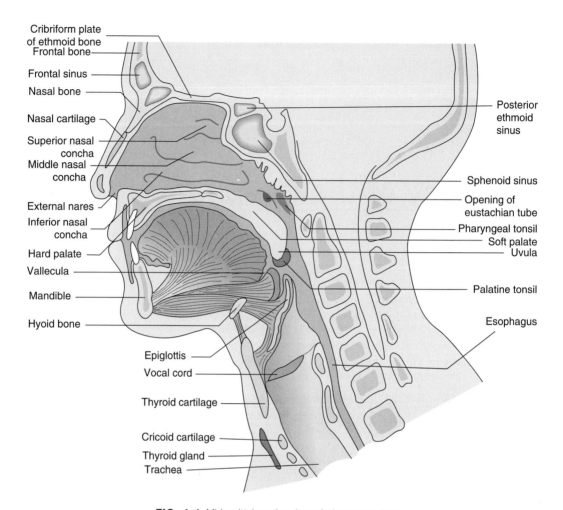

FIG. 4-1 Midsagittal section through the upper airway.

TABLE **4-1**

Anatomical Comparison of Epithelium in Upper Respiratory Tract

Structure	Epithelium
Vestibular region/nose	Stratified squamous
Olfactory region/nose	Pseudostratified columnar
Respiratory region/nose	Pseudostratified ciliated columnar
Paranasal sinuses	Pseudostratified ciliated columnar
Nasopharynx	Pseudostratified ciliated columnar
Oropharynx	Stratified squamous
Laryngopharynx	Stratified squamous
Larynx/above true cords	Stratified squamous

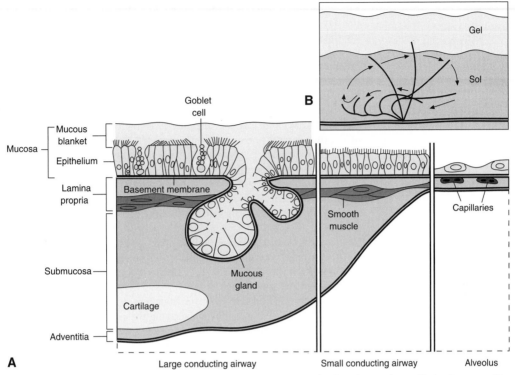

FIG. 4-2 A, The respiratory mucosal epithelium. Most airways contain ciliated, pseudostratified columnar epithelium. **B,** Detail of ciliary action. Cilia reach up into the gel mucous layer during the forward propulsive stroke, withdrawing and retracting in the sol layer.

    (3)   Largely because of the architecture of the nasal cavity, sniffing causes inspired gases to be drawn to the olfactory region and not much farther into the respiratory tract. This provides a protective mechanism for sampling potentially noxious environmental gases.

  c. Respiratory region: An area in each nasal cavity inferior to the olfactory region and posterior to the vestibular region. The respiratory region comprises most of the surface area of the nasal fossa.

    (1)   Contained in the respiratory region of each nasal fossa are three bony plates called turbinates or conchae. The turbinates extend in a medial and inferior direction from the lateral walls of the nasal fossa.

    (2)   The three turbinates or conchae (superior, middle, and inferior) overhang and define the three corresponding passageways through each nasal cavity, respectively, the superior, middle, and inferior meati (see Figure 4-1).

    (3)   Because of the arrangement of the turbinates and folded mucous membrane covering the turbinates in the nose, the respiratory region has a volume of approximately 20 ml and a remarkably large surface area of approximately 160 cm^2.

    (4)   Turbulent flow is created through this region.

    (5)   Heating, humidifying, and filtering of inspired gases are accomplished by the turbulent flow through this region of the nose. The turbulent flow produces a greater probability that each gas molecule will come in contact with the large surface area of the vascular nasal mucous membrane. This large gas-to-nasal surface interface allows the following:

      (a)   The abundant underlying vasculature to heat inspired gases to body temperature.

(b) The moist nasal mucous membrane to give up 650 to 1000 ml of H_2O per day in bringing inspired gases to a relative humidity of 80% on leaving the nose and entering the nasopharynx.

(c) Particles suspended in the inspired gas to contact the sticky mucous membrane, thus filtering out particles >5 µm by inertial impaction to an efficiency of approximately 100%.

(6) The epithelial lining of the respiratory region of the nasal cavity is pseudostratified ciliated columnar epithelium (see Figure 4-2).

(a) The cells are cylindrical and appear to be two cell layers thick because of the high lateral pressures compressing the cells. Actually, the epithelium is only one cell layer thick, with each columnar cell making contact with the basement membrane.

(b) Each columnar cell has 200 to 250 cilia on its surface. Each of the cilia contains two central and nine paired peripheral fibrils. It is the sliding interaction of these fibrils that is thought to cause the beating of the cilia.

(c) Goblet cells and submucosal glands are interspersed throughout the epithelium and, along with capillary seepage, are responsible for production of mucus (100 ml/day in health).

(d) Mucus exists in two layers:
(i) Sol layer: Fluid bottom layer housing the cilia.
(ii) Gel layer: A viscous layer overlying the cilia.

(e) On the forward stroke, the cilia become rigid. Their tips touch the undersurface of the gel layer and propel it toward the oropharynx. On the backward stroke, the cilia become flaccid, fold on themselves, and slide entirely through the sol layer to their resting position without producing a retrograde motion of the gel layer.

(f) The cilia of a particular cell and adjacent cells beat in a coordinated and sequential fashion that produces a motion similar to a wave. This allows a unidirectional flow of mucus. The cilia beat approximately 1000 to 1500 times/min and move the mucous layer at a rate of 2 cm/min.

(g) Functions of the mucus and pseudostratified ciliated columnar epithelium (mucociliary blanket) are:
(i) To entrap inspired particles.
(ii) To humidify inspired gas.
(iii) To transport debris-laden mucus out of the respiratory tract.

5. The nose is responsible for one half to two thirds of the total airway resistance during nasal breathing. Therefore, it is not surprising that mouth breathing predominates during stress (e.g., exercise or disease).

6. The nose ends with the outlet of the nasal cavity into the nasopharynx through the internal nares (posterior nares or choanae).

D. The oral cavity (see Figure 4-1)

1. The oral cavity extends from the lips to the palatine folds, a double web on each side of the oral cavity where the palatine tonsils reside.

2. The oral cavity is separated from the nasal cavity by the palate. The anterior two thirds is the bony hard palate, and the posterior one third, without bone, is the soft palate.

3. The oral cavity is considered an accessory respiratory passage because air usually only flows through it during stress and exercise.

4. The tongue attached to the floor of the cavity is involved in the mechanical aspects of swallowing, taste, and phonation.
a. The posterior surface is supplied by a nerve ending producing the vagal gag reflex.
b. The lingual tonsils are located at the base of the tongue.

5. The mucosal surface provides modest humidification and warming of inspired air.

6. Saliva is produced by groups of salivary glands.

E. Paranasal sinuses (see Figures 4-1 and 4-3)
   1. Sinuses are cavities of air in the bones of the cranium.
   2. The function of the sinuses is not clearly understood, but it may be twofold:
      a. To give the voice resonance (prolongation and intensification of sound).
      b. To lighten the head to some extent because the space occupied by the sinuses is filled with air rather than bone.
   3. The sinuses are absent or rudimentary at birth and grow almost simultaneously with the development of the permanent teeth. Formation of the sinuses is responsible for the alteration in facial shape that occurs at this time.
   4. All of the air sinuses are lined with pseudostratified ciliated columnar epithelium and produce mucus, which drains into the nasal meati.
   5. If nasogastric tubes or nasotracheal intubation blocks sinus drainage, sinusitis and sinus infection often result.
   6. Groups of paranasal sinuses: Frontal, maxillary, sphenoidal, and ethmoidal.
      a. The frontal sinuses appear as paired sinuses medial to the orbits of the eye and superior to the roof of the nasal cavity between the external and internal surfaces of the frontal bone. They drain into the anterior portion of the middle meati (middle passageway [cavity] formed by the turbinates).
      b. The maxillary sinuses appear as paired sinuses lateral to each nasal cavity and inferior to the orbits of the eye in the body of the maxilla. These sinuses, the largest of all the air sinuses, drain into the middle meati.
      c. The sphenoidal sinuses appear as paired sinuses posterior and inferior to the roof of the nasal cavity and superior to the internal nares (choanae) in the body of the sphenoid bone. They drain into the superior meati.
      d. The ethmoidal sinuses are paired sinuses that exist in three groups: anterior, medial, and posterior ethmoidal. They exist just lateral to the superior and middle conchae, medial to the orbits of the eyes, inferior to the frontal sinuses, and superior to the maxillary sinuses in the ethmoid bone. The ethmoidal sinuses drain into the superior and middle meati.
F. Pharynx
   1. The pharynx is a hollow muscular structure lined with epithelium (Figure 4-4).

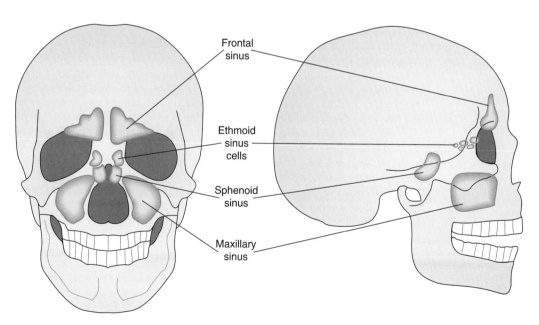

Frontal
sinus

Ethmoid
sinus
cells

Sphenoid
sinus

Maxillary
sinus

FIG. 4-3 Paranasal sinuses.

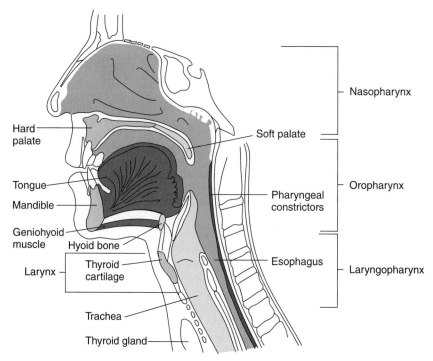

FIG. 4-4 Medial section of the pharynx showing the nasopharynx, oropharynx, and laryngopharynx and associated structures.

2. Major functions
   a. To produce the vowel sounds (phonation) by changing its shape.
   b. To serve as a common passageway for ventilatory gases, food, and liquid.
3. The pharynx is approximately 5 in. long and extends from the internal nares (choanae) inferiorly to the esophagus.
4. Sections of the pharynx: Nasopharynx, oropharynx, and laryngopharynx.
   a. The nasopharynx is located behind the nasal cavity and extends from the internal nares superiorly to the tip of the uvula inferiorly.
      (1) The epithelium is continuous with the epithelium of the nasal cavity and is pseudostratified ciliated columnar epithelium.
      (2) The eustachian or auditory tubes open into the nasopharynx on each of its lateral walls and communicate with the tympanic cavity or middle ear (see Figure 4-1).
         (a) This allows equilibration of pressure on each side of the tympanic membrane (eardrum) with environmental pressure changes.
         (b) Nasal intubation may block the eustachian tube openings and may cause otitis media (middle ear infection) or sinus infections.
      (3) The pharyngeal tonsil or adenoid is located in the superior and posterior wall of the nasopharynx.
         (a) The pharyngeal tonsil consists of a large concentration of lymphoid tissue comprising the superior portion of Waldeyer's ring. This ring of lymphoid tissue surrounds and guards the entrance to the respiratory and gastrointestinal tracts.
      (4) During the process of swallowing, the uvula and soft palate move in a posterior and superior direction to protect the nasopharynx and nasal cavity from the entrance of food, liquid, or both.

       (5) Major functions of the nasopharynx:
          (a) Gas conduction
          (b) Filtration of gases
          (c) Defense mechanism of the body (tonsils)

  b. The oropharynx is located behind the oral or buccal cavity and extends from the tip of the uvula superiorly to the tip of the epiglottis inferiorly.
       (1) The epithelial lining is stratified squamous epithelium.
       (2) The palatine tonsils are located lateral to the uvula on the lateral and anterior aspects of the oropharynx.
       (3) The lingual tonsil is located at the base of the tongue, superior and anterior to the vallecula (the space between the epiglottis and base of the tongue).
       (4) The two palatine tonsils, one lingual and one pharyngeal (adenoid), are the major components of Waldeyer's ring.
       (5) Major functions of the oropharynx:
          (a) Gas conduction
          (b) Food and fluid conduction
          (c) Filtration of inspired gases
          (d) Defense from microorganism entrance (Waldeyer's ring)

  c. The laryngopharynx or hypopharynx extends superiorly from the tip of the epiglottis to a point inferiorly where it bifurcates into the larynx and esophagus.
       (1) The epithelial lining is stratified squamous epithelium.
       (2) Major functions of the laryngopharynx:
          (a) Gas conduction
          (b) Food and fluid conduction
       (3) The laryngopharynx leads anteriorly into the larynx and posteriorly into the esophagus.
       (4) The larynx is considered the connection between the upper and lower airways, the exact division being the true vocal cords.
       (5) The larynx is considered part of the upper and lower respiratory tract. A complete description is given below.

II. Boundaries and Functions of the Lower Airway

  A. Boundaries: From the true vocal cords to the terminal air spaces (alveoli).

  B. Functions:
    1. Ventilation: To and fro movement of gas (gas conduction).
    2. External respiration: Actual gas exchange between body (pulmonary capillary blood) and external environment (alveolar gas).
    3. Sphincter or glottic mechanisms.
      a. Valsalva maneuver: Forced expiration against closed glottis.
      b. Müller maneuver: Forced inspiration against closed glottis.
      c. Cough.
      d. Protection of laryngeal inlet.
    4. Phonation: Production of sound.

  C. The larynx (Figures 4-5 and 4-6)
    1. The larynx is a boxlike structure made of cartilage connected by extrinsic and intrinsic muscles and ligaments. It is lined internally by a mucous membrane.
    2. Functions
      a. Gas conduction: Ventilation.
      b. Phonation: Production of sound.
      c. Sphincter or glottic mechanism.
    3. The larynx extends from the third to sixth cervical vertebrae in the anterior portion of the neck.
    4. Unpaired cartilages of the larynx: Epiglottis, thyroid, and cricoid (see Figure 4-5).
      a. Epiglottic cartilage
        (1) Leaf-shaped piece of fibrocartilage.

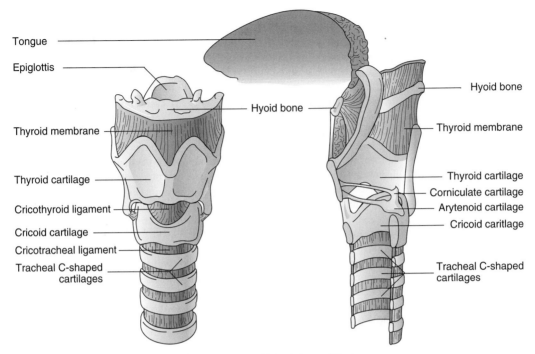

FIG. 4-5 Anterior and lateral views of the larynx.

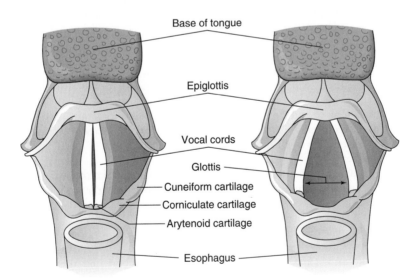

FIG. 4-6 Looking into the larynx from above and behind with the vocal cords closed and open.

(2) Anteriorly attached to thyroid cartilage just inferior to the thyroid notch.

(3) Laterally attached to folds of mucous membrane called aryepiglottic folds.

(4) On swallowing, the epiglottis is squeezed between the base of the tongue and thyroid cartilage, causing the epiglottis to pivot in a posterior and inferior direction to cover the laryngeal inlet.

    b.   Thyroid cartilage

       (1)   The largest laryngeal cartilage.

       (2)   The anterior aspect is called the laryngeal prominence or Adam's apple.

       (3)   Directly superior to the laryngeal prominence is the thyroid notch.

       (4)   The posterior and lateral aspects of this cartilage have two superior and two inferior projections: the superior and inferior cornua.

          (a)   The superior cornu articulates with the hyoid bone, which serves as a support from which the lower respiratory tract is suspended.

          (b)   The inferior cornu articulates with the cricoid cartilage below.

    c.   Cricoid cartilage

       (1)   Shaped like a signet ring, the smallest opening in the neonatal airway.

       (2)   Forms the entire inferior aspect and most of the posterior aspect of the larynx.

       (3)   There are articulating surfaces for the inferior cornu of the thyroid cartilage on the posterolateral surface.

       (4)   There are articulating surfaces for the paired arytenoid cartilages on the posterosuperior surface.

       (5)   Lies inferior to the thyroid and superior to the trachea, to which it attaches.

       (6)   Lies anterior to the esophagus; therefore, external cricoid pressure may facilitate viewing of the glottis during tracheal intubation and may prevent reflux from the stomach by compressing the esophagus.

5.   Paired cartilages of the larynx: Arytenoid, corniculate, and cuneiform (see Figure 4-6).

    a.   Arytenoid cartilages

       (1)   Shaped like upright pyramids.

       (2)   The base of each cartilage articulates with the posterosuperior surface of the cricoid cartilage.

       (3)   Each arytenoid cartilage has a ventral-medial projection from its base called the vocal process, to which the vocal ligaments attach.

       (4)   Arytenoid cartilages, along with the cricoid cartilage, make up the entire posterior surface of the larynx.

    b.   Corniculate cartilages

       (1)   Shaped like cones and are the smallest cartilages of the larynx.

       (2)   Articulate with the arytenoid cartilages on their superior surface, to which the corniculate cartilages are sometimes fused.

       (3)   When the larynx is viewed from above, the corniculate cartilages appear as two small elevations on the posteromedial aspect of the laryngeal inlet.

       (4)   Housed in mucosal folds called the aryepiglottic folds.

    c.   Cuneiform cartilages

       (1)   Shaped like small, elongated clubs.

       (2)   Located lateral and anterior to the corniculate cartilages.

       (3)   When the larynx is viewed from above, the cuneiform cartilages appear as two small elevations just lateral and anterior to the corniculate cartilages.

       (4)   Housed in the aryepiglottic folds.

       (5)   The cuneiforms, along with the aryepiglottic folds, form the lateral aspect of the laryngeal inlet. The epiglottis forms the anterior aspect, and the corniculates form the posterior aspect of the laryngeal inlet.

6.   Extrinsic ligaments of the larynx

    a.   Extrinsic ligaments attach cartilages of the larynx to structures outside the larynx.

    b.   The thyrohyoid membrane is a broad fibroelastic sheet that attaches the anterior and lateral superior aspects of the thyroid cartilage to the inferior surface of the hyoid bone (the posterior portion of the thyroid cartilage is attached to the hyoid bone by the superior cornu of the thyroid cartilage).

    c.   The hyoepiglottic ligament is an elastic band that attaches the anterior surface of the epiglottis to the hyoid bone.

    d.   The cricotracheal ligament connects the lower portion of the cricoid cartilage to the trachea by a broad fibrous membrane.

7. Intrinsic ligaments of the larynx
    a. Intrinsic ligaments attach cartilages of the larynx to one another.
    b. The thyroepiglottic ligament attaches the inferior aspect of the epiglottis to the thyroid cartilage on its internal surface below the thyroid notch.
    c. The aryepiglottic ligament attaches the arytenoid cartilages to the epiglottis and acts as a point of attachment for the aryepiglottic folds.
    d. The cricothyroid ligament attaches the anterior portion of the thyroid cartilage to the anterior portion of the cricoid cartilage. It is through this ligament that an emergency cricothyroidotomy is performed.
    e. The vocal ligament is a thick band that stretches from the vocal process of the arytenoid cartilages across the cavity of the larynx to attach to the thyroid cartilage just inferior to the thyroepiglottic ligament. The lateral borders of the vocal ligament attach to the inverted free borders of the cricothyroid ligament.
    f. The ventricular ligament is a thick band that stretches from the arytenoid cartilage across the cavity of the larynx to the thyroid cartilage. It exists superior and lateral to the vocal ligament.
8. Cavity of the larynx (see Figure 4-6)
    a. The larynx is divided into three sections by the pair of ventricular folds and vocal folds.
    b. The upper section, the vestibule of the larynx, extends from the laryngeal inlet to the level of the ventricular folds.
        (1) The ventricular folds are referred to as the false vocal cords.
        (2) The space between the ventricular folds is the rima vestibuli.
    c. The middle section, the ventricle of the larynx, extends from the ventricular folds to the vocal cords.
        (1) The vocal folds are the true vocal cords.
        (2) The space between the vocal folds is the rima glottidis or glottis.
            (a) The glottis is triangular, the base being posterior and the apex anterior.
            (b) It is the smallest opening of the adult airway (important when endotracheal tube size is selected).
            (c) The dimensions of the glottis are smaller in women than in men.
                (i) Average female transverse diameter: 7 to 8 mm.
                (ii) Average male transverse diameter: 9 to 10 mm.
                (iii) Average anteroposterior diameter in women: 17 mm.
                (iv) Average anteroposterior diameter in men: 24 mm.
        (3) The size of the rima glottidis also is variable, depending on the state of the vocal cords (see Figure 4-6).
            (a) Adduction is accomplished by medial rotation and approximation of the arytenoids, thus sealing the glottis.
            (b) Abduction is accomplished by lateral rotation of the arytenoids, thus increasing the size of the glottis.
        (4) The glottic or sphincter mechanism requires aryepiglottic folds, epiglottis, ventricular folds, and vocal folds to act in a coordinated fashion to seal the laryngeal inlet.
    d. The lower section, the subglottic cavity of the larynx, extends from the vocal folds to the cricoid cartilage.
    e. The epithelial lining of the larynx above the true vocal cords is continuous with the laryngopharynx and is stratified squamous epithelium (see Table 4-1).
    f. The epithelial lining of the larynx below the true vocal cords is pseudostratified ciliated columnar epithelium, the same as that in the trachea.
D. Tracheobronchial tree and lung parenchyma (Figure 4-7)
    1. The tracheobronchial tree functions in ventilation (to and fro movement of air) and is sometimes referred to as the conducting airway.
    2. The lung parenchyma functions in external respiration and is the area of the lung where actual gas exchange occurs.

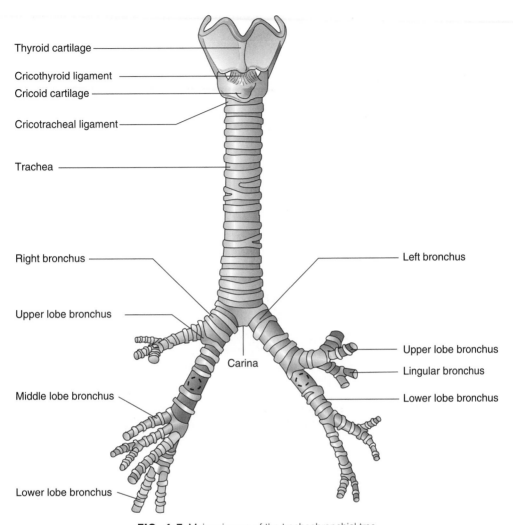

Thyroid cartilage

Cricothyroid ligament

Cricoid cartilage

Cricotracheal ligament

Trachea

Right bronchus

Left bronchus

Upper lobe bronchus

Carina

Upper lobe bronchus

Lingular bronchus

Middle lobe bronchus

Lower lobe bronchus

Lower lobe bronchus

FIG. 4-7 Major airways of the tracheobronchial tree.

3. As the lower airway subdivides, it gives way to additional airway generations. Each new generation of airway is assigned a number. The numbering system below begins with assigning generation 0 to the trachea. The first branching or division of the trachea constitutes the mainstem bronchi, which are assigned generation 1. Each subsequent branching of the lower airway is assigned the subsequent generation number.

E. Trachea (generation 0)
   1. The trachea is a cartilaginous, membranous tube 10 to 13 cm in length and 2 to 2.5 cm in diameter.
   2. The trachea extends from the cricoid cartilage at the sixth cervical vertebra to its point of bifurcation (carina) at the fifth thoracic vertebra.
   3. Sixteen to 20 incomplete (C-shaped) cartilaginous rings open posteriorly and are arranged horizontally. The open ends of the cartilage and the area between individual cartilages are joined by a combination of fibrous, elastic, and smooth muscle tissue.
      a. The smooth muscle is arranged longitudinally to shorten and elongate the trachea.
      b. The smooth muscle also is arranged transversely to constrict and dilate the trachea.
   4. The posterior wall of the trachea is separated from the anterior wall of the esophagus by loose connective tissue.

5. The trachea and following large airways (bronchi) contain three characteristic layers (Figure 4-8):
   a. Cartilaginous layer.
   b. Lamina propria, which contains small blood vessels, lymphatic vessels, nerve tracts, elastic fibers, smooth muscle, and submucosal glands.
   c. Epithelial, or intraluminal, layer, which is separated from the lamina propria by a noncellular basement membrane.
6. The epithelial lining of the trachea is continuous with the larynx above and consists of pseudostratified ciliated columnar epithelium (Table 4-2).

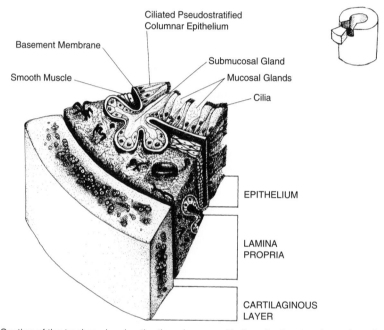

FIG. 4-8 Section of the trachea showing the three layers: epithelium, lamina propria, and cartilaginous layer.

TABLE **4-2**

Anatomical Comparison of Structures in the Lower Respiratory Tract

Structure	Epithelium	Division
Larynx/below true cords	Pseudostratified ciliated columnar	X
Trachea	Pseudostratified ciliated columnar	0
Mainstem bronchi	Pseudostratified ciliated columnar	1
Lobar bronchi	Pseudostratified ciliated columnar	2
Segmental bronchi	Pseudostratified ciliated columnar	3
Subsegmental bronchi	Pseudostratified ciliated columnar	4-9
Bronchioles	Pseudostratified ciliated columnar	10-15
Terminal bronchioles	Cuboidal to simple squamous	16
Respiratory bronchioles	Simple squamous	17-19
Alveolar ducts	Simple squamous	20-22
Alveolar sacs	Simple squamous	23
Alveoli	Type I; squamous	. . .
	Type II; granular	. . .
	Type III; macrophage	. . .

F. Mainstem bronchi (generation 1)
    1. The trachea bifurcates into two airways, the right and left mainstem bronchi, at the carina. The carina is generally located at the level of the fifth thoracic vertebra.
        a. Right mainstem bronchus
           (1) Branches off the trachea at an angle of approximately 20 to 30 degrees with respect to the midline.
           (2) Diameter: Approximately 1.4 cm.
           (3) Length: Approximately 2.5 cm.
        b. Left mainstem bronchus
           (1) Branches off the trachea at an angle of 40 to 55 degrees with respect to the midline.
           (2) Diameter: Appropriately 1.0 cm.
           (3) Length: Appropriately 5 cm.
    2. A portion of mainstem bronchi is extrapulmonary (exists outside the lung in the mediastinum), but the majority of it is intrapulmonary (inside the lung proper).
    3. The structural arrangement of the mainstem bronchi is the same as that of the trachea, with C-shaped pieces of cartilage, a lamina propria, and pseudostratified ciliated columnar epithelium (see Figure 4-8).
    4. The only structural difference between the mainstem bronchi and the trachea is that the intrapulmonary section of the mainstem bronchi is covered with a sheath of connective tissue, the peribronchiolar connective tissue.
        a. The function of peribronchiolar connective tissue is to encase large nerve, lymphatic, and bronchial blood vessels as they follow the branchings of the subdividing airways.
        b. The peribronchiolar connective tissue continues to follow the branching of the airways until the level of the bronchioles, where it disappears.
    5. Mainstem bronchi are sometimes referred to as primary bronchi.

G. Lobar bronchi (generation 2)
    1. Five lobar bronchi correspond, respectively, to the five lobes of the lung.
    2. The right mainstem bronchus trifurcates into the right upper, middle, and lower lobar bronchi.
    3. The left mainstem bronchus bifurcates into the left upper and lower lobar bronchi.
    4. The structural arrangement of lobar bronchi is the same as that of the mainstem bronchi (see Figure 4-8).
    5. The epithelial lining of lobar bronchi is pseudostratified ciliated columnar epithelium (see Table 4-2).
    6. Lobar bronchi are sometimes referred to as secondary bronchi.

H. Segmental bronchi (generation 3)
    1. There are 18 segmental bronchi, corresponding to the 18 segments of the lung, with diameters of approximately 4.5 to 13 mm.
    2. The structural arrangement of segmental bronchi is similar to that of lobar and mainstem bronchi, except that the C-shaped pieces of cartilage become less regular in shape and volume (Figure 4-9).
    3. The epithelial lining of segmental bronchi is pseudostratified ciliated columnar epithelium.
    4. Segmental bronchi are sometimes referred to as tertiary bronchi.

I. Subsegmental bronchi (generations 4-9)
    1. The diameter of subsegmental bronchi ranges from 1 to 6 mm.
    2. Cartilaginous rings give way to irregularly placed pieces of cartilage circumscribing the airway, the cartilaginous plaques (see Figure 4-9).
    3. By the ninth generation of airways, cartilage is only scantily present.
    4. As volume and regularity of cartilage have decreased from generation 0 to generation 9, so has the number of submucosal glands and goblet cells.
    5. The epithelial lining of subsegmental bronchi is pseudostratified ciliated columnar epithelium.

J. Bronchioles (generations 10-15)
    1. Diameter is characteristically approximately 1 mm.

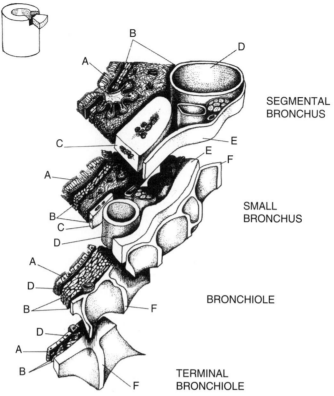

FIG. 4-9 Sections at various levels of the tracheobronchial tree. **A,** Pulmonary mucosa. **B,** Lamina propria. **C,** Cartilage. **D,** Blood vessels. **E,** Peribronchial connective tissue. **F,** Lung parenchyma.

    2. Cartilage is totally absent (see Figure 4-9).
    3. Peribronchiolar connective tissue is absent; the lamina propria of these airways is directly embedded in surrounding lung parenchyma.
    4. Airway patency is dependent not on the structural rigidity of surrounding cartilage but on fibrous, elastic, and smooth muscle tissue.
    5. The epithelial lining of bronchioles is pseudostratified ciliated cuboidal epithelium (short squat cells as opposed to the elongated columnar cells).
       a. This epithelium is functionally the same as pseudostratified ciliated columnar epithelium.
       b. It differs from pseudostratified ciliated columnar epithelium in three ways:
          (1) It is thinner, constructed of cuboidal cells rather than columnar cells.
          (2) The number of goblet cells and submucosal glands gradually decreases until they are almost nonexistent by generation 15.
          (3) The number of cilia also decreases, and cilia are all but gone by the end of generation 15.
  K. Terminal bronchioles (generation 16)
    1. Average diameter is 0.5 mm and represents a cross-sectional area of approximately 116 cm^2.
    2. Goblet cells and submucosal glands disappear, although mucus is found in these airways (see Figure 4-9).
    3. Cilia are absent from the epithelium of terminal bronchioles. This epithelium serves as a transition from the cuboidal epithelium of generation 15 to the squamous epithelium of generation 17.
    4. Clara cells are located in the terminal bronchioles.
       a. Plump columnar cells that bulge into the lumen of terminal bronchioles.

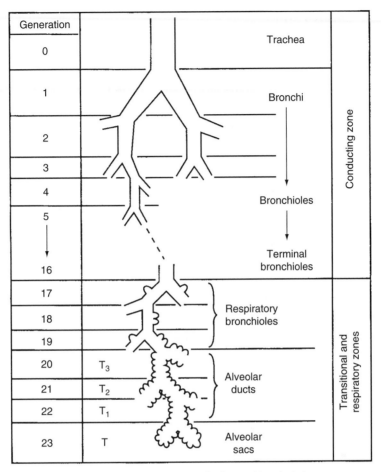

FIG. 4-10 Branching of the conducting and terminal airways.

    b. Probably responsible for production of mucus and surfactant found in terminal bronchioles.
  5. Terminal bronchioles mark the end of the conducting airways; all airway generations distal to the terminal bronchioles are considered part of the lung parenchyma (Figure 4-10).

L. Respiratory bronchioles (generations 17-19)
  1. Average diameter is <0.5 mm with a cross-sectional area of approximately 1000 cm^2.
  2. Alveoli originate from the external surface of the respiratory bronchioles, where a small portion of external respiration takes place.
  3. The epithelial lining of respiratory bronchioles is a low cuboidal epithelium interspersed with actual alveoli (simple squamous epithelium).

M. Alveolar ducts (generations 20-22)
  1. Alveolar ducts originate from respiratory bronchioles.
  2. The only difference between alveolar ducts and respiratory bronchioles is that the walls of the alveolar ducts are totally made up of alveoli.
  3. Approximately one half of the total number of alveoli originates from alveolar ducts.
  4. Alveolar ducts give way to alveolar sacs.

N. Alveolar sacs (generation 23)
  1. Alveolar sacs are the last generation of airways and are blind passageways.
  2. These appear functionally the same as alveolar ducts but differ because they form grapelike clusters having common walls with other alveoli.
  3. The remaining half of alveoli originates from alveolar sacs.

O. Alveoli (Figure 4-11)
    1. The alveoli are terminal air spaces that contain numerous capillaries in their septa, which serve as sites for gas exchange.
    2. The average number of total alveoli contained in both lungs combined is 300 million but varies directly with the height of the individual and may be as many as 600 million.
    3. The total cross-sectional area provided by the alveolar surface is approximately 80 m².
    4. The total cross-sectional area provided by the pulmonary capillaries is 70 m², thus constituting an alveolar gas-pulmonary blood interface of 70 m² (the size of a tennis court).
P. Alveolar capillary membrane or alveolar septum (Figure 4-12)

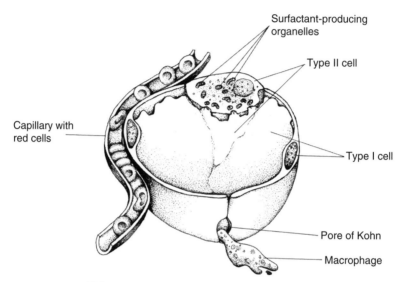

FIG. 4-11 Schematic representation of an alveoli.

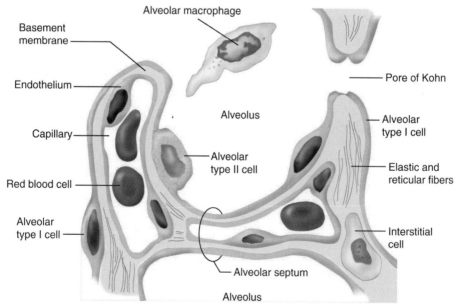

FIG. 4-12 Magnified view of an alveolus. Alveolar walls, or septa, are occupied mainly by capillaries. The basement membrane of the capillary is fused with that of the alveolar lining. The interstitium contains a few interstitial fibers composed mostly of reticular support fibers, elastic fibers, and one interstitial cell. An incomplete portion of the alveolar septum, called a *pore of Kohn,* is shown.

1. The alveolar capillary membrane has four components: surfactant layer, alveolar epithelium, interstitial space, and capillary endothelium.
   a. The surfactant is composed of a phospholipid attached to a lecithin molecule.
      (1) Surfactant lines the internal alveolar surface.
      (2) It reduces surface tension, facilitating inspiration and expiration.
   b. Alveolar epithelium (simple squamous epithelium) is a continuous layer of tissue made up of type I and II cells lying on a basement membrane (see Table 4-2).
      (1) Type I cells, or squamous pneumocytes: Flat, thin, simple squames making up 95% of alveolar surface.
      (2) Type II cells, or granular pneumocytes: Plump, highly metabolic cells credited with surfactant production and alveolar repair.
      (3) Type III cells, or alveolar macrophages: Free, wandering phagocytic cells that ingest foreign material on the alveolar surface.
   c. The interstitial space is the area that separates the basement membrane of alveolar epithelium from the basement membrane of capillary endothelium.
      (1) It contains interstitial fluid.
      (2) This space may be so small, especially where diffusion is to take place, that the basement membranes appear fused.
   d. Capillary endothelium is a continuous layer of tissue made up of flat, interlocking squames supported on a basement membrane.
2. Thickness of the alveolar capillary membrane varies from 0.35 to 1 μm.

III. The Lungs

A. The lungs are situated in the thoracic cavity separated by a structure (mediastinum) containing the heart, great vessels, esophagus, and trachea (Figure 4-13).
   1. Each thoracic cavity is lined with a fine serous membrane, the *parietal pleura*, which also covers the dome of each hemidiaphragm.
   2. The lung and each of its lobes are encased in a similar serous membrane called the visceral pleura.

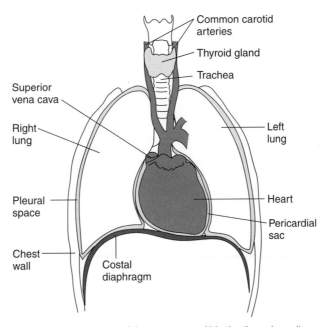

FIG. 4-13 Diagram of the structures within the thoracic cavity.

3. A potential space (intrapleural space) between the two pleura contains a small amount of fluid called pleural fluid.
   a. Pleural fluid allows cohesion of visceral and parietal pleura.
   b. Pleural fluid allows the two pleura to slide over each other with little frictional resistance.

B. The lung is a conical-shaped organ with four surfaces: apex, base, medial surface, and costal surface (Figure 4-14).
   1. The apices are rounded superior sections of the lung. They extend 1 to 2 in. above the clavicles.
   2. The bases are concave inferior surfaces of the lung. They rest on the hemidiaphragm. The right base lies higher in the thorax than the left to accommodate the large, underlying liver.
   3. The medial surface of each lung exhibits a deep concavity to accept the heart and great vessels. This concavity is called the cardiac impression. The left cardiac impression is deeper than the right because the heart projects to the left of the midline.
   4. The costal surface constitutes most of the lung surface in contact with the pleura lining the thoracic cavity.

C. The root of the lung enters the lung proper at the hilum.
   1. The root of the lung consists of a mainstem bronchus, a pulmonary artery, two pulmonary veins, major lymph vessels, and nerve tracts.
   2. The hilum is the area where the root enters the lung. There the mediastinal and visceral pleura become continuous, forming the pulmonary ligament. This arrangement keeps the pleural cavity sealed and allows the root to enter the sealed lung.

D. The right lung is divided into three lobes by the horizontal and oblique fissures (see Figure 4-14).
   1. The oblique fissure isolates the right lower lobe from the right middle and right upper lobe.
   2. The horizontal fissure divides the right upper lobe from the right middle lobe.

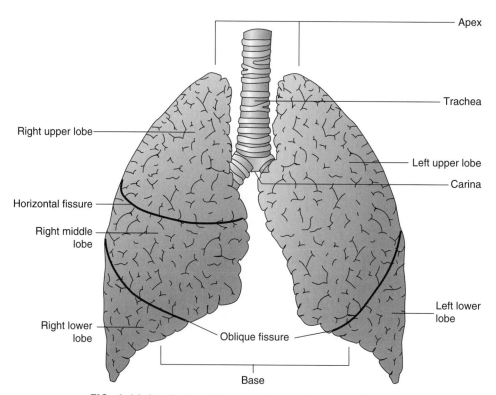

FIG. 4-14 Anterior view of the lungs showing the lobes and fissures.

3. Externally the oblique fissure courses through the following landmarks:
   a. Junction of the sixth rib and midclavicular line.
   b. Junction of the fifth rib and midaxillary line.
   c. Spinous process of the third thoracic vertebra.
4. Externally the horizontal fissure courses through the following landmarks:
   a. Junction of the fifth rib and midaxillary line.
   b. Follows the medial course of the fourth rib.
5. The right lung is larger than the left, and approximately 60% of gas exchange takes place in the right lung.

E. The left lung is divided into two lobes by the oblique fissure.
   1. The oblique fissure divides the left upper lobe from the left lower lobe.
   2. Externally the left oblique fissure courses through the same landmarks as the right oblique fissure.

F. The lobes of the lung are further subdivided into segments (Figure 4-15).
   1. Right upper lobe
      a. Anterior segment
      b. Apical segment
      c. Posterior segment
   2. Right middle lobe
      a. Lateral segment
      b. Medial segment
   3. Right lower lobe
      a. Superior segment
      b. Anterior basal segment
      c. Lateral basal segment
      d. Medial basal segment
      e. Posterior basal segment
   4. Left upper lobe
      a. Apical-posterior segment
      b. Anterior segment
      c. Superior segment lingula (anatomically corresponds to right middle lobe)
      d. Inferior segment
   5. Left lower lobe
      a. Superior segment
      b. Anteromedial basal segment
      c. Lateral basal segment
      d. Posterior basal segment
   6. Knowledge of bronchopulmonary segmentation becomes important when postural drainage, auscultation, radiographic findings, and bronchoscopy are considered.

G. The segments are further subdivided into secondary lobules.
   1. Secondary lobules consist of a 15th-order airway (bronchiole) and its associated three to five terminal bronchioles and their distal respiratory bronchioles, alveolar ducts, and alveolar sacs.
   2. The secondary lobule is the smallest self-contained unit of the lung that is surrounded by connective tissue.
   3. Secondary lobules appear as polyhedral masses observable on the lung surface and as dark intersecting lines between fissures.
   4. Secondary lobules have their own discrete single pulmonary arteriole, venule, lymphatic, and nerve supply.
   5. Secondary lobules are the building blocks of segments and are discernible on chest radiography.
   6. Each secondary lobule comprises 30 to 50 primary lobules and measures 1 to 2.5 cm in diameter.
      a. Primary lobules consist of a 19th-order respiratory bronchiole and every generation distal to it.

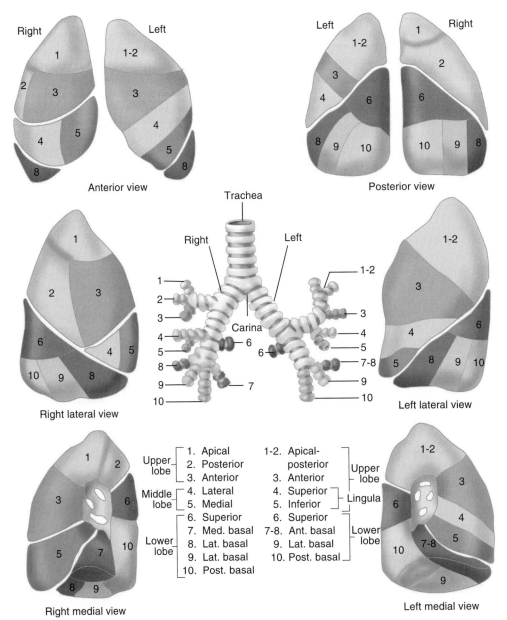

FIG. 4-15 Bronchopulmonary segments diagrammed in different views (anterior, posterior, lateral, and medial). Note similarities with minor variations between the right and left lungs.

b. Primary lobules are not self-contained in connective tissue.
c. There are approximately 23 million primary lobules in the lung.
7. Secondary lobules may be important in isolating and maintaining disease locally. They also may be responsible for local matching of ventilation to perfusion.
H. Bronchiolar and alveolar intercommunicating channels
1. The canals of Lambert, approximately 30 μm in size, provide collateral ventilation between primary lobules.
2. The pores of Kohn are interalveolar pores that allow collateral ventilation of alveoli. Their diameter varies from 3 to 13 μm.
3. A third channel connecting intersegmental respiratory bronchioles primarily in the lower lobes has been proposed, also providing collateral ventilation.

I. Innervation of the lungs
   1. Afferent and efferent pathways of the autonomic nervous system innervate the lungs.
   2. The afferent or sensory pathways originate in the epithelium of the bronchial walls, submucosa, interalveolar septa, and smooth muscles.
   3. Parasympathetic fibers via the vagus nerves arranged in three groups of sensory fibers have been identified.
      a. Pulmonary stretch receptors, which are slowly adapting.
        (1) Located in smooth muscles of intrapulmonary airways.
        (2) Stimulated by lung inflation or increased transpulmonary pressure.
        (3) Response to stimulation:
          (a) Hering-Breuer inflation reflex
          (b) Bronchodilation
          (c) Increased heart rate
          (d) Decreased peripheral vascular resistance
      b. Irritant, rapidly adapting
        (1) Located mainly in the epithelium of extrapulmonary airways.
        (2) Stimulated by:
          (a) Irritants
          (b) Mechanical stimulation
          (c) Anaphylaxis
          (d) Lung inflation or deflation
          (e) Hyperpnea
          (f) Pulmonary congestion
        (3) Response to stimulation
          (a) Bronchoconstriction
          (b) Hyperpnea
          (c) Expiratory constriction of larynx
          (d) Cough
          (e) Mucus secretion
      c. C-fiber–pulmonary type J receptors
        (1) Located in alveolar walls, airways, and blood vessels.
        (2) Stimulated by:
          (a) Increased interstitial volume (congestion)
          (b) Chemical injury
          (c) Microembolism
        (3) Response to stimulation:
          (a) Rapid shallow breathing
          (b) Laryngeal and tracheobronchial constriction
          (c) Bradycardia
          (d) Spinal reflex inhibition
          (e) Mucus secretion
        (4) Efferent or motor pathways reach the lung through the sympathetic and parasympathetic nervous system.
        (5) The sympathetic fibers terminate in the airway walls, vascular smooth muscle, and submucosal glands; stimulation causes:
          (a) Bronchial smooth muscle relaxation
          (b) Constriction of pulmonary arteries
          (c) Decreased glandular secretion
        (6) Stimulation of the parasympathetic motor fibers in the airways causes:
          (a) Airway constriction
          (b) Increased glandular secretion
J. Bronchial circulation
   1. The metabolic needs of the airways are provided by the bronchial arteries, which originate from the aorta or the upper intercostal arteries.
   2. These vessels accompany the bronchial tree down to the terminal bronchioles.

3. Structures distal to the terminal bronchioles are believed to obtain their nutrients from the mixed venous blood of the pulmonary circulation.
4. The bronchial circulation is approximately 1% to 2% of the cardiac output.
5. A portion of the venous blood from the capillaries of the bronchial circulation returns to the right heart by way of the:
   a. Azygos vein
   b. Hemiazygos vein
   c. Intercostal vein
6. The remainder of the bronchial circulation returns to the left heart by way of the:
   a. Bronchial artery plexuses
   b. Bronchopulmonary veins
7. Blood emptying into the left heart is termed venous admixture.

IV. **Bony Thorax (Figure 4-16)**
   A. It is a bony and cartilaginous frame within which lie the principal organs of circulation and respiration.
   B. It is conical and narrow above and broad below.
   C. Posteriorly, the thorax includes the 12 thoracic vertebrae and the posterior portion of the ribs.
   D. Laterally, the thorax is convex and formed by the ribs.
   E. Anteriorly, it is composed of the sternum, anterior ends of the ribs, and the costal cartilage.
   F. The superior opening into the thorax—defined by the manubrium, first rib, and first thoracic vertebra—is called the thoracic inlet or operculum.
   G. The inferior opening out of the thorax—defined by the 12th rib, costal cartilage of ribs 7 through 10, and 12th thoracic vertebra—is called the thoracic outlet.

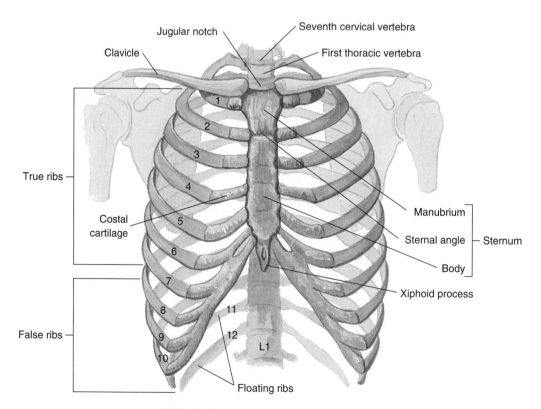

FIG. 4-16 Anterior view of the thoracic cage.

H. Functions of the bony thorax are to protect underlying organs, aid in ventilation, and provide a point of attachment for various bones and muscles.

I. Sternum (see Figure 4-16)
1. The sternum is approximately 17 cm long.
2. The sternum is divided into three sections:
    a. Manubrium: Superior portion
    b. Body: Middle portion
    c. Xiphoid process: Inferior portion
3. The manubrium articulates with the clavicle and the first and second ribs.
4. The junction of the manubrium and the body is called the angle of Louis. The trachea bifurcates beneath this junction.
5. The body of the sternum articulates with ribs 2 through 7.
6. The xiphoid process articulates with the seventh rib.

J. Ribs (see Figure 4-16)
1. Twelve elastic arches of bone, posteriorly connected to the vertebral column.
2. Types of ribs: True, false, and floating.
3. True ribs
    a. Rib pairs 1 through 7.
    b. Called vertebrosternal ribs because they connect to the sternum via costal cartilage and the vertebrae of the spinal column.
4. False ribs
    a. Rib pairs 8 through 10.
    b. Called vertebrocostal ribs because they connect to costal cartilage of superior rib and the vertebrae of the spinal column.
5. Floating ribs
    a. Rib pairs 11 and 12.
    b. Have no anterior attachment, lying free in abdominal musculature.
6. The space between the ribs is called the intercostal space.
    a. Wider anteriorly than posteriorly.
    b. Wider superiorly than inferiorly.
7. All 12 pairs of ribs are positioned in an inferior direction. Contraction of the intercostal muscles elevates the ribs from their natural inclined position.
    a. A superoinferior motion of the ribs causes an increase in the transverse diameter of the thorax and is called the bucket handle effect.
    b. An anteroposterior motion of the ribs causes an increase in the anteroposterior diameter of the thorax and is called the pump handle effect.

V. **Muscles of Inspiration (Figure 4-17)**
A. The diaphragm, external intercostal, parasternal intercostal, and scalene muscles are normally used for resting inspiration (Table 4-3).
1. Diaphragm: Dome-shaped muscle that separates the thoracic from the abdominal cavity.
    a. It is the major muscle of ventilation.
    b. It is composed of two parts:
        (1) Costal diaphragm
        (2) Crural diaphragm
    c. When standing, the dome of the diaphragm at functional residual capacity (FRC) on the right is located at the eighth thoracic vertebra and at the ninth thoracic vertebra on the left.
    d. During normal breathing the diaphragm moves 1.0 to 1.7 cm and may descend as much as 10 cm during stress.
    e. Normally at FRC part of the diaphragm lies along the rib cage (zone of opposition).
    f. Innervation: Cervical spinal motor nerves 3, 4, and 5 (phrenic nerve).
2. Intercostal muscles
    a. External and internal intercostal muscles are located between all ribs.
    b. The internal muscle is composed of two separate muscles:

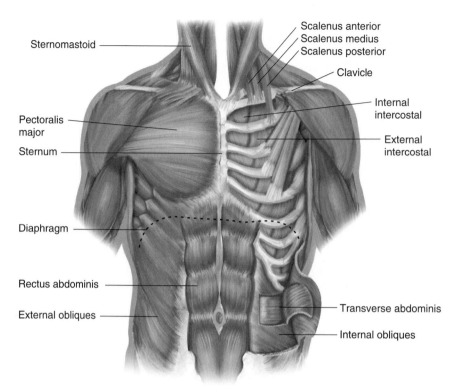

FIG. 4-17 The muscles of ventilation.

(1) Parasternal: An inspiratory muscle.
(2) Interosseous or internal intercostal muscle: An expiratory muscle.
c. External intercostal: An inspiratory muscle.
d. Innervation: Thoracic spinal motor nerves 1 through 11.
e. These muscles prevent the intercostal space from bulging and recessing with normal ventilatory efforts.
3. Scalene (scalenus) muscles
a. Three sets of muscles:
(1) Anterior
(2) Medius
(3) Posterior
b. All are active during normal breathing.
B. Accessory muscles of inspiration
1. Each tends to perform one of two actions, either raising the thorax or stabilizing the thorax so that other muscles can effectively raise the thorax.
a. Sternocleidomastoid (sternomastoid)
b. Pectoralis major
c. Pectoralis minor
2. It should be noted that use of accessory muscles for resting inspiration is abnormal and that accessory muscle use should occur only with deep or forced inspiration.

VI. **Accessory Muscles of Expiration (see Figures 4-17 and 4-18)**
A. There are no muscles of quiet resting expiration. Expiration is purely a passive process brought about by the normal elastic tendencies of the lung coupled with cessation of inspiratory muscle contraction. Therefore, any muscles used for expiration are termed accessory muscles of expiration.

TABLE 4-3

Muscles of Breathing

Muscle(s)	Phase	Use	Origin	Insertion	Action
Costal diaphragm	Inspiration	Normal	Inner surface of ribs 7-12 and sternum	Central tendon	Increases superior-inferior lung volume; lower lateral rib cage expansion
Crural diaphragm	Inspiration	Normal	First 3 lumbar vertebrae	Central tendon	Increases superior-inferior lung volume; lateral rib cage expansion
Parasternal intercostals	Inspiration	Normal	Costal cartilage	Costal cartilage, sternum	Lift ribs and sternum
Interosseous internal intercostals	Expiration	Accessory	Costal cartilage	Costal cartilage	Pull ribs downward
External intercostals	Inspiration	Accessory	Upper ribs	Lower ribs	Lift ribs forward and upward
Scalene, medius, and anterior	Inspiration	Normal	Lower 5 vertebrae	1st and 2nd ribs	Lift 1st and 2nd ribs and sternum
Sternomastoid	Inspiration	Accessory	Manubrium sterni and clavicle	Mastoid process and occipital bone	Lift upper ribs
External oblique	Expiratory	Accessory	Lower 8 ribs above the costal margins	Iliac crest and inguinal ligament	Constricts and compresses diaphragm
Internal oblique	Expiratory	Accessory	Lumbar fascia, iliac crest, inguinal ligament	Costal margin, pubis	Constricts and compresses diaphragm
Transverse abdominis	Expiratory	Accessory	Costal margin	Midline aponeurosis of the rectus sheath	Constricts and compresses diaphragm
Rectus abdominis	Expiratory	Accessory	Costal cartilage of ribs 5-7	Pubis	Constricts and compresses diaphragm
Pectoralis major	Inspiration	Accessory	Clavicle	Sternum, costal cartilage	Lifts upper chest wall
Pectoralis minor	Inspiration	Accessory	Ribs 3-5, near costal cartilage	Scapula	Lifts upper chest wall
Latissimus dorsi	Expiratory (controversial)	Accessory	Lumbar and sacral vertebrae	Humerus	Stabilizes back and vertebral column
Serratus anterior	Expiratory	Accessory	8 upper ribs	Scapula	Stabilizes back and vertebral column
Serratus, posterior superior	Expiratory	Accessory	Cervical and dorsal vertebrae	Ribs 2-5	Stabilizes back and vertebral column
Serratus, posterior inferior	Expiratory	Accessory	Dorsal and lumbar vertebrae	Ribs 9-12	Stabilizes back and vertebral column

From Pierson DJ, Kacmarek RM: *Foundations of Respiratory Care.* New York, Churchill Livingstone, 1992.

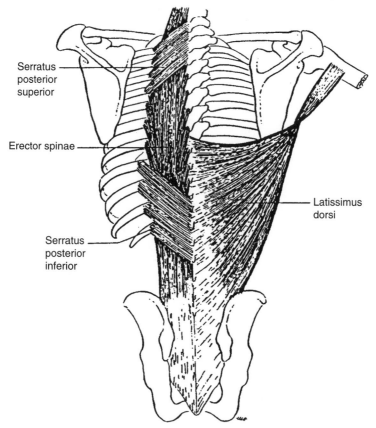

FIG. 4-18 Schematic illustration of the muscles of the back that play a role in ventilation.

B. Any muscle usage for quiet resting expiration is abnormal.
C. Accessory muscles of expiration are used only for forced expiration, making expiration an active process.
D. The accessory muscles of expiration are of the back, thorax, or abdomen and tend to either pull the thorax down or support the thorax so that other muscle groups can effectively pull down on the thorax.
   1. Interosseous internal intercostal
   2. Rectus abdominis
   3. External oblique
   4. Internal oblique
   5. Transverse abdominis
   6. Latissimus dorsi
   7. Serratus anterior
   8. Serratus, posterior superior
   9. Serratus, posterior interior

VII. **Other Functions of the Lung**
   A. Blood reservoir for the left ventricle.
      1. Approximately 600 ml is maintained in the lung.
      2. This volume is sufficient to maintain several cardiac cycles in the face of decreased venous return.
   B. The pulmonary circulation acts as a filter for the systemic circulation. Particles are trapped before they can enter the systemic circulation.

C. Metabolic function
1. The lungs are responsible for synthesis, activation, inactivation, and detoxification of many bioactive substances.
   a. Heparin
   b. Histamine
   c. Bradykinin
   d. Serotonin
   e. Prostaglandin
2. The lung activates angiotensin.
3. Adenosine triphosphate and norepinephrine are partially removed from the blood and inactivated by the lungs.

BIBLIOGRAPHY

Beachey W: *Respiratory Care Anatomy and Physiology: Foundations for Clinical Practice.* St. Louis, Mosby, 1998.

Comroe JH: *Physiology of Respiration,* ed 2. Chicago, Year Book Medical Publishers, 1974.

Guyton AC, Hall JE: *Textbook of Medical Physiology,* ed 10. Philadelphia, WB Saunders, 2000.

Hess DJ, MacIntyre NR, Mishoe SC, Galvin WF, Adams AB, Saposnick AB: *Respiratory Care Principles and Practice.* Philadelphia, WB Saunders, 2002.

Hicks GH: *Cardiopulmonary Anatomy and Physiology.* Philadelphia, WB Saunders, 2000.

Moser KM, Spragg RG, eds: *Respiratory Emergencies,* ed 2. St. Louis, CV Mosby, 1982.

Murray JF: *The Normal Lung.* Philadelphia, WB Saunders, 1976.

Osmond DG: Functional of anatomy of the chest wall. In Roussos C, ed: *The Thorax, Part A.* New York, Marcel Dekker, 1995, pp. 413-444.

Pierson DJ, Kacmarek RM: *Foundations of Respiratory Care.* New York, Churchill Livingstone, 1992.

Shapiro BA, Harrison RA, Kacmarek RM, et al: *Clinical Application of Respiratory Care,* ed 3. Chicago, Year Book Medical Publishers, 1985.

Shibel EM, Moser KM: *Respiratory Emergencies.* St Louis, CV Mosby, 1977.

Wilkins RL, Stoller JK, Scanlon CL: *Egan's Fundamentals of Respiratory Therapy,* ed 8. St. Louis, CV Mosby, 2003.

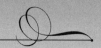
Mechanics of Ventilation

I. **The Lung-Thorax System**
   A. As described in Chapter 4, the lung and the thorax are lined by thin connective tissues sheets: the parietal pleura on the inside of the thoracic cage and the visceral pleura on the outside of the lung and mediastinum.
   B. These two pleurae are in contact with each other, separated by only a thin film of fluid.
   C. Because the lungs have a tendency to contract inward and the thorax expands outward during normal breathing, a negative (subatmospheric) pressure is maintained between the pleurae (Figure 5-1).
   D. A convenient way of viewing the lung-thorax system is to consider it a two-spring system held together by the pleura (Figure 5-2). The thorax can be conceptualized as a band spring tending to expand outward, and the lung can be described as a coil spring tending to contract inward.
   E. If the sternum is split and the pleura separated but not opened, the lung and thorax move to their independent resting positions (see Figure 5-1).
      1. The lung collapses.
      2. The thorax expands.
   F. If air is allowed to enter the potential pleural space, a pneumothorax develops.
   G. Any interference with the integrity of the pleura can interfere with ventilation.

II. **Pulmonary Pressures and Gradients**
   A. Six pressures are frequently referred to when discussing ventilation:
      1. Mouth pressure (P_{ao}): The pressure at the entry of the respiratory system, synonymous with end-expiratory pressure or airway opening pressure.
      2. Alveolar pressure (P_{alv}): The pressure within the alveoli; also referred to as intrapulmonary pressure. It is equal to mouth pressure, when all gas flow stops, is equilibrated, and the glottis is open.
      3. Pleural pressure (P_{pl}): The pressure within the potential pleural space; also referred to as intrathoracic pressure.
      4. Esophageal pressure (P_{es}): Pressure measured within the esophagus. When the pressure is properly determined, changes in esophageal pressure reflect changes in pleural pressure.
      5. Body surface pressure (P_{bs}): Equal to atmospheric pressure (P_{ATM}).
      6. Abdominal pressure (P_{ab}): Pressure measured in the abdominal cavity.
   B. When the mechanics of breathing are discussed, four pressure gradients are commonly defined (Figure 5-3):
      1. Transpulmonary pressure (P_l): The pressure difference across the lung (alveolar-pleural pressure, $P_l = P_{alv} - P_{pl}$).
         a. During resting spontaneous breathing maximally equals approximately 3 to 4 cm H_2O.

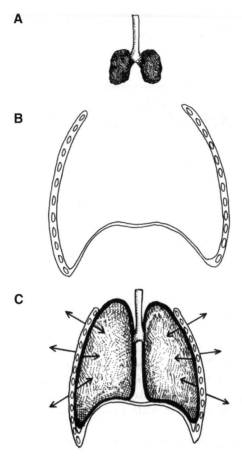

FIG. 5-1 A, Resting state of normal lungs when removed from the chest cavity (i.e., elasticity causes total collapse). **B,** Resting state of normal chest wall and diaphragm when apex is open to atmosphere and the thoracic contents removed. **C,** End-expiration in the normal, intact thorax. Note that elastic forces of lung and chest wall are in opposite directions. The pleural surfaces link these two opposing forces (see text).

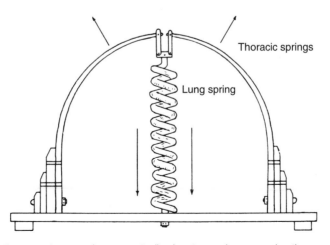

FIG. 5-2 The lung-thorax system may be conceptualized as two springs opposing the movement of each other, the thoracic band spring tending to expand and the lung coil spring tending to contract.

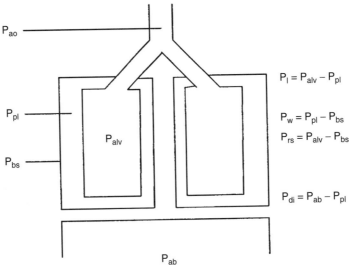

FIG. 5-3 Pressure gradients related to normal or stressed ventilation. P_{ao}, Airway opening pressure; P_{alv}, intrapulmonary or alveolar pressure; P_{pl}, pleural pressure; P_{bs}, body surface pressure; P_{ab}, abdominal pressure; P_l, transpulmonary pressure; P_w, transthoracic pressure; P_{rs}, transrespiratory pressure; and P_{di}, transdiaphragmatic pressure.

b. During forced spontaneous breathing maximally may exceed 25 cm H_2O.

c. During assisted ventilation may be from 1 to approximately 20 cm H_2O dependent on patient effort.

d. During controlled ventilation the value is approximately 5 cm H_2O under normal circumstances because alveolar and pleural pressures increase equal levels as inspiration continues.

e. The stiffer the lung, the greater the differences between alveolar and pleural pressures during spontaneous, assisted, and controlled ventilation.

f. The stiffer the chest, the smaller the differences between alveolar and pleural pressure during spontaneous, assisted, and controlled ventilation.

2. Transthoracic pressure (P_W): The pressure difference across the thorax (pleural-body surface pressure, $P_w = P_{pl} - P_{bs}$).

a. During spontaneous, assisted, and controlled breathing the transthoracic pressure is larger than the transpulmonary pressure by approximately 3 to 5 cm H_2O, depending on the stiffness of the lung and thorax and airway resistance.

b. The stiffer the lung and thorax or the greater the airway resistance, the greater the transthoracic pressure.

3. Transrespiratory pressure (P_{rs}): The pressure difference across the lung-thorax system; also referred to as the transairway pressure (alveolar-body surface pressure, $P_{rs} = P_{alv} - P_{bs}$).

a. During spontaneous, assisted, and controlled breathing the transrespiratory pressure is essentially equal to the change in alveolar pressure and tends to track transpulmonary pressures.

b. Transrespiratory pressure is most affected by changes in the chest wall (including abdominal pressure). The stiffer the chest wall the greater the transrespiratory pressure.

4. Transdiaphragmatic pressure (P_{di}): The pressure difference across the diaphragm (abdominal-pleural pressure, $P_{di} = P_{ab} - P_{pl}$).

a. During spontaneous breathing the transdiaphragmatic pressure is always greater than the transpulmonary pressure by a few cm H_2O. This is true because as the pleural pressure decreases, the abdominal pressure increases.

b. During assisted ventilation the transdiaphragmatic pressure is initially slightly greater than the transpulmonary pressure, but as positive pressure is delivered pleural and abdominal pressures increase to bring transdiaphragmatic pressure close to zero.

c. During controlled ventilation the transdiaphragmatic pressure changes little from zero because the diaphragm does not actively contract and pleural and abdominal pressures increase, thus there is little change in transdiaphragmatic pressure.

III. Inspiration

A. Figures 5-4 and 5-5 depict the intrapleural (intrathoracic) and intrapulmonary pressure curves during normal resting ventilation.

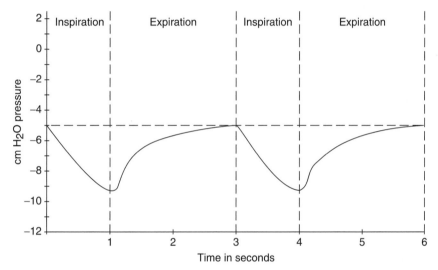

FIG. 5-4 Intrapleural (intrathoracic) pressure curve during normal spontaneous ventilation. Note that normal resting expiratory pressure is approximately –5 cm H_2O and decreases to –9 cm H_2O during inspiration.

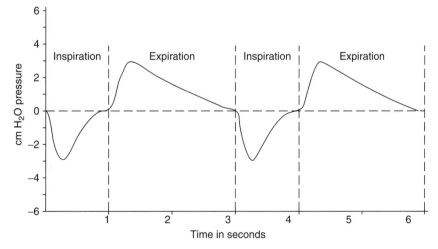

FIG. 5-5 Intrapulmonary pressure during normal spontaneous ventilation has a peak inspiratory pressure of approximately –3 cm H_2O and peak expiratory pressure of approximately +3 cm H_2O.

  B. At functional residual capacity (FRC) level or resting exhalation, the intrapleural pressure is approximately –5 cm H_2O, whereas the intrapulmonary pressure is zero (atmospheric; Figure 5-6).

    1. The transpulmonary pressure at FRC is thus equal to 5 cm H_2O.

    2. The transpulmonary pressure is also referred to as the alveolar distending pressure.

  C. Because the lung is a valveless pump, when gas flow stops and the glottis is open, intrapulmonary and atmospheric pressures are equal (i.e., the transrespiratory pressure gradient is zero).

    1. A negative transrespiratory pressure causes gas to enter the lung.

    2. A positive transrespiratory pressure causes gas to exit the lung.

  D. Pressure gradients causing inspiration are established by contraction of the diaphragm, intercostals, and scalene muscles.

  E. With inspiratory muscle contraction, the thoracic cavity expands, causing the intrapleural pressure to become more negative (approximately –9 cm H_2O).

  F. This pressure decrease increases the volume of the lung. Because of the relationship of the two pleura, the lungs must expand as the thorax expands.

  G. The expansion of the lung decreases the intrapulmonary pressure to approximately –3 cm H_2O.

  H. The decreased intrapulmonary pressure establishes a pressure gradient with atmosphere, causing gas to enter the lung.

  I. Once the intrapulmonary pressure is returned to normal by gas entering the lung, inspiration stops.

  J. Boyle's law explains all of the pressure-volume changes described in breathing.

 IV. **Exhalation**

  A. Exhalation is normally a passive process. The lung-thorax system is returned to its resting state as a result of the elastic recoil of the lung.

  B. Relaxation of the muscles of inspiration allows the intrapleural pressure to return to baseline (–5 cm H_2O); as a result, the intrapulmonary pressure increases to approximately +3 cm H_2O.

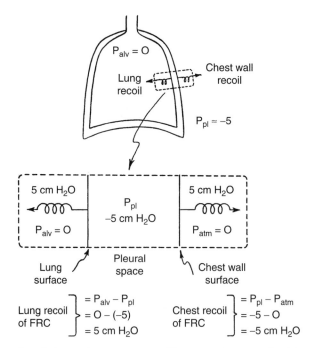

FIG. 5-6 The balance of respiratory system pressures and forces creates a negative intrapleural pressure at functional residual capacity (FRC).

C. Because the transrespiratory pressure is positive, gas leaves the lung.

D. Lung volume returns to the FRC level, and the transrespiratory pressure returns to zero.

V. **Resistance to Ventilation**
   A. Ventilation is opposed by three major factors:
      1. Elastic resistance
      2. Nonelastic resistance
      3. Inertia
   B. Elastic resistance is a result of distortion of pulmonary elastic tissue. Elastic resistance is established based on:
      1. Surface tension in the lung
      2. Lung elastance or compliance
   C. Nonelastic resistance is primarily the resistance to gas flow. It is equivalent to the frictional resistance of solids moving across each other. Overall nonelastic resistance is the combined effect of:
      1. Airway resistance
      2. Tissue viscous resistance
   D. Inertia is the tendency of a body in motion to stay in motion and a body at rest to stay at rest.
      1. During ventilation, effort is required to move the nonelastic structures of the lung thoracic system (e.g., bone and blood).
      2. In general, inertia contributes in only a minor degree to the resistance to ventilation.

VI. **Surface Tension**
   A. Surface tension is the force occurring at the interface between a liquid and another liquid or a gas that tends to cause the liquid to occupy the smallest volume possible (see Chapter 2).
   B. Surface tension causes alveoli to decrease in size and would cause collapse were it not for the presence of a pulmonary surfactant secreted by type II alveolar cells.
   C. The volume of surfactant produced by the respiratory tract is relatively constant. As a result, the effect the surfactant exerts is indirectly related to the surface area it covers.
   D. At FRC there is a large amount of surfactant applied per unit area. This causes a significant reduction in pressure as a result of surface tension, with the following results:
      1. Prevention of alveolar collapse on exhalation (preventing alveoli from reaching their critical volume).
      2. Reduction in pressure needed to overcome surface tension as inspiration begins.
   E. At maximum inspiration, a small volume of surfactant is applied per unit area. Thus, the pressure as a result of surface tension tending to collapse the alveoli is great. This pressure assists in normal passive exhalation.
   F. Pressures as a result of surface tension:
      1. At maximal inspiration: Approximately 40 dynes/cm^2.
      2. At maximal exhalation: Approximately 2 to 4 dynes/cm^2.
   G. As a result the pressure-volume relationship of the lung is different during inspiration and expiration; a hysteresis exists (Figure 5-7). Greater volume is maintained in the lung for a given pressure during exhalation than during inspiration.
   H. If the lung is filled with saline instead of air, much less pressure is needed to expand it with saline because the effect of surface tension is eliminated and the hysteresis disappears (see Figure 5-7).
   I. The effect of surface tension cannot be evaluated directly. Changes in surface tension cause a change in compliance or elastance of the lung.
   J. An increase in surface tension increases elastic resistance to ventilation and is reflected in a decrease in compliance, causing an increase in the work of breathing.

VII. **Compliance**
   A. Compliance is the ease of distention of the lung-thorax system and is inversely related to elastance (see Chapter 2).

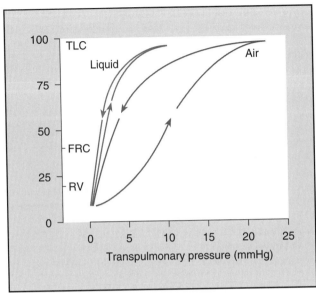

FIG. 5-7 Pressure-volume curve obtained on inflation and deflation of a normal air-filled lung and the same lung when filled with liquid to eliminate the forces caused by surface tension.

    B. Compliance is normally a static measurement so as to eliminate the effects of nonelastic resistance.

    C. Compliance is determined by comparing the change in volume in a system with the pressure necessary to maintain the volume change:

$$C = \frac{\Delta V}{\Delta P} \tag{1}$$

    D. In the respiratory system, there are basically three types of compliance (Figure 5-8):
        1. Pulmonary or lung (C_{pul})
        2. Thoracic or chest wall (C_{th})
        3. Total or respiratory system (C_{total})
    E. In the lung-thorax system, the tendency of the lung is to collapse to its resting position, and the tendency of the thorax is to expand to its resting position.
    F. The FRC is that volume maintained in the lung at the resting expiratory position as a result of the equal and opposing effects of pulmonary (lung) and thoracic (chest wall) compliance.
    G. Total compliance of the lung-thorax system is a result of the interaction of pulmonary and thoracic compliance (see Figure 5-8).
    H. Compliance is linear only at relatively normal tidal volumes. As the lung volume exceeds or falls below tidal levels, compliance decreases. Thus, the total compliance curve is significantly distorted as lung volume approaches residual volume (RV) or total lung capacity (TLC; see Figure 5-8).
        1. As lung volume approaches TLC, the tendency of the lung to collapse far outweighs the tendency of the thorax to expand. Specifically, the thorax reaches its resting position at 70% of TLC. Beyond this level the thorax tends to collapse. Because the lung has been distorted significantly beyond its resting position, continued pulmonary expansion requires greater force. At TLC an individual cannot exert sufficient force to continue lung expansion.
        2. As the lung volume approaches RV, the tendency of the thorax to expand far outweighs the tendency of the lung to collapse. This occurs because the lung is now near its resting point, whereas the thorax is significantly distorted from its resting point. At RV, the tendency of the thorax to expand is so great that the individual cannot voluntarily exhale a larger volume.

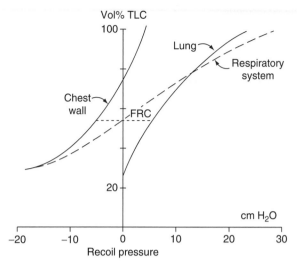

FIG. 5-8 The pressure-volume curves of the relaxed chest wall, the lungs, and the total respiratory system.

I. Total respiratory system compliance (C_{total}) is determined by dividing the tidal volume (V_T) by the static pressure necessary to maintain the V_T in the lung. Pressure should be measured at the patient's mouth. In the average young adult, total respiratory system compliance measured in the normal V_T range is typically equal to 0.08 to 0.1 L/cm H_2O, or 80 to 100 ml/cm H_2O.

J. Pulmonary compliance (C_{pul}) is determined by dividing the V_T by the static pressure necessary to maintain the V_T in the lung. The pressure measured should reflect changes in intrapleural pressures. Pressure recorded at the level of the midesophagus accurately reflects pleural pressure changes. In the average young adult, pulmonary compliance (C_{pul}) is typically equal to 0.16 to 0.2 L/cm H_2O, or 160 to 200 ml/cm H_2O.

K. Thoracic compliance (C_{th}) is a calculated value based on the following equation:

$$\frac{1}{C_{total}} = \frac{1}{C_{pul}} + \frac{1}{C_{th}} \tag{2}$$

In the average young adult, thoracic compliance is typically equal to 0.16 to 0.2 L/cm H_2O, or 100 to 200 ml/cm H_2O.

L. Changes in total respiratory system compliance (C_{total}) reflect total elastic resistance to ventilation.
   1. Total compliance reflects surface tension and tissue elastance.
   2. A decrease in total compliance results in a decrease in FRC.
   3. An increase in total compliance results in an increase in FRC.
   4. Alterations in pulmonary or thoracic compliance result in an alteration of total compliance.

M. With an increase in total respiratory system compliance, there is a corresponding decrease in elastance. This tends to make inspiration easier but also makes expiratory more difficult. In this situation a slow, deep ventilatory pattern minimizes the work of breathing.

N. With a decrease in total respiratory system compliance, there is a corresponding increase in elastance. This tends to make inspiration more difficult but makes exhalation easier. In this situation a rapid, shallow ventilatory pattern minimizes the work of breathing.

O. Total respiratory system compliance is decreased by any pathophysiologic change that inhibits lung or chest wall expansion:
   1. Pneumonitis
   2. Pulmonary consolidation
   3. Pulmonary edema
   4. Pneumothorax

     5. Abdominal distention

     6. Adult respiratory distress syndrome (ARDS)

     7. Pulmonary fibrosis

     8. Thoracic deformities

     9. Complete airway obstruction

  P. Total respiratory system compliance is increased by any factor that causes a loss of elastic lung tissue.

     1. Alveolar septal destruction

     2. Emphysema

  Q. Specific compliance is a method of comparing the compliance of individuals of different sizes or different lung units in the same individual.

     1. The formula for its determination takes into consideration the patient's measured FRC or local end-expiratory lung volume.

     2. Specific compliance (C_s) is equal to pulmonary compliance divided by the patient's FRC (or local end-expiratory lung volume) and normally is equal to approximately 0.08 (dimensionless number):

$$C_s = \frac{C_{pul}}{FRC} = 0.08 \qquad (3)$$

     3. Specific compliance can be determined for a lung segment or lobe (Figure 5-9).

VIII. Airway Resistance

  A. Airway resistance results from the movement of molecules of inspired gas over the surface of the airway.

  B. Airway resistance accounts for approximately 85% of nonelastic resistance to ventilation.

  C. Airway resistance (R) in laminar flow situations is equal to:

$$R = \frac{P}{\dot{V}} \qquad (4)$$

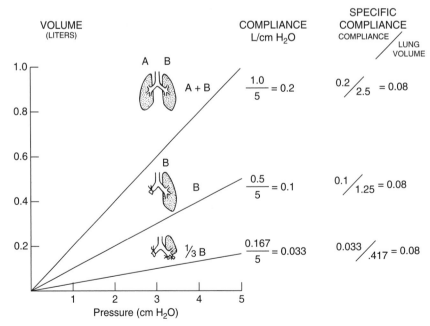

FIG. 5-9 Compliance and specific compliance for both lungs, one lung, and one lobe. Compliance decreases with decreasing lung volume; specific compliance does not.

whereas in turbulent flow situations the relationship is:

$$R = \frac{P}{\dot{V}^2} \tag{5}$$

    D. More than 60% of normal airway resistance is a result of turbulent gas flow through the nose, pharynx, and larynx.

    E. Resistance to gas flow decreases as gas moves into smaller generations of the airway. Because the cross-sectional area of the respiratory tract increases dramatically with increasing generations, flow through any single airway becomes progressively smaller. The pressure necessary to maintain flow decreases as airways become smaller because of the large airway surface area.

    F. At the level of the respiratory bronchioles, flow is almost absent, and gas movement basically is a result of diffusion.

    G. Airway resistance is increased when the lumen of the airway is decreased. The airway lumen is primarily decreased as a result of:
        1. Bronchospasm
        2. Mucosal edema
        3. Partial airway obstruction (e.g., retained secretions, foreign bodies, and tumors)

    H. Normal airway resistance is equal to approximately 0.6 to 2.4 cm H_2O/L/sec when measured at a standard flow rate of 0.5 L/sec.

IX. **Tissue Viscous Resistance**

    A. The force necessary to overcome the inertia of the nonelastic structures of the lung-thorax system (i.e., bone, pleurae sliding over each other).

    B. Tissue viscous resistance accounts for approximately 15% of the nonelastic resistance to ventilation.

X. **Equation of Motion**

    A. The equation of motion is used to describe the interactions between the ventilator, respiratory muscles, and the patient:

$$P_T = P_E + P_R \tag{6}$$

where P_T is the pressure required to deliver a volume of gas into the lung, P_E is the pressure needed to overcome elastic resistance, and P_R is the pressure needed to overcome nonelastic resistance.

    B. The elastic resistance of the respiratory system is determined by compliance (C) and tidal volume (V_T), and the nonelastic resistance is determined by flow ($\dot{V}$) and airway resistance (R).

$$P_E = \frac{V_T}{C} \tag{7}$$

$$P_R = \dot{V} \times R \tag{8}$$

    C. As a result the equation of motion is normally written as:

$$P_T = \frac{V_T}{C} + \dot{V} \times R \tag{9}$$

    D. The equation of motion states that tidal volume, compliance, flow, and airway resistance determine the pressure required to deliver a breath.

    E. The pressure required to deliver a breath is a result of the combined pressure applied to the proximal airway (P airway) and the pressure generated by the respiratory muscles (P muscle):

$$P_T = P \text{ airway} + P \text{ muscle} \tag{10}$$

F. Thus, during spontaneous breathing all of the pressure needed to deliver a breath is provided by the respiratory muscles (P muscle); during assisted ventilation the pressure needed to deliver a breath is provided by a combination of the respiratory muscles (P muscle) and the ventilator (P airway); and during controlled ventilation all of the pressure needed to deliver a breath is provided by the ventilator (P airway).

G. During volume ventilation, because flow and volume delivery from the ventilator are fixed, patient effort causes the airway pressure to decrease.

H. During pressure ventilation, because airway pressure is fixed, patient effort causes the tidal volume to increase.

XI. **Functional Residual Capacity**

A. As stated previously, the thorax tends to expand, whereas the lung tends to collapse. At the FRC level, the vector forces of pulmonary and thoracic elastance are equal in magnitude and opposite in direction.

B. The FRC is the most stable of all lung volumes and capacities because it is the level that is assumed when complete relaxation of ventilatory muscles occurs.

C. If the elastance of the thorax and/or the lung were to increase or decrease, the volume of FRC would be altered.

XII. **Ventilation/Perfusion Relationships**

A. Distribution of ventilation is unequal because of:

1. Respiratory time constants:

a. If the compliance of the lung or part of the lung is multiplied by resistance of that part of the lung, a time constant is determined:

$$\text{Compliance} \times \text{Resistance} = \text{Time constant} \qquad (11)$$

b. The time constant of a lung unit determines the amount of time it takes for the lung to fill or empty.

c. In healthy adults the respiratory time constant is approximately 0.25 second.

d. Approximately 3.5 to 4 time constants are required for inhalation or passive exhalation to be complete (Figure 5-10).

e. In the first time constant 63% of volume is delivered or exhaled.

f. In the second time constant 86.5% of volume is delivered or exhaled.

g. In the third time constant 95% of volume is delivered or exhaled.

h. In the fourth time constant 98.2% of volume is delivered or exhaled.

i. In the fifth time constant 99.3% of the volume is delivered or exhaled.

2. Regional variation in transpulmonary pressure in the respiratory tract:

a. In the standing position, the transpulmonary pressure gradient is greater in the apices than in the bases. As a result time constants are longer in the apices and shorter in the bases. The reasons for this variation are:

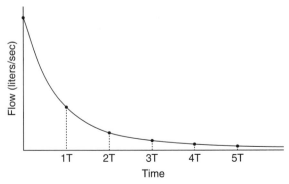

FIG. 5-10 The exponential decay curve of passive exhalation indicating the relationship to the number of respiratory time constants: 3.5 to 4 time constants necessary for complete passive exhalation to occur.

      (1)   The weight of the lung.

      (2)   The effect of gravity on the total system, forcing blood flow to dependent areas.

      (3)   Support of lung at the hilum.

  b. The transpulmonary pressure differences cause alveoli in the apices to contain a greater volume at FRC than alveoli in the bases.

  c. Increases in the respiratory time constant increase the likelihood of air trapping and auto-positive end-expiratory pressure.

  d. An increase in compliance or an increase in airway resistance increases the respiratory time constant.

  e. Local time constants vary throughout the lung based on actual position.

  f. These differences in alveolar size decrease as lung volume nears TLC.

3. As a result of differing transpulmonary pressure gradients and pulmonary time constants, when one inspires from FRC level:

  a. Alveoli in the apices fill slowly and empty slowly (slow alveoli).

  b. Alveoli in the bases fill rapidly and empty rapidly (fast alveoli).

  c. In normal tidal exchange most of the ventilation goes to the bases. Figure 5-11 illustrates the compliance curve of the total respiratory system. The position of the apices on the curve during tidal breathing is on the flatter aspect of the curve, whereas the bases are positioned on the steeper aspect of the curve. Points B to B′ indicate the volume change during normal ventilation in the bases; points A to A′ indicate the volume change during normal ventilation of the apices. There is a considerably larger volume change in the bases than in the apices per unit pressure change.

B. Distribution of pulmonary blood flow normally is greater in the bases than in the apices.

1. Perfusion of any aspect of the lung depends on a number of factors, the relationship between local pulmonary hydrostatic pressure and the local transpulmonary pressure gradient, oxygenation-induced vasoconstriction, and local hormone levels.

2. Because the pulmonary vascular system is a low-pressure system, when standing the apices of the lung receive virtually no blood flow, whereas the bases are engorged with blood because of the effect of gravity.

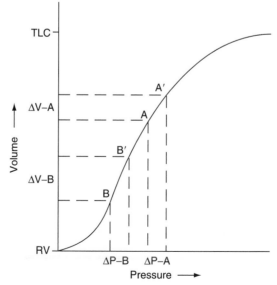

FIG. 5-11 Compliance curve of total lung at functional residual capacity. A to A′ indicates volume change in the apices during tidal exchange; B to B′ indicates volume change in the bases during tidal exchange. The change in volume of B (ΔV-B) is greater than the change in volume of A (ΔV-A) for the same pressure change (ΔP-B is equal to ΔP-A).

3. In general, the most gravity-dependent aspect of the lung receives the majority of the blood flow, whereas the least gravity-dependent areas receive little or no blood flow, although this difference is greatly reduced in the prone position.
4. Basically, in the upright lung, three zones exist (Figure 5-12):
   a. Zone 1: The extreme apex, where there is virtually no blood flow. Pulmonary vascular pressure is insufficient to overcome the effects of alveolar pressure compressing the blood vessels.
   b. Zone 2: The remainder of the apex and middle part of the lung, where blood flow is intermittent. Here blood flow depends on the relationship between pulmonary artery pressure and alveolar pressure. When pulmonary artery pressure exceeds alveolar pressure, blood flow is present.
   c. Zone 3: The bases, where blood flow is constant. Here blood flow is based on the difference between pulmonary artery and pulmonary venous pressures. A pulmonary artery catheter should always be placed in a Zone 3 blood vessel.
C. Ventilation/perfusion ratios ($\dot{V}/\dot{Q}$ ratios).
   1. The overall $\dot{V}/\dot{Q}$ ratio for the lung is 0.8.
   2. In the apices the $\dot{V}/\dot{Q}$ ratio is approximately 3.3; in the bases it is approximately 0.6.
   3. During normal ventilation and perfusion:
      a. The bases are better perfused than the apices.
      b. The bases are better ventilated than the apices.
      c. The apices are better ventilated than perfused.
      d. The bases are better perfused than ventilated.
D. Impact of position on gas exchange.
   1. In healthy patients gas exchange is essentially unaffected by position.
   2. In patients with ARDS in whom atelectasis and consolidation are common in the dependent lung when supine, positioning prone can be important.
   3. Oxygenation is generally improved in the prone position in those with ARDS because the $\dot{V}/\dot{Q}$ ratios throughout the lung are less varied.
   4. The distribution of ventilation and perfusion is not based solely on gravity (see Chapter 45).

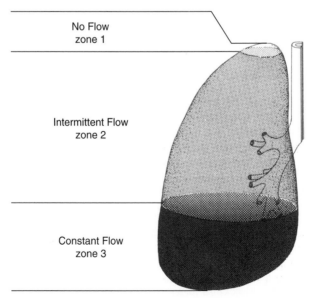

No Flow
zone 1

Intermittent Flow
zone 2

Constant Flow
zone 3

FIG. 5-12 The three-zone pulmonary blood flow model illustrating the effects of gravity on pulmonary perfusion (see text).

XIII. **Ideal Alveolar Gas Equation**
   A. In addition to the effects of P_{H_2O} on the partial pressure of gases in the alveoli, the carbon dioxide diffusing from the bloodstream into the alveoli further decreases alveolar P_{O_2}.
   B. Because carbon dioxide is leaving the bloodstream, a closed system, and entering the respiratory tract, an open system, there is an indirect relationship between the alveolar pressures of carbon dioxide and oxygen. Increases in alveolar P_{CO_2} result in decreases in alveolar P_{O_2}.
   C. This indirect relationship basically involves only carbon dioxide and oxygen because they are the only metabolically active gases.
   D. In addition, the amount of oxygen and carbon dioxide moving across the alveolar capillary membrane is unequal, 200 ml of carbon dioxide being produced for every 250 ml of oxygen consumed. Thus, the respiratory exchange ratio (R) CO_2 produced divided by O_2 consumed must be considered when estimating the alveolar P_{O_2}.
   E. The ideal alveolar gas equation is:

$$P_{AO_2} = (P_B - P_{H_2O})(F_IO_2) - (P_{aCO_2}) \left(F_IO_2 + \frac{1 - F_IO_2}{R} \right) \qquad (12)$$

   R normally equals 0.8. P_{aCO_2} is used instead of P_{ACO_2} because under physiologic conditions compatible with life they are equal, and P_{ACO_2} is impossible to determine clinically.
   F. A modification of equation (12) may be used for gross estimations of P_{AO_2}:

$$P_{AO_2} = (P_B - P_{H_2O})(F_IO_2) - \frac{P_{aCO_2}}{0.8} \qquad (13)$$

XIV. **Work of Breathing**
   A. Work associated with ventilation can be discussed from two perspectives:
      1. Total energy cost required for ventilatory work (cost of breathing).
      2. Mechanical performance of work.
   B. Metabolic cost of work of breathing:
      1. The normal oxygen cost of breathing is low, approximately 5% of total oxygen consumption (5 ml O_2/min or approximately 1 ml of O_2/L of ventilation).
      2. With mild to moderate increases in activity the oxygen cost of breathing is approximately 0.5 to 1.0 ml of O_2/L of increased ventilation.
      3. With marked increases in ventilation the oxygen cost of breathing can exceed 25% of total oxygen consumption and as a result limit overall activity.
      4. With cardiopulmonary disease baseline oxygen cost of breathing may be >10% to 15% of total oxygen consumption, significantly limiting any increase in overall activity.
      5. The more abnormal the airway resistance and compliance of the lung, the greater the increase in oxygen cost of breathing.
   C. Work (W) is defined as a force (F) applied to move an object a given distance (D):

$$W = F \times D \qquad (14)$$

   D. Thus, regardless of energy expenditure, no work is performed unless movement occurs.
   E. This relationship can be applied to the respiratory system because pressure (P) is a force per unit area and volume (V) represents a distance:

$$W = P \times V \qquad (15)$$

   F. Total mechanical work is equal to lung work plus chest wall work.
   G. Measurement of total mechanical work is illustrated in Figure 5-13.

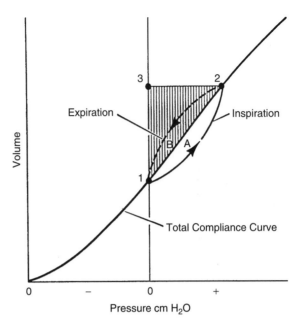

FIG. 5-13 Pressure-volume loop during tidal volume delivery via controlled positive pressure ventilation. The distance 1 to 3 equals tidal volume, and the distance 3 to 2 equals pressure change. Area A represents nonelastic inspiratory work; area B represents nonelastic expiratory work; and the shaded area represents elastic inspiratory work.

H. For measurement of total work, the lung-thorax system must be inflated with positive pressure in an apneic individual.
1. During inflation, pressure change in the airway or at the mouth is measured, as is V_T, and plotted against each other (see Figure 5-13).
2. Tidal ventilation is represented by the vertical distance 1 to 3, whereas pressure required to maintain thoracic expansion is represented by the horizontal distance 3 to 2.
3. The shaded triangle 1, 2, and 3 plus area A indicate the total mechanical work.
4. The shaded areas 1, 2, and 3 depict work required to overcome elastic forces.
5. Work required to overcome nonelastic forces is depicted by area A.
6. Work required to overcome inertial forces cannot be separated from elastic and nonelastic work by this method.
7. The elastic and nonelastic workloads are always additive.
8. Elastic work of inspiration is stored in the elastic structures of the thoracic cavity, whereas nonelastic work cannot be stored.
9. Nonelastic forces also are active only during gas movement.
10. Exhalation is normally passive as long as the work of exhalation does not exceed the stored elastic work. Area B is the nonelastic work required during passive exhalation. Exhalation will become active if the area of B exceeds the shaded areas 1, 2, and 3, which represent the elastic work stored during inspiration.

I. Figure 5-13 would also represent the work of the lung if the pressure gradient used were the transpulmonary pressure because the pleural pressure change represents the pressure required to move the lung.

J. Chest wall work (WOB_C) is not normally directly measured. It is usually calculated from lung work (WOB_L) and total mechanical work (WOB_T):

$$WOB_T = WOB_L + WOB_C \qquad (16)$$

K. During spontaneous unassisted breathing only lung work can be measured.

1. To measure lung work of breathing an esophageal balloon needs to be placed to reflect pleural pressure change.
2. Esophageal pressure is compared with atmospheric pressure to determine transpulmonary pressure change during normal tidal volume breathing.
3. Figure 5-13 also represents the methodology to determine spontaneous work of breathing of the lung.
   a. All that needs to be done is to reverse the signs on the pressure axis.
   b. To the right of zero the pressure would be negative, and to the left the pressure would be positive.
   c. During spontaneous inspiration esophageal pressure became more negative compared with baseline and tidal volume increases.
4. To measure total work of breathing and calculate chest wall work, the patient would have to be intubated, heavily sedated, and mechanically ventilated.

L. Pressure-time product
   1. Another approach to evaluate patient effort during spontaneous breathing or assisted ventilation is to determine the area of the esophageal pressure-time curve during inspiration.
   2. The larger the area the greater the effort.
   3. The value determined frequently is used to compare one set of circumstances (different levels of pressure support) with another set of circumstances.
   4. The pressure-time product is also used to evaluate the effort to trigger the ventilator during assisted ventilation. In this setting either airway pressure versus time or esophageal pressure versus time is evaluated.

M. The following are normal values for total lung and chest wall work in healthy individuals:

	Joules/L	kg × m/L
WOB_T	0.07-0.10	0.70-1.0
WOB_L	0.035-0.05	0.35-0.5
WOB_C	0.035-0.05	0.35-0.5

N. Workloads are also expressed for a 1-minute period. This is normally referred to as a representation of ventilatory power. If minute volume were equal to 6 L, the following values for power in kg × m/min and joules/min would be noted in normal adults:

	Joules/min	kg × m/min
Total ventilatory power	0.42-0.60	4.2-6.0
Lung power	0.21-0.30	2.1-3.0
Chest wall power	0.21-0.30	2.1-3.0

BIBLIOGRAPHY

Burton GC, Hodgkin JE, Ward JJ: *Respiratory Care,* ed 4. Philadelphia, JB Lippincott, 1997.

Cherniack RM, Cherniack L: *Respiration in Health and Disease,* ed 3. Philadelphia, WB Saunders, 1983.

Comroe JH: *Physiology of Respiration,* ed 2. Chicago, Year Book Medical Publishers, 1974.

Guyton AC, Hall JE: *Textbook of Medical Physiology,* ed 10. Philadelphia, WB Saunders, 2000.

Hess DJ, MacIntyre NR, Mishoe SC, Galvin WF, Adams AB, Saposnick AB: *Respiratory Care Principles and Practice.* Philadelphia, WB Saunders, 2002.

Kacmarek RM: The role of pressure support ventilation in reducing work of breathing. *Respir Care* 33: 99-120, 1988.

Kacmarek RM, Hess DJ, Stoller JK: *Monitoring in Respiratory Care.* St. Louis, Mosby–Year Book Publishers, 1993.

Murray JF: *The Normal Lung,* ed 2. Philadelphia, WB Saunders, 1987.

Pierson DJ, Kacmarek RM: *Foundations of Respiratory Care.* New York, Churchill Livingstone, 1992.

Roussos C: *The Thorax: Parts A and B,* ed 2. New York, Marcel Dekker, 1995.

Shapiro BA, Harrison RA, Kacmarek RM, et al: *Clinical Application of Respiratory Care,* ed 3. Chicago, Year Book Medical Publishers, 1985.

Wilkins RL, Stoller JK, Scanlan CL: *Egan's Fundamentals of Respiratory Therapy,* ed 8. St. Louis, CV Mosby, 2003.

Chapter **6**

Neurologic Control of Ventilation

I. The following areas located throughout the body each play a specific role in the neurologic control of ventilation. Two general regulatory mechanisms exist: automatic or involuntary control and voluntary or conscious control.
   A. Medulla oblongata
   B. Pons
   C. Peripheral chemoreceptors
   D. Central chemoreceptors
   E. Spinal cord
   F. Upper airway reflexes
   G. Vagus (cranial X) nerve
   H. Glossopharyngeal (cranial IX) nerve
   I. Cerebral cortex

II. Medulla Oblongata
   A. Located within the medulla oblongata is the respiratory control center, which receives afferent impulses from all other areas in the body (Figure 6-1).
   B. Afferent impulses are interpreted, and efferent impulses are initiated in the medulla oblongata.
   C. The medullary respiratory center maintains the normal rhythmic pattern of ventilation.
   D. The medullary respiratory center is located in the brain stem along with the pons and connects the midbrain and cerebellum with the spinal cord.
   E. Two fairly distinct areas in the medulla contain respiratory neurons (Figure 6-2).
      1. The dorsal respiratory group is located in two elongated bundles of neurons along the lateral walls of the medulla referred to as the nucleus tractus solitarius (NTS).
         a. Functions as initial processing centers of afferent impulses.
         b. Origin of inspiratory efferent impulses, which travel to ventral respiratory group neurons and spinal cord.
         c. The basic rhythm of respiration is generated by the dorsal respiratory group of neurons. Rhythmic ventilatory impulses are generated even when all peripheral nerves entering the medulla have been severed.
         d. Inspiration is normally (except during stressed breathing) a ramp signal, increasing steadily in force for approximately 2 seconds.
         e. Inspiration then ceases for approximately 3 seconds.
         f. The ramp signal is controlled in two ways:
            (1) The rate of increase in the ramp.
            (2) The length of the ramp signal.
         g. If the ramp signal ceases early the length of expiration is also decreased.
         h. As a result, the dorsal respiratory group is the primary controller of the depth and rate of inspiration.

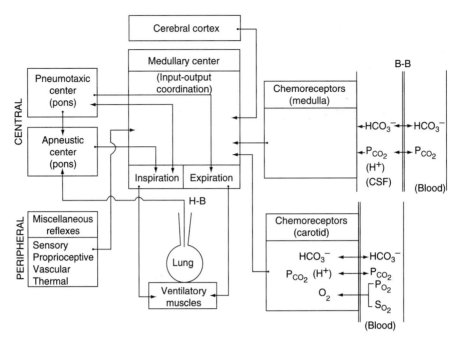

FIG. 6-1 Interrelationships among all areas responsible for ventilatory control (see text).

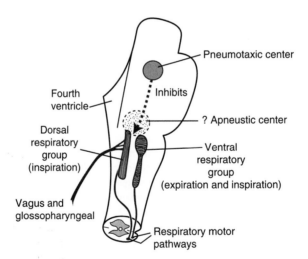

FIG. 6-2 Regions of the central nervous system where primary involuntary control of ventilation is coordinated.

2. The ventral respiratory group is located approximately 5 mm anterior and lateral to each dorsal respiratory group. These neurons are located in the nucleus ambiguus anteriorly and the nucleus retroambiguus caudally.
   a. Functions primarily by sending efferent impulses to all expiratory motor neurons during stressed ventilation.
   b. They are inactive during normal quiet breathing.
   c. Inspiratory efferent impulses are sent during stressed breathing.
   d. Important during exercise.
F. Areas from which afferent impulses are sent to the medulla oblongata:
   1. Cerebral cortex
   2. Pons
   3. Upper airway reflexes

    4. Vagus (cranial X) nerve
    5. Peripheral chemoreceptors
    6. Central chemoreceptors

III. Pons
  A. Two distinct centers in the pons contain afferent respiratory neurons.
    1. The pneumotaxic center is located dorsally in the nucleus parabrachialis of the upper pons (see Figure 6-2).
      a. Afferent impulses from the pneumotaxic center "fine tune" ventilatory rhythmicity by inhibiting length of inspiration.
      b. Maximum stimulation in adults can limit inspiration to 0.5 seconds, increasing rate to ≥40 breaths/min.
      c. A weak signal reduces respiratory rate to only 3 to 5 breaths/min.
      d. If the pneumotaxic center is destroyed, apneustic breathing (long, sustained inspirations) occurs.
    2. Apneustic center: Only *weak evidence* of its existence is available (see Figure 6-2).
      a. Located in the lower pons.
      b. Afferent impulses from the apneustic center cause a sustained inspiratory pattern with only short expiratory times; apneustic breathing.
      c. How and when these neurons are activated is unclear; the vagus nerve must be impaired for this center to be active.
      d. If the apneustic and pneumotaxic centers are destroyed, a rapid, irregular, gasping respiratory pattern develops.

VI. Spinal Cord
  A. Axons from the higher brain centers descend into the spinal cord.
  B. These projecting axons influence phrenic intercostal and abdominal motoneuron transmission.
  C. Thus ventilatory skeletal muscle is stimulated.
  D. Skeletal muscle is composed of two types of contractile fibers:
    1. Extrafusal fibers (main muscle): Contraction of these fibers is responsible for actual muscular contraction.
    2. Fusimotor fibers (muscle spindle fibers): These fibers are organs of proprioception that determine the extent of muscle contraction necessary to perform a certain workload.
  E. Ventilatory reflexes, such as cough and hiccup, are mediated by the spinal cord.
  F. Ascending spinal pathways transmit sensations of pain, touch, temperature, and proprioception to higher brain centers.

V. Upper Airway Reflexes
  A. Nose
    1. Stimulation of nasal mucosa may cause exhalation.
    2. Stimulated exhalation is frequently in the form of a sneeze.
    3. Apnea and bradycardia also may result from nasal stimulation.
  B. Nasopharynx
    1. Stimulation may cause the sniff or aspiration reflex.
    2. A rapid inspiration is initiated to move the irritant from the nasopharynx to the oropharynx.
    3. Stimulation may also cause bronchodilation and hypertension.
  C. Larynx
    1. Stimulation may result in afferent impulses, causing:
      a. Apnea
      b. Slow, deep breathing
      c. Coughing
      d. Hypertension
      e. Bronchoconstriction

- D. Trachea
  1. Stimulation may result in afferent impulses, causing:
     a. Coughing
     b. Bronchoconstriction
     c. Hypertension

VI. Vagus Nerve

- A. Afferent impulses via the vagus nerve originate from two areas:
  1. Baroreceptors
     a. Located in the aortic arch.
     b. Stimulated by variation in blood pressure.
     c. Afferent impulses from baroreceptors cause alteration of vascular tone to maintain normal blood pressure levels.
     d. Ventilatory response is minimal.
        (1) Hyperventilation may be caused by hypotension.
        (2) Hypoventilation may be caused by hypertension.
  2. Pulmonary reflexes
     a. Pulmonary stretch receptors (Hering-Breuer reflex)
        (1) Pulmonary stretch receptors are located in the smooth muscle of conducting airways.
        (2) Lung inflation and increased transpulmonary pressures stimulate these receptors.
        (3) They are slowly adaptive to changes in inflating pressure but do not appear to be active in humans until tidal volume exceeds 1.5 L.
        (4) Stimulation of these receptors may cause:
            (a) Increased inspiratory time
            (b) Increased respiratory rate
            (c) Bronchodilation
            (d) Tachycardia
            (e) Vasoconstriction
        (5) Integration of information from these receptors assists in determining the rate and depth of breathing.
     b. Deflation reflex
        (1) Lung collapse stimulates an increased force and frequency of inspiratory effort.
        (2) Mediated by the vagus nerve, but the specific receptors involved are unknown.
        (3) May be responsible for the hyperpnea of pneumothorax.
     c. Irritant receptors
        (1) Irritant receptors are located in the epithelium of the trachea, bronchi, larynx, nose, and pharynx.
        (2) They are rapidly adaptive.
        (3) Stimulation is caused by:
            (a) Inspired irritants (e.g., histamine and ammonia)
            (b) Mechanical factors (e.g., particulate matter)
            (c) Anaphylaxis
            (d) Pneumothorax
            (e) Pulmonary congestion
        (4) Stimulation may result in:
            (a) Bronchoconstriction
            (b) Hyperpnea
            (c) Constriction of larynx (e.g., laryngospasm)
            (d) Closure of glottis
            (e) Cough
     d. Type J (juxtapulmonary-capillary) receptors
        (1) Located in the walls of pulmonary capillaries

       (2) Stimulation is caused by:
          (a) Increased interstitial fluid volume
          (b) Pulmonary congestion
          (c) Chemical irritants
          (d) Microembolism
       (3) Stimulation of these receptors may result in:
          (a) Rapid, shallow breathing
          (b) Severe expiratory constriction of larynx
          (c) Hypoventilation and bradycardia
          (d) Inhibition of spinal reflexes

VII. **Glossopharyngeal Nerve**
    A. Innervates the peripheral chemoreceptor cells located in the carotid bodies.
    B. Conducts afferent impulses to the medullary respiratory center.

VIII. **Peripheral Chemoreceptors (Figure 6-3)**
    A. Chemoreceptor cells can differentiate between concentrations or pressures of various substances.
    B. Two primary groups of peripheral chemoreceptor cells have been identified.
       1. Carotid bodies
          a. Located at the bifurcation of the common carotid artery.
          b. Innervated by the glossopharyngeal (cranial IX) nerve.
          c. Stimulated by:
             (1) Decreased Pa_{O_2}
             (2) Decreased pH
             (3) Increased Pa_{CO_2}
       2. Aortic bodies
          a. Located in the arch of the aorta.
          b. Innervated by the vagus (crania X) nerve.
          c. Stimulated by:
             (1) Decreased Pa_{O_2}
             (2) Decreased pH
             (3) Increased Pa_{CO_2}
       3. Other less well-differentiated groups of cells are located in association with arteries in the thoracic and abdominal regions of the body.
    C. In general, a synergistic response from these receptors is noted in the presence of hypoxemia and acidosis.
    D. Effects of Pa_{O_2}
       1. Initial stimulation occurs at a Pa_{O_2} of 500 mm Hg and gradually increases as Pa_{O_2} decreases.
       2. Maximum stimulation occurs when Pa_{O_2} is between 40 and 60 mm Hg.
       3. A gradual decrease in stimulation is noted when Pa_{O_2} is <30 mm Hg.
       4. Additional sources of stimulation:
          a. Decreased blood flow
          b. Increased temperature
       5. These cells have a high blood flow for the size of tissue involved.
       6. They are primarily affected by oxygen delivery in the form of dissolved oxygen. Any pathophysiologic situation in which oxygen delivery is inadequate for the metabolic needs of these cells results in stimulation.
       7. Conditions having no stimulating effect:
          a. Carbon monoxide poisoning
          b. Anemia
    E. Effects of Pa_{CO_2} and H^+ concentrations
       1. The cell membrane is permeable to H^+ and Pa_{CO_2}.
       2. These cells are directly affected only by H^+ concentrations.

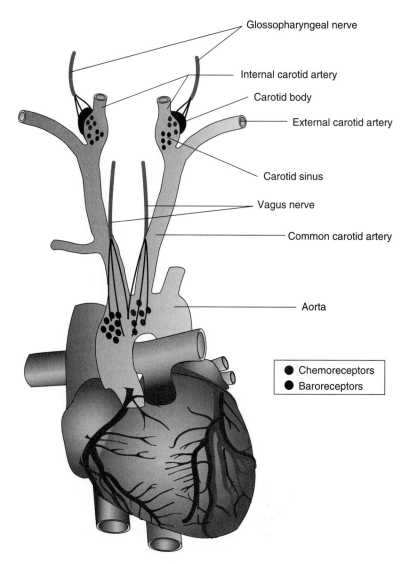

Glossopharyngeal nerve

Internal carotid artery

Carotid body

External carotid artery

Carotid sinus

Vagus nerve

Common carotid artery

Aorta

● Chemoreceptors
● Baroreceptors

FIG. 6-3 Location of the peripheral chemoreceptors at the bifurcation of the common carotid artery and in the wall of the arch of the aorta.

3. $Paco_2$ changes cause a change in H^+ concentration, which stimulates the receptor.
4. Thus, $Paco_2$ has an indirect effect on these cells.
5. Stimulation is primarily a result of an increase in H^+ concentration.
6. Decreases in H^+ concentration have only a minimal effect.
7. Stimulation of these receptors by an increase in $[H^+]$ causes:
   a. Increased respiratory rate
   b. Increased tidal volume
8. Stimulation of these receptors by a decrease in $[H^+]$ may cause:
   a. A slight decrease in respiratory rate
   b. A slight decrease in tidal volume
9. The magnitude of the response of the peripheral chemoreceptors to $[H^+]$ changes is less than that of the central chemoreceptors.
F. These receptors are adaptive over time.

IX. **Central Chemoreceptors (Figure 6-4)**
  A. Poorly defined groups of cells located near the ventrolateral surface of each side of the medulla oblongata.
  B. These cells are in contact with cerebral spinal fluid (CSF) and arterial blood.
  C. Actual stimulation is caused by $[H^+]$ of CSF.
  D. The composition of the CSF differs somewhat from that of blood.
    1. Electrolytes are similar in content to those in plasma.
    2. Protein content is low: 15 to 45 mg/100 ml
    3. P_{CO_2}: 50.2 ± 2.6 mm Hg
    4. pH: 7.336 ± 0.012
    5. HCO_3^-: 21.5 ± 1.2 mEq/L
  E. Diffusion across blood-brain barrier
    1. The only readily diffusible substanc across the blood-brain barrier is carbon dioxide.
    2. HCO_3^- and H^+ also move across the membrane but extremely slowly. Active transport mechanisms and diffusion are believed to be involved in the movement of these two substances.
  F. Mechanism of stimulation
    1. Changes in arterial P_{CO_2} alter diffusion of carbon dioxide across the blood-brain barrier, causing a change in P_{CO_2} of the CSF.
    2. The altered P_{CO_2} level effects a change in CSF $[H^+]$.
    3. The altered $[H^+]$ either stimulates or inhibits ventilation.
    4. Increased P_{CO_2} (increased H^+) stimulates ventilation, whereas decreased P_{CO_2} (decreased H^+) inhibits ventilation.
  G. Factors influencing CSF carbon dioxide levels:
    1. Cerebral blood flow
    2. CO_2 production
    3. CO_2 content of venous blood
    4. CO_2 content of arterial blood
    5. Alveolar ventilation

X. **Medullary Adjustments in Compensated Respiratory Acidosis**
  A. Acute increases in Pa_{CO_2} rapidly cause an increase in CSF P_{CO_2}. This occurs because the blood-CSF barrier is permeable to CO_2.
  B. The increased P_{CO_2} in the CSF causes the CSF pH to decrease, which stimulates the central chemoreceptors.

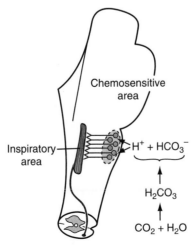

FIG. 6-4 Location of the central chemoreceptors in the medulla and the mechanism by which an increase in CO_2 causes stimulation.

C. If the body is unable to increase its level of ventilation, the elevated $Paco_2$ and CSF Pco_2 levels persist.

D. As a result, the kidney begins to retain HCO_3^-.

E. As the serum HCO_3^- level increases, active transport mechanisms and diffusion increase the CSF HCO_3^- level.

F. The CSF pH eventually returns to normal as the CSF HCO_3^- level increases.

G. When the CSF pH is returned to normal, the body responds to changes in $Paco_2$ at the newly elevated level.

H. Chronically elevated $Paco_2$ and CSF Pco_2 levels result in:
   1. Decreased central chemoreceptor drive to ventilate.
   2. Decreased sensitivity to carbon dioxide changes.

XI. **Medullary Adjustments in Compensated Respiratory Alkalosis**

A. Acute decreases in $Paco_2$ rapidly cause a decrease in CSF Pco_2.

B. This causes the CSF pH to increase, which inhibits the central chemoreceptors.

C. If the stimulus causing hyperventilation persists, the decreased $Paco_2$ and CSF Pco_2 levels also persist.

D. As a result, the kidney will begin to excrete more HCO_3^-.

E. As the serum HCO_3^- level decreases, active transport mechanisms and diffusion decrease the CSF HCO_3^- level.

F. The CSF pH eventually returns to normal as the CSF HCO_3^- decreases.

G. When the CSF pH is returned to normal, the body responds to changes in $Paco_2$ at the new decreased level.

XII. **Medullary Adjustments in Compensated Metabolic Acidosis**

A. Because H^+ does not readily cross the blood-brain barrier, decreases in plasma pH stimulate the peripheral chemoreceptors.

B. This is interpreted as an increase in $Paco_2$; thus, the peripheral chemoreceptors increase the level of ventilation, decreasing $Paco_2$.

C. The decreased $Paco_2$ decreases the CSF Pco_2, which increases the CSF pH, resulting in inhibition to ventilation via the central chemoreceptors.

D. As a result, the peripheral chemoreceptors stimulate ventilation, whereas the central chemoreceptors inhibit ventilation.

E. Because the effect on the peripheral chemoreceptors is the predominant stimulus, there is a stepwise readjustment (decrease) in CSF HCO_3^- levels. This allows normalization of CSF pH and a sustained increase in the drive to ventilate.

F. The maximum response of the respiratory system to a metabolic acidosis does not occur until the CSF pH is normalized.

XIII. **Medullary Adjustments in Compensated Metabolic Alkalosis**

A. Because neither H^+ nor HCO_3^- readily cross the blood-brain barrier and the peripheral chemoreceptors respond poorly to alkalosis, the respiratory system's response to a metabolic alkalosis is poor unless the alkalosis is significant.

B. A significant increase in plasma pH causes inhibition of the peripheral chemoreceptors, which inhibits ventilation, resulting in increased $Paco_2$.

C. The increased $Paco_2$ increases the CSF Pco_2, which stimulates ventilation via the central chemoreceptors.

D. As a result, the peripheral chemoreceptors inhibit ventilation, whereas the central chemoreceptors stimulate ventilation.

E. Because inhibition of the peripheral chemoreceptors is the predominant stimulus, there is a stepwise readjustment (increase) in the CSF HCO_3^-. This allows a normalization of the CSF pH and a sustained decrease in the drive to ventilate.

F. However, it is rare that the $Paco_2$ will increase above 50 mm Hg in an attempt to compensate unless the metabolic alkalosis is severe. Remember, if the $Paco_2$ increases, the alveolar Po_2 decreases, resulting in hypoxemia, which stimulates ventilation via the peripheral chemoreceptors.

XIV. **Voluntary Control of Ventilation**
    A. Most voluntary control of ventilation is initiated via the cerebral cortex.
       1. The cerebral cortex is responsible for ventilatory control during:
          a. Forceful inspiration
          b. Breath holding
          c. Forceful exhalation
          d. Speaking
          e. Laughing
          f. Swallowing
    B. The thalamus is involved in controlling breathing during emotional behavior:
       1. Fear
       2. Pain
       3. Anger
       4. Sorrow
       5. All intense emotions

XV. **Ventilatory Drive**
    A. The drive to breathe is affected by the numerous factors presented earlier. However, many individuals have varying responses to individual stimuli.
    B. In general, factors that stimulate ventilation include:
       1. Hypoxemia
       2. Hypercarbia
       3. Acidosis
       4. Fever
       5. Infection, sepsis
       6. Stimulation of type J receptors
       7. Pain (somatic)
       8. Fear, anxiety
       9. Pharmacologic stimulants
    C. Those factors depressing ventilation include:
       1. Hypocarbia
       2. Alkalosis
       3. Pain (visceral)
       4. Electrolyte imbalance
       5. Pharmacologic depressants
       6. Fatigue
       7. Mechanical inability of the thoracic cage

XVI. **Abnormal Breathing Patterns (Figures 6-5 and 6-6)**
    A. Normal breathing in adults at a rate of 10 to 20 breaths/min is referred to as *eupnea*.
    B. Rates >20 breaths/min are referred to as *tachypnea*.
    C. Rates <10 breaths/min are termed *bradypnea*.
    D. Tidal volumes greater than normal for an individual are termed *hyperpnea*.
    E. Tidal volumes smaller than normal for an individual are termed *hypopnea*.
    F. *Kussmaul breathing* is the rapid and deep breathing associated with a severe diabetic acidosis.
    G. *Cheyne-Stokes breathing* is a pattern of breathing associated with increasing and then decreasing tidal volumes, followed by a period of *apnea* (the absence of breathing). This pattern is associated with brain injury or severe cardiovascular disease.
    H. *Ataxic breathing* is a pattern of breathing with irregular tidal volumes and rates seen during respiratory muscle fatigue and impending respiratory failure.
    I. *Biot's breathing* is a highly irregular breathing pattern associated with periods of apnea; seen in individuals with severe brain stem injury unable to maintain control of breathing.
    J. *Apneustic breathing* is a pattern defined by long sustained inspirations and short expiratory times; seen when injury to the pons is present.

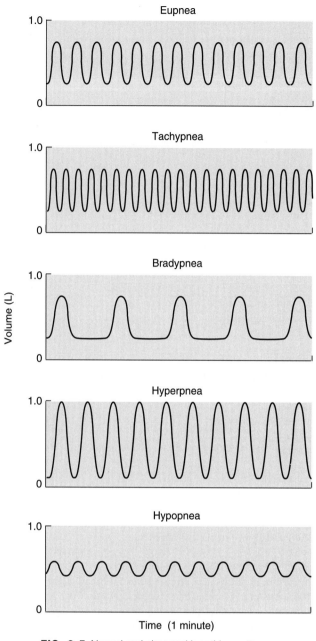

FIG. 6-5 Normal and abnormal breathing patterns.

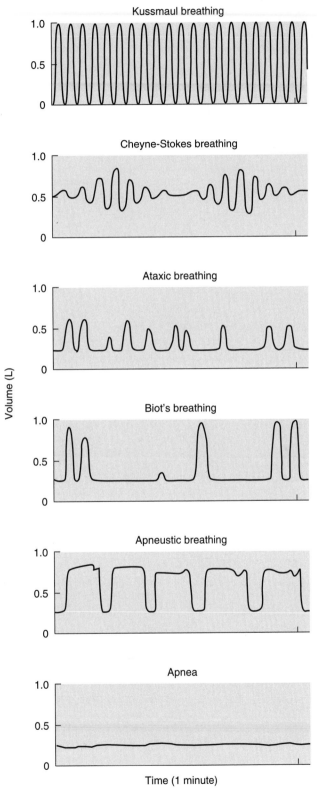

FIG. 6-6 Abnormal breathing patterns.

BIBLIOGRAPHY

Beachey W: *Respiratory Care Anatomy and Physiology: Foundations for Clinical Practice*. St. Louis, Mosby, 1998.

Burton GG, Hodgkin JE, Ward JJ: *Respiratory Care: A Guide to Clinical Practice,* ed 4. Philadelphia, JB Lippincott, 1997.

Comroe JH: *Physiology of Respiration,* ed 2. Chicago, Year Book Medical Publishers, 1974.

Fishman AP, Cherniack NS, Widdicombe JG: *Handbook of Physiology, The Respiratory System,* ed 2, vol II, parts 1 and 2. Baltimore, Williams & Wilkins, 1986.

Guyton AC, Hall JE: *Textbook of Medical Physiology,* ed 10. Philadelphia, WB Saunders, 2000.

Hicks GH: *Cardiopulmonary Anatomy and Physiology.* New York, WB Saunders, 2000.

Murray JF: *The Normal Lung,* ed 2. Philadelphia, WB Saunders, 1987.

Nunn JF: *Applied Respiratory Physiology,* ed 2. Stoneham, MA, Butterworth, 1977.

West JB: *Respiratory Physiology: The Essentials,* ed 2. Baltimore, Williams & Wilkins, 1979.

Wilkins RL, Stoller JK, Scanlon CL: *Egan's Fundamentals of Respiratory Care,* ed 8. St. Louis, Mosby, 2003.

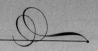
Oxygen and Carbon Dioxide Transport

I. **Oxygen Cascade**
   A. The partial pressure of oxygen (PO_2) decreases from 159.6 mm Hg in dry air at sea level to approximately 3 to 23 mm Hg in the mitochondria of the cell (Table 7-1).
   B. Four body systems are responsible for the movement of oxygen from the atmosphere to the mitochondria:
      1. Lungs
      2. Blood
      3. Circulation
      4. Body tissue
   C. Specifics regarding movement of oxygen from the atmosphere into the blood are detailed in Chapter 2.

II. **Role of Oxygen in the Cell**
   A. Approximately 90% of the oxygen consumed is used as the final electron acceptor of the electron transport chain in the mitochondria of the cell.
   B. The actual reaction produces H_2O:

$$\tfrac{1}{2} O_2 + 2 H^+ \rightarrow H_2O \tag{1}$$

   C. Without the presence of O_2, aerobic metabolism is stopped, whereas anaerobic metabolism continues, resulting in the production of lactic acid.
   D. The reaction of O_2 with H^+ to form H_2O allows the formation of the high-energy phosphate group adenosine triphosphate (ATP).
   E. The yield of ATP molecules from aerobic metabolism significantly exceeds that from anaerobic metabolism:

Aerobic Metabolism	Anaerobic Metabolism
Glucose	Glucose
↓	↓
Pyruvic acid	Pyruvic acid
↓	↓
$CO_2 + H_2O + 38$ moles of ATP	Lactic acid + 2 moles of ATP

   F. Mitochondrial PO_2 values of <2 mm Hg inhibit aerobic metabolism.

TABLE **7-1**

The Oxygen Cascade

Location	Partial Pressure (mm Hg)	Reason for Change
Dry atmospheric air	159.6	
Conducting airways	149.6	Addition of H_2O vapor
End-expiratory gas	114	Mixing of dead-space gas with alveolar gas
Ideal alveolar gas	101	Addition of CO_2
Arterial blood	97	Intrapulmonary shunting
Mean systemic capillary	40	O_2 diffusion into cell
Cellular cytoplasm	<40	O_2 diffusion into mitochondria
Mitochondria	3-23	Metabolic rate

III. **Carriage of Oxygen in the Blood**
   A. Oxygen is carried in two distinct compartments in the blood:
      1. Physically dissolved in plasma
      2. Chemically attached to hemoglobin molecules
   B. Volume physically dissolved in plasma
      1. According to the Bunsen solubility coefficient for oxygen, 0.023 ml of oxygen can be dissolved in 1 ml of plasma for every 760 mm Hg P_{O_2}.
      2. Simplifying the above factor to the number of milliliters of oxygen per milliliter of plasma per mm Hg P_{O_2} equals:

$$0.023 \text{ ml } O_2/760 \text{ mm Hg} = 0.00003 \text{ ml } O_2/1 \text{ ml plasma/mm Hg } P_{O_2} \qquad (2)$$

      3. Because the oxygen content normally is expressed in volumes percent, multiplying 0.00003 ml of oxygen per milliliter of plasma by 100 results in the common factor expressing the quantity of O_2 dissolved in plasma:

$$(0.00003 \text{ ml } O_2/\text{ml of plasma})(100)/1 \text{ mm Hg } P_{O_2}$$
$$= 0.003 \text{ ml } O_2/100 \text{ ml plasma/1 mm Hg } P_{O_2} \qquad (3)$$

      4. Thus, multiplying the P_{O_2} of blood by 0.003 will yield the number of milliliters of oxygen physically dissolved in every 100 ml of blood (vol%):

$$(P_{O_2})(0.003) = \text{ml of oxygen physically dissolved} \qquad (4)$$

   C. Hemoglobin: Structure and capacity to react with various substances:
      1. Composition of the normal hemoglobin molecule:
         a. Four porphyrin rings, called *hemes*, each with a central iron atom (Figure 7-1).
         b. Four polypeptide chains: two α chains and two β chains, called the *globin portion* of the molecule.
         c. Each chain is twisted and folded into a basket in which a heme is located.
         d. Each iron atom of the heme is bonded via four covalent bonds to the porphyrin ring and via one covalent bond to the globin portion of the molecule. One bond is available to combine with oxygen (Figure 7-2).
         e. The four chains are held together by chemical bonds between unlike chains (e.g., α to β and β to α).
         f. The hemoglobin molecule undergoes structural changes when it reacts with oxygen.
         g. The total molecule contracts when it combines with oxygen and expands when oxygen is released.
         h. The site of carbon dioxide attachment is the amino group (R-NH_2) on the porphyrin rings (R represents the rest of the molecule).

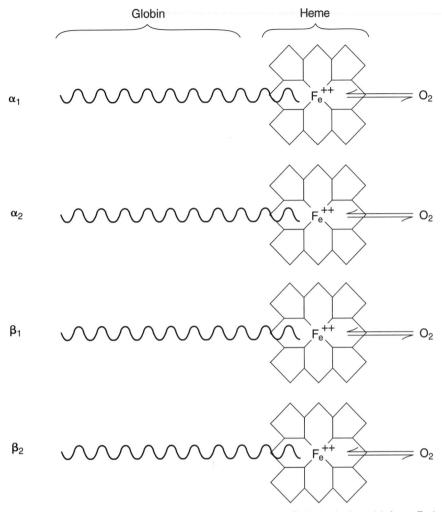

FIG. 7-1 Hemoglobin molecule comprises four polypeptide (2α and 2β) chains in the adult form. Each chain is attached to a porphyrin ring containing an iron ion in the ferrous state (Fe^{++}). O_2, Oxygen.

  i. The terminal imidazole (R-NH) groups also are available to buffer H^+ (see Chapter 15).
   (1) The importance of hemoglobin as a buffer is second only to that of the HCO_3^-/H_2CO_3 buffer system.
   (2) The buffering capacity of the hemoglobin molecule depends on attachment of oxygen to the iron portion of the heme.
   (3) Oxygenated hemoglobin (oxyhemoglobin) is a stronger acid but weaker buffer than unoxygenated hemoglobin (deoxyhemoglobin).
   (4) Thus the buffering capacity of venous blood is greater than that of arterial blood.
 2. The molecular weight of hemoglobin is approximately 64,500 g.
 3. Because oxygen attaches to each of the four iron atoms in the hemoglobin molecule, 4 gram molecular weights (GMWs) or 4 moles of oxygen combine with 64,500 g of hemoglobin (1 mole).

$$\frac{64,500 \text{ g of Hb}}{4 \text{ moles of } O_2} = 16,125 \text{ g of Hb/mole of } O_2 \qquad (5)$$

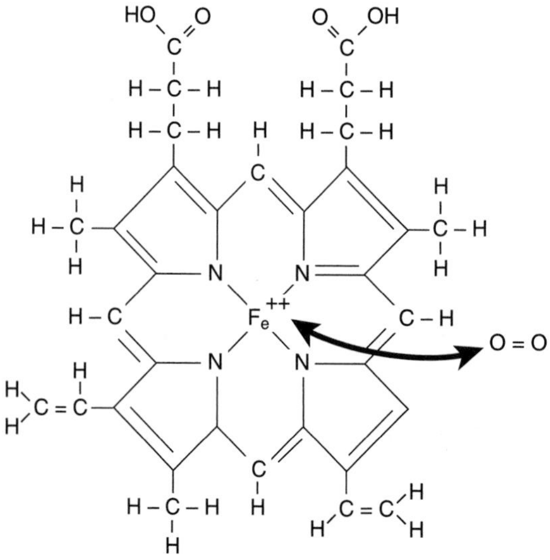

FIG. 7-2 Iron ion of the porphyrin ring is the loose binding site of oxygen.

4. One mole of oxygen can combine maximally with 16,126 g of hemoglobin.
5. Because 1 GMW of oxygen at standard temperature and pressure occupies 22.4 L:

$$\frac{22,400 \text{ ml of O}_2}{16,125 \text{ g of Hb}} = 1.34 \text{ ml of O}_2/\text{g of Hb} \qquad (6)$$

6. Thus at 100% saturation, 1.34 ml of oxygen can combine with each gram of hemoglobin.
7. The actual volume of oxygen carried attached to hemoglobin is equal to:

(Hb content)(1.34)(HbO$_2$% sat.) = vol% of O$_2$ carried attached to Hb   (7)

8. As hemoglobin combines with oxygen to form HbO$_2$, the complex takes on a negative charge, and as a result it forms a salt with K$^+$, or KHbO$_2$.
9. When O$_2$ is released at the tissue level, the K$^+$ is also released, and the Hb buffers H$^+$, forming HHb (reduced hemoglobin).
D. Oxygen content
   1. The total oxygen content of blood is equal to the volume of oxygen physically dissolved in plasma plus the amount chemically combined with hemoglobin (Figure 7-3).
   2. Mathematically this statement is equal to:

O$_2$ content in vol% = (Po$_2$)(0.003) + (Hb content)(1.34)(HbO$_2$% sat.)   (8)

E. Table 7-2 illustrates the effects of Po$_2$, Hb, and Sao$_2$ on oxygen content.
F. Oxyhemoglobin dissociation curve (Figure 7-4)
   1. The overall sigmoidal shape of the curve is a result of the varied affinities of the four oxygen-bonding sites on the hemoglobin molecule.
      a. The affinity of the last site bound generally is considerably less than the other three sites.
      b. The affinity of the first site also is less than that of the second or third sites.

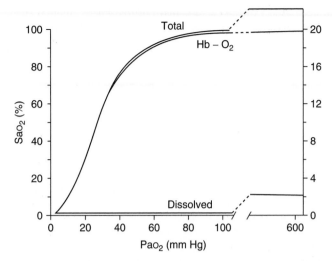

FIG. 7-3 The oxyhemoglobin dissociation curve showing the contribution of chemically bound and dissolved O_2 to the total O_2 content. Note that most of the O_2 by far is O_2 chemically bound to hemoglobin.

TABLE **7-2**

Effect of Po_2, Hb, and Sao_2 on Oxygen Content (Cao_2) *

Po₂ (mm Hg)	Hb (g%)	Sao₂ (%)	Cao₂ (vol%)
100	15	98	20.0
75	15	94	19.3
50	15	84	17.0
100	10	98	13.4
100	5	98	6.9

*A decrease in Hb has a greater effect on O_2 content than a decrease in Po_2.
From Pierson DJ, Kacmarek RM: *Foundations of Respiratory Care*, Churchill Livingstone, New York, 1992.

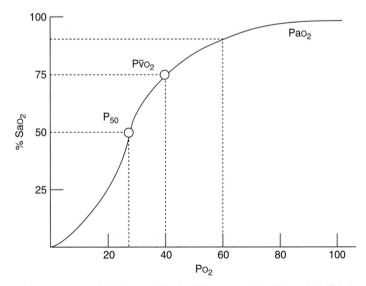

FIG. 7-4 The partial pressure at which hemoglobin is 50% saturated is 27 mm Hg. This is referred to as P_{50}. Normal venous Po_2 of 40 mm Hg and 75% oxyhemoglobin saturation are also indicated. A Po_2 of 60 mm Hg results in 90% saturation of the hemoglobin, whereas the normal arterial Po_2 of 97 mm Hg results in 97% saturation of the hemoglobin.

2. The steep aspect of the curve is that portion where minimal changes in P_{O_2} normally result in large increases in $HbO_2\%$ saturation and therefore oxygen content.
   a. Increasing the saturation from 50% to 75% normally necessitates only a 13-mm Hg P_{O_2} increase, whereas increasing the saturation from 75% to 100% normally necessitates well over a 100-mm Hg P_{O_2} increase.
3. P_{50} is defined as that P_{O_2} at which the hemoglobin is 50% saturated with oxygen. Normally the P_{50} is equal to 27 mm Hg (see Figure 7-4).
   a. An increased P_{50} indicates a shift of the oxyhemoglobin dissociation curve to the right, resulting in a decreased hemoglobin affinity for oxygen (greater unloading of oxygen at the tissue and decreased loading at the alveoli).
   b. A decreased P_{50} indicates a shift of the oxyhemoglobin dissociation curve to the left, resulting in an increased hemoglobin affinity for oxygen (decreased unloading of oxygen at the tissue and increased loading at the alveoli).
   c. Hemoglobin is considered an allosteric enzyme because of the two conformational structures it assumes (deoxyhemoglobin and oxyhemoglobin). Allosteric enzymes are substances with two binding sites: one active site and one secondary site. The binding of substances at the secondary site can affect the affinity of binding at the active site.
   d. Box 7-1 lists factors that alter the affinity of hemoglobin for oxygen by affecting the secondary site.
4. Various substances affect the shape of the oxyhemoglobin dissociation curve. Shifting the position of the curve alters the binding capabilities of hemoglobin. A shift to the right decreases the affinity of hemoglobin for oxygen, whereas a shift to the left increases affinity of hemoglobin for oxygen.

G. *Bohr effect*: The effect of carbon dioxide or $[H^+]$ on uptake and release of oxygen from the hemoglobin molecule. The effect is relatively mild.
   1. As seen earlier, carbon dioxide and $[H^+]$ cause a shift in the oxyhemoglobin dissociation curve.
   2. At the systemic capillary bed, increased carbon dioxide and $[H^+]$ moving into the blood decrease hemoglobin affinity for oxygen and increase the volume of oxygen released at the tissue level.
   3. At the pulmonary capillary bed, decreased carbon dioxide and $[H^+]$ levels increase hemoglobin affinity for oxygen, thus increasing the volume of oxygen picked up at the pulmonary level.

H. Carbon monoxide
   1. Carbon monoxide attaches to hemoglobin at the same site as O_2.
   2. The affinity of hemoglobin for carbon monoxide is 200 times greater than its affinity for O_2.
   3. In addition, carboxyhemoglobin (HbCO) shifts the oxyhemoglobin dissociation curve to the left, decreasing the ability of hemoglobin to unload oxygen.

I. Abnormal hemoglobins
   1. There are >100 abnormal forms of hemoglobins.
   2. Twelve of these have an effect on the affinity of hemoglobin for oxygen. However, the two most important are fetal hemoglobin and methemoglobin.

BOX 7-1

Factors Affecting Hb Affinity for O_2

Increased Affinity (shifted to left)	**Decreased Affinity (shifted to right)**
Decreased P_{CO_2}	Increased P_{CO_2}
Decreased $[H^+]$ or increased pH	Increased $[H^+]$ or decreased pH
Decreased temperature	Increased temperature
Decreased 2,3-DPG	Increased 2,3-DPG
Carboxyhemoglobin	
Fetal hemoglobin	
Methemoglobin	

3. Fetal hemoglobin has two γ chains instead of β chains, which results in a decreased P_{50} (shift to the left).
4. Fe atoms oxidized from the ferrous to the ferric state form methemoglobin; this also results in a decreased P_{50} (shift to the left).

J. An increased affinity of Hb for O_2 means that the hemoglobin carries more O_2, but the hemoglobin *does not* readily release O_2 at the tissue level. Conversely, a decreased affinity of Hb for O_2 means that the hemoglobin carries less O_2, but the hemoglobin *does* readily release O_2 at the tissue level.

IV. **Oxygen Availability**
   A. The quantity of oxygen available to the tissue depends on oxygen content and cardiac output (see Figure 7-4).
   B. The amount of oxygen transported to tissue is equal to:

$$(O_2 \text{ content in vol\%})(10)(\text{Cardiac output in L/min}) \qquad (9)$$

   C. In the normal healthy adult, oxygen content equals approximately 20 vol%, and cardiac output is approximately 5 L/min. Thus:

$$O_2 \text{ transport} = (20 \text{ vol\%})(10)(5 \text{ L/min}) = 1000 \text{ ml/min}$$

   D. Oxygen availability is most significantly affected by the hemoglobin level and cardiac output.
   E. Normal oxygen transport ranges from approximately 900 to 1200 ml/min at rest.
   F. Oxygen transport may be decreased by any of the following (Table 7-3):
      1. Decreased cardiac output
      2. Decreased oxygen content
         a. Decreased Po_2
         b. Decreased hemoglobin
         c. Rightward shift of the oxyhemoglobin dissociation curve

V. **Oxygen Consumption**
   A. The normal arterial oxygen content is 20 vol%.
   B. The normal mixed venous oxygen content is approximately 15 vol%.
   C. Thus $Cao_2 - C\bar{v}o_2$ is 5 vol%.
   D. If the cardiac output is 5 L/min, the body consumes 250 ml/min of oxygen.
   E. Oxygen consumption in the adult varies from approximately 150 to 350 ml/min (basal metabolic level), depending on body size and metabolic rate.

TABLE 7-3

Effect of Cardiac Output and O_2 Content on Oxygen Transport*

Cao_2 (vol%)	Cardiac Output (L/min)	O_2 Transport (ml/min)
20	5	1000
15	5	750
10	5	500
20	10	2000
20	2.5	500
15	10	1500
15	2.5	375
10	10	1000
10	2.5	250

*Reductions in Cao_2 and cardiac output can affect O_2 transport. Marked reductions in O_2 transport occur if Cao_2 and cardiac output are simultaneously reduced.
From Pierson DJ, Kacmarek RM: *Foundations of Respiratory Care,* Churchill Livingstone, New York, 1992.

F.   Oxygen consumption is altered by:
1.   Physical activity (metabolic rate)
2.   Physiologic stress
3.   Temperature
4.   Alterations in microcirculation
G.   In the adequately perfused normothermic patient who is not shivering or seizing, oxygen consumption is equal to approximately 3.0 ml/kg body weight/min.

VI.   **Production of Carbon Dioxide**
A.   Carbon dioxide is produced by the metabolism of all food.
B.   In addition, carbon dioxide is produced in the conversion of glucose to fatty acids.
C.   Normal carbon dioxide production is approximately 120 to 280 ml/min, depending on body size and metabolic rate, or approximately 2.4 ml/kg/min.

VII.   **Carriage of Carbon Dioxide in the Blood**
A.   Carriage in plasma occurs in three distinct ways (Figure 7-5):
1.   Carbon dioxide is dissolved in plasma as P_{CO_2}, which is in equilibrium with the P_{CO_2} in red blood cells (RBCs).
2.   Carbon dioxide is carried predominantly as bicarbonate (HCO_3^-) formed in the RBCs and by the kidney. The HCO_3^- levels in plasma are in equilibrium with the HCO_3^- in RBCs.
   a.   Plasma carbon dioxide reacts minimally with water, forming carbonic acid, which dissociates into H^+ and HCO_3^-:

$$CO_2 + H_2O \rightleftharpoons H_2CO_3 \rightleftharpoons H^+ + HCO_3^- \tag{10}$$

   b.   The H^+ formed is buffered in the plasma and therefore causes a mild decrease in pH (venous blood).
   c.   The previous reaction's point of equilibrium (equation 10) is shifted to the left in the plasma, therefore favoring formation of the reactants.
   d.   The mathematical relationship between dissolved CO_2 and H_2CO_3 is:

$$(P_{CO_2} \text{ mm Hg})(0.0301) = H_2CO_3 \text{ mEq/L, or mmol/L} \tag{11}$$

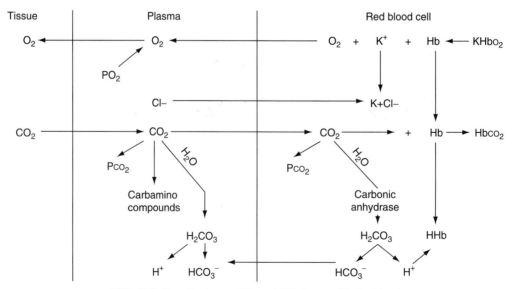

FIG. 7-5 Overall scheme of O_2 and CO_2 transport in the blood.

3. Carbon dioxide is attached to plasma proteins, forming carbamino compounds similar to those formed when CO_2 combines with hemoglobin.
    a. Carbon dioxide reacts with the terminal amino groups on the plasma proteins (R-NH_2):

$$R-N\underset{H}{\overset{H}{\big<}} + CO_2 \rightleftharpoons R-N\underset{COO^-}{\overset{H}{\big<}} + H^+ \tag{12}$$

(R indicates the remainder of the plasma protein)

    b. Most of the H^+ liberated is buffered and therefore causes a mild decrease in the pH (venous blood).

    c. The ionization state of the amino groups affects their ability to bond with carbon dioxide. If the NH_2 groups are oxidized to NH_3^+, their ability to combine with carbon dioxide is significantly decreased.

B. Carriage of carbon dioxide in RBCs occurs in three distinct ways (see Figure 7-5):

1. As dissolved P_{CO_2} in equilibrium with plasma P_{CO_2}.

2. As HCO_3^- formed in the RBC.
    a. The rate of the reaction shown in equation 10 is significantly increased as a result of the presence of the enzyme carbonic anhydrase (CA). The point of equilibrium is shifted to the right, favoring formation of the products:

$$CO_2 + H_2O \overset{CA}{\rightleftharpoons} H_2CO_3 \rightleftharpoons H^+ + HCO_3^- \tag{13}$$

    b. As increasing levels of HCO_3^- are formed in the RBC, HCO_3^- diffuses into the plasma. As HCO_3^- diffuses, there is an imbalance of electric charges inside the RBC, causing Cl^- to move into the RBC. This process is referred to as the *chloride shift* or *Hamburger phenomenon*. The Cl^- diffusing into the RBC associates with the K^+ released as the hemoglobin molecule gives up O_2 and buffers H^+.

3. As carbon dioxide attached to the terminal amino (R-NH_2) groups of the hemoglobin molecule. This reaction is the same as that shown in equation 12. The H^+ released from the formation of HCO_3^- again must be buffered.
    a. In RBCs, the imidazole groups on the hemoglobin molecule are the primary buffer.
    b. The ability of the imidazole groups to buffer is affected by oxyhemoglobin saturation. With oxygen bound to the heme, the imidazole groups are poor buffers. Without oxygen attached to the heme, the imidazole groups are good buffers.
    c. As oxygen attaches to the heme, more R-NH_2 groups will exist in the R-NH_3^+ form. The tendency for carbon dioxide to attach to the R-NH_3^+ form is less than to the R-NH_2 form.

VIII. **Haldane Effect**

    A. Figure 7-6 illustrates the Haldane effect, which is defined as the effect of oxygen on carbon dioxide uptake and release.

    B. As P_{O_2} increases at the pulmonary capillary bed, the ability of hemoglobin to carry carbon dioxide is decreased because more amino groups exist in the oxidized R-NH_3^+ state. This allows large volumes of carbon dioxide to be released at the pulmonary capillary bed.

    C. As the P_{O_2} decreases at the tissue level, the ability of hemoglobin to carry carbon dioxide is increased because more amino groups exist in the reduced R-NH_2 form. This allows large volumes of carbon dioxide to be picked up at the systemic capillary bed (see Figure 7-6).

    D. The Haldane effect facilitates carriage of the normal 4 vol% (200 ml/min) of carbon dioxide picked up from the tissue and released at the lung.

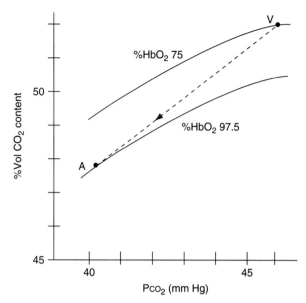

FIG. 7-6 Effect of oxyhemoglobin saturation on volume of CO_2 carried in blood. The carrying capacity of blood for CO_2 is decreased as oxyhemoglobin saturation is increased (Haldane effect). The arrow from V to A depicts change of CO_2 content from venous to arterial blood.

IX. **Quantitative Distribution of Carbon Dioxide**
   A. Percentage of carbon dioxide carried in each compartment:
      1. Approximately 90% of carbon dioxide in blood exists as HCO_3^-.
      2. Approximately 5% of carbon dioxide in blood exists as carbamino compounds.
      3. Approximately 5% of carbon dioxide in blood exists as dissolved P_{CO_2}.
   B. Percentage of carbon dioxide exhaled from various compartments:
      1. Approximately 60% of the carbon dioxide exhaled is carried as HCO_3^-.
      2. Approximately 30% of the carbon dioxide exhaled is carried as carbamino compounds.
      3. Approximately 10% of the carbon dioxide exhaled is carried as dissolved P_{CO_2}.

X. **Total Carbon Dioxide**
   A. Total carbon dioxide is an expression of the sum of HCO_3^- plus dissolved CO_2.
   B. Total carbon dioxide may be expressed in millimoles per liter (mmol/L), milliequivalents per liter (mEq/L), or vol%.

$$(P_{CO_2})(0.0301) = \text{mmol/L or mEq/L of } H_2CO_3 \qquad (14)$$

$$\text{Vol\% of } CO_2 = (\text{mEq/L})(2.23) \text{ or } (\text{mmol/L})(2.23) \qquad (15)$$

$$\text{mmol/L or mEq/L of } CO_2 = \text{vol\%}/2.23 \qquad (16)$$

   C. In arterial blood:

$$\text{Total } CO_2 = [HCO_3^-] + [\text{dissolved } P_{CO_2}] \qquad (17)$$

   1. 25.2 mmol/L = 24 mmol/L + 1.2 mmol/L
   2. 56.2 vol% = 53.52 vol% + 2.68 vol%

XI. **Respiratory Quotient, Respiratory Exchange Ratio, and Ventilation/Perfusion Ratio**
  A. The respiratory quotient (RQ) is defined as the volume of carbon dioxide produced divided by the volume of oxygen consumed per minute; normally the RQ equals:

$$RQ = \frac{4\, vol\%\ CO_2}{5\, vol\%\ O_2} \text{ or } \frac{200\, ml\ CO_2}{250\, ml\ O_2} = 0.8 \qquad (18)$$

  B. The RQ is an expression of *internal* respiration.
  C. The respiratory exchange ratio (R) is defined as the volume of carbon dioxide moving from the pulmonary capillaries into the lung divided by the volume of oxygen moving from the lung into the pulmonary capillaries:

$$R = \frac{4\, vol\%\ CO_2}{5\, vol\%\ O_2} = \frac{200\, ml\ CO_2}{250\, ml\ O_2} = 0.8 \qquad (19)$$

  D. R is an expression of *external* respiration.
  E. Under normal circumstances RQ and R are equal, with a mean value of approximately 0.8.
  F. The ventilation/perfusion ($\dot{V}/\dot{Q}$) ratio is equal to the minute alveolar ventilation divided by the minute cardiac output:

$$\dot{V}/\dot{Q} = \frac{4\, L\ alveolar\ minute\ volume}{5\, L\ minute\ cardiac\ output} = 0.8 \qquad (20)$$

  G. $\dot{V}/\dot{Q}$ is equal to RQ and R under normal circumstances.
  H. It is the alveolar ventilation and the cardiac output that maintain the RQ and R equal.

BIBLIOGRAPHY

Beachey W: *Respiratory Care Anatomy and Physiology.* St. Louis, Mosby, 1998.

Bendixen HH, Pontoppidan H, Laver MB, et al: *Respiratory Care.* St. Louis, CV Mosby, 1965.

Burton GG, Hodgkin JE, Ward JJ: *Respiratory Care: A Guide to Clinical Practice*, ed 4. Philadelphia, JB Lippincott, 1997.

Comroe JH: *Physiology of Respiration,* ed 2. Chicago, Year Book Medical Publishers, 1974.

Guyton AC, Hall JE: *Textbook of Medical Physiology*, ed 10. Philadelphia, WB Saunders, 2000.

Hess D, MacIntyre N, Mishoe SC, et al: *Respiratory Care: Principles and Practices.* St. Louis, Mosby, 2002.

Hicks GH: *Cardiopulmonary Anatomy and Physiology.* Philadelphia, WB Saunders, 2000.

Murray JF: *The Normal Lung.* Philadelphia, WB Saunders, 1976.

Shapiro BA, Harrison RA, Cane R, et al: *Clinical Application of Blood Gases*, ed 4. Chicago, Year Book Medical Publishers, 1989.

Shapiro BA, Harrison RA, Kacmarek RM, et al: *Clinical Application of Respiratory Care*, ed 4. Chicago, Year Book Medical Publishers, 1991.

West JB: *Respiratory Physiology: The Essentials*, ed 4. Baltimore, Williams & Wilkins, 1990.

Wilkins RL, Stoller JK, Scanlan CL, Egan DF: *Egan's Fundamentals of Respiratory Therapy*, ed 8. St. Louis, CV Mosby Co, 2003.

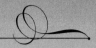

Chapter 8

Intrapulmonary Shunting and Deadspace

I. **Spectrum of Ventilation/Perfusion ($\dot{V}/\dot{Q}$) Abnormalities (Figure 8-1)**
   A. **Ideal alveolar-capillary unit:** An alveolar-capillary unit in which perfusion and ventilation are normal; theoretically, a unit with a $\dot{V}/\dot{Q}$ ratio of 1.0.
   B. **Deadspace unit:** An alveolar-capillary unit in which ventilation is normal but perfusion is diminished or absent; a unit with a $\dot{V}/\dot{Q}$ ratio >1.0.
   C. **Shunt unit:** An alveolar-capillary unit in which perfusion is normal but ventilation is diminished or absent; a unit with a $\dot{V}/\dot{Q}$ ratio <1.0.
   D. **Silent unit:** An alveolar-capillary unit without perfusion or ventilation and therefore a $\dot{V}/\dot{Q}$ ratio of 0.0.

II. **Intrapulmonary Shunting**
   A. A pathophysiologic process in which blood enters the left side of the heart without having been oxygenated by the lungs. The mixing of venous blood with oxygenated blood from the pulmonary capillaries to form arterial blood.
   B. The total quantity of shunted blood is the *physiologic shunt*, which is composed of three subdivisions (Figure 8-2).
      1. **Anatomic shunt:** The portion of the total cardiac output that bypasses the pulmonary capillary bed.
         a. Normally approximately 2% to 5% of the cardiac output bypasses the pulmonary capillaries because the following veins empty into the left side of the heart:
            (1) Bronchial
            (2) Pleural
            (3) Thebesian
         b. Increases in anatomic shunt may occur as a result of:
            (1) Vascular pulmonary tumors
            (2) Arterial venous anastomosis
            (3) Congenital cardiac anomalies
            (4) Severe liver disease
      2. **Capillary shunt:** The portion of the total cardiac output that perfuses nonventilated alveoli (Figure 8-3).
         a. Normally capillary shunting does not exist.
         b. Capillary shunting is caused by:
            (1) Atelectasis
            (2) Consolidating pneumonia
            (3) Complete airway obstruction
            (4) Pneumothorax

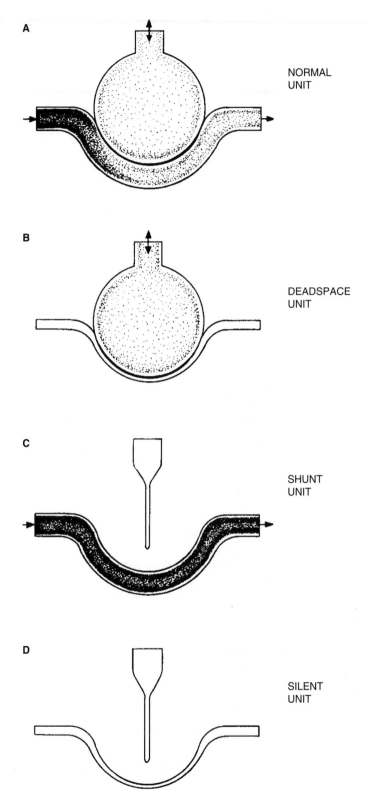

FIG. 8-1 The theoretical respiratory unit. **A,** Normal ventilation, normal perfusion. **B,** Normal ventilation, no perfusion. **C,** No ventilation, normal perfusion. **D,** No ventilation, no perfusion.

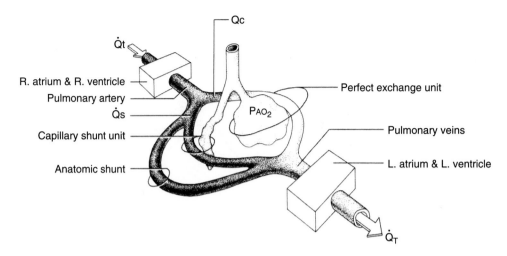

FIG. 8-2 Concept of physiologic shunting (see text). $\dot{Q}t$ is cardiac output per unit time; $\dot{Q}c$ is the portion of the cardiac output that exchanges perfectly with alveolar air; $\dot{Q}s$ is the portion of the cardiac output that does not exchange with alveolar air; and P_{AO_2} is the alveolar oxygen tension.

    (5) Pulmonary edema
    (6) Any pathophysiologic process that eliminates ventilation to perfused alveoli
  3. Shunt effect (ventilation/perfusion inequality, low $\dot{V}/\dot{Q}$, venous admixture): Any pathophysiologic process in which perfusion is in excess of ventilation; however, some ventilation is still present (Figure 8-4).
    a. Under normal conditions, shunt effect occurs in the bases of the lung, where $\dot{V}/\dot{Q}$ ratios are <1.0.
    b. Venous admixture may be increased by:
      (1) Retained secretions
      (2) Bronchospasm
      (3) Partial airway obstruction
      (4) Regional increases in fibrotic tissue
      (5) Decreased tidal volumes
      (6) Mucosal edema at the bronchiolar level
      (7) Interstitial edema

III. Derivation of Classic Shunt Equation
  A. Definition of abbreviations
    1. $\dot{V}O_2$: Volume of oxygen consumed per minute
    2. $\dot{Q}s$: Shunted cardiac output
    3. $\dot{Q}c$: Capillary cardiac output
    4. $\dot{Q}t$: Total cardiac output
    5. Cc_{O_2}: Capillary oxygen content
    6. Ca_{O_2}: Arterial oxygen content
    7. $C\bar{v}_{O_2}$: Mixed venous oxygen content
    8. P_{AO_2}: Alveolar oxygen partial pressure
    9. Pa_{O_2}: Arterial oxygen partial pressure
  B. The shunt equation is based on the Fick equation, which normally is used to calculate oxygen consumption or cardiac output:

$$\dot{V}O_2 = \dot{Q}t(Ca_{O_2} - C\bar{v}_{O_2})\tag{1}$$

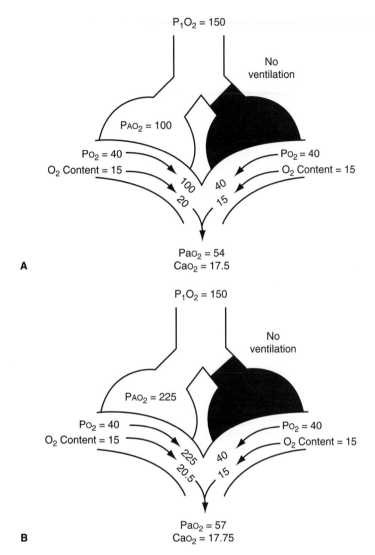

FIG. 8-3 Alveolar-capillary diagram of intrapulmonary (capillary) shunting showing why supplemental O_2 fails to correct hypoxemia. Only O_2 exchange is shown, and $P_{(A-a)O_2}$ is assumed to be zero. **A,** With room air, although blood leaving the normal alveolar-capillary unit is normally saturated, blood passing the capillary on the right "sees" no O_2 because its alveolus is unventilated and it leaves the unit unsaturated. When the two streams of blood mix, the resulting Pa_{O_2} is determined by the average of their O_2 contents, not by their Po_2 values. **B,** Addition of 40% oxygen fails to correct the hypoxemia because O_2 content is not significantly increased in the normal unit and capillary blood in the unventilated unit still "sees" no O_2. Even 100% O_2 could not completely reverse the oxygenation defect in this example; very different from the effect with a low $\dot{V}/\dot{Q}$ as illustrated in Figure 8-4.

C. Because actual capillary blood flow ($\dot{Q}c$) represents the portion of the cardiac output that actually perfuses ventilated alveoli and Cc_{O_2} is the oxygen content of blood leaving those perfused and ventilated alveoli, this equation may be rewritten as:

$$\dot{V}_{O_2} = \dot{Q}c(Cc_{O_2} - C\bar{v}_{O_2})\qquad(2)$$

D. Thus total cardiac output is equal to shunted cardiac output plus capillary cardiac output:

$$\dot{Q}t = \dot{Q}s + \dot{Q}c\qquad(3)$$

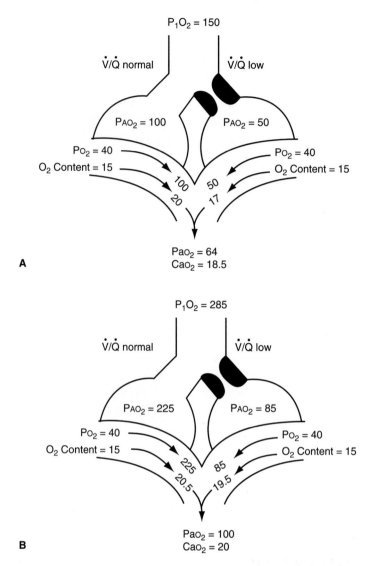

FIG. 8-4 Hypoxemia caused by $\dot{V}/\dot{Q}$ mismatch showing the effect of supplemental O_2. $\dot{V}/\dot{Q}$ is normal on the left side of each idealized lung unit and low on the right. Only O_2 exchange is shown, and the $P(A-a)O_2$ is assumed to be zero. **A,** With room air, not enough O_2 reaches the poorly ventilated alveolus to fully saturate its capillary blood. **B,** With 40% O_2, PAO_2 in this alveolus is increased enough to make its capillary PO_2 nearly normal. Note that the PaO_2 in the mixed blood from the two capillaries is determined by the average of the O_2 contents of the two blood streams, not by their PaO_2 values.

E. Solving equation 3 for $\dot{Q}c$:

$$\dot{Q}c = \dot{Q}t - \dot{Q}s \qquad (4)$$

F. Substituting into equation 2 the equivalent of $\dot{V}O_2$ from equation 1:

$$\dot{Q}t(CaO_2 - C\bar{v}O_2) = \dot{Q}c(CcO_2 - C\bar{v}O_2) \qquad (5)$$

G. Substituting into equation 5 the equivalent of $\dot{Q}c$ from equation 4:

$$\dot{Q}t(Cao_2 - C\bar{v}o_2) = (\dot{Q}t - \dot{Q}s)(Cco_2 - C\bar{v}o_2) \tag{6}$$

H. Rearranging equation 6:

$$\dot{Q}tCao_2 - \dot{Q}tC\bar{v}o_2 = \dot{Q}tCco_2 - \dot{Q}tC\bar{v}o_2 - \dot{Q}sCco_2 + \dot{Q}sC\bar{v}o_2 \tag{7}$$

I. Eliminating $-\dot{Q}tC\bar{v}o_2$ from both sides of equation 7:

$$\dot{Q}tCao_2 = \dot{Q}tCco_2 - \dot{Q}sCco_2 + \dot{Q}sC\bar{v}o_2 \tag{8}$$

J. Rearranging equation 8:

$$\dot{Q}sCco_2 - \dot{Q}sC\bar{v}o_2 = \dot{Q}tCco_2 + \dot{Q}tCao_2 \tag{9}$$

K. Simplifying equation 9:

$$\dot{Q}s(Cco_2 - C\bar{v}o_2) = \dot{Q}t(Cco_2 - Cao_2) \tag{10}$$

L. Rearranging equation 10:

$$\dot{Q}s/\dot{Q}t = \frac{Cco_2 - Cao_2}{Cco_2 - C\bar{v}o_2} \tag{11}$$

M. Equation 11 is the classic shunt equation, which states that the difference between the capillary oxygen content and arterial oxygen content divided by the difference between the capillary oxygen content and the mixed venous oxygen content equals the intrapulmonary shunt fraction.

N. This equation is used to calculate the total physiologic shunt.

IV. Calculation of the Total Physiologic (or Intrapulmonary) Shunt

A. The intrapulmonary shunt is determined by calculating the capillary oxygen content, arterial oxygen content, and mixed venous oxygen content.

B. All oxygen content determinations are based on the following equation:

$$O_2 \text{ content (vol\%)} = (\text{Hb cont})(HbO_2\% \text{ sat})(1.34) + (0.003)(Po_2) \tag{12}$$

C. Calculation of the arterial oxygen content requires data from an arterial blood gas.

D. Calculation of the mixed venous oxygen content requires data from a pulmonary artery blood gas.

E. Capillary oxygen content

1. Because a blood sample from an *ideally functioning alveolar-capillary* unit is impossible to obtain, this calculation is based on the assumption that the end pulmonary capillary oxygen tension (Pco_2) is equal to the alveolar oxygen tension (PAo_2) in an ideally ventilated and perfused alveolar-capillary unit.

2. The PAo_2 is obtained by calculation, using the ideal alveolar gas equation (see Chapter 5):

$$PAo_2 = (PB - PH_2O)(F_Io_2) - (Paco_2)\left(F_Io_2 + \frac{1 - F_Io_2}{R}\right) \tag{13}$$

3. Hemoglobin content is the same as that measured in arterial blood or mixed venous blood.

4. Oxyhemoglobin percent saturation ($HbO_2\%$ sat)
   a. If the PAo_2 is $\geq$150 mm Hg, it is assumed that the $HbO_2\%$ saturation is 100%.
   b. For PAo_2 values of <150 mm Hg, an oxyhemoglobin dissociation curve is used to estimate the $HbO_2\%$ saturation.

c. The capillary $HbO_2\%$ saturation is also corrected for the $HbCO\%$ saturation present in the arterial blood.

F. *Example:*

$$Cao_2 = 17.5 \text{ vol}\%$$
$$Cco_2 = 19.5 \text{ vol}\%$$
$$C\bar{v}o_2 = 13.0 \text{ vol}\%$$

$$\frac{\dot{Q}s}{\dot{Q}t} = \frac{Cco_2 - Cao_2}{Cco_2 - C\bar{v}o_2}$$

$$\frac{\dot{Q}s}{\dot{Q}t} = \frac{19.5 - 17.5}{19.5 - 13.0} = 0.31$$

or 31% intrapulmonary shunt.

V. **Estimated Intrapulmonary Shunt Calculation**
   A. In patients without a pulmonary artery catheter, it is impossible to measure the $C\bar{v}o_2$.
   B. However, in the majority of critically ill patients with cardiovascular stability, it has been determined that the $Cao_2 - C\bar{v}o_2$ is approximately 3.5 vol%.
   C. Thus in these patients 3.5 vol% may be used as an estimate of $Cao_2 - C\bar{v}o_2$.
   D. The denominator of the classic shunt equation may be expressed as follows:

$$Cco_2 - C\bar{v}o_2 = (Cco_2 - Cao_2) + (Cao_2 - C\bar{v}o_2) \tag{14}$$

   E. Because $Cao_2 - C\bar{v}o_2$ is estimated at 3.5 vol%, the denominator in equation 11 can be expressed as:

$$(Cco_2 - Cao_2) + 3.5 \tag{15}$$

   F. The modified shunt equation used to estimate intrapulmonary shunt is:

$$\frac{\dot{Q}s}{\dot{Q}t} = \frac{Cco_2 - Cao_2}{(Cco_2 - Cao_2) + 3.5} \tag{16}$$

   G. Equation 16 should be used only if pulmonary artery blood is unavailable and the patient is cardiovascularly stable.

VI. **F_IO_2 Used to Calculate Percent Intrapulmonary Shunt**
   A. Historically shunt fractions were determined at an F_IO_2 of 1.0.
   B. However, it has been demonstrated that the shunt fraction is increased at an F_IO_2 of 1.0.
   C. This occurs secondary to:
      1. Nitrogen washout atelectasis
         a. Areas of the lung that are ventilated poorly tend to collapse if the nitrogen is removed.
         b. Nitrogen normally maintains alveolar stability. When nitrogen is removed and replaced by oxygen, the blood absorbs the oxygen faster than it can be replaced because of the poor ventilation.
         c. As a result, alveolar size decreases, eventually falling below its critical volume, and collapse occurs (Figure 8-5).
      2. Redistribution of pulmonary blood flow
         a. If an area of lung is poorly ventilated or not ventilated at all, the decreased Po_2 in the area causes the pulmonary vasculature surrounding the alveoli to constrict.
         b. This decreases blood flow to poorly ventilated areas and increases blood flow to areas more appropriately ventilated.
         c. When a high F_IO_2 is administered, this autoregulatory mechanism is abated because the Po_2 throughout the lung is elevated and capillaries that were previously constricted are now dilated.

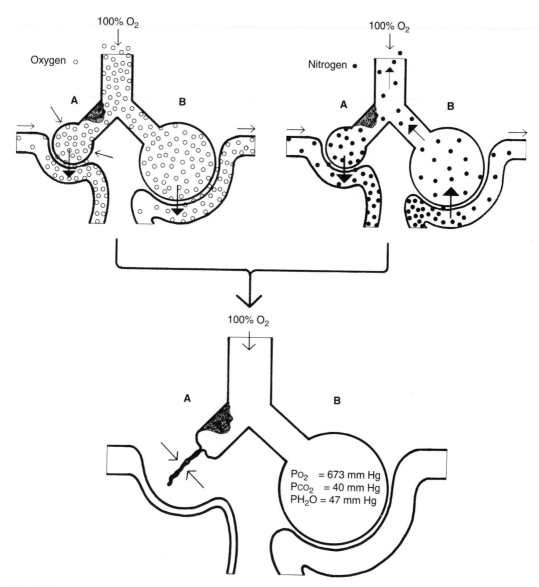

FIG. 8-5 Schematic representation of primary mechanisms causing denitrogenation absorption atelectasis. *Top drawings* represent alveolar capillary units shortly after administration of 100% inspired oxygen. *White circles* represent oxygen molecules that have increased in concentration in both units *A* and *B*. The elimination of alveolar hypoxia in unit *A* results in loss of vasoconstriction with considerably increased blood flow. The increased blood flow to this still poorly ventilated alveolus results in significantly increased oxygen extraction, which results in decreased gas volume. *Black circles* represent nitrogen, which is rapidly depleted from all units secondary to the fact that inspired nitrogen concentration is now zero. Initially more nitrogen leaves the blood and the body via unit *B* because it is better ventilated. However, as the blood P_{N_2} level progressively decreases, nitrogen will start to leave alveolus *A* via the blood. This results in further loss of gas volume from alveolus *A* because it remains poorly ventilated but well perfused. Thus nitrogen is depleted from all units within 5 to 15 min. *Bottom drawing* represents the final steady state, in which increased oxygen and nitrogen extraction has caused the alveolus to collapse. Thus a poorly ventilated, poorly perfused unit *A* becomes a nonventilated, poorly perfused unit after administration of 100% inspired oxygen.

d. This results in increased blood being shunted past nonventilated and poorly ventilated alveoli.

D. Figure 8-6 represents the relationship between F_IO_2 and percent shunt. Clinically it appears
that the lowest measured shunt occurs at approximately 50% oxygen.
1. The percent shunt increases as the F_IO_2 decreases <0.5 because of the effect of venous
admixture.
2. The percent shunt increases as the F_IO_2 increases >0.5 because of nitrogen washout
atelectasis and redistribution of pulmonary blood flow.

E. Percent intrapulmonary shunts should be calculated at the F_IO_2 the patient is maintained
and at 100% oxygen so that the quantity of venous admixture contributing to the total
shunt faction can be determined by the difference between the two.

VII. **Clinical Use of the Shunt Calculation**
A. Differentiating causes of hypoxemia
1. Hypoxemia is caused by:
a. True shunting: A combination of anatomic and capillary shunting.
b. Shunt effect or venous admixture ($\dot{V}/\dot{Q}$ mismatch): A decrease in local alveolar
oxygen tension.
c. Decreased mixed venous oxygen content.
(1) This causes hypoxemia or an increase in hypoxemia only if intrapulmonary
shunting also exists.
(2) Essentially it accentuates the effect of a preexisting shunt because the blood
that is shunted is now more deoxygenated than normal.
2. The numerator of the shunt equation, $Cc_{O_2} - Ca_{O_2}$, can be considered a reflection of
intrapulmonary pathology (i.e., hypoxemia of pulmonary origin will increase the Cc_{O_2}
$- Ca_{O_2}$ value, increasing the calculated shunt fraction).
3. The denominator in the shunt equation, $Cc_{O_2} - Ca_{O_2}$, can be considered a reflection of
the relationship of cardiac output to oxygen demand.

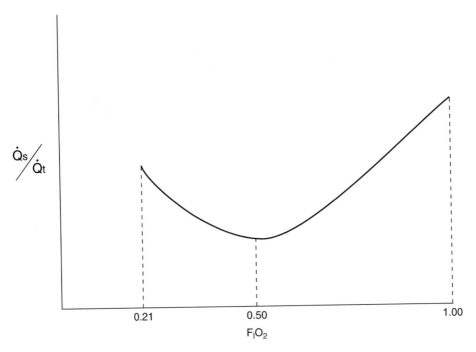

FIG. 8-6 Schematic representation of intrapulmonary shunt calculations ($\dot{Q}s/\dot{Q}t$) versus inspired oxygen concentration (F_IO_2) in normal and diseased lungs.

    a. This is true because $CaO_2 - C\bar{v}O_2$ is contained in the denominator.

    b. If hypoxemia is a result of cardiovascular pathology, it is primarily reflected in a widening of the $CcO_2 - C\bar{v}O_2$ but may not be accompanied by a proportional widening of the numerator.

  4. Hypoxemia accompanied by an increased shunt measurement generally denotes an increase in intrapulmonary pathology.

  5. Hypoxemia without a major increase in shunt fraction usually denotes cardiovascular causes of hypoxemia.

B. Assessment of spontaneous ventilatory capabilities in patients being mechanically ventilated

  1. An intrapulmonary shunt determination of <10% during mechanical ventilation is clinically comparable with normal lungs.

  2. An intrapulmonary shunt determination of 10% to 19% should not represent sufficient pulmonary disease to interfere with spontaneous ventilation.

  3. An intrapulmonary shunt of 20% to 30% may result in ventilatory failure in patients with central nervous system or cardiovascular dysfunction if spontaneous ventilation is attempted. However, many patients are able to sustain spontaneous ventilation with this level of shunt.

  4. An intrapulmonary shunt of >30% represents a degree of pulmonary disease that normally requires aggressive cardiopulmonary support (i.e., increased positive end-expiratory pressure [PEEP], lung recruitment, fluid therapy, and prone positioning).

C. Assessment of specific cardiopulmonary abnormalities

  1. Performance of intrapulmonary shunt studies while a patient is in different positions may delineate the locale and extent of certain pulmonary pathology.

    a. This is true because of the effects of gravity on pulmonary blood flow.

    b. If the diseased area is gravity dependent, the percent intrapulmonary shunt is increased and may be a strong indication for prone positioning.

  2. In the neonate the extent of right-to-left shunting is increased in the presence of the following congenital anomalies:

    a. Ventricular septal defects

    b. Atrial septal defects

    c. Patent ductus arteriosus

D. Monitoring of oxygen and PEEP therapy

  1. If the hypoxemia is of pulmonary origin and caused primarily by shunt effect, the appropriate application of oxygen therapy should demonstrate a decrease in intrapulmonary shunt.

  2. If the hypoxemia is of pulmonary origin and caused primarily by capillary shunting of a generalized diffuse nature (e.g., acute respiratory distress syndrome [ARDS]), lung recruitment maneuvers, PEEP therapy, and prone positioning are primarily indicated, along with appropriate adjustment of F_IO_2.

  3. However, the greater the percent intrapulmonary shunt, the less effect increasing F_IO_2 has on PaO_2 (Figure 8-7).

  4. In patients with >30% $\dot{Q}s/\dot{Q}t$, F_IO_2 of 1.0 may not increase the PO_2 to a clinically acceptable level.

VIII. **Other Methods of Estimating Shunting and Oxygenation Status (Table 8-1)**

A. Alveolar-arterial PO_2 difference: $P(A-a)O_2$

  1. The $P(A-a)O_2$ gradient has been used to estimate the percent intrapulmonary shunt.

  2. The normal $P(A-a)O_2$ when room air is breathed is 7 to 14 mm Hg.

  3. However, at an F_IO_2 of 1.0, it increases to 31 to 56 mm Hg.

  4. During 100% oxygen breathing, some estimate the shunt fraction as 1% for every 10 to 15 mm Hg of $P(A-a)O_2$.

  5. The fact that $P(A-a)O_2$ exhibits variability with changes in F_IO_2 limits its usefulness as an indicator of overall cardiopulmonary function.

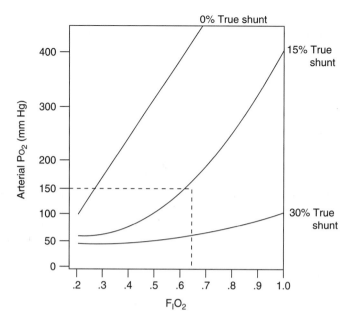

FIG. 8-7 Comparison of the theoretical F_IO_2–PaO_2 relationships in 0%, 15%, and 30% true shunts. These relationships were calculated assuming normal lung ventilation, hemoglobin of 15 g%, arteriovenous oxygen content difference of 5 vol%, and normal cardiac output, metabolic rate, pH, and PCO_2. This schema assumes that only true shunting exists (i.e., no shunt effect is present). The 0% true shunt line reveals a PaO_2 of 100 mm Hg at room air. There is a predictable increase in PaO_2 for incremental increases in F_IO_2 because the arterial hemoglobin is nearly fully saturated at room air. Because all the blood exchanges with alveolar gas, incremental increases in alveolar oxygen tensions produce similar increases in arterial oxygen tensions. Note that with 15% true shunt, the arterial PO_2 is approximately 60 mm Hg (90% saturation) because 15% of the cardiac output enters the left side of the heart with approximately 75% hemoglobin saturation. Incremental increases in alveolar PO_2 result in small increases in oxygen content (dissolved oxygen) in 85% of the cardiac output, whereas 15% of the cardiac output continues to enter the left side of the heart with a hemoglobin saturation of approximately 75%. Note that the arterial blood does not approach 100 mm Hg (near complete hemoglobin saturation) until the F_IO_2 approaches 0.5. With incremental F_IO_2 increases >0.5, near linear increases in PaO_2 occur but at a slightly lesser slope than with 0% true shunt. Thirty percent true shunt produces an arterial PO_2 of approximately 45 mm Hg at room air. This degree of true shunt does not allow an arterial PO_2 of 100 mm Hg, even at 100% inspired oxygen concentration.

TABLE 8-1
Methods of Calculating or Estimating Shunt

Index	Normal Value	Abnormal Value	Limitations
$\dot{Q}s/\dot{Q}t$	2-5%	>10%	Invasive
$P(A–a)O_2$	7-14 mm Hg (RA)	100-150 at F_IO_2 1.0	Varies with F_IO_2
	31-56 mm Hg (1.0)		
PaO_2/PAO_2	>0.75	<0.75	_____
PaO_2/F_IO_2	450-500	<300-350	Varies with $PaCO_2$ and F_IO_2

RA, Room air; *1.0*, 100% O_2.

 B. Arterial-alveolar ratio: PaO_2/PAO_2
  1. The lower limit of normal for PaO_2/PAO_2, regardless of F_IO_2, is ≥0.75.
  2. The lower the PaO_2/PAO_2, the greater the cardiopulmonary abnormality.
  3. Because PaO_2/PAO_2 is not affected by changes in F_IO_2, it is a more reliable index of abnormality than $P(A–a)O_2$.
 C. Arterial-F_IO_2 ratio: PaO_2/F_IO_2
  1. The normal PaO_2/F_IO_2 is approximately 450 to 500.

2. A $Pa_{O_2}/F_{I}O_2$ <200 has been associated with a shunt fraction of >20%.
3. Pa_{CO_2} and increasing F_IO_2 inversely affect the Pa_{O_2}/F_IO_2.
4. As a result, it is a much cruder index of cardiopulmonary dysfunction than $P(A-a)O_2$ or Pa_{O_2}/PA_{O_2}.
5. The Pa_{O_2}/F_IO_2 is the most commonly used index because it is easy to calculate.

IX. **Pulmonary Deadspace**
   A. Pulmonary deadspace is the portion of the total ventilation that does not undergo external respiration.
   B. The total quantity of pulmonary deadspace is the *physiologic deadspace* and is composed of three subdivisions:
      1. Anatomic deadspace: The portion of the total ventilation that does not contact the alveolar epithelium.
         a. Normally the anatomic deadspace is equal to approximately 1.0 ml/lb of ideal body weight.
         b. The relationship between anatomic deadspace and tidal volume is increased by small tidal volumes and rapid rates.
         c. The absolute quantity of anatomic deadspace is increased by:
            (1) Positive pressure ventilation
            (2) Mechanical circuit deadspace
         d. Anatomic deadspace is decreased by:
            (1) Tracheostomy/endotracheal tubes
            (2) Pneumothorax
      2. Alveolar deadspace: The portion of the total ventilation that contacts the alveolar epithelium but does not participate in gas exchange because of a lack of pulmonary capillary blood flow (Figure 8-8).
         a. Alveolar deadspace accounts for a small amount of the total physiologic deadspace in the healthy individual.
         b. Alveolar deadspace is increased by:
            (1) Pulmonary emboli
            (2) Vascular tumors
      3. Deadspace effect (ventilation/perfusion inequality): Any pathophysiologic process in which ventilation is in excess of perfusion but some perfusion does exist (i.e., $\dot{V}/\dot{Q}$ ratio >1.0) (see Figure 8-8).
         a. In the standing individual, deadspace effect occurs in the apices of the lungs because blood flow to this region is greatly diminished.
         b. Deadspace effect is increased by:
            (1) Positive pressure ventilation
            (2) Decreased cardiac output
            (3) Alveolar septal wall destruction

X. **Derivation of the Deadspace Equation**
   A. Definition of abbreviations
      1. V_T: Tidal volume
      2. V_D: Deadspace volume
      3. V_A: Alveolar volume
      4. FA_{CO_2}: Fractional concentration of CO_2 in alveolar gas
      5. $F\bar{E}_{CO_2}$: Mean fractional concentration of CO_2 in mixed expired gas
      6. Pa_{CO_2}: Partial pressure of arterial CO_2
      7. $P\bar{E}_{CO_2}$: Partial pressure of mean expired CO_2
      8. FD_{CO_2}: Fractional concentration of deadspace CO_2
   B. Tidal volume is equal to deadspace volume plus alveolar volume.

$$V_T = V_D + V_A \qquad (17)$$

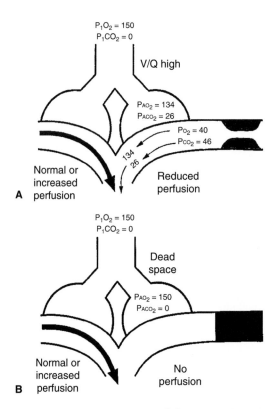

FIG. 8-8 Alveolar diagrams depicting lung units with (**A**) high $\dot{V}/\dot{Q}$ and (**B**) alveolar deadspace. Areas of high $\dot{V}/\dot{Q}$ experience alveolar hyperventilation, and capillary blood leaves them with higher PaO_2 and lower $PaCO_2$ than in the normal units. Because these areas are poorly perfused, they impair the efficiency of overall gas exchange. When some alveoli are not perfused at all (alveolar deadspace), their ventilation is wasted, and overall ventilation must be increased to maintain normal CO_2 elimination.

C. The total volume of CO_2 in exhaled gas is equal to V_T times the fractional concentration of CO_2 in the exhaled gas.

$$(V_T)(F\bar{E}_{CO_2}) = \text{total } CO_2 \text{ exhaled} \tag{18}$$

D. This volume can be subdivided into the amount of CO_2 exhaled from deadspace and alveoli:

$$(V_T)(F\bar{E}_{CO_2}) = (V_A)(F_{A_{CO_2}}) + (V_D)(F_{D_{CO_2}}) \tag{19}$$

E. Because the concentration of CO_2 in exhaled deadspace gas is approximately zero, equation 19 can be rewritten as:

$$(V_T)(F\bar{E}_{CO_2}) = (V_A)(F_{A_{CO_2}}) \tag{20}$$

F. Because $V_A = V_T - V_D$, equation 20 may be rewritten as:

$$(V_T)(F\bar{E}_{CO_2}) = (V_T)(F_{A_{CO_2}}) - (V_D)(F_{A_{CO_2}}) \tag{21}$$

G. By rearrangement of and simplification of equation 21, the Bohr equation for the determination of the deadspace/tidal volume ratio (V_D/V_T ratio) is generated.

$$VD/VT = \frac{FACO_2 - \overline{FE}CO_2}{FACO_2} \qquad (22)$$

H. Because the concentration of CO_2 in the alveoli is equal to the concentration of CO_2 in the arterial blood and because the partial pressures of gases are proportional to their concentration, equation 22 may be rewritten as the Enghoff modification of the Bohr equation:

$$VD/VT = \frac{PaCO_2 - \overline{PE}CO_2}{PaCO_2} \qquad (23)$$

I. In all circumstances, as the deadspace increases, there is a widening of the $PaCO_2 - \overline{PE}CO_2$ gradient.
J. Normal VD/VT ratios are approximately 20% to 40%.

XI. **Calculation of the Deadspace/Tidal Volume Ratio**
  A. A *simultaneous* sampling of arterial blood and exhaled gas is obtained.
    1. The exhaled gas sample must be large enough to reflect a mean exhaled PCO_2 value.
    2. In spontaneously breathing patients, approximately 40 L of exhaled gas is collected. This is done to compensate for tidal volume variations.
    3. If a patient is being mechanically ventilated without spontaneous efforts with consistent tidal volumes, a 5-L sample is sufficient.
  B. The patient should be stable and quiet at the time the sample is obtained.
      Example:

$$VD/VT = \frac{PaCO_2 - \overline{PE}CO_2}{PaCO_2}$$

$$0.52 = \frac{42 - 20}{42}$$

XII. **Minute Volume–$PaCO_2$ Relationship**
  A. Because the arterial $PaCO_2$ level clinically defines the physiologic adequacy of ventilation, a relationship between total minute volume and arterial $PaCO_2$ must exist.
  B. In the average adult, a minute volume of 4 to 6 L maintains a $PaCO_2$ of 40 mm Hg.
  C. If the minute volume increases, the $PaCO_2$ should decrease, and if the minute volume decreases, the $PaCO_2$ should increase.
  D. It is generally accepted that with each doubling of the minute volume, the $PaCO_2$ decreases by approximately 10 mm Hg (Table 8-2).
  E. If there is a disparity between the minute volume and the expected $PaCO_2$, deadspace is most probably increased.
      Example:
      If the $PaCO_2$ is 42 mm Hg and the minute volume is 20 L, deadspace ventilation is increased. A $PaCO_2$ of approximately 20 mm Hg would be expected with a minute ventilation of 20 L.

TABLE **8-2**	
Normal Minute Volume–$PaCO_2$ Relationship	
VA(L/min)	$PaCO_2$ (mm Hg)
1.25	60
2.50	50
5.00	40
10.00	30
20.00	20

XIII. **Clinical Use of the Deadspace/Tidal Volume Ratios**
 A. Assessment of spontaneous ventilatory capabilities in patients being mechanically ventilated
  1. The V_D/V_T ratio is typically increased during mechanical ventilation and is considered normal up to 0.50.
  2. A V_D/V_T ratio <0.60 normally does not represent pulmonary pathology of sufficient magnitude to interfere with spontaneous ventilation.
  3. A V_D/V_T ratio of 0.60 to 0.80 represents significant disease and frequently interferes with an individual's ability to maintain prolonged spontaneous ventilation.
  4. A V_D/V_T ratio >0.80 normally requires mechanical ventilatory support.
 B. Evaluation of the presence of pulmonary embolism
  1. An increase in deadspace supports the diagnosis of pulmonary embolism.
  2. However, a definitive diagnosis cannot be made by deadspace studies alone.

XIV. **Guidelines for Differentiating Shunt-Producing From Deadspace-Producing Diseases**
 A. Deadspace-producing diseases
  1. Minute volume greatly increased with little or no decrease in Pa_{CO_2}.
  2. Although hypoxemia is present and correctable by oxygen therapy, minute ventilation changes are minimal when hypoxemia is corrected.
 B. Shunt-producing diseases
  1. Pa_{CO_2} decreases as minute volume increases.
  2. Assuming the hypoxemia is responsive, oxygen therapy will decrease myocardial and ventilatory work and relieve hypoxemia. Thus minute volume and Pa_{CO_2} return to normal.
  3. If hypoxemia is refractory, caused by true shunting, the application of PEEP or prone positioning is necessary to reverse the hypoxemia.

BIBLIOGRAPHY

Beachey W: *Respiratory Care Anatomy and Physiology: Foundations for Clinical Practice.* St. Louis, Mosby, 1998.

Burton GG, Hodgkin JE, Ward JJ: *Respiratory Care: A Guide to Clinical Practice,* ed 4. Philadelphia, JB Lippincott Co, 1997.

Cane RD, Shapiro BA, Harrison RA, et al: Minimizing errors in intrapulmonary shunt calculation. *Crit Care Med* 8:294-297, 1980.

Comroe JH: *Physiology of Respiration,* ed 2. Chicago, Year Book Medical Publishers, 1974.

Comroe JH, Forster RE II, Dubois AB, et al: *The Lung: Clinical Physiology and Pulmonary Function Tests,* ed 2. Chicago, Year Book Medical Publishers, 1962.

Guyton AC, Hall JE: *Textbook of Medical Physiology,* ed 10. Philadelphia, WB Saunders, 2000.

Hess D, MacIntyre N, Mishoe S, et al: *Respiratory Care: Principles and Practices.* St. Louis, Mosby, 2002.

Hicks GH: *Cardiopulmonary Anatomy and Physiology.* Philadelphia, WB Saunders, 2000.

Maxwell C, Hess D, Shefet D: Use of the arterial/alveolar oxygen tension ratio to predict the inspired oxygen concentration needed for a desired arterial oxygen tension. *Respir Care* 29:1135-1139, 1984.

Shapiro BA, Cane RD, Harrison RA, et al: Changes in intrapulmonary shunting with administration of 100 percent oxygen. *Chest* 77:138-141, 1980.

Shapiro BA, Harrison RA, Cane R, et al: *Clinical Application of Blood Gases,* ed 4. Chicago, Year Book Medical Publishers, 1989.

Shapiro BA, Harrison RA, Kacmarek RM, et al: *Clinical Application of Respiratory Care,* ed 4. Chicago, Year Book Medical Publishers, 1990.

Wilkins RL, Stoller JK, Scanlan CL: *Egan's Fundamentals of Respiratory Therapy,* ed 8. St. Louis, Mosby, 2003.

Chapter 9

Anatomy of the Cardiovascular System

I. Blood
   A. A heterogeneous substance composed of a fluid (plasma) and a cellular component (Figure 9-1).
   B. Plasma: Whole blood minus the cellular component.
      1. It is a pale yellow (strawlike) color.
      2. The three major body fluids are plasma, the interstitial fluid, and the intracellular fluid.
      3. Major constituents are water and chemical compounds (solutes).
         a. Water, the solvent, constitutes approximately 90% of plasma.
         b. The major solutes protein, foodstuffs, and electrolytes constitute approximately 10% of plasma.
      4. Plasma minus clotting factors is called *blood serum*.
   C. Cellular components: Red blood cells (RBCs), white blood cells (WBCs), and platelets are all generated in the red bone marrow from a common stem cell, the hemocytoblast (Figure 9-2).
      1. RBCs, also called erythrocytes, are biconcave disks with a diameter of 7 to 8 μm and a thickness of approximately 2 μm.
         a. Mature RBCs are anucleated (have no nucleus).
         b. A semipermeable membrane surrounds RBCs.
            (1) Placed in a hypotonic solution (<0.9% NaCl), they will swell and can rupture (hemolysis).
            (2) Placed in a hypertonic solution (>0.9% NaCl), they will shrivel (crenation).
         c. RBCs are relatively flexible and are able to accommodate changes in shape without rupturing. This becomes important when they pass through tight and/or irregular spots in the circulation (e.g., capillaries or sinusoids).
         d. RBCs are produced in myeloid tissue (red bone marrow), a process termed *erythropoiesis*.
         e. The normal number of RBCs is higher in males than in females.
            (1) Female: 4.1 to 5.1 million RBCs/mm^3
            (2) Male: 4.8 to 6.0 million RBCs/mm^3
         f. Reticulocytes are newly released RBCs that retain a small portion of the hemoglobin-forming endoplasmic reticulum.
            (1) In 2 to 3 days, formation of hemoglobin will be complete. At this point, the endoplasmic reticulum disappears, and the cell is a mature erythrocyte.
            (2) The percentage of total RBCs that are reticulocytes indicates the rate of erythropoiesis.

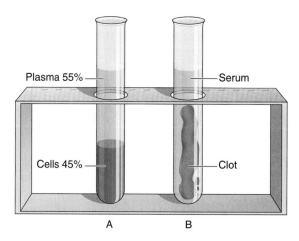

FIG. 9-1 Blood in a test tube. **A,** Shows the proportions of plasma and cells. **B,** Shows the presence of a blood clot in serum.

   (3) The normal range (percentage) of reticulocytes is 0.5% to 1.5% of the total number of RBCs.

    (a) More than 1.5% usually indicates increased erythropoiesis.

    (b) Less than 0.5% usually indicates decreased erythropoiesis.

  g. Hemoglobin is the major solute contained within the RBC.

   (1) The normal amount of hemoglobin contained in the blood is higher in males than in females:

    (a) Female: 12 to 14 g of hemoglobin/100 ml of blood

    (b) Male: 13 to 16 g of hemoglobin/100 ml of blood

  h. The hematocrit is the volume percentage of RBCs in whole blood (e.g., a hematocrit equal to 45 means that 45% of whole blood is RBCs by volume) (see Figure 9-1).

   (1) The normal hematocrit is higher in males than in females:

    (a) Female: 37 to 47

    (b) Male: 40 to 54

  i. Normally the RBC count is approximately one third the hemoglobin levels, and the hemoglobin levels are equal to approximately one third of the hematocrit. Hence given a hematocrit of 45%, an approximation of hemoglobin of 15 gm% and an RBC count of 5 million/mm^3 is made.

 2. WBCs, also called leukocytes, are of the following five types: polymorphonuclear neutrophils, eosinophils, and basophils and mononuclear monocytes and lymphocytes.

  a. Polymorphonuclear leukocytes

   (1) Are formed in myeloid tissue.

   (2) Have a multilobed nucleus.

   (3) Are collectively called *polys.*

   (4) Appear histologically to possess granulated cytoplasm and are collectively termed *granulocytes.*

   (5) All can perform phagocytosis.

   (6) Polymorphonuclear neutrophils

    (a) Have a diameter of approximately 10 μm.

    (b) Have a nucleus that contains one to five lobes.

    (c) Are highly phagocytic.

    (d) Make up 50% to 75% of the total number of leukocytes.

   (7) Polymorphonuclear eosinophils

    (a) Readily absorb an acid stain.

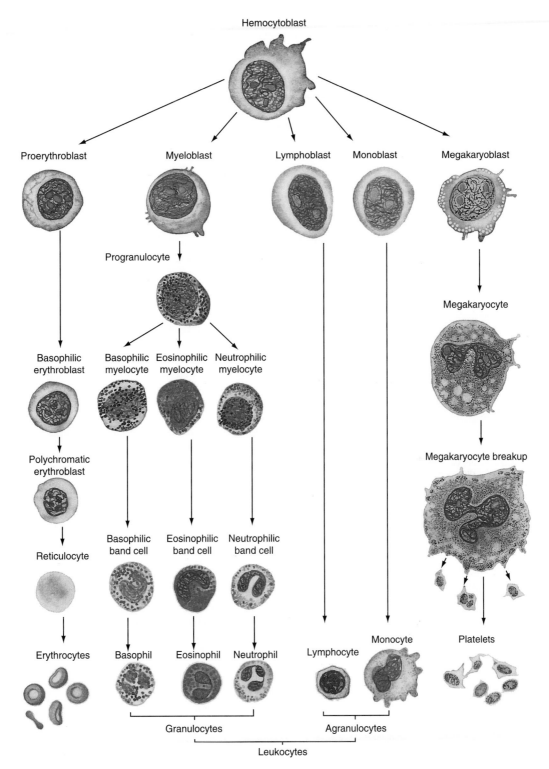

FIG. 9-2 Normal generation of the blood cell types (see text).

    (b) Have a bilobed nucleus.

    (c) Are implicated in parasitic and allergic processes.

    (d) Make up 2% to 4% of the total number of leukocytes.

    (e) Have a diameter of approximately 10 μm.

   (8) Polymorphonuclear basophils

    (a) Readily absorb a basic stain.

    (b) Have a nucleus that contains three to four lobes.

    (c) Contain heparin, which may serve to prevent coagulation of blood at sites of inflammation.

    (d) Make up <0.5% of the total number of leukocytes.

    (e) Have a diameter of approximately 10 μm.

  b. Mononuclear leukocytes

   (1) Are formed in lymphoid tissue.

   (2) Mononuclear monocytes

    (a) Have a diameter of 10 to 15 μm.

    (b) Have a crescent-shaped nucleus.

    (c) Have cytoplasm containing fine granules.

    (d) Are highly phagocytic cells.

    (e) Make up 3% to 8% of the total number of leukocytes.

   (3) Mononuclear lymphocytes

    (a) Have a diameter of approximately 6 to 9 μm.

    (b) Have a round nucleus.

    (c) Have cytoplasm that appears clear.

    (d) Form antibodies that remain intracellular (cellular antibodies) or form antibodies that are released into the bloodstream (circulating antibodies).

    (e) Make up 20% to 40% of the total number of leukocytes.

 c. Total WBC count has the normal range of 5,000 to 10,000 WBCs/mm^3.

 d. A differential count identifies the percentage of the total WBC count that each WBC type comprises (Table 9-1). (Note normal range [percent] in each of the WBC types previously described.)

 e. Megakaryocyte: A special type of blood cell.

  (1) Formed in myeloid tissue.

  (2) Fragments into small irregular pieces of protoplasm called *thrombocytes* or *platelets.*

   (a) Are 2 to 4 μm in diameter.

   (b) Have no nucleus.

   (c) Have a granular cytoplasm.

   (d) Normal platelet count is 200,000 to 350,000/mm^3.

   (e) Function in clot formation (hemostasis).

D. Total blood volume of an individual

 1. The total blood volume of an individual is equal to approximately 60 to 80 ml of blood/kg of body weight, which is equal to approximately 5 L in a normal man.

TABLE **9-1**

Normal Function and Percentage Composition of Leukocytes

Type	Function	Percentage Composition
Neutrophil	Phagocytosis	50-75
Eosinophil	Hypersensitivity reaction	2-4
Basophil	Anticoagulation	<0.5
Monocyte	Phagocytosis	3-8
Lymphocyte	Antibody formation	20-40

2. This relationship varies inversely with the amount of excess body fat; in other words, an obese individual has less blood volume per kilogram than a slender individual and vice versa.

II. **The Blood Vessels (Figure 9-3)**
   A. The blood vessels consist of a closed system of connected arteries, arterioles, capillaries, venules, and veins.
   B. *Arteries* contain three characteristic layers: tunica adventitia, tunica media, and tunica intima.
      1. Tunica adventitia (external layer)
         a. It consists of connective tissue surrounding a network of collagenous and elastic fibers.
         b. It supports and protects the blood vessels.

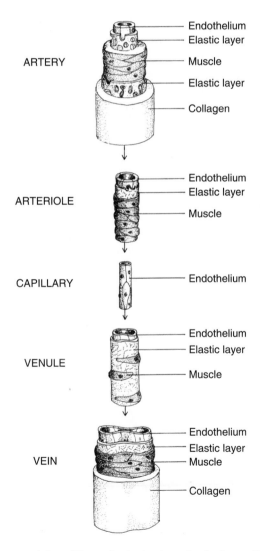

FIG. 9-3 Schematic representation of the anatomic structure of major types of blood vessels (see text).

    c. It contains vasa vasorum, fine vessels that serve the tunica adventitia with its blood supply.

    d. It contains lymphatic vessels and nerve fibers.

  2. Tunica media (middle layer)

    a. It is the thickest layer of the artery.

    b. It is composed of concentrically arranged smooth muscle and elastic fibers.

    c. Nerve fibers contained in tunica adventitia terminate in the smooth muscle layer of the tunica media.

  3. Tunica intima (internal layer)

    a. It is the thinnest layer of the artery.

    b. It consists of a flat layer of simple squamous cells called the *endothelium*:

      (1) A fine layer of connective tissue supports the endothelium.

      (2) A longitudinally placed network of elastic fibers surrounds the connective tissue.

    c. Common to all blood vessels, the endothelium is even continuous with the endocardium of the heart, providing a smooth containment for blood travel.

C. Large arteries: Termed *elastic arteries* because the tunica media has less smooth muscle and more elastic fibers.

D. Medium-sized arteries: Sometimes called *nutrient arteries* because they control the flow of blood to various regional areas of the body. Their ability to regulate blood flow lies in a tunica media, which is composed almost entirely of smooth muscle.

E. *Arterioles* (small arteries)

  1. The arterioles have a thin tunica intima and adventitia but have a thick, smooth muscle layer in the tunica media.

  2. The arterioles range in diameter from 20 to 50 μm.

  3. The tunica media is extensively innervated by postsynaptic sympathetic nerve fibers (Figure 9-4).

  4. Because of the extensive innervation and abundance of smooth muscle, the arterioles control local blood flow to the capillary beds.

  5. The arterioles are frequently called the *resistance vessels*. By vasomotion, they control the rate of arterial runoff (the rate at which blood leaves the arterial tree) and thereby arterial blood volume and, to a great extent, blood pressure.

  6. The arterioles terminate in either metarterioles or capillaries.

    a. Metarterioles range in diameter from 10 to 20 μm.

    b. Metarterioles can bypass a capillary bed entirely by shunting blood directly to the venules.

    c. Metarterioles can also allow blood to pass from arterioles to capillaries.

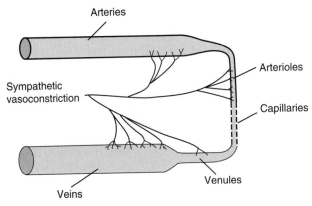

FIG. 9-4 Sympathetic innervation of the systemic circulation.

F. *Capillaries*
  1. Capillaries consist only of tunica intima.
  2. They vary in diameter from 5 to 10 μm.
  3. Where capillaries originate from arterioles or metarterioles, there frequently is a small band of smooth muscle called the *precapillary sphincter.*
     a. This sphincter controls blood flow through the distal capillary.
     b. It is responsive (vasoactive) to local P_{CO_2}, P_{O_2}, pH, and temperature.
  4. Capillaries frequently are called *exchange vessels* because they are the site of gas, fluid, nutrient, and waste exchange (Figure 9-5).
     a. An intracellular cleft lies between the individual squames comprising the endothelium.
        (1) They are approximately 50 to 60 Å wide.
        (2) They act as pores through which substances can move into and out of the capillaries.
     b. The basement membrane usually is continuous in the capillaries and may limit movement of substances into and out of the capillaries.
G. *Veins* consist of a tunica adventitia, media, and intima, but each layer is thinner than its counterpart in the arteries.
  1. Tunica adventitia
     a. Is one to five times as thick as the tunica media.
     b. Is made up of connective, elastic, and smooth muscle tissue.
  2. Tunica media
     a. Is made up of concentrically arranged smooth muscle, collagenous, and elastic tissue.
     b. Is innervated by postsynaptic fibers of the sympathetic nervous system (see Figure 9-4).
        (1) Veins are not as extensively innervated as arteries.
        (2) By venodilation or venoconstriction, veins can alter venous blood volume and "venous return."
  3. Tunica intima
     a. Consists of endothelial cells supported by delicate elastic fibers and connective tissue.

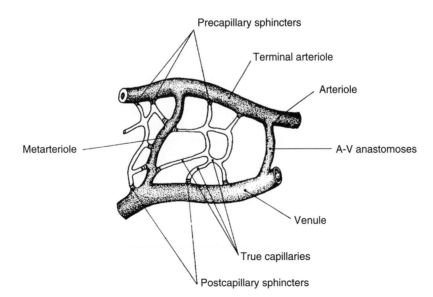

FIG. 9-5 Schematic representation of the vascular components involved in the regulation of blood flow through the systemic capillary beds (the microcirculation).

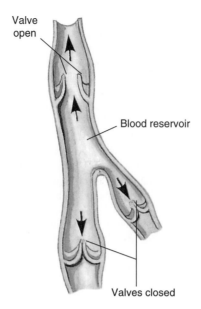

Valve
open

Blood reservoir

Valves closed

FIG. 9-6 Interior of vein.

   H. All vessels of the venous system generally have smaller amounts of elastic and smooth muscle tissue than their arterial counterparts.

   I. *Venules* (small veins) have the three characteristic layers, but they are thin and almost indistinguishable.

   J. Veins are called *capacitance vessels*, or *reservoir vessels*, because 70% to 75% of the blood volume exists in the venous system.

   K. Veins contained in the periphery of the body contain one-way valves (Figure 9-6).
      1. Valves are formed by duplication of endothelial lining of veins.
      2. Valves are semilunar and prevent retrograde flow of blood.
      3. Valves are found in veins >2 mm in diameter and exist in areas subjected to muscular pressure (e.g., arms and legs).
      4. Valves are absent in veins <1 mm in diameter and in areas such as the abdominal and thoracic cavities.

III. The Lymphatic Vessels
   A. These vessels are a type of circulatory system that collects fluid, protein, lipids, and other material in the interstitial space and returns them to the venous vasculature.

   B. Lymphatic vessels originate as blindly ending vessels called *lymphatic capillaries.*
      1. They have no basement membrane and consist only of loosely fitting endothelial cells.
      2. They are invested in every tissue of the body except for cartilage, bone, and epithelium and are importantly absent in the central nervous system.

   C. Lymphatic capillaries drain into larger lymphatic vessels, which take on three characteristic layers similar to those of the veins.
      1. Larger lymphatic channels contain smooth muscle, elastic, fibrous, and connective tissue.
      2. These vessels resemble the veins except that the three layers composing the lymphatic vessels are thinner and less developed.
      3. One-way semilunar valves are found approximately every millimeter and are more frequent in the lymphatic vessels than in the veins.

   D. The larger lymphatic vessels drain into lymph nodes (Figure 9-7).
      1. Lymph nodes are found in the neck, axilla, groin, thorax, breast, arms, and mouth.
      2. Lymph nodes are bean or oval shaped.
      3. Lymph moves into the lymph nodes via afferent lymphatic channels.

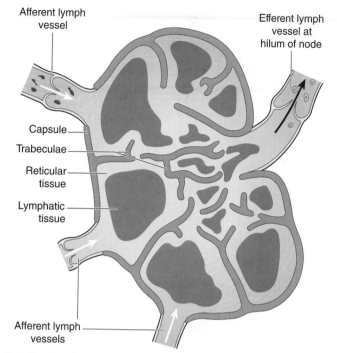

FIG. 9-7 Section of a lymph node. Arrows show the direction of flow of the lymph.

    a. The lymph is exposed to resident phagocytic reticular endothelial cells lining the sinus of the nodes.

    b. The lymph is filtered and exits from the lymph node via efferent lymphatic channels.

E. The large efferent lymphatic vessels join one of two major lymphatic ducts, either the right lymphatic duct or the thoracic duct (Figure 9-8):

  1. Right lymphatic duct

    a. Drains right upper quadrant of the trunk.

    b. Drains right side of the head and neck.

    c. Drains filtered lymph into the right subclavian vein.

  2. Thoracic duct

    a. Drains remainder of the body.

    b. Is the largest lymphatic vessel but is smaller than either vena cava.

      (1) The duct is 15 to 18 in. long.

      (2) It originates in the lumbar region of the abdominal cavity and ascends to the neck.

    c. Drains filtered lymph into the left subclavian vein.

F. Total lymphatic flow varies from 2 to 4 L/day, an amount roughly equal to the total plasma volume. This suggests that 50% to 100% of the plasma fluid volume leaves the vascular proper daily and is ultimately returned to the venous circulation.

G. Having no true pump to create lymphatic flow, the lymphatic system depends on the contraction of skeletal muscle, intrathoracic pressure changes, and the pulsation of neighboring arteries to assist the movement of lymph.

IV. The Heart

  A. The heart is a muscular pump that maintains circulation of the blood through the vessels to all parts of the body.

  B. The heart is located between the lungs in the mediastinum (Figure 9-9).

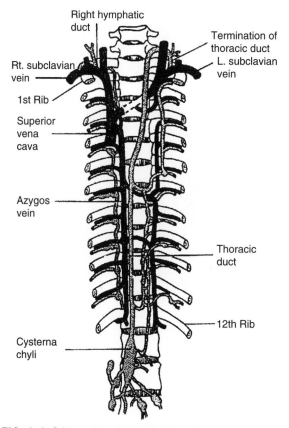

FIG. 9-8 Origin and position of the thoracic duct and right lymphatic duct.

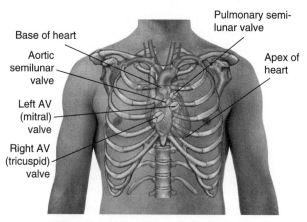

FIG. 9-9 Location of the heart in the thorax.

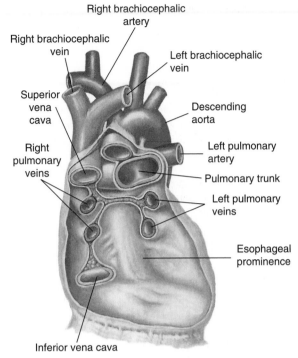

Right brachiocephalic artery

Right brachiocephalic vein

Left brachiocephalic vein

Superior vena cava

Descending aorta

Right pulmonary veins

Left pulmonary artery

Pulmonary trunk

Left pulmonary veins

Esophageal prominence

Inferior vena cava

FIG. 9-10 Heart removed from the pericardial sac.

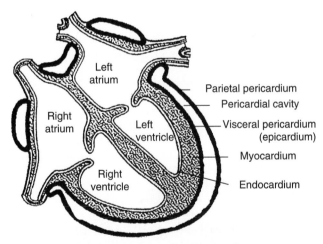

Left atrium

Right atrium

Left ventricle

Right ventricle

Parietal pericardium

Pericardial cavity

Visceral pericardium (epicardium)

Myocardium

Endocardium

FIG. 9-11 Heart wall and pericardium.

C. The apex is the inferior portion of the heart and is directed inferiorly, anteriorly, and to the left, with the majority of it located left of the midline.
D. The base is the superior aspect of the heart.
E. The heart is approximately the size of the clenched fist.
F. A loose nondistensible sac called the *pericardium* encases the heart (Figure 9-10).
G. Layers of pericardium (Figure 9-11)
　1. *Fibrous pericardium*
　　a. Is the outermost layer of pericardium.

b. Attaches to the great vessels (major vessels entering and exiting from the heart) of the heart and loosely encases the heart proper.

c. Is made of white fibrous tissue that protects and anchors the heart to some extent.

d. Is externally attached to the sternum, vertebral column, central tendon, and left hemidiaphragm.

2. *Parietal serous pericardium*

a. Lines the fibrous pericardium, to which it is closely adherent.

b. A moist serous membrane that forms a smooth surface to reduce frictional resistances.

c. Produces a small volume of serous fluid called *pericardial fluid.*

d. Becomes continuous with the visceral serous pericardium.

3. *Visceral serous pericardium*

a. The visceral serous pericardium is directly adherent to the heart.

b. It is also known as the *epicardium* of the heart.

c. It is a serous membrane that produces serous pericardial fluid.

d. The small space between visceral and parietal serous pericardial layers is called the *pericardial space.*

4. The fact that the visceral and parietal serous pericardial layers are smooth membranes with a small volume of lubricating pericardial fluid between them allows the heart to move freely in the pericardial sac opposed by reduced frictional forces.

5. Abnormal fluid and/or blood accumulation in the pericardial space may impede normal filling of the heart and hence compromise cardiac output, a condition called *cardiac tamponade.*

H. The heart wall has three distinctive layers (see Figure 9-11):

1. *Epicardium*, or visceral serous pericardium

a. Is the most superficial layer.

b. Is a transparent serous sheet lying on a delicate network of connective tissue.

c. Contains fat, coronary blood vessels, and coronary nerves, which are observable on the cardiac surface.

2. *Myocardium*

a. Is located just deep to the epicardium and is the middle layer of the heart wall.

b. Is composed almost exclusively of cardiac muscle with the exception of coronary blood vessels.

c. Is the thickest and most substantial of the three cardiac layers.

3. *Endocardium*

a. It is the deepest cardiac layer, the internal lining of the heart.

b. It is a smooth layer of squamous epithelium.

c. It is continuous with endothelial lining of all blood vessels.

d. Duplication of this layer in the heart forms the cardiac valves.

I. The heart has four chambers (Figure 9-12).

1. It has two superior chambers, or atria.

2. It has two inferior chambers, or ventricles.

3. Externally the two atria are separated from the two ventricles by a groove that circumscribes the heart, the coronary sulcus.

4. The roots of the aorta and the pulmonary artery externally separate the two atria from each other.

5. Externally the two ventricles are separated from each other by a groove, the interventricular sulcus.

6. A wall, the interatrial septum, internally separates the two atria from each other.

a. The fossa ovalis, a depression in the atrial septal wall, is the remnant of the fetal foramen ovale.

7. Internally the two ventricles are separated from each other by a fibrous and muscular interventricular septum. It is continuous with the interatrial septum through its fibrous portion (see Figures 9-11 and 9-12).

8. Internally the atria are separated from the ventricles by a structure known as the *fibroskeleton* of the heart (Figure 9-13).

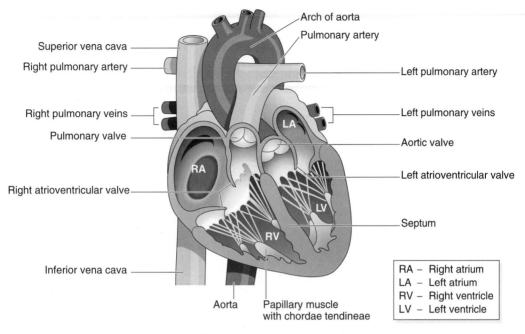

Superior vena cava

Right pulmonary artery

Right pulmonary veins

Pulmonary valve

Right atrioventricular valve

Inferior vena cava

Arch of aorta

Pulmonary artery

Left pulmonary artery

Left pulmonary veins

Aortic valve

Left atrioventricular valve

Septum

Aorta

Papillary muscle with chordae tendineae

RA – Right atrium
LA – Left atrium
RV – Right ventricle
LV – Left ventricle

FIG. 9-12 Interior of the heart.

Anatomic components of the heart

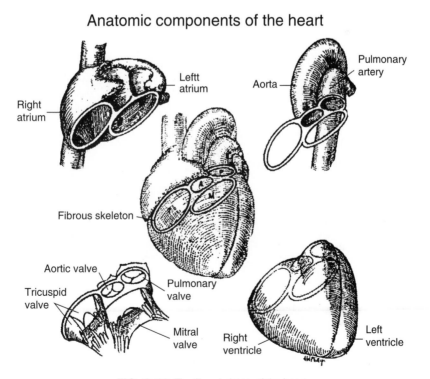

Right atrium

Leftt atrium

Aorta

Pulmonary artery

Fibrous skeleton

Aortic valve

Tricuspid valve

Pulmonary valve

Mitral valve

Right ventricle

Left ventricle

FIG. 9-13 The fibroskeleton of the heart.

a. The fibroskeleton consists of fibrous rings (which surround the two atrioventricular [AV] cardiac valves, the pulmonic semilunar and aortic semilunar valves), fibrous interventricular septum, right and left trigone, and tendon of conus.
   (1) The right fibrous trigone consists of fibrous tissue that connects the two AV rings, fibrous interventricular septum, and ring of the aortic semilunar valve.
   (2) The left fibrous trigone consists of fibrous tissue that connects the fibrous ring of the left AV valve with the aortic semilunar valve.
   (3) The tendon of conus is fibrous tissue that connects the fibrous ring of the pulmonic semilunar valve with the ring surrounding the aortic semilunar valve.
b. Functions of the fibroskeleton
   (1) Houses the four cardiac valves.
   (2) Serves as the origin of and point of insertion for atrial and ventricular bands of muscle.
   (3) Electrically isolates atrial muscle bundles from ventricular muscle bundles.
      (a) The fibroskeleton is bridged (penetrated) only by the common bundle branch of the electrical conduction system of the heart, called the *bundle of His.*
      (b) This arrangement allows repolarization and depolarization of the atria separate from the ventricles.
9. The *right atrium* is positioned atop the right ventricle (Figure 9-14).
   a. It is anterior to the left atrium because the heart is rotated to the left.
      (1) Thus the bulk of the anterior surface of the heart is composed of the right side of the heart (i.e., right atrium and ventricle).
      (2) Most of the posterior surface of the heart is composed of the left side of the heart (i.e., left atrium and ventricle).
   b. The right atrium is larger than the left atrium and has a thinner wall.
      (1) The right atrial wall is approximately 2 mm thick.

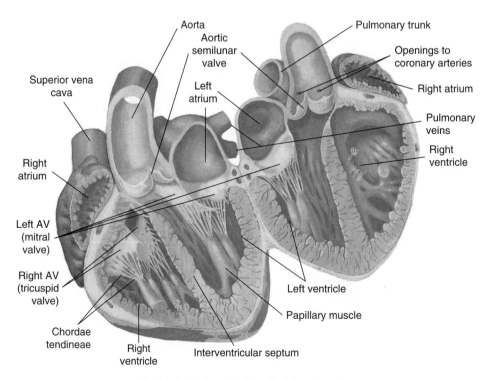

FIG. 9-14 Heart cut to show the internal anatomy.

      (2) The atrial musculature is divided into deep atrial muscle, which encircles each atrium individually, and superficial atrial muscle, which encircles both atria.

      (3) The deep and superficial muscle fibers run perpendicularly to one another and originate and insert on the fibroskeleton of the heart.

      (4) Therefore contraction of the two major groups of atrial muscle fibers tends to decrease the size of the respective atria in all dimensions.

  c. The cavity of the right atrium consists of two parts:

      (1) The major cavity of the right atrium, or sinus venarum.

      (2) The smaller cavity, which appears externally as a pouch, called the *right auricle*. (*Note:* Auricle is a term formerly used to denote the entire atrium.)

  d. The right atrium accepts venous blood from the following veins:

      (1) The superior vena cava, which opens into the superior and posterior portions of the major cavity of the right atrium.

      (2) The inferior vena cava, which opens into the most inferior portion of the right atrium near the interatrial septal wall.

      (3) The coronary sinus (of the coronary circulation), which opens into the right atrium between the tricuspid valve and the opening of the inferior vena cava.

10. The *left atrium* is positioned atop the left ventricle (see Figure 9-14).

  a. The left atrium is smaller than the right atrium and has a thicker wall.

      (1) The left atrial wall is approximately 3 mm thick.

      (2) The left atrial muscle fibers are divided into deep and superficial muscle groups and have an arrangement similar to that of the right atrium.

  b. The cavity of the left atrium consists of two parts:

      (1) The major cavity of the left atrium.

      (2) The left auricle, which appears externally as a pouchlike structure.

  c. The left atrium accepts arterial blood from the four pulmonary veins, which open into its superior and posterior aspects.

11. Right ventricle (see Figure 9-14).

  a. It constitutes most of the anterior surface of heart.

  b. The right ventricular wall is one third the thickness of the left ventricular wall.

  c. The ventricular musculature is classically separated into superficial and deep muscle groups.

      (1) Superficial and deep muscle groups appear to originate on the fibroskeleton of the heart.

      (2) Superficial fibers follow a clockwise spiral course to the apex of the heart. At the apex, these fibers turn inward and follow a spiraled course counterclockwise and upward toward the base of the heart to insert on the fibroskeleton.

      (3) Deep fibers follow a similar course to the superficial ventricular fibers, with three exceptions:

         (a) The spiraled course of the deep fibers is in a direction opposite to that of the superficial fibers.

         (b) Deep fibers may not follow a course all the way to the apex of the heart before starting to ascend.

         (c) Deep fibers may insert into the cardiac fibroskeleton, papillary muscles, or trabeculae carneae.

            (i) Papillary muscles are fingerlike projections of cardiac muscle located in the cavity of each ventricle.

            (ii) Trabeculae carneae are irregular bundles of muscle that form ridges along the internal wall of the ventricular cavity.

      (4) Contraction of ventricular muscle fibers tends to decrease the internal anteroposterior and transverse diameters significantly but leaves the vertical diameter virtually unchanged (Figure 9-15).

  d. The right ventricle receives venous blood from the right atrium through an opening called the *right AV orifice*.

      (1) A fibrous ring that is a part of the cardiac fibroskeleton surrounds this orifice.

(2) The right AV orifice is approximately 4 cm in diameter.
(3) The right AV orifice contains the tricuspid valve.
    (a) The tricuspid valve contains three cusps, each fused at its origin in the circumference of the AV ring.
    (b) The cusps are formed by a duplication of the endocardial layer of the heart and are supported with fibrous tissue.
    (c) The three cusps collectively have a funnel shape that projects into the cavity of the right ventricle.
    (d) The free borders (inferior border) of each cusp have an attached fibrous cordlike structure, the chordae tendineae.
    (e) The chordae tendineae are in turn attached to the intraventricular papillary muscles.
    (f) The chordae tendineae commonly cross, passing from one of the cusps to a group of papillary muscles on the opposite side of the ventricle.

e. The cavity of the right ventricle is lined with muscular ridges (trabeculae carneae) and papillary muscle covered by endocardium.
  (1) The cavity of the right ventricle has a bellows or U shape (see Figure 9-15).
  (2) The muscular arrangement and shape of the right ventricle are well suited to its function of pumping blood under low pressure.

f. Blood exits from the cavity of the right ventricle by passing into the pulmonary artery via an opening called the *orifice of the pulmonary trunk.*
  (1) A fibrous ring, a component of the cardiac fibroskeleton, surrounds this orifice.
  (2) The pulmonary orifice is located in the superior, anterior, and medial sections of the right ventricle.
  (3) The pulmonary orifice contains the pulmonic semilunar valve.
    (a) The pulmonic semilunar valve is composed of three half-moon–shaped cusps.

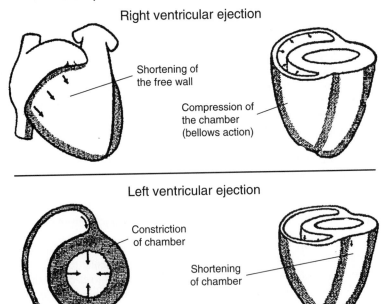

Components of ventricular contraction

Right ventricular ejection

Shortening of the free wall

Compression of the chamber (bellows action)

Left ventricular ejection

Constriction of chamber

Shortening of chamber

Traction on right ventricular wall

FIG. 9-15 Components of ventricular contraction.

(b) This valve resembles the type found in the large veins of the periphery.

(c) This valve, like the AV valves, is formed by duplication of the endocardial layer and is supported by fibrous tissue.

12. Left ventricle (see Figure 9-14)

a. It constitutes most of the posterior surface of the heart.

b. The left ventricular wall is three times the thickness of the right ventricular wall.

c. Left ventricular muscle fibers are part of the continuum of muscle circumscribing both ventricles and cannot be anatomically separated from right ventricular fibers. (*Note:* The arrangement of the ventricular muscle fibers is described in the foregoing section on the right ventricle.)

d. The left ventricle receives arterial blood from the left atrium through the left AV orifice.

(1) A fibrous ring, which is one of the components of the cardiac fibroskeleton, surrounds this orifice.

(2) Contained in the left AV orifice is the bicuspid or mitral valve.

(a) The mitral valve is composed of two cusps.

(b) The anatomic structure is similar to that of the previously discussed tricuspid valve except that the chordae tendineae are thicker and stronger in the left ventricle.

e. The cavity of the left ventricle is lined with muscular ridges (trabeculae carneae), which appear in a more numerous and dense arrangement than in the right ventricle. The endocardial layer covers the papillary muscles with the corresponding thick chordae tendineae, along with the trabeculae carneae.

(1) The cavity of the left ventricle is conical.

(2) The arrangement of the more developed left ventricular musculature coupled with its conical shape lends well to its function of pumping blood under high pressure (see Figure 9-15).

f. Blood exits from the cavity of the left ventricle into the root of the aorta by passing through the aortic opening.

(1) A fibrous ring, a component of the cardiac fibroskeleton, surrounds this opening.

(2) The aortic opening exists in the superior, posterior, and medial sections of the left ventricle.

(3) The aortic opening contains the aortic semilunar valve.

(a) The aortic semilunar valve is anatomically similar to the pulmonic semilunar valve except that the aortic cusps are stronger, larger, and thicker.

J. The coronary circulation (Figure 9-16)

1. Blood supply to the heart is delivered via the right and left coronary arteries, which have their origins in the root of the aorta just distal to the aortic semilunar valve.

a. The right coronary artery bifurcates into the posterior (interventricular) descending and marginal arteries serving the majority of the right side of the heart with its blood supply.

b. The left coronary artery bifurcates into the anterior (interventricular) descending and circumflex arteries serving the majority of the left side of the heart with its blood supply.

c. The aforementioned four arteries divide numerous times over the epicardial layer of the heart and ultimately penetrate the myocardium, giving way to a typical vascular bed and providing the myocardial perfusion.

d. The coronary circulation terminates in the large coronary veins and the anterior cardiac vein that drain into the coronary sinus and right auricle, respectively. The thebesian veins of the coronary circulation empty a minor amount of venous blood directly into the right and left ventricles.

e. It is worth noting that the normal coronary circulation, despite having a significant cardiac distribution, does not possess many anastomoses, hence making the tissue it serves (the myocardium) prone to ischemia and infarction should the local arterial vessels be compromised.

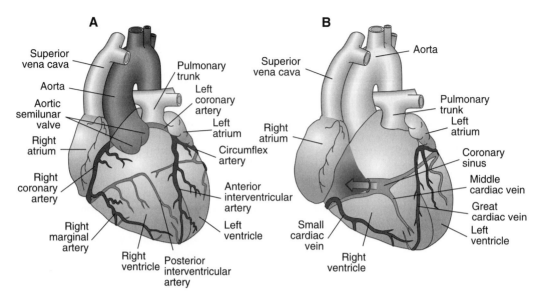

FIG. 9-16 Coronary circulation. **A,** Arteries. **B,** Veins. Both illustrations are anterior views of the heart. Vessels near the anterior surface are more darkly colored than vessels of the posterior surface seen through the heart.

BIBLIOGRAPHY

Ayres SM, Gafford F, Sterling M, Adler D: *Care of the Critically Ill*, ed 3. St. Louis, Mosby, 1987.

Cottrell GP: *Cardiopulmonary Anatomy and Physiology for Respiratory Care Practitioners*. Philadelphia, FA Davis, 2000.

DesJardins TR: *Cardiopulmonary Anatomy and Physiology: Essentials for Respiratory Care*, ed 4. New York, Delmar Publishers, 2001.

Feneis H: *Pocket Atlas of Human Anatomy*, ed 4. New York, Thieme Medical Publishers, 2000.

Gosling JA: *Human Anatomy*, ed 4. St. Louis, Mosby, 2002.

Grant JCB: *Grant's Atlas of Anatomy*, ed 9. Baltimore, Williams & Wilkins, 1994.

Grindel CG, Crowley LV: *Anatomy and Physiology*. Baltimore, Lippincott Williams & Wilkins, 1997.

Guyton AJ, Hall JE: *Textbook of Medical Physiology*, ed 10. Philadelphia, Elsevier Health Sciences Division, 2000.

Hicks GH: *Cardiopulmonary Anatomy and Physiology*. Philadelphia, Elsevier Health Sciences Division, 1999.

Jacob SW, Francone CA, Lossow WJ: *Structure and Function in Man*, ed 5. Philadelphia, Elsevier Health Sciences Division, 1982.

Little RC: *Physiology of the Heart and Circulation*. St. Louis, Mosby, 1988.

Matthews LR: *Cardiopulmonary Anatomy and Physiology*. Philadelphia, Lippincott Williams & Wilkins, 1996.

McLaughlin AJ: *Essentials of Physiology for Advanced Respiratory Therapy*. St. Louis, Mosby, 1977.

Moffett DF, Moffett SB, Schauf CL: *Human Physiology: Foundations and Frontiers*, ed 2. St. Louis, Mosby-Yearbook Inc., 1993.

Moore KL, Agur AMR: *Essential Clinical Anatomy*, ed 2. Philadelphia, Lippincott Williams & Wilkins, 2002.

Shapiro BA, Harrison RA, Kacmarek RM, et al: *Clinical Applications of Respiratory Care*, ed 4. Philadelphia, Elsevier Health Sciences Division, 1990.

Sheldon RL, Spearman CB: *Egan's Fundamentals of Respiratory Therapy*, ed 4. St. Louis, Mosby, 1982.

Shier D: *Human Anatomy and Physiology*, ed 9. New York, McGraw-Hill, 2002.

Srebnik HH: *Concepts in Anatomy*. New York, Kluwer Academic Publishers, 2002.

Thibodeau GA, Patton KT: *Anthony's Textbook of Anatomy & Physiology*, ed 15. St. Louis, Mosby-Yearbook, Inc., 1994.

Waugh A, Grant A: *Anatomy and Physiology in Health and Illness*, ed 9. Philadelphia, Elsevier Health Sciences Division, 2001.

Williams PL: *Gray's Anatomy: The Anatomical Basis of Medicine and Surgery*, ed 38. Philadelphia, Elsevier Health Sciences Division, 1995.

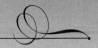
Physiology of the Cardiovascular System

I. **Functions of the Blood**
   A. Primary vehicle of transport of substances in the body.
      1. Respiratory gases (e.g., oxygen and carbon dioxide)
      2. Circulating antibodies and leukocytes involved in the body's defense mechanisms
      3. Platelets and clotting factors involved in hemostasis
      4. Cellular nutrients to all of the cells
      5. Cellular waste products away from the cells
      6. Electrolytes, proteins, water, and hormones, all of which contribute to the numerous complex functions of blood.

II. **Anatomic Classification of the Vascular Bed (Figure 10-1)**
   A. The typical vascular bed begins with the aorta or pulmonary artery.
   B. Branches from either of these main arteries are called *large arteries*.
   C. The larger arteries continue to branch to medium arteries.
   D. The medium arteries branch further to the arterioles.
   E. The end of the arteriolar bed is marked by a thick band of smooth muscle called the *precapillary sphincter*, which marks the initial portion of the microcirculation.
   F. The arterioles branch to metarterioles or directly to capillaries.
   G. Distal to the precapillary sphincter are the capillaries.
   H. Many capillaries join to form venules.
   I. Numerous venules join to form small veins, which in turn join to form large veins.
   J. Large veins join the major veins of the body, either the superior vena cava, inferior vena cava, or pulmonary veins.

III. **Functional Divisions of the Vascular Bed**
   A. Distribution, resistance, exchange, and capacitance vessels
      1. Distribution vessels begin with the major arteries and include the large and medium arteries.
         a. These vessels distribute the cardiac output (CO) to the various organ systems.
         b. These vessels typically are under an elevated pressure, contain a relatively small percentage of total blood volume, and are highly elastic.
      2. Resistance vessels begin with the arterioles and end with the precapillary sphincter.
         a. These vessels have the largest proportion of smooth muscle constituting the vascular wall of any of the blood vessels.
         b. Through contraction and relaxation of the smooth muscle, the resistance vessels can regulate the distribution of blood to the various capillary beds.

169

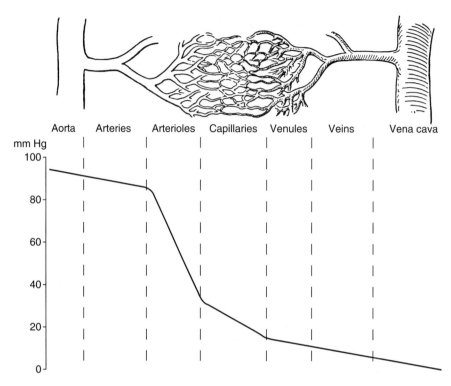

FIG. 10-1 Typical vascular bed with graphic representation of pressure decrease across the systemic circulation.

      c. The resistance vessels are the major source of peripheral resistance and predominantly function in arterial blood pressure regulation.

   3. The exchange vessels are the capillaries.

      a. Fluid, gas, nutrient, and waste exchange occurs in these vessels.

      b. Exchange of these substances occurs between capillary blood and interstitial fluid. Exchange then occurs from the interstitial fluid to the cells that make up the tissue.

      c. The major process underlying exchange in the capillaries is diffusion.

      d. Because of the vast distribution of capillary beds, the process of diffusion is sufficiently fast enough to maintain cellular metabolism.

   4. Capacitance vessels include the venules through the large veins and encompass the total venous system.

      a. Capacitance vessels serve as channels for blood return to the heart from the various capillary beds.

      b. These vessels are called *capacitance*, or *reservoir, vessels* because they contain most (70% to 75%) of the total blood volume.

      c. The capacitance vessels are typically under low pressure, contain a large blood volume, and are relatively inelastic compared with their arterial counterparts.

   5. Distribution (volume) of blood in the components of the vascular system varies widely depending on the function of the component (Table 10-1).

IV. Vascular System: Systemic and Pulmonary Circulations (Figure 10-2)

  A. Systemic circulation

   1. Systemic circulation begins with the systemic pump, the left ventricle, and continues to a typical vascular bed, ending with the right atrium.

      a. Functions of systemic circulation:

TABLE **10-1**		
Estimated Distribution of Blood in Vascular System of the Hypothetical Adult Man		

	Volume	
Region	ml	%
Heart (diastole)	360	7.2
Pulmonary		
Arteries	130	2.6
Capillaries	110	2.2
Veins	200	4.0
Subtotal	440	8.8
Systemic		
Aorta and large arteries	300	6.0
Small arteries	400	8.0
Capillaries	300	6.0
Small veins	2300	46.0
Large veins	900	18.0
Subtotal	4200	84.0
Grand total	5000	100

Age, 40 years; weight, 75 kg; surface area, 1.85 m².
From Mountcastle VB: *Medical Physiology*, ed 14. St. Louis, Mosby, 1980.

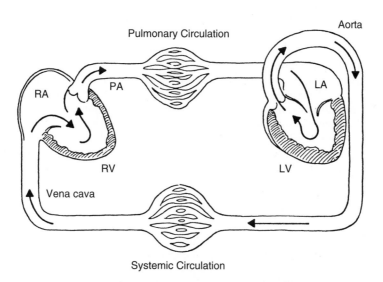

FIG. 10-2 The pulmonary and systemic circulation.

    (1)   To distribute left ventricular CO so that each region of the body receives an adequate volume of blood per unit time.
    (2)   To perfuse individual tissues so that cellular metabolism is maintained.
    (3)   To return venous blood to the right side of the heart to maintain right ventricular output.
  b. The velocity of the blood flow varies inversely with the total cross-sectional area through which blood flows at a given time (Figure 10-3). This physical law, coupled with the architecture of the vascular system, nicely accomplishes the three functions of the systemic circulation.
    (1)   The velocity of the blood flowing through the aorta is fast.

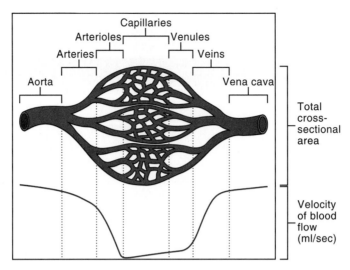

FIG. 10-3 The estimated cross-sectional area and linear velocity for the cardiovascular tree. The total flow is the same throughout the system, but the linear velocity in a segment depends on the total cross-sectional area of the many parallel branches.

(2) The velocity of blood flow progressively slows from the arteries to arterioles.

(3) As the extraordinarily large cross-sectional area of the systemic capillaries is encountered, the velocity of blood flow attains it slowest rate.

(4) The velocity of the blood flow progressively increases from venules to veins as the cross-sectional area markedly decreases.

(5) As a result blood is quickly distributed (arteries), spends the greatest amount of time in the parenchymal tissue of the circulation (capillaries) serving the metabolic needs of the tissues, and then is quickly returned (veins) for recirculation.

2. Control of systemic circulation is governed by four major mechanisms: autonomic control, hormonal control, local control, and mechanical factors.

   a. The arterial portion of the systemic circulation is basically governed by three mechanisms: autonomic nervous system, hormonal control, and local control.

     (1) Arteries and arterioles are innervated extensively and virtually exclusively by postganglionic fibers of the sympathetic nervous system.

     (2) The arterial vasculature of different tissues varies in the degree of sympathetic innervation.

       (a) The largest degree of sympathetic innervation is to the arterial vasculature perfusing the skin.

       (b) The degree of sympathetic innervation steadily decreases through the arterial vasculature perfusing spleen, mesenteric vessels, and kidneys.

       (c) A smaller degree of sympathetic innervation exists in the muscles.

       (d) The least degree of sympathetic innervation exists in the vessels perfusing the heart and brain. Furthermore, these vessels have a small degree of parasympathetic innervation.

     (3) Sympathetic stimulation of blood vessels results in smooth muscle contraction and vasoconstriction.

       (a) This principally affects the resistance vessels because of their large component of smooth muscle.

       (b) Tonic sympathetic stimulation of arterial blood vessels results in a given arteriolar caliber.

         (i) Increased sympathetic stimulation above this tonic level results in vasoconstriction and an increase in resistance to flow through these vessels.

(ii)   Decreased sympathetic stimulation below this tonic level results in vasodilation and a decrease in resistance to flow through these vessels.

(iii)   Because of differing degrees of sympathetic innervation in the different tissues, general sympathetic stimulation results in varying degrees of vasoconstriction and varying vascular resistance from tissue to tissue and hence a corresponding varying amount of blood flow from tissue to tissue (Table 10-2).

(4)   Parasympathetic stimulation of the arterial vasculature of the brain and heart results in smooth muscle relaxation and vasodilation. This phenomenon results in a decrease in resistance to blood flow.

(5)   The adrenomedullary hormones norepinephrine and epinephrine stimulate the α (alpha) receptors and produce vasoconstriction.

(6)   Acidosis, hypoxemia, hypercarbia, and increased temperature produce local relaxation of smooth muscle in resistance vessels and resultant vasodilation.

b.   The capillary bed of the systemic circulation is governed almost exclusively by local factors.

(1)   In tissues where capillary blood flow is limited by arteriolar constriction, there is local accumulation of acid and carbon dioxide and a deficiency of oxygen.

(2)   These local factors result in relaxation of the smooth muscle and local arteriolar dilation, which reestablishes blood flow.

(3)   Blood flow removes the local accumulation of waste products and replenishes oxygen and nutrient supply, resulting in arteriolar constriction, which in turn limits blood flow.

(4)   Thus the cycle repeats itself, providing blood flow to tissues intermittently to maintain cellular metabolism.

c.   The veins of the systemic circulation are governed by the autonomic nervous system, hormonal factors, and mechanical factors.

(1)   The veins are exclusively innervated by postganglionic fibers of the sympathetic nervous system.

(2)   The veins have a less extensive innervation than do their arterial counterparts. However, unlike that of the arteries, sympathetic innervation of the venous vasculature does not vary from one tissue to the next.

(a)   Thus sympathetic stimulation causes venoconstriction of all veins of the body.

TABLE 10-2

Estimated Distribution of Cardiac Output and Oxygen Consumption in Normal Human Subject* at Rest Under Usual Indoor Conditions

Circulation	Blood Flow		Arteriovenous Oxygen Difference (vol%)	Oxygen Uptake	
	ml/min	% Total		ml/min	% Total
Splanchnic	1400	24	4.1	58	25
Renal	1100	19	1.3	16	7
Cerebral	750	13	6.3	46	20
Coronary	250	4	11.4	27	11
Skeletal muscle	1200	21	8.0	70	30
Skin	500	9	1.0	5	2
Other organs	600	10	3.0	12	5
Total	5800	100	4.0*	234	100

*Average value.

From Mountcastle VB: *Medical Physiology,* ed 14. St. Louis, Mosby, 1980.

(b) Generalized venoconstriction decreases the venous vascular space, resulting in increased venous return to the heart.

(c) Conversely, decreased sympathetic stimulation results in a decrease in venous tone and venodilation.

(d) Generalized venodilation increases the venous vascular space and decreases venous return to the heart.

(3) Adrenomedullary hormones epinephrine and norepinephrine mimic sympathetic stimulation and produce venoconstriction.

(4) Mechanical factors that affect the veins of the systemic venous system are the thoracoabdominal pump, skeletal muscle pump, and semilunar valves.

(a) The thoracoabdominal pump affects the veins by aiding venous return. This is accomplished by exposing the intrathoracic veins to the fluctuating subatmospheric pressure produced by spontaneous ventilation. Coupled with the fact that extrathoracic veins are surrounded by atmospheric or supraatmospheric pressure, venous return is enhanced.

(b) The veins in the limbs contain semilunar valves that prevent retrograde flow of blood. When skeletal muscle contracts, it compresses the veins, increasing venous pressure. Because these veins have valves, compression of vessels can squeeze blood in only one direction. This mechanism also is responsible for enhancing venous return.

3. Specific regional systemic circulations

a. Coronary circulation is most influenced by local and mechanical factors.

(1) Local metabolites are major determinants of perfusion.

(2) Seventy-five percent of coronary perfusion takes place during ventricular diastole when the myocardium is in a state of mechanical relaxation. Hence diastolic arterial pressure is the value most often monitored to assess the perfusion pressure at the openings of the coronary arteries. Diastolic pressures <60 mm Hg directly reduce coronary blood flow.

(3) Sympathetic influences are minor.

b. Cerebral circulation is most influenced by local factors.

(1) Local metabolites are the major determinant of perfusion.

(2) Sympathetic influences are minor.

c. Gastrointestinal/splanchnic/pancreatic/hepatic circulations

(1) Sympathetic influences are dominant.

(2) Venous systems of these circulations contain significant blood volumes and respond by increasing and decreasing venous return directly as a result of the amount of venomotor tone exerted by sympathetic input.

(3) Local factors and hormones exert minor influence.

d. Renal and epidermal circulation are principally under significant sympathetic influence.

e. Skeletal muscular circulation

(1) Local metabolites are major determinants of perfusion, especially in exercise.

(2) Sympathetic influences are significant.

B. Pulmonary circulation (see Figure 10-2)

1. Pulmonary circulation begins with the pulmonary pump (the right ventricle) and continues to a typical vascular bed, ending with the left atrium.

a. Functions of pulmonary circulation:

(1) To distribute right ventricular output to pulmonary capillaries, matching the alveolar ventilation with an adequate volume of blood per unit time (external respiration).

(2) To perfuse the cells of the lung parenchyma with nutrients and rid them of waste products.

(3) To return blood to the left side of the heart to maintain left ventricular output.

b. The velocity of the blood flow varies inversely with the total cross-sectional area through which blood flows at a given time. This physical law, coupled with the

architecture of the vascular system, nicely accomplishes the three functions of the pulmonary circulation (see Figure 10-3).
(1) The velocity of the blood flowing through the pulmonary artery is fast.
(2) The velocity of blood flow progressively slows from the arteries to arterioles.
(3) As the extraordinarily large cross-sectional area of the pulmonary capillaries is encountered, the velocity of blood flow attains it slowest rate.
(4) The velocity of the blood flow progressively increases from venules to veins as the cross-sectional area markedly decreases.
(5) As a result blood is quickly distributed (arteries), spends the greatest amount of time in the parenchymal tissue of the pulmonary circulation (capillaries) performing external respiration, and then is quickly returned (veins) to the heart for recirculation.

2. Control of pulmonary circulation is governed by the same four mechanisms that affect systemic circulation.
   a. The pulmonary vasculature generally has less smooth muscle and thinner walls than its counterpart in the systemic circulation.
   b. This makes pulmonary circulation susceptible to mechanical factors (e.g., intrathoracic and alveolar pressures) and the effects of gravity (secondary to alterations in bodily position) on the distribution of blood flow.
   c. Pulmonary vasculature responds to sympathetic stimulation just as does the systemic circulation but to a much lesser extent.
   d. Three local factors that have profound effects on pulmonary resistance vessels are decreased alveolar P_{O_2}, hypoxemia, and acidemia. All three cause pulmonary vasoconstriction, with increased resistance to blood flow.
   e. Adrenomedullary hormones produce pulmonary vasoconstriction but to a milder degree than in systemic circulation.
   f. Thus most of the control of pulmonary circulation depends on passive response to mechanical factors and on local factors. This is in contrast to the dominance that the sympathetic nervous system displays in controlling systemic circulation.
3. Systemic vascular resistance is normally 6 to 10 times pulmonary vascular resistance.

V. **Basic Functions of the Heart (Figure 10-4)**
   A. To impart sufficient energy to the blood to provide circulation through the vascular system.

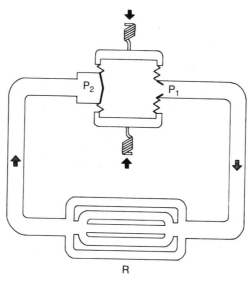

R

FIG. 10-4 Schematic representation of circulation depicting the heart's function of establishing the pressure gradient.

1. As has been discussed, the vascular resistance of systemic circulation is much greater than that of pulmonary circulation. Therefore, the left side of the heart must create greater pressures than the right side to bring about a given flow.
2. The major principle of circulation (blood flow) is that for circulation to exist, there must be a pressure gradient. The heart must create the pressure head (P_1) for the pressure gradient ($P_1 - P_2$) across the respective parts of the vasculature. Therefore for a given vascular resistance, blood flow is a direct function of the pressure head generated by the heart.

VI. **Mechanical Events of the Cardiac Cycle (Figure 10-5)**
   A. Electrical events of the heart are precursors to the mechanical events of the heart.
      1. If the heart is normal, depolarization of the atria causes atrial contraction (systole).
      2. Depolarization of the ventricles causes ventricular contraction (systole).
      3. Repolarization of the atria causes atrial relaxation (diastole).
      4. Repolarization of the ventricles causes ventricular relaxation (diastole).
   B. Atrial systole (Figure 10-6).
      1. Mechanical left and right atrial systole begins at the peak of the P wave of the electrocardiogram (ECG).
      2. The decrease in size of the respective atria causes left atrial pressure to increase approximately 7 to 8 mm Hg and right atrial pressure to increase 5 to 6 mm Hg concurrently. The pressure differential from atria to ventricles causes blood to flow from the atria through the respective atrioventricular (AV) orifices to the ventricles.
      3. Normal mean right and left atrial pressures are 0 to 8 mm Hg and 2 to 12 mm Hg, respectively.
      4. Atrial systole accounts for 20% to 40% of the total ventricular volume. This figure depends on heart rate (HR) and atrial contractility. The remaining 60% to 80% of ventricular volume is a result of passive filling by venous return, highlighting its critical importance in maintaining adequate CO.
      5. The atria are weak pumps compared with the ventricles and should be thought of as thin-walled blood reservoirs for the respective ventricles. The 20% to 40% of ventricular volume added by atrial systole is simply a priming of the ventricles before ventricular

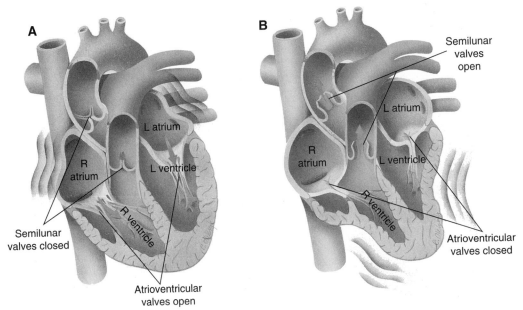

FIG. 10-5 Chambers and valves of the heart. Action of the heart chambers and valves when atria contract **(A)** and when the ventricles contract **(B)**.

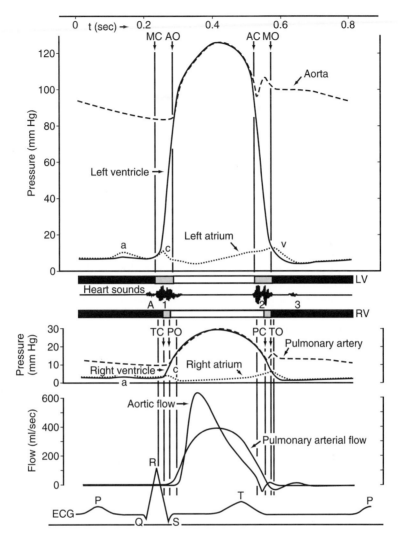

FIG. 10-6 Diagrammatic representation of the events in the cardiac cycle.

systole. Atrial systole is not essential for adequate ventricular filling, as can be demonstrated by atrial fibrillation or complete heart block.

6. Atrial systole increases the end-diastolic volume of each ventricle to approximately 145 ml. It also increases the end-diastolic pressure of the right and left ventricles to 2 to 8 mm Hg and 4 to 12 mm Hg, respectively. The ventricles are now prepared (loaded) for their subsequent contraction.

C. Ventricular systole and atrial diastole (see Figure 10-6).

1. Mechanical left and right ventricular systole begins at the peak of the R wave of the ECG and coincides with atrial diastole.

2. Ventricular contraction increases intraventricular pressure. When pressure in the respective ventricles exceeds atrial pressure, the tricuspid and mitral valves close, producing the first, or S_1, heart sound.

3. Aortic and pulmonic semilunar valves have been closed during ventricular diastole because pressure in the aorta and pulmonary artery has exceeded left and right ventricular pressure.

4. With AV and semilunar valves closed, the ventricles are functionally closed chambers. Contraction of the ventricle decreases their size and rapidly increases intraventricular pressure.
5. The first portion of ventricular systole is called *isovolumetric contraction*. It is characterized by the AV and semilunar valves being closed and by a rapid increase in intraventricular pressure without a concomitant change in intraventricular blood volume.
6. The second portion of ventricular systole is called the *period of ejection*. Ejection begins when left and right intraventricular pressure exceeds the pressure in the aorta and pulmonary artery, respectively. It should be noted that this point is the diastolic pulmonary artery and aortic pressure. Previous to ventricular systole, blood has been steadily leaving the pulmonary and systemic (aortic) arterial systems, and intraarterial pressures have been steadily decreasing in both. The lowest intraarterial pressure is attained just before actual ventricular ejection and is called *diastolic pressure* of the respective arteries. Normal diastolic pressure for the aorta and pulmonary artery is 60 to 90 mm Hg and 5 to 16 mm Hg, respectively.
7. The period of ejection is characterized by opening of the semilunar valves.
   a. During this time intraventricular pressure steadily increases above intraarterial pressure, causing blood to leave the ventricles.
   b. Intraventricular pressure attains its maximum value (ventricular systolic pressure), followed by a resultant increase in intraarterial pressure to its maximum value (arterial systolic pressure).
   c. Normal right and left ventricular systolic pressure is 15 to 28 mm Hg and 90 to 140 mm Hg, respectively.
   d. Normal pulmonary artery and aortic systolic pressure is 15 to 28 mm Hg and 90 to 140 mm Hg, respectively.
   e. When ejection is complete, intraarterial pressure and retrograde blood flow cause closing of aortic and pulmonic semilunar valves. This produces the second, or S_2, heart sound.
8. The total period of ejection causes a stroke volume (SV) of 70 ml to be added to each arterial system by the respective ventricles.
9. It should be noted that the end-diastolic volume of each ventricle is 145 ml and the SV is 70 ml. This results in a residual blood volume of each ventricle equal to 75 ml. The residual volume is called the *end-systolic volume*. The percentage of the end-diastolic volume that is ejected as the SV is termed the *ejection fraction* (EF). Expressed as an equation:

$$EF = \frac{SV}{EDV} \times 100\% \tag{1}$$

10. All previous blood pressure and volume values are based on the normal resting heart.
11. Closure of aortic and pulmonic semilunar valves marks the beginning of ventricular diastole.
D. Ventricular diastole (see Figure 10-6).
   1. Mechanical left and right ventricular diastole begins after completion of the T wave of the ECG.
   2. Ventricular diastole begins with closure of the pulmonic and aortic semilunar valves and ends with onset of atrial systole.
   3. Tricuspid and mitral valves have remained closed through the preceding ventricular systole and remain closed in early ventricular diastole. This is because intraventricular pressure exceeds intraatrial pressure.
   4. The ventricles are functionally closed chambers with all cardiac valves remaining closed. Relaxation of the ventricular myocardium precipitates a large decrease in intraventricular pressure without a change in intraventricular blood volume, called *isovolumetric relaxation*.
   5. When right and left intraventricular pressures decrease below the respective intraatrial pressures, the tricuspid and mitral valves open. This results in a rapid filling of each

ventricle by intraatrial blood, followed by passive distention of the ventricles by blood returning from the lung and periphery.

6. It should be noted that blood will continue to passively fill the ventricles through the AV valves, which remain open until the onset of ventricular systole. This slow but steady addition to ventricular volume is evidenced by a small increase in intraatrial and intraventricular pressures.

7. The ventricular filling occurring during ventricular diastole accounts for 60% to 80% of the end-diastolic volume.

8. The entire myocardium remains relaxed until the onset of the P wave and atrial systole initiate another cardiac cycle.

E. Summary of mechanical events of the cardiac cycle (Figure 10-7).

1. After the P wave of the ECG, the atria contract, propelling blood through the open AV valves to the ventricles.

2. During the height of the subsequent QRS complex, the ventricles contract in unison. It is during this same time that atrial relaxation occurs.

3. Intraventricular pressure soon increases above atrial pressure and causes the AV valves to close. This prevents retrograde flow of the blood from the ventricles to atria. Closure of the AV valves produces the S_1 heart sound.

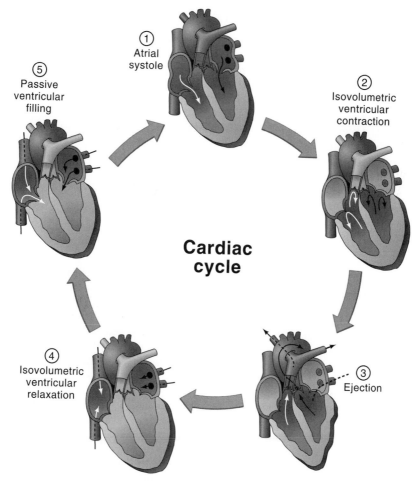

FIG. 10-7 The five steps of the heart's pumping cycle described in the text are shown as a series of changes in the heart wall and valves.

4. Intraventricular pressure continues to increase rapidly and soon exceeds intraarterial pressure. This causes the semilunar valves to open and provides blood flow from the ventricles to the arteries.
5. Relaxation of the ventricles occurs after completion of the T wave of the ECG.
6. As the ventricles relax, intraventricular pressure decreases below the respective intraarterial pressures. This causes the semilunar valves to close, preventing retrograde flow of blood from arteries to respective ventricles. Closure of the semilunar valves produces the S_2 heart sound.
7. Intraventricular pressure continues to decrease until intraventricular pressure decreases below the intraatrial pressure. This causes the respective AV valves to open and provides blood flow from atria to ventricles.
8. Blood returning from pulmonary and systemic circulation continues to flow through the atria and open AV valves passively, filling the relaxed ventricles. This passive filling continues until the onset of the subsequent atrial contraction, which begins the next cardiac cycle.

VII. **Cardiac Output**
   A. CO is the amount of blood pumped out of each ventricle over time.
   B. The CO of the right and left ventricles is equal and identical for a given period of time.
   C. The CO is equal to the SV times the HR:

$$CO = SV \times HR \qquad (2)$$

   1. The CO is conventionally expressed in liters per minute.
      a. The normal range of CO in a resting individual is 4 to 8 L/min.
      b. *With stress or exercise, the CO can increase five to six times its normal resting value.*
   2. The SV is the amount of blood ejected from the ventricle with each ventricular systole.
      a. The SV is expressed in milliliters per contraction.
      b. The normal range for the SV of a resting individual is 60 to 130 ml per contraction.
   3. The HR is the number of times the heart contracts per minute. The normal range for the HR of a resting individual is 60 to 100 contractions per minute.
   4. *Example:*
      An individual with an SV equal to 70 ml per contraction and an HR of 80 contractions per minute would have a CO of 5600 ml/min, or 5.6 L/min, by the following calculation:

$$\frac{70 \text{ ml}}{\text{contraction}} \times \frac{80 \text{ contractions}}{\text{min}} = \frac{5,600 \text{ ml}}{\text{min}} \text{ or } \frac{5.6 \text{ L}}{\text{min}} \qquad (3)$$

   5. It should be clear that increases in CO are brought about by increases in the HR and/or SV and that decreases in CO are brought about by decreases in HR and/or SV.
   D. Control of HR
   1. The pacemaker of the heart (SA node) sets the HR. The number of times per minute that the SA node depolarizes is largely governed by neural and chemical factors.
   2. The neural factors that affect HR are mediated through the two divisions of the autonomic nervous system, namely, the parasympathetic and sympathetic nervous systems.
      a. Parasympathetic impulses are conducted to the SA node through cranial nerve X (vagus nerve).
         (1) Parasympathetic effects on the SA node are inhibitory and decrease the HR.
         (2) Decreasing the HR is called *negative chronotropism*. Thus the parasympathetic nervous system exhibits negative chronotropic effects.
      b. Sympathetic impulses are conducted to the SA node through sympathetic nerve fibers originating from the upper thoracic (T1 to T5) segment of the spinal cord.
         (1) Sympathetic effects on the SA node are excitatory and increase the HR.
         (2) Increasing the HR is called *positive chronotropism*. Thus, the sympathetic nervous system exhibits positive chronotropic effects.

      c. The sympathetic and parasympathetic nervous systems are generally considered antagonists. However, in bringing about changes in HR, the two divisions of the autonomic nervous system complement each other.

         (1) However, each nervous system can perform positive and negative chronotropism. Under certain clinical conditions, HR is altered by selective activities of one division of the autonomic nervous system.

         (2) The parasympathetic nervous system generally is the dominant division of the neural input into the SA node. This is evidenced by total autonomic blockade, resulting in mild tachycardia.

      d. Neural control of HR also is mediated through higher brain centers, such as the cerebral cortex and hypothalamus.

         (1) The cerebral cortex is responsible for changes in HR in response to emotional factors, such as anxiety, fear, anger, and grief.

         (2) The hypothalamus appears responsible for changes in HR in response to alterations in local and environmental temperature.

  3. Major chemical factors that affect HR: electrolytes, exogenously administered drugs, and hormones.

      a. The three major electrolytes affecting the HR are potassium, sodium, and calcium.

         (1) Excess potassium and sodium decrease the HR.

         (2) Excess calcium increases the HR.

         (3) Potassium and sodium imbalance can alter cardiac membrane permeability and thus slow or speed the rate of electric conduction through the myocardium. However, only electrolyte imbalance brings about such changes in HR.

      b. Classes of drugs that affect HR by either mimicking or inhibiting the activity of the sympathetic or parasympathetic nervous system:

         (1) Sympathomimetics, such as isoproterenol, epinephrine, dobutamine, and dopamine, mimic the activity of the sympathetic nervous system and cause positive chronotropism.

         (2) Sympatholytics, such as propranolol and metoprolol, inhibit the activity of the sympathetic nervous system and cause negative chronotropism.

         (3) Parasympathomimetics, such as methacholine, pilocarpine, and neostigmine, mimic the activity of the parasympathetic nervous system and cause negative chronotropism.

         (4) Parasympatholytics, such as atropine, inhibit the activity of the parasympathetic nervous system and cause positive chronotropism.

      c. The major hormones that affect the HR are the adrenomedullary hormones.

         (1) The adrenal medulla secretes epinephrine and norepinephrine into the circulating blood.

         (2) These two naturally occurring catecholamines have direct positive chronotropic effects on the heart.

  4. *HR is under many influences*, ranging from conscious control by the cerebral cortex to exogenously administered pharmacologic agents. However, the most important regulatory control of HR is mediated through the autonomic nervous system.

E. Control of SV

  1. Size of SV: Governed by preload, afterload, and state of contractility of ventricles.

      a. *Preload*: Degree of ventricular diastolic filling before ejection begins, or the presystolic ventricular loading force.

         (1) The Frank-Starling law states that the more the heart is filled during diastole, the greater the subsequent force of contraction. This results in increased SV (Figure 10-8), all other variables being equal.

         (2) This relationship is related primarily to presystolic myocardial fiber length.

         (3) Presystolic myocardial fiber length is directly related to end-diastolic volume because it is the actual intraventricular blood volume coupled with the compliance characteristics of the ventricle that results in myocardial fiber stretch.

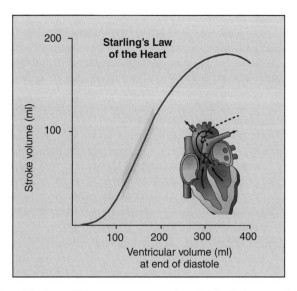

FIG. 10-8 Starling's law of the heart. This curve represents the relationship between the stroke volume (SV) and the ventricular volume at the end of diastole. The range of values observed in a typical heart is shaded. Notice that if the ventricle has an abnormally large volume at the end of diastole (far right portion of the curve), the SV cannot compensate.

(4) Because myocardial fiber length is virtually impossible to measure in the intact heart, it would seem that end-diastolic volume is an appropriate parameter to assess preload.

(a) The first factor affecting end-diastolic volume is the presence of a total blood volume sufficient for an effective vascular volume to vascular space relationship. There must be an adequate blood volume within the vascular space for the heart to circulate blood effectively. It is the *relationship* between vascular volume to vascular space that is crucial, not the absolute values of either vascular volume or vascular space.

(b) The state of the venous tone is the second factor affecting end-diastolic volume. The relationship between vascular volume and vascular space is essential to ensure adequate venous return and ventricular filling. Sixty percent to 80% of ventricular filling is accomplished by passive return of blood from the veins. The state of venous tone regulates venous vascular space, and it is therefore as crucial as blood volume in determining adequacy of venous return.

(c) The third major factor that affects end-diastolic volume is force of atrial systole. As mentioned, 20% to 40% of ventricular filling is accomplished by atrial systole. This is not of critical importance in the normal heart but becomes paramount in any cardiac dysfunction where ventricular compliance is decreased (i.e., ventricular hypertrophy or myocardial infarction).

(d) The fourth major factor that affects end-diastolic volume is compliance of the ventricle. As mentioned, this factor is not of importance in the normal heart, but decreases in ventricular compliance require a greater filling pressure per unit volume change. Thus increased filling pressure is necessary or the end-diastolic volume will have a reduced value.

(e) End-diastolic volume is an acceptable parameter for assessing preload; however, this too is difficult to measure with any accuracy in the intact heart. The most easily measured parameter that reflects preload is ventricular end-diastolic pressure.

(5) Given a constant ventricular compliance, it may be inferred that ventricular end-diastolic pressure should correlate well with ventricular end-diastolic volume. Accepting the latter as true, myocardial fiber length can be expressed as a function of end-diastolic pressure.

    (a) In clinical practice, preload is assessed by measuring ventricular end-diastolic pressure.

    (b) Right ventricular preload is assessed by end-diastolic pressure measurements taken from a central venous pressure (CVP) catheter as CVP (see Chapter 12).

    (c) Left ventricular preload is assessed by end-diastolic pressure measurements taken from a pulmonary artery catheter as pulmonary wedge pressure (PWP; see Chapter 12).

    (d) In general, the higher the end-diastolic pressure (preload), the greater the subsequent ventricular contraction and resulting SV.

(6) The Frank-Starling relationship is the basis for matching CO to venous return and balancing the output of right and left ventricles. For example, if venous return to the right atrium has suddenly increased because increased venous tone has altered the vascular volume/vascular space relationship:

    (a) Increased venous return to the right ventricle would increase the right ventricular end-diastolic volume.

    (b) Increased end-diastolic volume would result in an increased myocardial fiber length.

    (c) Increased myocardial fiber length would in turn result in an increased force of contraction of the right ventricle.

    (d) Increased force of contraction of the right ventricle would result in an increased right ventricular SV, all other factors remaining equal.

    (e) Two phenomena have occurred. First venous blood has been mobilized back to the heart, and the increased venous return has been matched by an increase in right ventricular SV. This is one of the major ways that CO is increased. Second right ventricular output transiently exceeds left ventricular output.

    (f) Increased right ventricular output will result in increased venous return to the left atrium and left ventricle.

    (g) In similar fashion increased venous return to the left ventricle increases left ventricular end-diastolic volume.

    (h) The increased end-diastolic volume would result in increasing the left ventricular myocardial fiber length. This in turn would result in an increase in the force of contraction of the left ventricle.

    (i) The increased force of contraction of the left ventricle would result in an increased left ventricular SV.

    (j) At this point venous blood has been mobilized from the venous reservoirs and has resulted in increased output from the right and left sides of the heart. Furthermore left ventricular output is in equilibrium with right ventricular output, all in accordance with the Frank-Starling relationship.

    (k) The regulatory function of the Frank-Starling mechanism is frequently referred to as *autoregulation* because it is an intrinsic factor based on the architecture of the myocardial fibers, which automatically regulate CO to equal venous return. Thus it has led physiologists over the years to make the statement that within the physiologic limits of the heart, it will pump out all the blood it receives without allowing a backup of blood into the venous system.

b. *Afterload*: Resistance to flow from the ventricles.

(1) The work the heart must perform to pump blood out of the ventricles and into the circulation depends on three major factors: resistance of the semilunar valves, blood viscosity, and arterial blood pressure.

    (a)   As resistance of the semilunar valves (i.e., pulmonic or aortic stenosis) increases, afterload will be increased.

    (b)   As blood viscosity increases (i.e., hyperproteinemia or polycythemia), afterload will be increased.

    (c)   As arterial blood pressure increases (pulmonary or systemic hypertension), afterload will be increased.

    (d)   Decreases in any of these three parameters result in decreasing the afterload.

(2)   Increases in afterload result in increases of ventricular work.

    (a)   The greater the resistance against which the ventricle must contract to eject blood, the more slowly it contracts.

    (b)   Increased afterload results in a decreased SV, which initially increases end-systolic volume. The normal venous return will then be added to the already increased end-systolic volume and increase the end-diastolic volume above normal. This allows a more forceful contraction against an increased afterload as a result of the Frank-Starling mechanism. This enables the ventricle to pump a given SV against an increased afterload. *This compensation is at the expense of an increase in ventricular size.* The larger the heart, the greater the work necessary to develop the myocardial tension required to produce a given intraventricular pressure (Laplace's law).

    (c)   The slower rate of contraction and the increased ventricular size result in greater oxygen requirements to perform a given amount of work compared with that of the normal heart.

(3)   Thus increases in afterload may or may not cause a decrease in SV but will cause increases in myocardial work.

(4)   Decreases in afterload, commonly called *afterload reduction*, may or may not cause an increase in SV but will cause decreases in myocardial work (a cornerstone of post–myocardial infarction management).

(5)   In general, the poorer the cardiac function, the more dependent the SV is on afterload.

    (a)   Increases in afterload tend to decrease SV in the patient with poor cardiac function.

    (b)   Increases in afterload do not cause decreases in SV in the patient with normal cardiac function.

    (c)   Decreases in afterload tend to increase SV in the patient with poor cardiac function.

    (d)   Decreases in afterload generally do not cause increases in SV in the patient with normal cardiac function.

(6)   In the absence of valvular disease, afterload is clinically assessed by measuring mean arterial blood pressure.

    (a)   Right ventricular afterload is assessed by mean pulmonary artery pressure ($\overline{PAP}$) measurements taken via a pulmonary artery catheter.

    (b)   Left ventricular afterload is assessed by mean systemic arterial pressure (MAP) measurements taken via a (systemic) intraarterial catheter.

c. *State of ventricular contractility*: Force with which the ventricles contract.

(1)   The force of contraction of the ventricles at any given preload and afterload depends on the state of contractility (Figure 10-9).

    (a)   An increase in the state of ventricular contractility for a given preload and afterload is termed *positive inotropism* (see Figure 10-9, *B*).

    (b)   A decrease in the state of ventricular contractility for a given preload and afterload is termed *negative inotropism* (see Figure 10-9, *C*).

    (c)   The net effect of positive inotropism is generally a greater volume output per unit time.

    (d)   The net effect of negative inotropism is generally a smaller volume output per unit time.

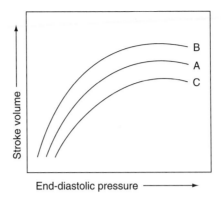

FIG. 10-9 The Frank-Starling relationship. **A,** Control. **B,** Positive inotropism. **C,** Negative inotropism (see text).

(2) Ventricular contractility is altered by the sympathetic and parasympathetic nervous systems, blood gases (Po_2, Pco_2), pH, hormones, and exogenously administered drugs.

(3) The sympathetic nervous system extensively innervates the atrial and ventricular myocardium.

  (a) Postganglionic nerve fibers of the sympathetic nervous system release norepinephrine to β (beta) receptor sites in the atrial and ventricular myocardium.

  (b) This increases contractility of the myocardium (positive inotropism). Thus the sympathetic nervous system displays positive inotropic effects.

  (c) Alterations in sympathetic discharge to the myocardium are believed to constitute the most important regulatory control of ventricular contractility.

(4) The parasympathetic nervous system only minutely innervates the atrial myocardium, and the ventricular myocardium is so innervated even more sparsely.

  (a) Postganglionic nerve fibers of the parasympathetic nervous system release acetylcholine to the muscarinic receptor sites of the atrial and ventricular myocardium.

  (b) As previously mentioned, because of the scantiness of parasympathetic innervation, the result is only a mild decrease in myocardial contractility or a slight negative inotropism. Thus the parasympathetic nervous system displays minor negative inotropic effects.

(5) Effects of blood gases on myocardial contractility:

  (a) Mild decreases in Po_2 result in increased contractility, whereas severe decreases in Po_2 result in decreased myocardial contractility.

  (b) Increases in Pco_2 result in decreased contractility, whereas decreases in Pco_2 result in increased myocardial contractility.

  (c) Metabolic or respiratory acidosis results directly in decreased contractility, whereas metabolic and respiratory alkalosis may alter contractility through electric conduction dysfunction and arrhythmia.

(6) The most important hormones affecting myocardial contractility are the adrenomedullary hormones.

  (a) The adrenal medulla secretes epinephrine and norepinephrine into the circulating blood.

  (b) These two naturally occurring catecholamines have direct positive inotropic effects on the myocardium.

  (c) The major differences between the effects of the catecholamines and direct sympathetic stimulation are that the effects of catecholamines take longer to establish but are longer lasting.

    (d) The aforementioned statement is true of the effect of catecholamines on contractility and HR.

  (7) The following exogenously administered drugs can alter myocardial contractility:

    (a) The sympatholytics (e.g., propranolol and metoprolol) produce negative inotropic effects through β-receptor blockade.

    (b) The sympathomimetics (e.g., isoproterenol, epinephrine, dobutamine, and dopamine) produce positive inotropic effects through β-receptor stimulation.

    (c) Some antiarrhythmic agents (e.g., quinidine and procainamide) produce negative inotropic effects.

    (d) Derivatives of digitalis produce positive inotropic effects.

    (e) Calcium channel blockers (e.g., verapamil and nifedipine) produce negative inotropic effects.

  (8) Myocardial contractility is an elusive parameter to assess clinically. However, controversial attempts have been made to quantitate it.

  (9) It should be remembered that the SV is under a gamut of influences. However, any SV is determined by the interrelation of preload, afterload, and the state of ventricular contractility.

F. Increases in CO

  1. Increases in CO are normally achieved by an increase in HR and SV via the interplay of the aforementioned mechanisms.

    a. HR increases first and in a linear relationship with demand.

    b. SV initially increases according to the Frank-Starling relationship but eventually decreases (descending limb of the ventricular performance curve), thus becoming the ultimate limiting factor in maximal CO.

VIII. Control of Arterial Blood Pressure

A. Under normal circumstances, arterial blood volume exceeds arterial vascular space. This relationship results in an intravascular pressure dictated by the absolute arterial blood volume and the elastic properties of the arterial vasculature.

B. The arterial system is continually receiving blood (inflow) from the left ventricle as CO and continually allowing blood to leave the arterial system (outflow) as arterial runoff.

C. It is the balance or imbalance between CO (inflow) and arterial runoff (outflow) that results in any given arterial blood volume.

D. The relationship between arterial blood volume and arterial vascular space is the primary determinant of arterial blood pressure.

E. Thus by the equation $P = \dot{Q} \times R$, it can be demonstrated that CO ($\dot{Q}$) and peripheral resistance (R) are directly related to arterial blood pressure (P). Arterial blood pressure depends on alteration of the blood volume to vascular space relationship by CO and/or peripheral resistance, as follows (Figure 10-10):

  1. Increases in peripheral resistance (i.e., vasoconstriction) result in decreasing arterial runoff. If CO remains the same, inflow exceeds outflow from the arterial vasculature. This results in an increase in the arterial blood volume to vascular space relationship and a concomitant increase in arterial blood pressure.

  2. Decreases in peripheral resistance (i.e., vasodilation) result in decreasing arterial blood pressure by the exact opposite mechanism.

  3. Increases in CO result in increasing the rate of inflow to the arterial system. If peripheral resistance remains the same, inflow exceeds outflow from the arterial vasculature. This results in an increase in the arterial blood volume to vascular space relationship and an increase in arterial blood pressure.

  4. Decreases in CO result in decreasing arterial blood pressure by the exact opposite mechanism.

  5. It should be noted that in the previous four examples the imbalance between inflow and outflow is only temporary. It is by these mechanisms that arterial blood pressure can be increased or decreased. Once the desired arterial pressure is attained, the balance between inflow and outflow will maintain the pressure at that level.

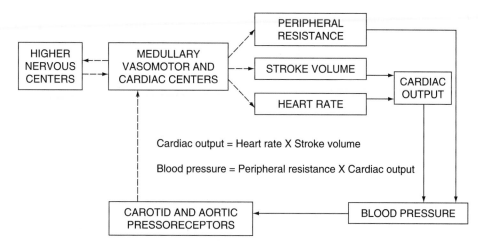

FIG. 10-10 Schematic representing regulatory control of arterial blood pressure. Blood pressure is sensed by the pressoreceptors, which send impulses to the medulla. The medullary centers send impulses to motor fibers of the sympathetic and parasympathetic nervous system. When pressure at the receptor increases or decreases, it is reflexly corrected by an alteration of heart rate, stroke volume, and peripheral resistance. Dotted lines indicate neural connections.

F. As has been described, CO and peripheral resistance are for a large part under neural control. Therefore it becomes apparent that regulation of arterial blood pressure is mediated through neural alterations in CO and peripheral resistance.

G. Neural regulation of arterial blood pressure is mediated through autonomic fibers that originate from an area of the medulla oblongata. This area of the medulla is sometimes called the *cardiovascular center*.

H. The cardiovascular center may be functionally divided into four subcenters: the vasomotor excitatory (vasoconstrictor) center, vasomotor inhibitory (vasodilator) center, cardiac excitatory center, and cardiac inhibitory center (Figure 10-11).

  1. The vasomotor excitatory center influences the arterioles through the sympathetic nervous system. The degree of vasoconstriction or vasodilation is directly related to the amount of sympathetic stimulation.

  2. The vasomotor inhibitory center does not influence the arterioles directly but acts by inhibiting the activity of the vasomotor excitatory center.

  3. The cardiac excitatory center influences the heart through the sympathetic nervous system. Sympathetic stimulation originating from this center results in positive inotropic and chronotropic effects.

  4. The cardiac inhibitory center influences the heart through the parasympathetic nervous system. Parasympathetic stimulation originating from this center results in a negative chronotropic effect and a mild negative inotropic effect.

I. The cardiovascular center in the medulla receives sensory input from the entire body. The most important sources of sensory input are the exteroceptors, higher brain centers, local factors, peripheral chemoreceptors, and baroreceptors (see Figure 10-10).

  1. Exteroceptors (e.g., proprioceptors, thermal receptors, and pain receptors) are sources of sensory input. Stimulation of the proprioceptors, pain receptors, and thermal receptors through muscular activation, pain, and heat, respectively, results in an increase in HR. This potentially will increase arterial blood pressure. Cold and muscular inactivity slow the HR and potentially decrease arterial blood pressure.

  2. Higher brain centers (e.g., the cerebral cortex and hypothalamus) have medullary input.

    a. Emotional factors alter blood pressure by mediation through the cerebral cortex. Fear or anger usually increases the blood pressure by stimulating the vasomotor and cardiac excitatory centers. This stimulation results in vasoconstriction and an increase in

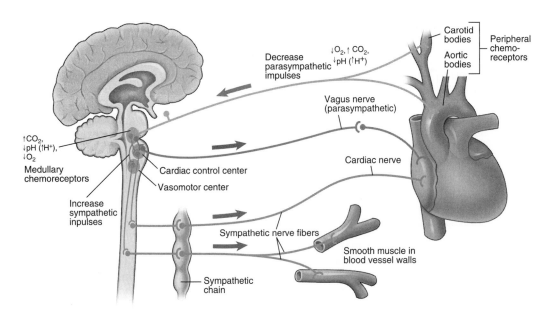

FIG. 10-11 Vasomotor chemoreflexes. Chemoreceptors in the carotid and aortic bodies, as well as chemoreceptive neurons in the vasomotor center of the medulla itself, detect increases in carbon dioxide (CO_2), decreases in blood oxygen (O_2), and decreases in pH (which is really an increase in H^+). This information feeds back to the cardiac control center and the vasomotor control center of the medulla, which in turn alter the ratio of parasympathetic and sympathetic output. When O_2 decreases, CO_2 increases, and/or pH decreases, a dominance of sympathetic impulses increases heart rate and stroke volume and constricts reservoir vessels, in response.

HR. However, decreases in blood pressure can be mediated through the cerebrum by stimulation of the vasomotor inhibitory center, as in fainting or blushing.

b. The hypothalamus mediates its control on the vasomotor inhibitory center in response to increases in body temperature. This causes vasodilation of the vessels of the skin and loss of body heat. A decrease in body temperature will result in vasoconstriction of the vessels of the skin with heat conservation as mediated through the hypothalamus.

c. Direct stimulation of the anterior portion of the hypothalamus produces bradycardia and a decrease in arterial blood pressure, whereas stimulation of the posterior portion of the hypothalamus produces tachycardia and an increase in arterial blood pressure.

3. The vasomotor inhibitory and excitatory centers are sensitive to local and direct effects of pH and P_{CO_2} of arterial blood perfusing these centers.

a. Local increases in arterial pH and decreases in P_{CO_2} cause depression of the vasomotor excitatory center by the vasomotor inhibitory center. This results in vasodilation, a decrease in peripheral resistance, and a decrease in arterial blood pressure.

b. Local decreases in arterial pH and increases in P_{CO_2} cause direct excitation of the vasomotor excitatory center. This results in vasoconstriction, an increase in peripheral resistance, and an increase in arterial blood pressure.

c. A local decrease in P_{O_2} of arterial blood potentiates the vasoconstrictor effect but alone has no local effect.

4. Peripheral chemoreceptors (aortic and carotid bodies) are responsible for initiating the vasomotor chemoreflex.

a. Hypoxemia, hypercapnia, and acidemia each stimulate the peripheral chemoreceptors.

b. The stimulated chemoreceptors in turn send an increased number of afferent impulses to the vasomotor excitatory center, with resultant vasoconstriction. This increases peripheral resistance and arterial blood pressure.

c. When hypoxemia and hypercapnia or hypoxemia and acidemia exist, the chemore-ceptors display a synergistic effect (i.e., the stimulation originating from the chemoreceptors secondary to two simultaneous stimuli is greater than the mathe-matical sum of the two stimuli when they act alone). This results in a more pro-found vasoconstriction and an increase in blood pressure.

5. Baroreceptors are by far the most important short-acting regulator of arterial blood pressure.

   a. Baroreceptors (pressoreceptors) are stretch receptors located in the arch of the aorta and carotid sinus.

   b. They respond to changes in pressure, which stretch them to different degrees. The greater the pressure, the greater the number of impulses the baroreceptors will send.

   c. With a decrease in arterial blood pressure, the number of impulses sent by the baroreceptors decreases. This decreased number of inhibitory impulses causes the vasomotor excitatory and cardiac excitatory centers to become more active. This results in increased CO and increased peripheral resistance, thus restoring arterial blood pressure to normal.

   d. With an increase in arterial blood pressure, the number of impulses sent out by the baroreceptors increases. This increased number of inhibitory impulses causes the vasomotor excitatory center to become depressed directly and indirectly through increased activity of the vasomotor inhibitory center. The increased number of inhibitory impulses also depresses the cardiac excitatory center and stimulates the cardiac inhibitory center, resulting in a decreased HR. Thus peripheral resistance and CO decrease, restoring normal blood pressure.

J. Long-term regulation of arterial blood pressure is accomplished by maintenance or alter-ations in the total blood volume.

   1. Increases in total blood volume accomplished by renal fluid retention increase the venous vascular volume to space relationship and result in increased venous return.

      a. Increased venous return increases end-diastolic volume and the resulting SV and CO.

      b. The increased CO increases arterial blood volume and hence arterial blood pres-sure.

   2. Conversely, decreases in total blood volume by renal fluid excretion decrease the venous vascular volume to space relationship and result in decreased venous return.

      a. Decreased venous return decreases end-diastolic volume and the resulting SV and CO.

      b. The decreased CO decreases arterial blood volume and hence arterial blood pres-sure.

      c. This physiologic concept is the basis for the use of diuretics in the long-term main-tenance of systemic hypertension.

BIBLIOGRAPHY

Cottrell GP: *Cardiopulmonary Anatomy and Physiology for Respiratory Care Practitioners.* Philadelphia, FA Davis, 2000.

DesJardins TR: *Cardiopulmonary Anatomy and Physiology: Essentials for Respiratory Care,* ed 4. New York, Delmar Publishers, 2001.

Ganong WF: *Review of Medical Physiology,* ed 2. New York, McGraw-Hill, 2003.

Grindel CG, Crowley LV: *Anatomy and Physiology.* Baltimore, Lippincott Williams & Wilkins, 1997.

Guyton AJ, Hall JE: *Textbook of Medical Physiology,* ed 10. Philadelphia, Elsevier Health Sciences Division, 2000.

Hicks GH: *Cardiopulmonary Anatomy and Physiology.* Philadelphia, Elsevier Health Sciences Division, 1999.

Little RC: *Physiology of the Heart and Circulation.* St. Louis, Mosby, 1988.

Matthews LR: *Cardiopulmonary Anatomy and Physiology.* Philadelphia, Lippincott Williams & Wilkins, 1996.

Mountcastle VB: *Medical Physiology,* ed 14. St. Louis, Mosby, 1980.

Ross G: *The Essentials of Human Physiology,* ed 2. St. Louis, Mosby, 1982.

Ruch TC, Patton HD: *Physiology and Biophysics,* ed 20. Philadelphia, WB Saunders, 1982.

Shapiro BA, Harrison RA, Kacmarek RM: *Clinical Applications of Respiratory Care*, ed 4. Philadelphia, Elsevier Health Sciences Division, 1990.

Shier D: *Human Anatomy and Physiology*, ed 9. New York, McGraw-Hill, 2002.

Thibodeau GA, Patton KT: *Anthony's Textbook of Anatomy & Physiology*, ed 15. St. Louis, Mosby-Yearbook, Inc., 1994.

Williams PL: *Gray's Anatomy: The Anatomical Basis of Medicine and Surgery,* ed 38. Philadelphia, Elsevier Health Sciences Division, 1995.

Chapter 11

Cardiac Electrophysiology and ECG Interpretation

I. **The electric conduction system of the heart functions in the:**
   A. Provision of electric excitation of the myocardial fibers without extrinsic stimuli (automaticity).
   B. Conduction of electric impulses through the myocardium.
   C. Organized distribution of the electric impulses to the myocardium in a repetitive, sequential fashion.

II. **Electroconduction System of the Heart (Figure 11-1)**
   A. Sinoatrial (SA) node
      1. The SA node is located in the right atrium just inferior and posterior to the entrance of the superior vena cava.
      2. It is commonly referred to as the *pacemaker of the heart*, its *primary function*.
      3. The SA node has an intrinsic rate of depolarization of 60 to 100/min.
      4. The rate of depolarization ordinarily is under the control of the sympathetic and parasympathetic nervous systems.
         a. Sympathetic stimulation of the SA node increases the rate of depolarization-positive chronotropism.
         b. Parasympathetic stimulation of the SA node decreases the rate of depolarization-negative chronotropism.
      5. The wave of depolarization initiated from the SA node travels outwardly through the atrial musculature in concentric circles, thus depolarizing the atria and ultimately the atrioventricular (AV) node.
      6. For all practical purposes, the left and right atria depolarize simultaneously.
   B. Atrioventricular node
      1. The AV node is located in the right atrium between the opening of the coronary sinus and interatrial septum.
      2. Histologically it comprises cells identical to those of the SA node.
      3. The *function* of the AV node is threefold:
         a. Backup cardiac pacemaker because of its intrinsic depolarization rate of 40 to 60/min.
         b. The only electrical bridge between atria and ventricles.
         c. Responsible for delaying impulses from atria to ventricles.
      4. The AV node becomes continuous with the common bundle branch (bundle of His) and is the only normal pathway for electric conduction between atria and ventricles. The fibroskeleton of the heart electrically separates atrial from ventricular muscle. The AV node and common bundle penetrate the cardiac fibroskeleton.

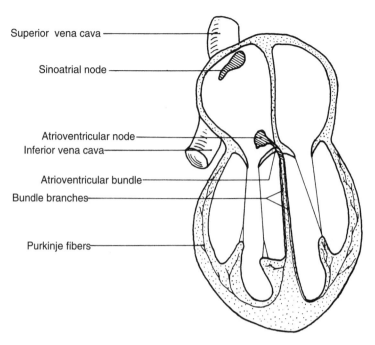

Superior vena cava

Sinoatrial node

Atrioventricular node
Inferior vena cava

Atrioventricular bundle
Bundle branches

Purkinje fibers

FIG. 11-1 The electrical conduction system of the heart (see text).

5. The tissue of the AV node slows the rate of electrical conduction and accounts for the time delay between atrial and ventricular depolarization. This time delay also allows optimal ventricular filling before ventricular contraction (systole).
6. The rate of conduction of electrical impulses through the AV node is under the control of the sympathetic and parasympathetic nervous systems.
   a. Sympathetic stimulation decreases conduction time and allows overall increases in cardiac rate.
   b. Parasympathetic stimulation increases conduction time of the AV node. Strong parasympathetic stimulation may actually block all or a portion of the impulses originating from the atria.
C. Common bundle branch
   1. It is also known as the *AV bundle* or *bundle of His*.
   2. It is located on the right side of the interventricular septum and penetrates the right fibrous trigone.
   3. Its *function* is twofold:
      a. To conduct impulses from the AV node to the left and right bundle branches.
      b. To penetrate the fibroskeleton of the heart, electrically bridging the atrial conduction system to the ventricular conduction system.
   4. The common bundle branch travels inferiorly in the interventricular septum for approximately 10 to 12 mm and then divides into one right and two left bundle branches.
D. Right and left bundle branches
   1. The right bundle branch appears simply as a continuation of the common bundle branch and follows an inferior course toward the apex of the heart.
   2. The left bundle branch penetrates the interventricular septum and divides into an anterior and posterior left bundle branch. Both bundle branches course inferiorly on the left side of the interventricular septum.
   3. The *function* of the three major bundle branches is to conduct electric impulses from the common bundle branch to the Purkinje fibers.

E. Purkinje fibers
   1. The Purkinje fibers are fine ramifications of the bundle branches, which terminate on the endocardial layer of the heart.
   2. They are located throughout the entire endocardial layer of both ventricles and conduct the electrical impulses from the bundle branches to the ventricles. Depolarization of the ventricles begins when impulses leaving the Purkinje fibers invade the endocardial layer.
   3. The wave of depolarization travels from the endocardial layer outward toward the epicardium and also from the apex toward the base of the ventricles.
F. Summary of pathway of normal electrical conduction
   1. Impulses originate in the right atrium by spontaneous depolarization of the SA node.
   2. Impulses are conducted through atrial muscle, which results in depolarization of right and left atria and AV node.
   3. The impulse is delayed at the AV node and then conducted through the cardiac fibroskeleton by the AV node and common bundle branch.
   4. The impulse is then conducted from the common bundle branch through the right and left bundle branches to the Purkinje fibers.
   5. The impulses exit the Purkinje fibers and cause depolarization of the ventricle from inside out and from apex to base.
   6. Design of the electrical conduction system of the heart allows simultaneous depolarization of the right and left atria totally separate from simultaneous depolarization of the right and left ventricles. This fact has important implications for the mechanical function of the heart (Figure 11-2).

III. **Electrocardiogram**
   A. Electrocardiography (ECG) provides a graphic display of current generated by the heart at the surface of the body. It depicts depolarization and repolarization of atria and ventricles.
   B. ECG is used to assess the electrical activity of the heart and should be clearly delineated from the mechanical activity of the heart. However, the electrical activity possesses significant potential implications in the mechanical activity of the heart.
   C. Each portion of the cardiac cycle generates a specific type of electrical impulse. These impulses are repetitious and produce characteristic patterns on an ECG recording.
   D. The four major electrical cardiac events are atrial depolarization, atrial repolarization, ventricular depolarization, and ventricular repolarization.
      1. The polarized state is the normal resting state of cardiac muscle fiber. The extracellular charge is positive with respect to the intracellular charge (Figure 11-3, *A*).
      2. Depolarization is the process of reversing the normal state of polarity. Thus depolarization causes the extracellular charge to be negative with respect to the intracellular charge. This is largely because inflow of extracellular sodium ions is faster than outflow of intracellular potassium ions. Reversal of the cellular membrane charge is transmitted along cardiac muscle fiber, depolarizing subsequent fibers (see Figure 11-3, *B*). If the muscle

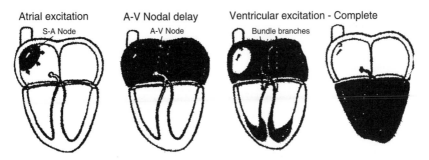

FIG. 11-2 Sequence of cardiac excitation.

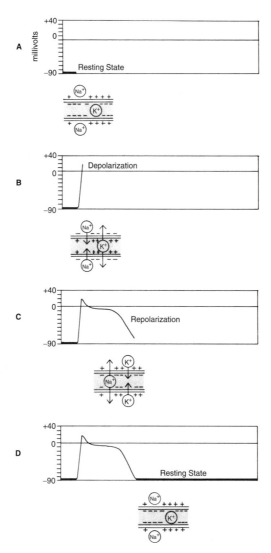

FIG. 11-3 Schematic diagram of the electrophysiology of a single myocardial cell, depicting electrical activity and the electrolytic cellular environment. Note the horizontal axis represents time. **A,** The resting state of repolarization, the –90-mV intracellular state is primarily caused by sodium (Na+) and potassium (K+) ion distribution. **B,** Depolarization occurs in response to appropriate stimulus; the intracellular state becomes positive in relation to extracellular environment caused by ion changes. **C,** Repolarization occurs as ionic distribution returns to predepolarization state. **D,** The resting state in which the cell is capable of repeating process.

      fibers are normal, this electrochemical stimulation results in mechanical activity (e.g., shortening of muscle fibers and cardiac contraction).

3. Repolarization is the process of reestablishing the normal state of polarity (i.e., reestablishing a positive extracellular charge with respect to the intracellular charge). The reestablishment of the resting cellular membrane charge is transmitted along the cardiac muscle fiber, repolarizing subsequent fibers (see Figure 11-3, C). If muscle fibers are normal, this electrochemical stimulation results in lengthening of muscle fibers and cardiac relaxation. (*Note:* It is a mistake to assume that the mechanical activity of the heart is normal simply because the electric activity [ECG] is normal.)

E. The electric deflections of the ECG in normal sequence are P wave, QRS complex, and T wave when measured by electrodes with specific polarities placed in standardized positions on the chest and limbs (Figure 11-4).
   1. The P wave is produced by atrial depolarization and normally is 0.06 to 0.11 second in duration.
   2. The QRS complex is produced by ventricular depolarization and normally is 0.03 to 0.12 second in duration. Repolarization of the atria occurs simultaneously with ventricular depolarization and is masked by the overwhelming electric event of the QRS complex.
   3. The T wave is produced by ventricular repolarization and normally is 0.14 to 0.26 second in duration.
F. PR, RR, and PP intervals
   1. PR interval: Time from the beginning of atrial depolarization to the beginning of ventricular depolarization. The PR interval normally is 0.12 to 0.20 second in duration.
   2. RR interval: Time from the peak of one QRS complex to the next QRS complex. It is used to measure the total cardiac cycle and normally is 0.6 to 1.0 second in duration.
   3. PP interval: Time from the beginning of one P wave to the beginning of the next P wave. It can be used to measure the total cardiac cycle time and hence the cardiac rate. It is normally equal to the RR interval (0.6 to 1.0 second in duration).
G. Summary of normal time values for ECG events (Table 11-1)
H. Standard leads for measuring/monitoring ECG events
   1. The three standard limb leads are lead I, lead II, and lead III (Figure 11-5).
      a. Lead I has the negative (−) electrode on the right arm and the positive (+) electrode on the left arm.
      b. Lead II has the negative (−) electrode on the right arm and the positive (+) electrode on the left leg.
      c. Lead III has the (−) electrode on the left arm and the positive (+) electrode on the left leg.
      d. The three standard limb leads comprise Einthoven's triangle and measure the electrical activity of the heart from three different orientations each in the coronal (plane) dimension.

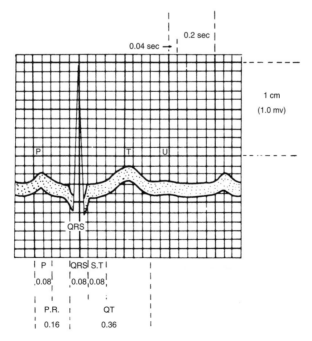

FIG. 11-4 Schematic representation of electrocardiographic (ECG) tracing (see text).

TABLE **11–1**

Normal Time Values for Electrocardiographic (ECG) Events

ECG Event	Time
P wave	0.06-0.11 second
PR interval	0.12-0.20 second
QRS complex	0.03-0.12 second
T wave	0.14-0.26 second
PP/RR intervals	0.60-1.00 second

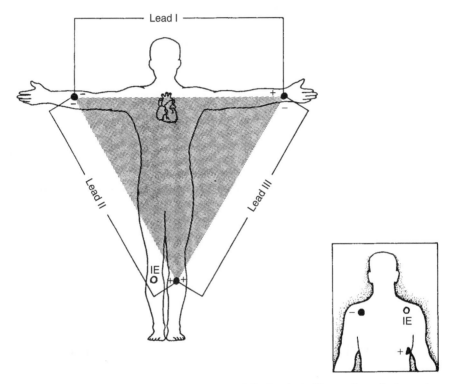

FIG. 11-5 Standard limb leads of the electrocardiogram (ECG). IE is the indifferent electrode. Insert demonstrates the simplified ECG monitoring used for acutely ill patients. These "chest leads" may be used in various positions to accomplish continuous ECG monitoring.

2. The six standard unipolar precordial leads are V_1, V_2, V_3, V_4, V_5, and V_6, where the V represents voltage and each of the numbers 1 through 6 designates a standard position on the chest of the positive (+) electrode (Figure 11-6).
   a. The V_1 lead has the positive electrode placed at the right sternal margin and the fourth intercostal space.
   b. Successive positioning for V_2 through V_6 is located laterally left all at the same transverse level, with V_6 being positioned at the left midaxillary line.
   c. The six precordial leads measure the electrical activity of the heart from six different orientations each in the transverse (plane) dimension.
3. Therefore the same consistently generated electrical activity of the heart will be depicted graphically differently for each lead (Figure 11-7).
4. The standard monitoring lead for acutely ill patients is typically a modified lead II position with the electrodes moved onto the chest and somewhat arbitrarily placed to generate the clearest, consistent representation of ECG events (see Figure 11-5, insert).

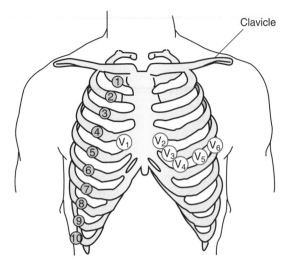

FIG. 11-6 Positions of unipolar precordial (chest) leads as routinely recorded in electrocardiography. V_1 is immediately to the right of the sternum in the fourth intercostal space. V_2 is just to the left of the sternum in the fourth intercostal space. V_4, in the fifth intercostal space, is at the midclavicular line. V_3 is between V_2 and V_4 in the fifth intercostal space and the anterior axillary line. V_6, in the fifth intercostal space, is at the midaxillary line.

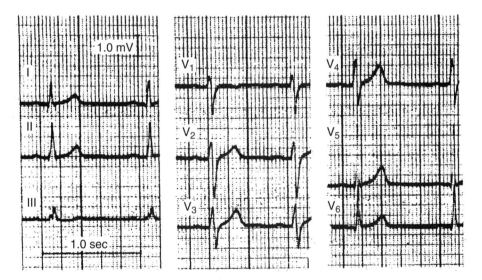

FIG. 11-7 Electrocardiogram from normal adult man showing three standard limb leads recorded simultaneously and six precordial leads.

5. There are three more unipolar extremity leads, V_R, V_L, and V_F, which along with the aforementioned nine standard leads comprise the diagnostic 12-lead ECG. Each of the V_R, V_L, and V_F leads has the positive electrode placed on the right arm, left arm, and left leg, respectively. These leads measure the electrical activity of the heart in the coronal (plane) dimension and provide an orientation similar to that of the standard limb leads.

6. *The P wave, QRS complex, and T wave each represent the collective amount of electrical current and instantaneous direction of that current as measured by a single lead (unidimensional orientation).*

   a. For example, depolarization of the atria proceeds from the superior aspect of the atria and heads in an inferior and slightly leftward direction with successively more collective current generated by greater amounts of atrial muscle fibers depolarized, then decreasing current because there are fewer fibers involved, and eventually no current when depolarization is complete. When measured at a monitoring lead (modified lead II) there is a steadily increasing, then steadily decreasing, collective wave of positive charges heading toward the positive (+) electrode and away from the negative (−) electrode. This is represented on the ECG as a positive deflection (wave) above the baseline or the classic P wave. When depolarization of the atria is complete there is no electrical current, and the ECG tracing returns to baseline, generating the flat PR segment.

b. Depolarization of the ventricles is a little more complex, initially heading from the apex toward the base with septal emphasis. The majority of ventricular depolarization then heads from the base toward the apex, followed by a small portion of depolarization heading in the initial apex to base direction. When measured at a monitoring lead there is a small initial wave of positive charges heading toward the negative (−) electrode, generating the small negative deflection from baseline (Q wave). This is followed by a steadily increasing (and eventually large) wave of positive charges heading toward the positive (+) electrode, which generates the large R wave on the ECG. The collective end of ventricular depolarization heads toward the base of the heart, generating a small wave of positive charges toward the negative (−) electrode and a small negative deflection (S wave). Collectively these ventricular events are represented on the ECG as the classic QRS complex.

c. ECG representation of the repolarization of the atria is masked by the large electrical event of ventricular depolarization as it occurs simultaneously.

d. Repolarization of the ventricles proceeds interestingly from the apex to the base and is characterized by a steadily increasing, then steadily decreasing, collective wave of negative charges heading toward the negative (−) electrode. This is represented on the ECG as a positive deflection (wave) above the baseline or the classic T wave.

e. Note that if the orientation of the lead was changed with the positive electrode placed on the upper right chest and the negative electrode placed on the lower left chest, the same electrical current generated by the heart would generate negative deflections from the baseline for the P, R, and T waves and positive deflections for the Q and S waves, all with the same general configuration and magnitude as compared with what was previously described.

IV. ECG Interpretation

A. The following system represents one simple, organized approach to the evaluation of ECG tracings. There exists a multitude of approaches to the evaluation of ECGs. No matter which one is used, it should provide an organized, repetitive system, which evaluates, at the very least, the following aspects of the ECG.

1. P waves
   a. Should be present.
   b. Should have a configuration similar to that of other P waves.
   c. Should be related on a one-to-one basis to the QRS complex.
2. PR intervals
   a. Should have a normal duration of 0.12 to 0.20 second.
   b. Should have consistent duration when compared with other PR intervals.
3. QRS complexes
   a. Should have a duration of <0.12 second.
   b. Should have a similar configuration when compared with other QRS complexes.
4. RR and PP intervals
   a. RR intervals should have a consistent duration when compared with other RR intervals.
   b. PP intervals should have a consistent duration when compared with other PP intervals.
   c. RR interval should be approximately equal to the PP interval in duration.

5. Cardiac rate
   a. Should be 60 to 100 events/min.
      (1) Rates <60 events/min denote bradycardia.
      (2) Rates >100 events/min denote tachycardia.
   b. Atrial rate should be equal to the ventricular rate.
   c. The atrial and ventricular rates can be determined by using the PP and RR interval measurements on calibrated ECG paper (see Figure 11-4).
      (1) The ECG paper is divided into small (fine-lined) and large (bold-lined) squares that measure 1 mm and 5 mm, respectively, on each side.
         (a) The horizontal (x) axis represents time.
         (b) The vertical (y) axis represents electrical voltage.
      (2) Each small (1 mm) horizontal square represents 0.04 second, and each larger (5 mm) horizontal square represents 0.2 second.
      (3) Therefore if the RR interval spans four large boxes, it measures 0.8 second; 60 sec/min divided by 0.8 sec/ventricular cycle = 75 ventricular cycles/min. If the PP and RR intervals are equal, then the cardiac rate = 75 events/min.
      (4) The resulting rate for the RR interval spanning one large box is 300/min. The RR interval spanning two large boxes is 150/min; three large boxes is 100/min; four large boxes is 75/min; five large boxes is 60/min; six large boxes is 50/min; seven large boxes is 43/min; and eight large boxes is 37/min. This provides for a quick estimate of rate of any cardiac event by simply memorizing and counting off large (bold-lined) boxes spanned by cardiac events, with the descending rates of 300, 150, 100, 75, 60, 50, 43, and 37/min.
      (5) The small (1 mm) vertical square represents 0.1 mV, and each larger (5 mm) vertical square represents 0.5 mV of electrical amplitude. This measurement is of little importance in the clinical setting when the ECG is being used on a continuous monitoring basis. Further the amplitude is commonly amplified to generate a large R wave that will easily be recognized by the monitor and therefore provide an accurate heart rate.
6. After careful evaluation of the previous five steps, the underlying aberration, if any, should be revealed and the rhythm easily identified.
7. Treatment, if any, should then be guided by the existent and/or potential mechanical consequences of the identified cardiac rhythm.

B. Normal sinus rhythm (Figure 11-8)
   1. P waves are present, have similar configurations, and are related to QRS complexes.
   2. PR interval is 0.12 to 0.20 second and equal to other PR intervals.
   3. QRS complex is <0.12 second and similar in configuration to other QRS complexes.
   4. RR intervals are regular and equal to PP intervals.
   5. Cardiac rate is 60 to 100 events/min.
   6. No treatment is warranted.

C. Sinus arrhythmia (Figure 11-9)
   1. P waves are present, have similar configuration, and are related to the QRS complexes.
   2. PR interval is normal in duration and equal to other PR intervals.
   3. QRS complex is normal in duration and similar in configuration to other QRS complexes.

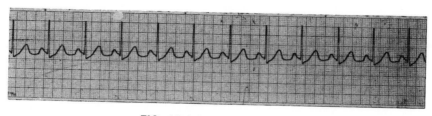

FIG. 11-8 Normal sinus rhythm.

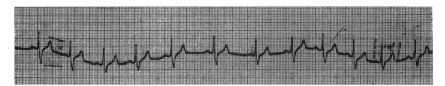

FIG. 11-9 Sinus arrhythmia.

4. PP and RR intervals vary (typically with the ventilatory cycle); however, they are equal to one another for a given cardiac cycle.
5. Cardiac rate varies; however, it generally averages 60 to 100 events/min.
6. Generally no treatment is warranted unless there are significant alterations in arterial blood pressure (i.e., symptomatic hypotension), in which (rare) case, atropine may be used to accelerate cardiac rate.

D. Sinus bradycardia (Figure 11-10)
1. P waves are present, have similar configuration, and are related to QRS complexes.
2. PR interval is normal in duration and equal to other PR intervals.
3. QRS complex is normal in duration and similar in configuration to other QRS complexes.
4. RR intervals are regular and equal to PP intervals.
5. Cardiac rate is <60 events/min.
6. Generally no treatment is warranted unless there are significant alterations in arterial blood pressure (i.e., symptomatic hypotension). Treatment is aimed at increasing the heart rate, in which case intravenous atropine is the drug of choice. Further therapies include transcutaneous and transvenous pacing and epinephrine, dopamine, and isoproterenol administration.

E. Sinus tachycardia (Figure 11-11)
1. P waves are present, have similar configuration, and are related to QRS complexes.
2. PR interval is normal in duration (lower limits of normal) and equal to other PR intervals.
3. QRS complex is normal in duration and similar in configuration to other QRS complexes.
4. RR intervals are regular and equal to PP intervals.
5. Cardiac rate is >100 events/min.

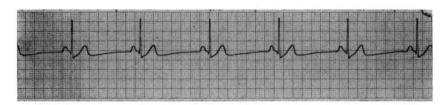

FIG. 11-10 Sinus bradycardia.

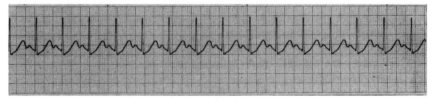

FIG. 11-11 Sinus tachycardia.

6. This rhythm is the normal physiologic response to stress and occurs with infection, hypovolemia, hypoxemia, and myocardial infarction and in response to stimulant drugs; therefore, intervention should be aimed at treating the underlying cause. The rate usually has a gradual onset and elimination.

F. Premature atrial contraction (PAC) (Figure 11-12)
   1. P wave occurs earlier than expected and may have a normal or abnormal configuration.
   2. PR interval is usually normal and equal in duration to other PR intervals.
   3. QRS complex is usually normal in duration and similar in configuration to other QRS complexes; however, it may be absent if the P wave is not conducted through the AV node.
   4. PP and RR intervals vary with the PAC; however, they are equal to one another for a given cardiac cycle.
   5. Cardiac rate: PACs can occur at any rate.
   6. No treatment is warranted if the PACs are infrequent. There are many causes, including increased sympathetic stimulation, exogenous stimulants, drug interactions, cardiac ischemia, and acute myocardial infarction. PACs indicate increased automaticity; therefore, when they are frequent, discontinuation of stimulants such as tobacco, caffeine, and/or sympathomimetics is generally indicated.

G. Atrial tachycardia (Figure 11-13)
   1. P waves are present; however, they may be superimposed on a preceding T wave.
   2. PR interval is usually normal in duration and equal to other PR intervals. However, with rapid rates it may be difficult to determine.
   3. QRS complex is usually normal in duration and similar in configuration to other QRS complexes.
   4. PP and RR intervals are regular and usually equal to each other.
   5. Rate: Atrial rate is usually 160 to 220/min, and ventricular rate is 160 to 220/min with 1:1 conduction; however, it may be 80 to 110/min with 2:1 conduction.
   6. Conservative treatment, such as vagal stimulation (i.e., carotid sinus massage or Valsalva maneuver), should be used for the symptomatic but hemodynamically stable patient, followed by intravenous adenosine administration to allow identification of the tachycardic source, underlying cause, and appropriate treatment. If cardiac function remains good, sequential priority-based administration of β-blockers, Ca^{2+} channel blockers, and amiodarone is warranted. Conversely, for patients with poor cardiac function (e.g., congestive heart failure or ejection fraction <40%), amiodarone and diltiazem, without synchronized direct current (DC) countershock, are used. When the arrhythmia has resulted in significant hemodynamic instability, synchronized DC countershock with sequentially increasing power (50, 100, 200, 300, and 360 J) is the treatment of choice.

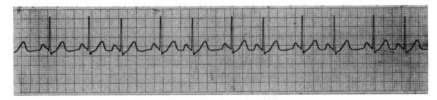

FIG. 11-12 Premature atrial contraction.

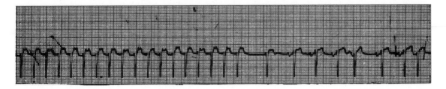

FIG. 11-13 Atrial tachycardia.

H. Atrial flutter (Figure 11-14)
1. P waves are present, have similar configuration, and resemble a saw-tooth or picket fence pattern.
2. PR interval is usually normal and equal in duration to other PR intervals; however, it may be difficult to measure.
3. QRS complex is usually normal in duration and similar in configuration to other QRS complexes.
4. PP interval is regular and equal to other PP intervals; RR interval is regular and equal to other RR intervals; PP interval is usually not equal to RR interval as a result of AV nodal block.
5. Atrial rate is typically 220 to 350/min; ventricular rate depends on the degree of conduction through the AV node (i.e., 2:1, 3:1, or 4:1 conduction).
6. When a rapid ventricular rate has resulted in hemodynamic instability, synchronized DC countershock is the treatment of choice. If cardiac function is poor and/or the patient is not a candidate for cardioversion, a course of digoxin, esmolol HCL, or amiodarone is used. Controlled, definitive treatment is surgical or catheter ablation.

I. Atrial fibrillation (Figure 11-15)
1. P waves are not truly present; rather, fine or coarse irregular rapid baseline undulations called *fibrillatory waves* (f waves) occur, characterized by an undulating baseline replacing P waves and an irregularly irregular ventricular response.
2. PR interval is not present.
3. QRS complex is usually normal in duration and similar in configuration to other QRS complexes.
4. PP interval is not measurable; RR interval is irregular and not equal to other RR intervals.
5. Atrial rate is approximately 350 to 700/min; ventricular rate is 100 to 200/min.
6. Initial treatment typically consists of anticoagulation and increasing doses of digoxin, esmolol HCL, or amiodarone in an attempt to block the number of impulses reaching the ventricles. However, as for atrial flutter, the treatment of choice is synchronized DC countershock when the individual is manifesting hemodynamic compromise.

J. First-degree heart block (Figure 11-16)
1. P waves are present, are similar in configuration to other P waves, and are related to the QRS complex.
2. PR interval is >0.20 second and usually equal in duration to other PR intervals but may vary.

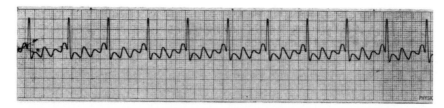

FIG. 11-14 Atrial flutter.

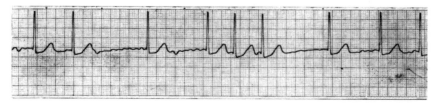

FIG. 11-15 Atrial fibrillation.

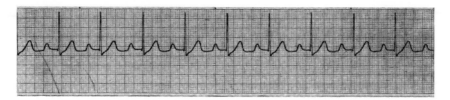

FIG. 11-16 First-degree heart block.

3. QRS complex is normal in duration and similar in configuration to other QRS complexes.
4. RR intervals are regular and equal to PP intervals.
5. Rate: First-degree heart block can occur at any rate.
6. Is seen in normal patients, however, may occur as a result of insult to AV node, hypoxemia, myocardial infarction, digitalis toxicity, ischemia of the conduction system, and/or increased vagal tone. No treatment is warranted with the exception of monitoring for the occurrence of higher order forms of heart block (i.e., second or third degree).

K. Type I (Wenckebach) second-degree heart block (Figure 11-17)
1. P waves are present, are similar in configuration to other P waves, and are related to QRS complexes, except for the nonconducted P waves.
2. PR interval may begin with normal duration but lengthens progressively until one P wave is not conducted.
3. QRS complex is normal in duration and similar in configuration to other QRS complexes.
4. PP interval is regular and equal to other PP intervals. RR intervals vary with absent QRS complexes.
5. Atrial rate is typically 60 to 100/min; ventricular rate varies with degree of block (i.e., 2:1, 3:2, or 4:3 conduction).
6. Generally no treatment is warranted unless there are significant alterations in arterial blood pressure (i.e., symptomatic hypotension), in which case atropine, dopamine, and epinephrine should be used to accelerate cardiac rate. A transcutaneous pacemaker is indicated when pharmacologic intervention is either not effective or contraindicated. In any case, monitoring for higher order heart block is advised but rarely does this conduction abnormality progress to higher degree heart blocks.

L. Type II (Mobitz II) second-degree heart block (Figure 11-18)
1. P waves are present, are similar in configuration to other P waves, and are related to QRS complexes, except for the nonconducted P waves.

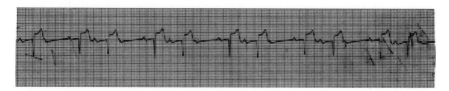

FIG. 11-17 Type I second-degree heart block.

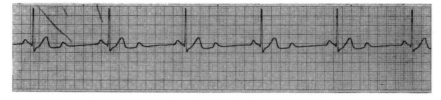

FIG. 11-18 Type II second-degree heart block.

2. PR interval may be normal or prolonged; however, it is equal in duration to other PR intervals.
3. QRS complex is usually normal in duration and similar in configuration to other QRS complexes.
4. PP interval is regular and equal to other PP intervals. RR intervals vary with absent QRS complexes; however, the PP and RR intervals are equal in cardiac cycles where the P wave is conducted.
5. Atrial rate is typically 60 to 100/min; ventricular rate varies with the degree of block.
6. A permanent pacemaker is the treatment of choice to ensure adequate ventricular rate. Intravenous atropine, transcutaneous pacing, dopamine, epinephrine, and lastly transvenous pacing are used to ensure an adequate ventricular rate in the interim.

M. Third-degree or complete heart block (Figure 11-19)
1. P waves are present, are similar in configuration to other P waves, but are unrelated to the QRS complexes.
2. PR interval is completely variable and of no consequence.
3. QRS complexes are normal in configuration and duration when block occurs at the AV node or bundle of His. QRS complexes are wide and aberrant when block occurs at the bundle branches.
4. PP and RR intervals are regular but are not equal to each other.
5. Atrial rate is typically 60 to 100/min; ventricular rate is typically 40 to 60/min with block at the AV node and <40/min with infranodal block.
6. Left alone it may progress to ventricular standstill. A permanent pacemaker is the treatment of choice to ensure adequate ventricular rate. Intravenous atropine, transcutaneous pacing, dopamine, epinephrine, and lastly transvenous pacing are used to ensure an adequate ventricular rate in the interim.

N. Junctional or nodal rhythm (Figure 11-20)
1. P waves are typically absent; however, they may be conducted retrogradely and appear anywhere in the cardiac cycle.
2. PR interval is usually not measurable.
3. QRS is usually normal in duration and is similar in configuration to other QRS complexes.
4. PP interval usually not measurable. RR interval is regular.
5. Ventricular rate is typically 40 to 60/min.
6. This arrhythmia occurs with increased vagal tone to the SA node, hypoxemia, and/or digitalis toxicity. Atropine, dopamine, and epinephrine should be used to accelerate cardiac rate and maintain blood pressure. A transcutaneous pacemaker is indicated when pharmacologic intervention is either not effective or contraindicated.

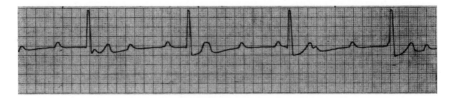

FIG. 11-19 Third-degree or complete heart block.

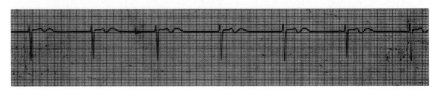

FIG. 11-20 Junctional or nodal rhythm.

O. Supraventricular tachycardia (Figure 11-21)
   1. P waves are usually indiscernible. They may be absent, conducted retrogradely, or buried in the preceding T wave.
   2. PR interval cannot be measured.
   3. QRS complex is normal in duration and similar in configuration to other QRS complexes.
   4. PP interval is not measurable. RR interval is regular and equal to other RR intervals.
   5. Rate is typically >150/min.
   6. Intervention for the hemodynamically stable patient commonly includes vagal maneuvers, followed by intravenous adenosine administration to allow identification of the tachycardic source, underlying cause, and appropriate treatment. However, in the instance of hemodynamic compromise, synchronized DC countershock with sequentially increasing power (50, 100, 200, 300, and 360 J) is the treatment of choice.

P. Premature ventricular contraction (PVC) (Figure 11-22)
   1. P waves are typically absent.
   2. PR interval with PVC is not measurable.
   3. QRS complex is wide (>0.12 second), bizarre, and unlike normal QRS complexes. It appears earlier in the cardiac cycle than expected and has a T wave on the opposite side of the baseline from the terminal portion of the QRS (PVC) complex.
   4. PP interval with PVC is not measurable. RR interval varies with the occurrence of PVC.
   5. PVCs can occur at any rate.
   6. In the healthy heart no treatment is warranted. However, with impaired cardiac function, increased frequency, or multiform variations, treatment is indicated. PVCs may indicate acute myocardial ischemia requiring rapid intervention, including oxygen, nitroglycerin, or morphine. However, intravenous procainamide or lidocaine is the treatment of choice along with eventual identification and treatment of the underlying cause.

Q. Ventricular tachycardia (Figure 11-23)
   1. P waves are generally indiscernible.
   2. PR interval is not measurable.
   3. QRS complex is wide, bizarre, and generally similar in configuration to other QRS complexes.
   4. PP interval is not measurable. RR interval is regular or slightly irregular.
   5. Ventricular rate is 100 to 250/min.
   6. Intravenous procainamide is the treatment of choice for the hemodynamically stable patient. For the hemodynamically unstable (with pulse) patient, synchronized DC cardioversion with sequentially increasing power (100, 200, 300, and 360 J) is indicated. In

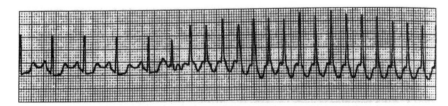

FIG. 11-21 Supraventricular tachycardia.

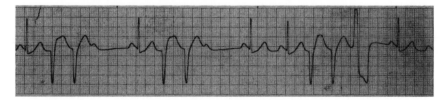

FIG. 11-22 Premature ventricular contraction.

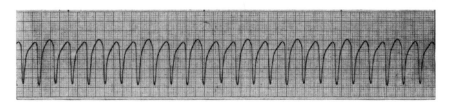

FIG. 11-23 Ventricular tachycardia.

contrast, for the pulseless patient, a precordial thump is initiated if witnessed; support with cardiopulmonary resuscitation (CPR) until defibrillation can be implemented sequentially at progressively higher power (200 J, 200 to 300 J, and 360 J) and is successful.

R. Ventricular flutter (Figure 11-24)
1. P waves are absent.
2. PR interval is absent.
3. QRS complex appears as a smooth sinusoidal wave with QRS complex and T waves merged and no clear separation of cardiac cycles.
4. PP interval is absent. RR interval is regular.
5. Ventricular rate is typically 200 to 300/min.
6. Initially support with CPR (if witnessed, initiate a precordial thump) until defibrillation can be implemented at progressively higher power (200 J, 200 to 300 J, and 360 J) and is successful.

S. Ventricular fibrillation (Figure 11-25)
1. P waves are absent.
2. PR interval is absent.
3. QRS complexes are absent; however, there is low (fine) or high (coarse) amplitude undulation from the baseline that varies in shape and represents varying degrees of depolarization and repolarization.
4. PP and RR intervals are absent.
5. Rate is absent.
6. Treat with CPR (if witnessed, initiate a precordial thump) until defibrillation can be implemented at progressively higher power (200 J, 200 to 300 J, and 360 J) and is successful.

T. Asystole (Figure 11-26)

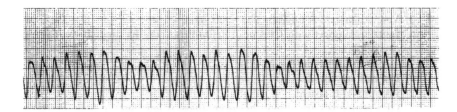

FIG. 11-24 Ventricular flutter.

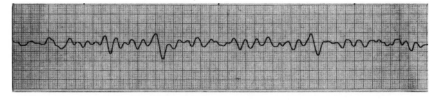

FIG. 11-25 Ventricular fibrillation.

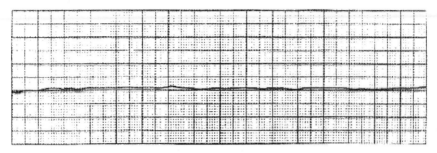

FIG. 11-26 Asystole.

1. Represented by the total absence of electrical activity; however, there may be erratic undulations from baseline.
2. Treat with CPR, confirm true asystole (versus fine ventricular fibrillation) with second ECG lead, and then implement transcutaneous pacemaker and intravenous epinephrine and atropine.

BIBLIOGRAPHY

Conover MB: *Exercise in Diagnosing ECG Tracings,* ed 3. St. Louis, Mosby, 1984.

Cummins RO: *Textbook of Advanced Cardiac Life Support.* Dallas, American Heart Association Incorporated, 1994.

Daily EF: *Techniques in Hemodynamic Monitoring,* ed 5. St. Louis, Mosby, 1994.

Dubin D: *Rapid Interpretation of EKGs,* ed 3. Tampa, Cover Publishing, 1979.

George RB, Light RW, Matthay MA, Matthay RA: *Chest Medicine—Essentials of Pulmonary and Critical Care Medicine,* ed 3. Baltimore, Williams & Wilkins, 1995.

Grauer K: *Practical Guide to ECG Interpretation,* ed 2. St. Louis, Mosby, 1998.

Guyton AJ, Hall JE: *Textbook of Medical Physiology,* ed 10. Philadelphia, Elsevier Health Sciences Division, 2000.

Marriott HJL: *Practical Electrocardiography,* ed 6. Baltimore, Williams & Wilkins, 1980.

Morris F: *ECG Interpretation for Emergency Medicine: A Self Assessment Guide,* Philadelphia, Elsevier Science & Technology Books, 1997.

Mountcastle VB: *Medical Physiology,* ed 14. St. Louis, Mosby, 1980.

Netter FH: *Section II, The Electrocardiogram, The CIBA Collection of Medical Illustrations, vol 5.* New York, CIBA, 1978.

Ochs G: *Recognition and Interpretation of ECG Rhythms,* ed 3. New York, Prentice Hall, 1997.

Phillips RE, Feeney MK: *The Cardiac Rhythms: A Systematic Approach to Interpretation,* ed 3. Philadelphia, Elsevier Health Sciences Division, 1990.

Randall M: *ECG Interpretation,* ed 2. Raleigh, Hayes Barton Press, 2000.

Ruch TC, Patton HD: *Physiology and Biophysics,* ed 20. Philadelphia, WB Saunders, 1982.

Rushmer RF: *Cardiovascular Dynamics,* ed 4. Philadelphia, Elsevier Health Sciences Division, 1976.

Shapiro BA, Harrison RA, Kacmarek RM, et al: *Clinical Applications of Respiratory Care,* ed 3. Chicago, Year Book Medical Publishers, 1985.

Spearman CB, Sheldon RL, Egan DF: *Egan's Fundamentals of Respiratory Therapy,* ed 4. St. Louis, Mosby, 1982.

Springhouse Corporation Staff: *ECG Interpretation Made Incredibly Easy!* ed 2. Philadelphia, Lippincott Williams & Wilkins, 2001.

Tobin MJ: *Principles and Practices in Intensive Care Monitoring.* New York, McGraw-Hill, 1997.

Wagner GS: *Practical Electrocardiography,* ed 9. Baltimore, Williams & Wilkins, 1994.

Chapter 12

Hemodynamic Monitoring

I. **Systemic Arterial Blood Pressure**
   Systemic arterial blood pressure is expressed as a systolic pressure over a diastolic pressure (Figure 12-1).
   A. Systolic pressure is the highest pressure attained in the artery and is determined by three major factors:
      1. Stroke volume of left ventricle
         a. Increased stroke volume generally causes increased systolic pressure.
         b. Decreased stroke volume generally causes decreased systolic pressure.
      2. Rate of blood ejection from left ventricle
         a. An increased rate of left ventricular ejection generally results in increased systolic pressure.
         b. A decrease in the rate of ejection generally results in decreased systolic pressure.
      3. Elasticity of the arterial tree
         a. Increased arterial elasticity generally results in increased systolic pressure.
         b. Decreased arterial elasticity generally results in decreased systolic pressure.
   B. Diastolic pressure is the lowest pressure attained in the artery and is determined by three major factors:
      1. Magnitude of preceding systolic pressure
         a. In general, the higher the preceding systolic pressure, the higher the resulting diastolic pressure.
         b. The lower the preceding systolic pressure, the lower the resulting diastolic pressure.
      2. Length of ventricular diastolic interval
         a. The longer the diastolic interval, the greater the time available for blood to leave the arterial system and the lower the resultant diastolic pressure.
         b. The shorter the diastolic interval, the higher the diastolic pressure by the opposite mechanism.
      3. State of peripheral resistance
         a. The greater the peripheral resistance, the lower the rate of arterial runoff and the higher the resultant diastolic pressure.
         b. The lower the peripheral resistance, the higher the rate of arterial runoff and the lower the resultant diastolic pressure.
   C. Measurement of arterial blood pressure generally assesses left ventricular function by systolic pressure and peripheral resistance by diastolic pressure. The most significant factor responsible for systolic pressure is stroke volume, and the factor principally responsible for diastolic pressure is the state of peripheral resistance.
   D. Thus it is assumed that the greater the difference between systolic and diastolic pressures, the greater the resultant flow. The difference between systolic and diastolic pressures is called the *pulse pressure*.

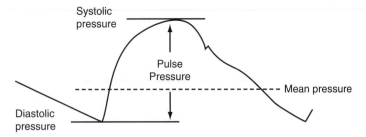

FIG. 12-1 Graphic representation of arterial pressure tracing depicting systolic, diastolic, mean, and pulse pressure (see text).

1. By the equation:

$$\dot{Q} = P \times \frac{1}{R} \tag{1}$$

   increases in systolic pressure indicate increases in the pressure gradient (P) across the systemic circulation, and decreases in diastolic pressure indicate decreases in peripheral resistance (R).
2. Therefore widening of pulse pressure is generally thought to indicate increased blood flow ($\dot{Q}$).
3. By the opposite mechanism, narrowing of pulse pressure is generally thought to indicate decreased flow.
4. It should be noted that widening of pulse pressure could occur without increased blood flow. Normal blood flow also can exist with a narrow pulse pressure. These phenomena occur by alterations in the other factors (i.e., diastolic interval and arterial elasticity) that determine systolic and diastolic pressure. Therefore it is imperative to assess all factors responsible for systolic and diastolic pressure before blindly stating that an increased or decreased pulse pressure represents increased or decreased blood flow in a given patient.
5. In the absence of pulmonary artery catheterization and/or serial cardiac output measurements, the trend in pulse pressure is used as a gross indicator of trends in cardiac output.
   E. The mean arterial pressure (MAP) represents the average pressure over one complete systolic and diastolic interval.
   1. The MAP can be directly measured via a systemic arterial line or estimated by the following formula:

$$MAP = \frac{(2 \times diastolic\,pressure) + (systolic\,pressure)}{3} \tag{2}$$

   2. The MAP is the average pressure in the arterial tree over a given time and therefore generally is used to assess the average pressure to which the arterial system is exposed.
   3. The pressure gradient across the systemic circulation is generally expressed as MAP – central venous pressure (CVP; see Section II, Central Venous Pressure).
   4. The MAP is also commonly used as an indicator of left ventricular afterload, thus representing the resistance (in terms of pressure) against which the left ventricle must pump.
      a. Afterload generally reflects an inverse relationship with stroke volume the more compromised the state of the left ventricle.
      b. Afterload always represents a direct relationship with myocardial oxygen consumption and therefore myocardial work.
   F. Arterial blood pressure and mean arterial blood pressure can be directly measured by an intraarterial line (catheter). Alternately arterial blood pressure can be indirectly measured using a sphygmomanometer (Figure 12-2), and the MAP can be calculated from the obtained systolic and diastolic values.

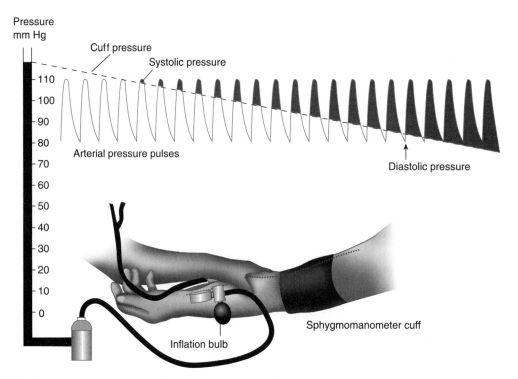

FIG. 12-2 Sphygmomanometry. When the pressure within the sphygmomanometer cuff is increased above arterial blood pressure, the arteries under the cuff are occluded and no pulse can be palpated at the wrist. As the cuff pressure is gradually released, the systolic peaks of pressure finally exceed cuff pressure and blood spurts into the arteries below the cuff, producing palpable pulses at the wrist. The sudden acceleration of blood below the cuff produces vibrations that are audible through a stethoscope. The pressure in the mercury manometer at the time the pulse is heard or felt indicates systolic pressure. As cuff pressure is further diminished, the sounds increase in intensity and then rather suddenly become muffled at the level of diastolic pressure where the arteries remain open throughout the entire pulse wave. At still lower pressures, the sounds disappear completely when laminar flow is reestablished.

    G. Normal values for arterial blood pressure in the adult are as follows:

Systolic:	90 to 140 mm Hg
Diastolic:	60 to 90 mm Hg
Mean:	70 to 105 mm Hg

II. Central Venous Pressure

The CVP usually is expressed as a single number representing the mean right atrial pressure ($\overline{RAP}$).

  A. The numerical pressure value of CVP is the result of the following factors:

    1. The pump capabilities of the right side of the heart in part determine the CVP. If the right ventricle pumps what it receives, blood will not back up in the atrium, and the CVP should be normal. If the right side of the heart is not pumping adequately, there will be a backup of blood in the atrium that will be reflected in elevated CVP.

    2. The venous tone determines CVP because venous tone is responsible for determining the venous vascular space. It thus has major implications in venous return and filling pressure of the right atrium.

    3. Blood volume, which in part determines CVP, must be adequate to fill the venous vascular space, or venous return to the heart will be impeded.

4. *If the pump capabilities of the right side of the heart are adequate, the CVP will directly reflect the venous vascular volume (blood volume)-to-venous vascular space relationship.* Fluid therapy and diuresis are frequently gauged in terms of the CVP's reflection of this relationship.

B. The CVP is commonly used as an indicator of right ventricular preload when measured as the right ventricular end-diastolic pressure (RVEDP).
    1. The RVEDP represents compliance of the right ventricle.
    2. The RVEDP also represents the filling pressure necessary for the ensuing right ventricular contraction.
C. The CVP is measured directly through a catheter inserted in a peripheral vein that traverses the vena cava with its tip resting in the right atrium (Figure 12-3) or from a four-lumen pulmonary artery catheter having a proximally located open channel in the right atrium (see Figure 12-8).
D. Normal values for CVP in the adult are 0 to 8 mm Hg.

III. **Pulmonary Artery Pressure (PAP)**
   The PAP is expressed as systolic pressure over diastolic pressure.
   A. Systolic pressure is the highest pressure attained in the pulmonary artery and is determined by the same three factors that determine systolic pressure in the systemic arterial system:
       1. Size of right ventricular stroke volume
       2. Rate of blood ejection from right ventricle
       3. Elasticity of pulmonary arterial tree
   B. Diastolic pressure is the lowest pressure attained in the pulmonary artery and is determined by the same three factors that determine diastolic pressure in the systemic arterial system:
       1. Magnitude of preceding systolic pressure
       2. Length of ventricular diastolic interval
       3. State of peripheral resistance of the pulmonary arterial tree
   C. Measurement of PAP generally assesses right ventricular function by systolic pressure and pulmonary arterial resistance by diastolic pressure. Thus PAP is used in precisely the same fashion as systemic arterial pressure. In this light it should be noted that all factors contributing to systolic and diastolic PAP should be fully assessed before inferences concerning blood flow are made from these values.

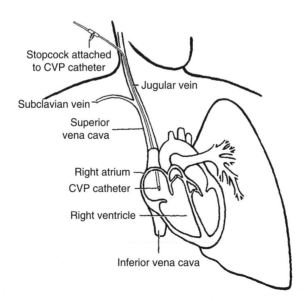

FIG. 12-3 Central venous pressure (CVP) catheter inserted through the jugular vein with the tip positioned in the right atrium.

D. The mean pulmonary artery pressure ($\overline{\text{PAP}}$) represents the average pressure over one complete systolic and diastolic interval.

  1. The $\overline{\text{PAP}}$ is the average pressure in the pulmonary artery over a given time and is used to assess the average pressure head (or front) to which the pulmonary arterial system is exposed.
  2. Thus the pressure gradient across the pulmonary circulation is generally represented by the expression $\overline{\text{PAP}}$ – pulmonary wedge pressure (PWP), or mean left atrial pressure, also referred to as the pulmonary artery opening pressure (PAOP) or pulmonary capillary wedge pressure (PCWP; see Section IV, Pulmonary Wedge Pressure).
  3. The $\overline{\text{PAP}}$ is commonly used to assess right ventricular afterload, thus representing the resistance (in terms of pressure) against which the right ventricle must pump.
      a. Afterload generally reflects an inverse relationship with stroke volume the more compromised the state of the right ventricle.
      b. Afterload always represents a direct relationship with myocardial oxygen consumption and therefore myocardial work.
      c. Afterload of the right and left ventricles may vary dramatically and, when monitoring allows, should be independently evaluated.

E. The PAP and $\overline{\text{PAP}}$ are directly measured using a pulmonary artery catheter. The pulmonary artery catheter is inserted through a peripheral vein and traverses the vena cava, right atrium, and ventricle, with its tip resting in the pulmonary artery. As the catheter is advanced, the typical pressure curves (deflection) generated on an oscilloscope are observed to monitor its distal location (Figure 12-4).

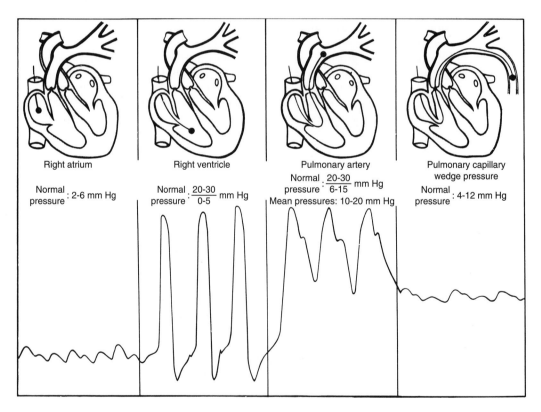

FIG. 12-4 From left to right: Right atrial pressure; right ventricular pressure—note that diastolic pressure is zero baseline or below; pulmonary artery pressure—note that diastolic pressure is significantly above zero baseline; pulmonary wedge pressure—catheter tip senses only pulmonary capillary back pressure since balloon obstructs arterial flow. Deflation of the balloon should result in immediate return of the pulmonary artery pressure pattern (see text).

F. Normal values for pulmonary arterial blood pressure in the adult are as follows:

Systolic:	15 to 28 mm Hg
Diastolic:	5 to 16 mm Hg
Mean:	10 to 22 mm Hg

IV. Pulmonary Wedge Pressure (PAOP or PCWP)

PWP is expressed as a single number representing the mean left atrial pressure ($\overline{LAP}$).

A. The numerical pressure value of the PWP will be the result of the following factors:
1. The pump capabilities of the left side of the heart in part determine the PWP. If the left ventricle pumps what it receives, blood will not back up into the atrium, and the PWP should be normal. If the left ventricle is not pumping adequately, there will be a backup of blood into the atrium that will be reflected as elevated PWP.
2. Blood return to the left atrium is largely the result of an adequate blood volume-to-pulmonary venous (venomotor tone) vascular space relationship.
3. If the left ventricle is pumping adequately, the PWP depends on the aforementioned vascular volume-to-vascular space relationship.

B. The PWP is commonly used as an indicator of left ventricular preload when measured as the left ventricular end-diastolic pressure (LVEDP).
1. The LVEDP represents compliance of the left ventricle.
2. The LVEDP also represents the filling pressure necessary for the ensuing left ventricular contraction.
3. Preload generally varies directly with the size of the ensuing stroke volume and therefore cardiac output as may be experienced with fluid therapy.
4. However, in the failing ventricle or fluid-overloaded patient, preload varies inversely with stroke volume and cardiac output. Such a situation also represents increases in myocardial oxygen consumption and work.
5. Preload of the left and right ventricles may also vary dramatically and therefore should be separately assessed with the availability of a pulmonary artery catheter.

C. The PWP is measured directly through a pulmonary artery catheter by the intermittent inflation of a balloon that occludes the local branch of the pulmonary artery (Figure 12-5). Pressure readings are taken from the tip of the catheter, which is distal to the balloon. The inflated balloon obstructs the systolic and diastolic pulmonary artery pressures (the characteristic pressure contour should be absent). Therefore the pressure measurement reflects backpressure (through a low resistance system) from the left atrium.

D. Normal values for the PWP in the adult are 2 to 12 mm Hg.

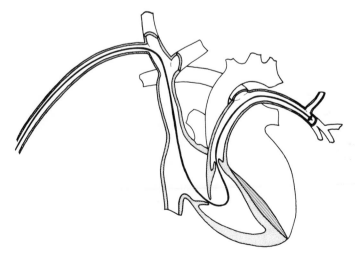

FIG. 12-5 Location of a pulmonary artery catheter.

V. **Calculation and Comparison of Systemic and Pulmonary Vascular Resistance**
A.

$$R = \frac{\Delta P}{\dot{Q}} \tag{3}$$

where R = vascular resistance expressed in mm Hg/L/min; ΔP = change in pressure across the circulation or pressure gradient, expressed in mm Hg; and Q̇ = cardiac output or flow expressed in L/min.

B. Systemic vascular resistance (SVR) (Figure 12-6) equals:
1.

$$SVR = \frac{MAP - \overline{RAP}}{\dot{Q}} \tag{4}$$

where MAP = mean arterial pressure; $\overline{RAP}$ = mean right atrial pressure (CVP); and Q̇ = cardiac output.

2. Replacing the factors with representative normal values results in

$$SVR = \frac{(100 - 5)\,mm\,Hg}{5\,L/min} = 19\,mm\,Hg/L/min \tag{5}$$

C. Pulmonary vascular resistance (PVR) (see Figure 12-6) equals:
1.

$$PVR = \frac{\overline{PAP} - \overline{LAP}}{\dot{Q}} \tag{6}$$

where $\overline{PAP}$ = mean pulmonary arterial pressure; $\overline{LAP}$ = mean left atrial pressure (PWP); and Q̇ = cardiac output.

2. Replacing the factors with representative normal values results in

$$R = \frac{(15 - 5)\,mm\,Hg}{5\,L/min} = 2\,mm\,Hg/L/min \tag{7}$$

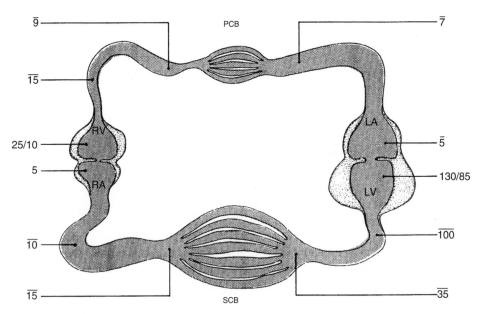

FIG. 12-6 Schema of circulatory mechanics in the human cardiopulmonary system. *LA,* Left atrium; *RA,* right atrium; *LV,* left ventricle; *RV,* right ventricle; *SCB,* systemic capillary bed; *PCB,* pulmonary capillary bed. The numbers represent mean pressure except in the ventricles where systolic and diastolic pressures are noted (see text).

D. In this example, SVR equals 19 mm Hg/L/min and PVR equals 2 mm Hg/L/min. This relationship results in SVR being approximately 9.5 times the PVR. Stated otherwise, a pressure gradient 9.5 times as great is required of the left ventricle when compared with the right ventricle to create the same (5 L) left and right cardiac output (Figure 12-7).

E. In the aforementioned example, vascular resistance is represented by an arbitrary vascular resistance unit (VRU) for simplicity. Vascular resistance in the clinical and research setting is reported as a proper scientific representation of resistance expressed as dyne-sec/cm^5 with a conversion factor of 1 VRU = 80 dyne-sec/cm^5. Hence in the aforementioned example, PVR = 2 VRU × 80 dyne-sec/cm^5 or 160 dyne-sec/cm^5 and SVR = 19 VRU × 80 dyne-sec/cm^5 or 1520 dyne-sec/cm^5.

F. Vascular resistance should be independently assessed and serially tracked as indices of the effectiveness or necessities of interventional therapies, such as:
1. Administration of vasoactive drugs (e.g., dopamine and dobutamine)
2. Fluid or diuretic therapy
3. Administration of adequate oxygenation levels
4. Optimization of mean intrathoracic pressures during mechanical ventilation

VI. **Summary of Normal Hemodynamic Values (Table 12-1)**

VII. **Techniques of Measuring Cardiac Output**
A. Fick method
1. The total amount of oxygen available for tissue utilization must be equal to arterial oxygen content (CaO_2), expressed in vol%, times the volume of blood presented to the tissues per unit time ($\dot{Q}$ or cardiac output), expressed in L/min:

$$\text{Total } O_2 \text{ available} = (\dot{Q}) \times (CaO_2) \tag{8}$$

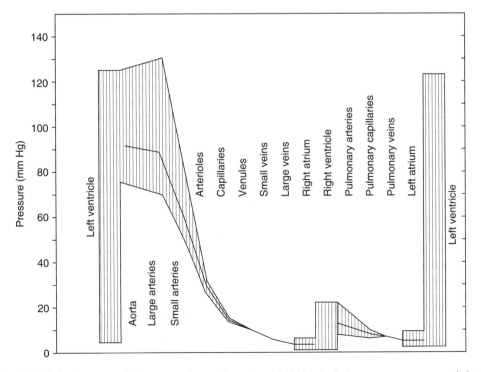

FIG. 12-7 Typical pressures in human cardiovascular system. Solid line indicates mean pressures, and shaded area indicates pulsations in systole and diastole.

TABLE **12-1**		
Normal Ranges of Systemic and Pulmonary Hemodynamic Values		
	Systemic	**Pulmonary**
Systolic	90-140 mm Hg	15-28 mm Hg
Diastolic	60-90 mm Hg	5-16 mm Hg
Mean	70-105 mm Hg	10-22 mm Hg
CVP or PWP	0-8 mm Hg	2-12 mm Hg
Vascular R	1200-2000 dyne-sec/cm^5	160-400 dyne-sec/cm^5
Cardiac index	2.5-4 L/min/m^2	2.5-4 L/min/m^2

CVP, Central venous pressure; *PWP,* pulmonary wedge pressure; *R,* resistance.

2. The total amount of oxygen returned to the lung from the tissues must be equal to the mixed venous oxygen content ($C\bar{v}o_2$) times the volume of blood presented to the lung per unit time ($\dot{Q}$ or cardiac output):

$$\text{Total } O_2 \text{ returned} = (\dot{Q}) \times (C\bar{v}o_2) \tag{9}$$

3. Therefore total tissue extraction of oxygen per unit time ($\dot{V}o_2$) must be equal to the total oxygen available minus the total oxygen returned:

$$\dot{V}o_2 = [(\dot{Q}) \times (Cao_2)] - [(\dot{Q}) \times C\bar{v}o_2)] \tag{10}$$

4. Equation 10 may be simplified by extracting the common factor of ($\dot{Q}$) and rewriting it as follows:

$$\dot{V}o_2 = (\dot{Q}) \times (Cao_2 - C\bar{v}o_2) \tag{11}$$

5. Equation 11 is called the *Fick equation*, and by solving for cardiac output ($\dot{Q}$), it becomes:

$$\dot{Q} = \frac{\dot{V}o_2}{Cao_2 - C\bar{v}o_2} \tag{12}$$

6. Thus by measuring total oxygen consumption per minute and arterial and mixed venous oxygen content in vol%, the cardiac output can be easily calculated by equation 12.
   a. Total oxygen consumption generally is calculated by analysis of exhaled gases.
   b. Arterial oxygen content requires systemic arterial blood sampling.
   c. Mixed venous oxygen content requires pulmonary arterial blood sampling.
7. *Example:* Given the following values:

$$\dot{V}o_2 = \frac{280 \text{ ml of } O_2}{\text{min}}$$

$$Cao_2 = \frac{20 \text{ ml of } O_2}{100 \text{ ml of blood}} \text{ or } 20 \text{ vol\%}$$

$$C\bar{v}o_2 = \frac{15 \text{ ml of } O_2}{100 \text{ ml of blood}} \text{ or } 15 \text{ vol\%}$$

the cardiac output must equal 5.6 L/min by the following calculation:

$$\dot{Q} = \frac{\dfrac{280 \text{ ml of } O_2}{\text{min}}}{\dfrac{20 \text{ ml of } O_2}{100 \text{ ml of blood}} - \dfrac{15 \text{ ml of } O_2}{100 \text{ ml of blood}}}$$

$$= \frac{5600 \text{ ml of blood}}{\text{min}} \text{ or } \frac{5.6 \text{ L of blood}}{\text{min}}$$

8. The cardiac output determination obtained by using the Fick equation is considered the most accurate. The Fick method is therefore the standard by which other methods of cardiac output determinations are compared for accuracy.

B. Dye dilution method

1. A dye (typically indocyanine green) that can be analyzed by a spectrophotometer is used as an indicator.
2. A known amount (milligrams) of dye is injected rapidly into the right atrium or pulmonary artery.
3. The dye is allowed to mix in the pulmonary circulation, and a continuous representative sampling of blood is drawn from the sampling catheter located in a major systemic artery.
4. Blood samples are analyzed by spectrophotometry for concentration of dye, and the concentrations are plotted on a graph against time.
5. Knowing the number of milligrams of dye injected and plotting the measured concentrations against time allow calculation of the cardiac output ($\dot{Q}$) by the following equation using a computer normally associated with the device:

$$\dot{Q} = \frac{d_o}{\overline{d}_c \times t} \tag{13}$$

where $\dot{Q}$ = cardiac output; d_o = mg of dye injected; $\overline{d}_c$ = mean concentration of dye; and t = time from appearance to disappearance of dye at sampling site.

C. Thermal dilution method

1. This technique uses a four-lumen pulmonary artery catheter (Swan-Ganz catheter) with a port approximately 30 cm proximal from the end of the catheter (Figure 12-8).
2. This proximal port usually lies in the right atrium and is used for injection of a known volume (usually 10 ml) of fluid (D_5W) at a known temperature (usually 0° C).
3. At the distal end of the catheter is a thermistor, which senses changes in temperature. This device normally resides in a branch of the pulmonary artery.
4. The bolus of cold solution is injected into the right atrium. The right ventricle is used as the mixing chamber, and the blood is continually sampled by the thermistor for changes in temperature.
5. The changes in blood temperature can be plotted on a graph against time.
6. The principle underlying cardiac output determination by thermal dilution is identical to that previously described for dye dilution.
7. Knowing the volume of the injected solution and the blood and solution temperatures and plotting the changes in blood temperature against time allow calculation of the cardiac output by the following equation using a computer that is normally attached to the device:

$$\dot{Q} = \frac{V \times (T_b - T_s)}{\overline{T}_b \times t} \tag{14}$$

where $\dot{Q}$ = cardiac output; V = volume of solution injected; T_b = temperature of blood; T_s = temperature of solution injected; $\overline{T}_b$ = mean change in temperature of blood; and t = time from appearance to disappearance of temperature change at sampling site.

8. The measurement typically is made using a bedside computer and integrated software to instantaneously provide the calculation. Three sequential measurements are customarily taken, and if all are within a given range of variance (<20%), the mean of the three measurements will be recorded as the cardiac output.
9. The simplicity of the thermal dilution method, along with the unrequired simultaneous sampling of systemic and pulmonary arterial blood, makes this the standard method used to serially measure cardiac output (Table 12-2).

D. The cardiac output of different individuals varies greatly according to body size. Therefore cardiac output is frequently expressed in terms of body size and is then called the *cardiac index* (CI).

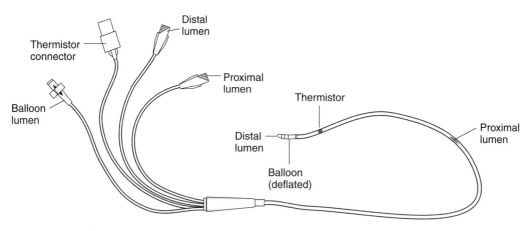

FIG. 12-8 Four-channel pulmonary artery catheter.

TABLE **12-2**

Comparison of Fick versus Thermodilution Cardiac Output Measurement

	Fick	Thermodilution
Accuracy in low cardiac output, high intrapulmonary shunt, or cardiac valvular insufficiencies	Accurate	Not accurate
Simplicity of measurement	Complex	Simple
Availability of data	Protracted	Immediate
Reproducibility	Excellent	Good

1. The CI is equal to the cardiac output in liters per minute per body surface area (BSA) in square meters.
2. The BSA is obtained from a standardized chart using the individual's height and body weight in the determination.
3. The CI becomes a more meaningful value when comparing cardiac outputs of different individuals.
4. Because the CI is a more consistent value among different individuals, it has a narrow normal range of 2.5 to 4 L/min/m².
5. Some prefer to monitor stroke index (SI), which is derived from the CI as follows:

$$SI = \frac{CI}{HR} \qquad (15)$$

   where SI = stroke index expressed in ml/contraction/m²; CI = cardiac index; and HR = heart (contraction) rate.
6. Normal values for SI range from 30 to 70 ml/contraction/m².

VIII. **Assessing Myocardial Contractility**
   A. Ventricular performance curves (Figure 12-9)
      1. Typically these graphs have some index of preload (PWP) on the horizontal (x) axis and some index of cardiac output on the vertical (y) axis.
      2. As increases in preload are made by incremental additions of fluid administration, the resulting cardiac output is measured and graphically plotted.

3. The resulting curve is a representation of the ventricular performance and captures the state of contractility at that moment. By itself it represents a small amount of data; however, when compared with other curves it provides relative changes in contractility.
    a. Increased contractility is represented by an upward and left shift of the ventricular performance curve.
    b. Decreased contractility is represented by a downward and right shift of the ventricular performance curve.

B. Ejection fraction (EF)
    1. Defined as the percentage of blood ejected by the ventricle with each contraction. In equation form:

$$EF = \frac{SV}{EDV} \times 100\% \tag{16}$$

   a. Generally measured by two-dimensional echocardiography at the bedside and performed on the left ventricle, although either can be assessed.
   b. Normal EFs range from 55% to 75%.
   c. EFs < 40% demonstrate heart failure or cardiac myopathy.
    2. Nuclear ventriculogram (MUGA scan) using a radioactive isotope and a gamma camera provides more reproducible results. The gamma cameras have built-in microprocessors and a generator that provides for bedside studies.

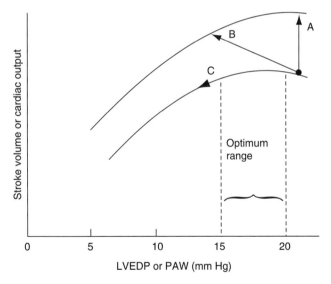

FIG. 12-9 Schematic left ventricular (LV) function curves showing an index of LV performance such as stroke volume or cardiac output on the vertical axis and pulmonary artery wedge (PAW) pressure as a reflection of LV filling pressure on the horizontal axis. As the PAW (or LV end-diastolic [LVED]) pressure increases, myocardial fiber shortening increases (Frank-Starling law), resulting in increased CO. Increases in PAW pressure >20 mm Hg usually produce little or no improvement in CO, as reflected by flattening of the curve. Arrow A reflects a shift to a higher ventricular function curve and stroke volume without a change in preload (this occurs with positive inotropic therapy). Arrow B reflects a shift to a higher ventricular function curve and stroke volume at a lower preload level (this occurs with vasodilator therapy). Arrow C reflects a shift to a lower preload and stroke volume while remaining on the same ventricular function curve (this occurs with diuretic therapy).

3. Right EF (REF) catheter
   a. Modified thermodilution pulmonary artery catheter to sense rapid temperature changes
      (1) Rapid thermistor at the distal tip
      (2) Two sensitive electrocardiographic electrodes for R wave detection
   b. Using a rapid beat-to-beat thermodilution technique the computer provides a derived measurement of right ventricular EF and right ventricular end-diastolic volume and right ventricular stroke volume.
   c. This monitoring technique, although less accurate than traditional quantification of EF, is easily integrated into the critical care setting because of its:
      (1) Familiarity (using a pulmonary artery catheter)
      (2) Simplicity (thermodilution technique)
      (3) Rapidly and serially available results
C. Systolic arterial pressure
   1. In the absence of more sophisticated measures, the arterial systolic pressure can be used as a rough index of ventricular contractility because its numeric value is almost identical to ventricular systolic pressure.
   2. The systolic pressure varies directly with ventricular contractility.

IX. **Continuous Monitoring of Oxygenation Status**
   A. Monitoring oxygenation of venous blood at the pulmonary capillary bed.
      1. Noninvasive continuous monitoring of the oxygen saturation of arterial blood (SaO_2) is easily accomplished using a pulse oximeter and sensor attached to the finger or bridge of the nose. The SpO_2 is essentially equivalent to the SaO_2.
      2. This is commonly integrated into a computer module with display of the arterial pulse contour and numeric value for SpO_2.
      3. The respective SpO_2 is a result of the collective oxygenation of venous blood in the pulmonary capillary bed.
      4. The SpO_2 is a reflection of PaO_2 as displayed by the oxyhemoglobin dissociation curve.
      5. Therefore the easily measured SpO_2 is used as a continuous monitor of impending hypoxemia and pulmonary function.
      6. Normally SpO_2 <90% is considered abnormal.
      7. Clearly it does not replace the necessity of arterial blood gas analysis for complete oxygenation and acid-base status.
   B. Monitoring deoxygenation of arterial blood at the systemic capillary bed
      1. Invasive continuous monitoring of the oxygen saturation of mixed venous blood ($S\bar{v}O_2$) is accomplished using a specialized pulmonary artery catheter with a channel containing optical fibers, which will transmit and collect light wavelength data from its distal tip in similar fashion to a standard oximetry probe.
      2. These data are commonly integrated into a computer module and displayed as a continuous graph and instantaneous numeric value.
      3. The respective $S\bar{v}O_2$ is a result of the collective deoxygenation of arterial blood in the systemic capillary bed.
      4. The $S\bar{v}O_2$ is a reflection of the $P\bar{v}O_2$ as displayed by the oxyhemoglobin dissociation curve.
      5. Therefore $S\bar{v}O_2$ is used as a continuous monitor of gross tissue oxygen demand and is the average resultant of oxygen supply versus oxygen demand.
      6. However, $S\bar{v}O_2$ is also affected by metabolic rate and cardiac output.
      7. Many use changes in $S\bar{v}O_2$ to reflect changes in CO: decreased $S\bar{v}O_2$, decreased CO; increased $S\bar{v}O_2$, increased CO.
      8. Normally the range for $S\bar{v}O_2$ is 60% to 80%.
      9. $S\bar{v}O_2$ < 60% generally represents an oxygen demand that exceeds the oxygen supply.
      10. Note that a normal $S\bar{v}O_2$ does not ensure adequate oxygenation of all tissue beds because the $S\bar{v}O_2$ is the result of the collective average oxygen use of all tissue beds, allowing for the possibility of some being underperfused and others being overperfused.

X. Hemodynamic monitoring via a pulmonary artery catheter continues to be the mainstay used to evaluate the physiologic status and/or response to therapy in critical care. However, increased efforts have been made to develop less invasive or noninvasive monitoring methods of hemodynamic monitoring such as:
   A. Arterial transpulmonary thermodilution and arterial pulse contour analysis
      1. Uses a CVP line and a noncardiac thermodilution arterial line with the thermistor normally placed in the femoral artery.
      2. Intermittent injection of cold saline into the CVP and the resulting measurement by the thermistor in the femoral arterial line using a computer-executed algorithm generate a cardiac output measurement.
      3. An arterial pressure curve is concurrently generated, and correlation of the cardiac output to the curve is performed using the computer.
      4. Changes in the area under subsequently generated pressure curves are compared with the reference (measured cardiac output) arterial pressure curve and are computer interpolated as changes in cardiac output.
      5. This provides for continuous, non–personnel-driven generation and monitoring of cardiac output.
   B. Transesophageal echocardiography derives cardiac output from ultrasound echo Doppler shift reflected by red blood cell flow in the left ventricular outflow tract using an intraesophageal probe.
   C. Inductive plethysmography derives cardiac output from two thoracic surface electrodes, which measure electrical resistance changes across the chest. By subtracting the resistance generated by normal ventilatory (motion) fluctuations, the remaining changes in resistance are attributed to the volume of blood entering and leaving the heart and are correlated with a cardiac output measurement. Although not accurate as yet, this is a totally noninvasive means of continuously measuring cardiac output.
   D. Lithium dilution using a CVP and arterial line: injection of lithium solution and subsequent measurement at the arterial site generate a dye dilution curve. Analysis of the area under the curve provides a cardiac output measurement. Concurrent generation of the arterial pulse contour (reference) is correlated to the cardiac output measurement. The cardiac output can be continuously measured and displayed by an ongoing computer comparison of subsequent arterial pulse contours with the reference contour. The amount of radiation exposure from this technique is approximately the same as standard chest x-ray.

XI. **Data Obtained from Arterial and Venous Lines**
   A. Arterial line measurements
      1. Systemic systolic pressure
      2. Systemic diastolic pressure
      3. Systemic mean arterial blood pressure
      4. Arterial blood gases
      5. Arterial oxygen content CaO_2
      6. Pulmonary deadspace study
   B. Central venous line measurements
      1. Central venous pressure
      2. Venous blood sample
   C. Pulmonary arterial line (catheter) measurements
      1. Pulmonary systolic pressure
      2. Pulmonary diastolic pressure
      3. Mean pulmonary arterial pressure
      4. PWP
      5. Mixed venous blood gases
      6. Mixed venous oxygen content $C\bar{v}O_2$
      7. Intrapulmonary shunt study
      8. Cardiac output
      9. Central venous pressure (on catheters so equipped)

XII. **Complications of Arterial and Venous Lines**
  A. Arterial lines
    1. Thrombosis
    2. Embolism
    3. Hemorrhage
    4. Infection
  B. Central venous line
    1. Thrombosis
    2. Thromboembolism and/or air embolism
    3. Infection/sepsis
  C. Pulmonary arterial line
    1. Thrombosis
    2. Thromboembolism and/or catheter embolism
    3. Pulmonary hemorrhage
    4. Knotting of line in the cardiac chambers
    5. Cardiac dysrhythmias
    6. Endocarditis
    7. Infection/sepsis

XIII. **Effects of Ventilation on Intrathoracic Hemodynamic Pressure Values**
  A. Alterations during spontaneous ventilation
    1. Pulmonary and CVPs follow intrathoracic pressure changes.
    2. During spontaneous inspiration, intrathoracic pressure decreases and thereby decreases all pulmonary arterial and CVPs.
      a. This phenomenon is exaggerated by deep inspiratory efforts and in patients who are experiencing increased work of breathing.
    3. During spontaneous exhalation, intrathoracic pressure increases and thereby increases all pulmonary arterial and CVPs.
      a. This phenomenon is exaggerated by forced expiratory efforts (i.e., Valsalva maneuver) and in patients who are experiencing increased work of breathing.
  B. Alterations during spontaneous ventilation with positive end-expiratory pressure (PEEP; continuous positive airway pressure)
    1. As in spontaneous ventilation, intrathoracic pressure, pulmonary arterial pressure, and CVP decrease on inspiration and increase on exhalation.
    2. However, as a result of the increased intrathoracic pressure transmitted by PEEP, the measured pulmonary arterial pressure and CVP will be elevated by that factor.
  C. Alterations during positive pressure ventilation
    1. As in spontaneous ventilation, pulmonary arterial and CVPs follow intrathoracic pressure changes; however, they are influenced to a greater degree.
      a. The extent of the influence depends on the combination of transmitted intrathoracic and intraairway pressures resulting from the following factors:
        (1) Ventilatory rate
        (2) Size of the tidal volume
        (3) Elastic resistance to ventilation
        (4) Nonelastic resistance to ventilation
        (5) Amount of PEEP
    2. During positive pressure inspiration, intrathoracic pressure increases and thereby increases all pulmonary arterial and CVPs.
      a. High ventilatory pressures, ventilatory rates, and/or any PEEP exaggerate this phenomenon.
    3. During positive pressure exhalation, intrathoracic pressure decreases and thereby decreases all pulmonary arterial and CVPs.
      a. Low ventilatory rates and/or lack of PEEP exaggerate this phenomenon.
  D. Whether the patient is breathing spontaneously or receiving continuous positive airway pressure, intermittent mandatory ventilation, intermittent positive pressure ventilation, or

continuous positive pressure ventilation, the aforementioned effects on intrathoracic and subsequent hemodynamic pressures need to be considered. However, minimizing the artifact of positive-negative intrathoracic pressure swings is best accomplished by *making the hemodynamic pressure recording at end exhalation regardless of the mode of ventilation.*

XIV. **Representative Hemodynamic Profiles**

Note: The following examples represent numeric data consistent with the listed disorders; however, it should be fully appreciated that wide variations exist, and it is dangerous at best to come to any conclusions without viewing first hand the patient's clinical presentation. Further the real value of using hemodynamic monitoring lies not with individual values or measurements. Rather most significant are the sequential measurements that compare the delta (change) factor over time against any interventional therapeutics and/or changing hemodynamic status.

   A. Pulmonary hypertension

BP = 127/88	MAP = 101	CVP = 7	SVR = 1880
PAP = 42/28	$\overline{PAP}$ = 33	PWP = 4	PVR = 580
HR = 105	CI = 3.2		

   B. Systemic hypertension

BP = 175/105	MAP = 128	CVP = 5	SVR = 2480
PAP = 26/14	$\overline{PAP}$ = 18	PWP = 7	PVR = 224
HR = 110	CI = 3.0		

   C. Right ventricular failure

BP = 120/100	MAP = 107	CVP = 28	SVR = 2080
PAP = 36/8	$\overline{PAP}$ = 17	PWP = 4	PVR = 344
HR = 130	CI = 1.9		

   D. Left ventricular failure

BP = 100/40	MAP = 93	CVP = 6	SVR = 2320
PAP = 42/30	$\overline{PAP}$ = 34	PWP = 28	PVR = 160
HR = 140	CI = 1.8		

   E. Hypervolemia

BP = 160/118	MAP = 132	CVP = 18	SVR = 1520
PAP = 42/28	$\overline{PAP}$ = 33	PWP = 26	PVR = 960
HR = 100	CI = 4.4		

   F. Hypovolemia

BP = 85/70	MAP = 75	CVP = 2	SVR = 1920
PAP = 17/12	$\overline{PAP}$ = 14	PWP = 4	PVR = 264
HR = 165	CI = 1.7		

   G. Normovolemia with continuous positive pressure ventilation

BP = 135/70	MAP = 91	CVP = 8	SVR = 1760
PAP = 32/24	$\overline{PAP}$ = 27	PWP = 18	PVR = 192
HR = 100	CI = 2.1		

BIBLIOGRAPHY

Cummins RO: *Textbook of Advanced Cardiac Life Support.* Dallas, American Heart Association Incorporated, 1994.

Daily EF: *Techniques in Hemodynamic Monitoring,* ed 5. St. Louis, Mosby, 1994.

Darovic GO: *Handbook of Hemodynamic Monitoring,* ed 2. Philadelphia, Elsevier Health Sciences Division, 2003.

Guyton AJ, Hall JE: *Textbook of Medical Physiology,* ed 10. Philadelphia, Elsevier Health Sciences Division, 2000.

Little RC: *Physiology of the Heart and Circulation.* St. Louis, Mosby, 1988.

Mountcastle VB: *Medical Physiology,* ed 14. St. Louis, Mosby, 1980.

Murray JF: *The Normal Lung,* ed 2. Philadelphia, WB Saunders, 1987.

Oakes D: *Hemodynamic Monitoring: A Bedside Reference,* ed 3. Orono, ME, Health Educator Publications Inc., 2000.

Otto SE, Blitt CD: *Percutaneous Invasive Hemodynamic Monitoring.* St. Louis, Mosby, 2000.

Ross G: *The Essentials of Human Physiology,* ed 2. St. Louis, Mosby, 1982.

Ruch TC, Patton HD: *Physiology and Biophysics,* ed 20. Philadelphia, WB Saunders, 1982.

Rushmer RF: *Cardiovascular Dynamics,* ed 4. Philadelphia, Elsevier Health Sciences Division, 1976.

Schactman M, Wolff C, Silva V, Scott C: *Hemodynamic Monitoring.* New York, Delmar Learning, 1995.

Schroeder JS, Daily EK: *Techniques in Bedside Hemodynamic Monitoring,* ed 2. St. Louis, Mosby, 1981.

Shapiro BA, Harrison RA, Kacmarek RM, et al: *Clinical Applications of Respiratory Care,* ed 3. Chicago, Year Book Medical Publishers, 1985.

Spearman CB, Sheldon RL, Egan DF: *Egan's Fundamentals of Respiratory Therapy,* ed 4. St. Louis, Mosby, 1982.

Tobin MJ: *Principles and Practices in Intensive Care Monitoring.* New York, McGraw-Hill, 1997.

Chapter 13

Renal Anatomy and Physiology

I. **Gross Anatomy (Figure 13-1)**
   A. The kidneys are located outside the peritoneal cavity on each side of the spinal column within the posterior abdominal wall.
   B. Renal vessels and nerves enter on the medial border.
   C. A single ureter that conducts urine to the bladder exits each kidney from the medial border.
   D. A single urethra leaves the bladder.
   E. The renal pelvis is a continuation of the ureter and forms the urine-collecting area of each kidney.
      1. The outer border of the renal pelvis is divided into major calices.
      2. Each major calyx is further subdivided into minor calices.
      3. Each minor calyx is formed about a renal pyramid.
      4. Nephrons, the functional aspect of the kidney, are located within each renal pyramid (Figure 13-2).
   F. A dissection of the kidney from top to bottom demonstrates two major regions:
      1. The outer region, called the *renal cortex*
      2. The inner region, called the *renal medulla*

II. **The Nephron (Figure 13-3)**
   A. The nephron is the functional unit of the kidney.
   B. Each kidney is composed of approximately 1.3 million nephrons.
   C. Each nephron is composed of a kidney tubule and its corresponding blood supply.
   D. The site of initial formation of urine is the glomerulus. The glomerulus filters blood into Bowman's capsule, forming the glomerular filtrate.
   E. The kidney tubule itself begins with Bowman's capsule and continues sequentially with the following structures:
      1. Proximal convoluted tubule
      2. Loop of Henle
         a. Descending limb
            (1) Thick section
            (2) Thin section
         b. Ascending limb
            (1) Thin section
            (2) Thick section
      3. Distal convoluted tubule
      4. Collecting duct
   F. The arcuate artery provides the circulatory supply of the nephron.
      1. This artery becomes the interlobular artery, which leads to an afferent arteriole leading to the glomerulus.

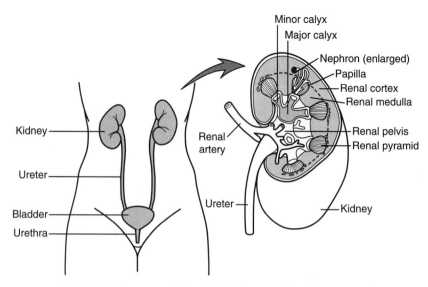

FIG. 13-1 Gross organization of the kidneys and the urinary system.

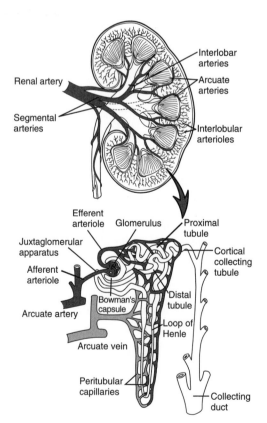

FIG. 13-2 Section of the human kidney showing the major vessels that supply the blood flow to the kidney and schematic of the microcirculation of each nephron.

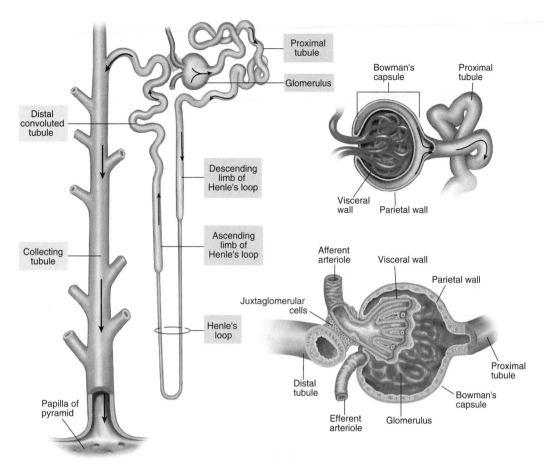

FIG. 13-3 Components of nephron showing direction of fluid flow; schematic of Bowman's capsule showing parietal and visceral walls and relationship of glomerulus to Bowman's capsule and adjacent structures.

2. Blood exits the glomerulus via an efferent arteriole.
3. The efferent arteriole forms the peritubular capillaries, which intertwine about the distal and proximal convoluted tubules.
4. The efferent arterioles also form the vasa recta, a long looping capillary that forms about the loop of Henle.
5. Blood leaves the peritubular capillaries and the vasa recta via the interlobular veins and then the arcuate veins.

III. **Major Functions of the Kidney**
A. The primary function of the kidney is twofold:
1. Excretion of end products of bodily metabolism
2. Control of the concentration of constituents of the body fluids
B. These primary functions are performed by a number of interrelated processes.
1. Filtration: Formation of the glomerular filtrate (see Section IV, Glomerular Filtration)
2. Tubular reabsorption (see Section V, Tubular Reabsorption)
3. Tubular secretion (see Section VI, Tubular Secretion)
4. Renin secretion (see Section XI, Renin-Angiotensin)
5. Erythropoietic factor secretion: In the presence of hypoxemia, the kidney secretes erythropoietic factor, which stimulates red blood cell production.
6. Activation of vitamin D: Vitamin D is necessary for appropriate absorption of calcium via the gastrointestinal tract.

7. Gluconeogenesis: The formation of glucose from fats and protein during periods of significant physiologic stress.
8. Excretion of urine.

IV. Glomerular Filtration

A. Filtration of fluid and electrolytes at the glomerulus follows Starling's law of fluid exchange (see Chapter 14).
B. However, because protein is poorly filterable across the glomerulus, except under pathologic conditions, only three forces normally control fluid exchange.

   1. Forces moving fluid out of the glomerulus

Glomerular hydrostatic pressure	60 mm Hg
Total outward force	60 mm Hg

   2. Forces maintaining fluid in the glomerulus

Glomerular colloid osmotic pressure	32 mm Hg
Bowman's capsule hydrostatic pressure	+18 mm Hg
Total inward force	50 mm Hg

   3. Net filtration pressure

Total outward force	60 mm Hg
Total inward force	− 50 mm Hg
Filtration pressure	10 mm Hg

C. In the average adult approximately 125 ml/min of fluid is filtered across the glomerulus.
D. This filtrate is essentially protein free and has concentrations of dissolved crystalloids similar to that of plasma (Table 13-1).
E. The kidney receives approximately 20% of the cardiac output, of which approximately 55% is fluid.

   1. If cardiac output is 5.5 L, 1.1 L perfuses the kidney each minute.
   2. Fifty-five percent of 1.1 L is 605 ml/min of fluid.
   3. From this fluid volume, 125 ml/min of glomerular filtrate is formed.
   4. The glomerular filtration fraction is the percent of the plasma volume filtered:

$$\frac{125 \text{ ml/min}}{605 \text{ ml/min}} \text{ or approximately } 20\%$$

   5. Normally 20% of the fluid presented to the kidney is filtered.

F. Alterations in the tone of the afferent arteriole and the efferent arteriole affect the volume of glomerular filtrate formed.

TABLE 13-1

Approximate Concentrations of Substances in the Glomerular Filtrate and in the Urine

Substance	Urine	Glomerular Filtrate
Glucose (mg%)	100	0
Creatinine (mEq/L)	196	1.1
Uric acid (mEq/L)	3	42
Urea (mEq/L)	26	1820
SO_4^{-2} (mEq/L)	0.7	33
$H_2PO_4^{-1}/HPO_4^{-2}$ (mEq/L)	2	50
HCO_3^- (mEq/L)	28	14
Cl^- (mEq/L)	103	134
Mg^{+2} (mEq/L)	3	15
Ca^{+2} (mEq/L)	4	4.8
K^+ (mEq/L)	5	60
Na^+ (mEq/L)	142	128

1. Increased tone of the afferent arteriole decreases glomerular hydrostatic pressure and thus filtration volume.
2. Increased tone of the efferent arteriole increases glomerular hydrostatic pressure and thus filtration volume.

V. **Tubular Reabsorption: The movement of filtered substances back into the bloodstream**
   A. Of the 125 ml/min of glomerular filtrate formed, only 1 ml/min of urine is formed; the remainder is reabsorbed. Normally urinary output is approximately 40 to 60 ml/hr.
   B. Reabsorption occurs via simple diffusion, facilitated diffusion, and active transport mechanisms (see Chapter 14).
   C. The vast majority of the electrolytes in the glomerular filtrate are reabsorbed (see Table 13-1).
   D. All filtered glucose is reabsorbed unless the blood glucose level is >375 mg/dl (mg%), the threshold for the spillage of glucose in the urine.
   E. Approximately 50% of the urea filtered is reabsorbed.
   F. Little of the creatinine and creatine filtered is reabsorbed.

VI. **Tubular Secretion**
   A. Tubular secretion is the movement of substances from the blood into the kidney tubule.
   B. The following substances are secreted into the kidney tubule:
      1. Potassium
      2. Hydrogen
      3. Urea
      4. Creatinine
   C. The urinary excretion rate of a substance is equal to its filtration rate: its reabsorption rate + its secretion rate.
   D. Figure 13-4 depicts the potential outcome of all substances in the blood as they pass through the kidney.

VII. **Renal Clearance**
   A. Clearance of a substance refers to the volume of plasma cleared of the substance per unit time.
   B. Every substance in the blood has its own clearance rate.
   C. Renal clearance of a substance is equal to the glomerular filtration rate (GFR) if the substance is:
      1. Freely diffusible at the glomerulus.
      2. Not chemically altered in the kidney.

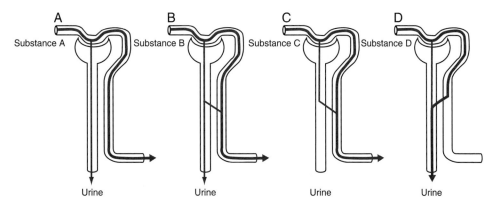

FIG. 13-4 Renal handling of four hypothetical substances. The substance in **A** is freely filtered but not reabsorbed. The substance in **B** is freely filtered, but part of the filtered load is reabsorbed back in the blood. The substance in **C** is freely filtered but is not excreted in the urine because all the filtered substance is reabsorbed from the tubules into the blood. The substance in **D** is freely filtered and is not reabsorbed but is secreted from the peritubular capillary blood into the renal tubes.

3. Not secreted.
4. Not reabsorbed.
5. Thus all of the substance that is filtered is excreted.
D. Renal clearance is equal to:

$$C = \frac{(U)(V)}{P} \tag{1}$$

where C = clearance of the substance, U = urine concentration of the substance, V = urine volume per unit time, and P = arterial plasma concentration of the substance.
E. Normally renal clearance is determined from a 24-hour urine sample.
F. Inulin, an inert polysaccharide, is the standard to determine the GFR because its renal clearance is equal to the GFR.
G. Clinically plasma creatinine and urea levels are used as indicators of GFR changes.
   1. Creatinine results from the breakdown of voluntary muscle. As muscle breaks down, creatine is produced, which is converted to creatinine in the blood.
   2. Urea is produced from the metabolism of amino acids.
   3. Plasma creatinine levels are indirectly affected by the GFR.
   4. All creatinine filtered is excreted.
   5. A small quantity of creatinine also is secreted.
   6. Plasma concentration of creatinine is usually approximately 1.3 mEq/L but can increase 10-fold during renal failure.
   7. Plasma concentration of urea is 26 mEq/L and may increase to 200 mEq/L during renal failure.
   8. Thus as the GFR decreases, the plasma creatinine and urea levels increase.
   9. Plasma concentrations of creatinine are affected by the following:
      a. GFR
      b. Breakdown of voluntary muscle
      c. Hypermetabolic states
   10. Plasma concentrations of urea are affected by the following:
      a. GFR
      b. Breakdown of voluntary muscle
      c. Hypermetabolic state
      d. Metabolism of sequestered (third space) blood

VIII. **Counter Current Multiplier**
   A. The configuration of the nephron allows for the concentrating of urine.
   B. In the descending limb of the loop of Henle, water is reabsorbed. However, Na^+ and Cl^- are not reabsorbed. Thus the concentration of the filtrate increases toward the tip of the nephron.
   C. In the ascending limb of the loop of Henle, Na^+ and Cl^- are reabsorbed. However, water is not reabsorbed. Thus the concentration of the filtrate decreases toward the top of the loop of Henle.
   D. This arrangement causes a variation in the osmolarity of the interstitium from the top to the bottom of the loop of Henle. This variation is maintained by the arrangement of the circulatory system.
   E. The collecting duct passes through the interstitium parallel to the loop of Henle. As a result, fluid moving through the collecting duct can be concentrated if the permeability of the collecting duct to water and Na^+ reabsorption are increased.

IX. **Antidiuretic Hormone (ADH)**
   A. ADH affects the reabsorption of water in the distal convoluted tubule and the collecting duct.
   B. Increased ADH increases the reabsorption of water.
   C. Decreased ADH decreases the reabsorption of water.
   D. ADH levels are controlled by the hypothalamus.

E. ADH is released by the posterior pituitary via stimulation from the hypothalamus.
F. ADH levels are affected by:
1. Pressure in the atria
    a. The body views increased atrial pressure as an increased extracellular fluid volume; therefore, ADH levels are decreased.
    b. The body views decreased atrial pressure as a decreased extracellular fluid volume; therefore, ADH levels are increased. (Positive pressure ventilation and positive end-expiratory pressure [PEEP] normally decrease atrial pressure.)
2. Osmolarity of the extracellular fluid
    a. The body views decreased osmolarity as an increase in extracellular fluid volume; therefore, ADH levels are decreased.
    b. The body views increased osmolarity as a decrease in extracellular fluid volume; therefore, ADH levels are increased.
3. Urine specific gravity provides an index of how concentrated the urine is.
    a. Normally the specific gravity is approximately 1.020, but it may range between 1.002 and 1.045.
    b. Decreased specific gravity is associated with decreased ADH production and increased vascular volume.
    c. Increased specific gravity is associated with increased ADH production and decreased vascular volume.

X. **Aldosterone**
A. Aldosterone controls the reabsorption of Na^+ and the secretion of K^+.
B. Increased aldosterone increases the reabsorption of Na^+ and the secretion of K^+.
C. Decreased aldosterone decreases the reabsorption of Na^+ and the secretion of K^+.
D. Aldosterone affects Na^+ and K^+ movement at the distal convoluted tubule and the collecting duct.
E. Aldosterone is secreted by the adrenal cortex. Its levels are increased by:
1. Decreased serum Na^+
2. Increased serum K^+
3. Increased adrenocorticotropic hormone
4. Increased angiotensin II

XI. **Renin-Angiotensin**
A. Renin is secreted by the kidney in response to a decrease in the delivery of sodium chloride to a group of cells located between the afferent and efferent arterioles, the macula densa cells.
B. Primarily a decrease in perfusion of the kidney increases the release of renin.
C. Renin converts angiotensinogen formed by the liver to angiotensin I.
D. Angiotensin I is converted to angiotensin II by the pulmonary endothelium.
E. Figure 13-5 summarizes the effects of angiotensin II.
F. Angiotensin II is converted to angiotensin III. Most of the effects in Figure 13-5 can also be attributed to angiotensin III.
G. Angiotensin levels facilitate Na^+ and H_2O retention and elevate arterial blood pressure. Angiotensin is the strongest vasopressor produced by the body.
H. Angiotensin levels increase in response to physiologic stress.

XII. **Secretion of H^+ and Reabsorption of HCO_3^-**
A. Figure 13-6 illustrates the sequence of reactions maintaining normal H^+ secretion and HCO_3^- reabsorption.
B. Carbonic anhydrase is present in kidney tubule cells, increasing the hydration of CO_2, which dissociates into H^+ and HCO_3^-.
C. As CO_2 enters the kidney cell, H^+ and HCO_3^- are formed. The HCO_3^- formed moves into the blood, and the H^+ moves into the glomerular filtrate. As each H^+ moves into the glomerular filtrate, a Na^+ is reabsorbed into the bloodstream.

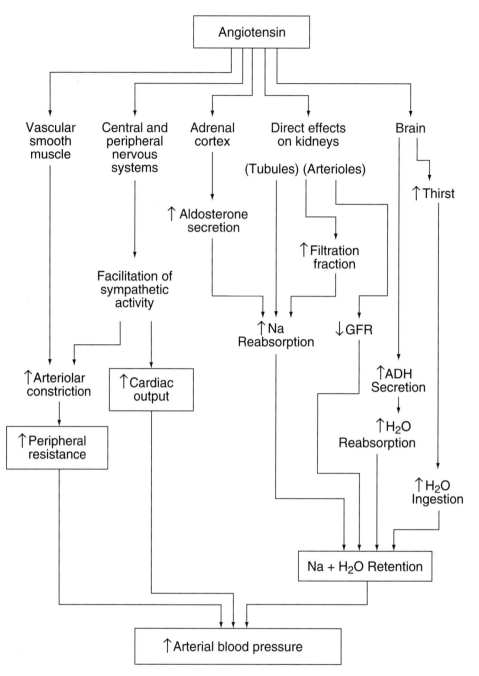

FIG. 13-5 The direct and indirect effects of an increase in angiotensin. Note that all responses are directed toward an increase in Na$^+$ and H$_2$O retention and an increase in arterial blood pressure.

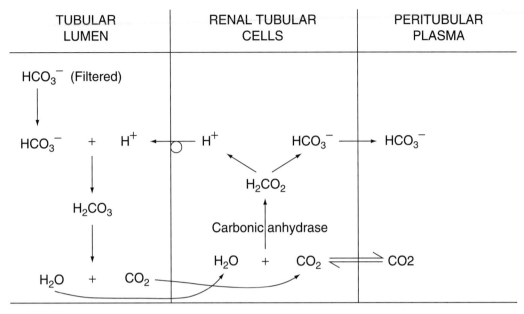

TUBULAR LUMEN	RENAL TUBULAR CELLS	PERITUBULAR PLASMA

FIG. 13-6 The normal mechanism for the reabsorption of filtered HCO_3^-. For every HCO_3^- reabsorbed, one H^+ ion is secreted. O under the arrow indicates that movement of H^+ is via an active transport mechanism.

D. In the glomerular filtrate, the H^+ is buffered by:
   1. HCO_3^-
   2. HPO_4^{-2} (dibasic phosphate)
   3. NH_3 (ammonia)
E. Note that for every HCO_3^- reabsorbed, one H^+ is secreted.
F. This series of reactions (see Figure 13-6) continues in the presence of normal acid-base balance.
G. If a decrease in plasma $Paco_2$ occurs, there is a decrease in the amount of HCO_3^- reabsorbed and H^+ excreted.
H. If $Paco_2$ levels are increased, there is an increase in the amount of HCO_3^- reabsorbed and H^+ excreted.
I. When this occurs, the HCO_3^- in the tubular lumen is rapidly depleted; HPO_4^{-2} and NH_3 are used to buffer the excess H^+ excreted (Figures 13-7 and 13-8).
J. The kidney can continue to buffer acid until the pH of the urine decreases to approximately 4.0.
K. Normal pH of the urine is approximately 7.33 to 7.37.
L. The quantity of HCO_3^- reabsorbed over normal is equal to the amount of acid excreted in the form of $H_2PO_4^{-1}$ and NH_4^+.
M. Renal compensation for respiratory acid-base imbalances:
   1. If Pco_2 level increases, more HCO_3^- is formed and moved into the blood. This normalizes the acidic pH caused by the increased Pco_2 level.
   2. If Pco_2 level decreases, less HCO_3^- is formed and moved into the blood. This normalizes the alkalotic pH caused by the decreased Pco_2 level.
   3. Compensation by the kidney is relatively complete, but the mechanism may take a long time to normalize the pH (24 to 48 hours or longer).

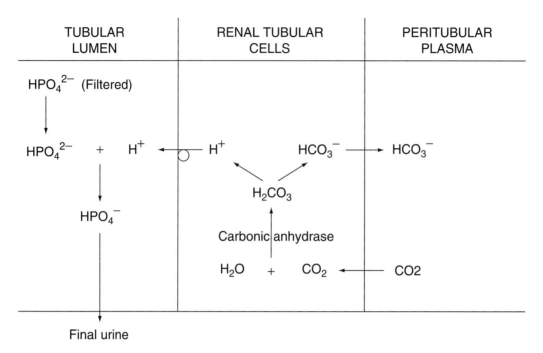

FIG. 13-7 The use of HPO_4^{-2} as a buffer of secreted H^+. This system is active primarily in the presence of excess $Paco_2$, creating a larger quantity of H^+ to be secreted than normal. With each H^+ ion secreted, a HCO_3^- is reabsorbed, thus increasing total extracellular $[HCO_3^-]$. O under the arrow indicates active transport.

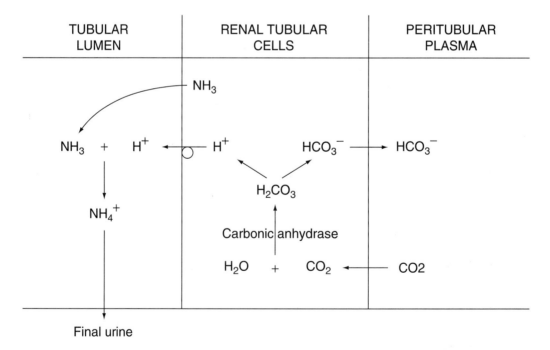

FIG. 13-8 The reaction of secreted H^+ with NH_3. This system is active primarily in the presence of excess $Paco_2$. The additional H^+ formed is buffered, and HCO_3^- is reabsorbed, increasing the total extracellular $[HCO_3^-]$. O under the arrow indicates active transport.

BIBLIOGRAPHY

Beachey W: *Respiratory Care Anatomy and Physiology: Foundations of Clinical Practice*. St. Louis, Mosby, 1998.

Ellerbe S: *Fluid and Blood Component Therapy in the Critically Ill and Injured*. New York, Churchill Livingstone, 1981.

Gabow PA: *Fluids and Electrolytes: Clinical Problems and Their Solution*. Boston, Little, Brown & Co, 1983.

Guyton AC, Hall JE: *Textbook of Medical Physiology*, ed 10. New York, WB Saunders, 2000.

Hicks GH: *Cardiopulmonary Anatomy and Physiology*. New York, WB Saunders, 2000.

Pierson DJ, Kacmarek RM: *Foundations of Respiratory Care*. New York, Churchill Livingstone, 1992.

Schrier RW (ed): *Renal and Electrolyte Disorders,* ed 2. Boston, Little, Brown & Co, 1980.

Smith K: *Fluids and Electrolytes: A Conceptual Approach*. New York, Churchill Livingstone, 1980.

Vander AJ: *Renal Physiology,* ed 2. New York, McGraw-Hill, 1980.

Weldy NJ: *Body Fluids and Electrolytes: A Programmed Presentation,* ed 3. St. Louis, Mosby, 1980.

Wilkins RL, Stoller JK, Scanlon CL: *Egan's Fundamentals of Respiratory Care,* ed 8. St. Louis, Mosby, 2003.

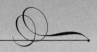

Chapter 14

Fluid and Electrolyte Balance

I. **Distribution of Body Fluids**
   A. Percentage of body weight made up by water (Table 14-1):
      1. Adult men: 60 ± 15%.
      2. Adult women: 50 ± 15%.
      3. Newborn: 80%.
      4. Obese persons: ≤45%. Fat is much less vascular than muscle, thus the greater the fat content, the lower the water content.
   B. In the average adult, total body fluid volume is approximately 40 L.
      1. Intracellular (approximately two thirds of total body fluid): 25 L
         a. Red blood cell (RBC) volume: 2 L
         b. Other cellular compartments: 23 L
      2. Extracellular (approximately one third of total body fluid): 15 L
         a. Plasma volume: 3 L
         b. Other extracellular fluid: 12 L

II. **Normal Intake and Output of Fluids**
   A. In the healthy individual, intake and output should be in complete balance.
   B. Normal intake:
1. Drink	1200 ml/day
2. Food	1000 ml/day
3. Metabolically produced	350 ml/day
4. Total intake	2550 ml/day
   C. Normal output (Table 14-2)
1. Evaporation (lung and skin)	900 ml/day
2. Sweat (on hot, humid days this can increase markedly)	50 ml/day
3. Feces	100 ml/day
4. Urine	1500 ml/day
5. Total output	2550 ml/day

III. **Composition of the Intravascular Space (Figure 14-1)**
   A. Normally all fluid compartments in the body are in electrostatic balance as described by the law of electroneutrality (i.e., cation and anion concentrations are equal).
      1. Cation mean values (mEq/L):

Na^+	142
K^+	5
Ca^{+2}	5
Mg^{+2}	3
Total	155

TABLE 14-1

Distribution of Body Fluids

Body Water	Adult Male (% body weight)	Adult Female (% body weight)	Infant (% body weight)
Total body water	60 ± 15	50 ± 15	80
Intracellular	45	40	50
Extracellular	15-20	15-20	30
Interstitial	11-15	11-15	24
Intravascular	4.5	4.5	5.0

From Wilkins RL, et al: *Egan's Fundamentals of Respiratory Care,* ed 8. St. Louis, Mosby, 2003.

TABLE 14-2

Daily Water Exchange

Regulation	Average Daily Volume (mL)	Maximum Daily Volume
Water Losses		
Insensible		
Skin	700	1500 ml
Lung	200	
Sensible		
Urine	1000-1200	2000+ ml/hr
Intestinal	200	8000 ml
Sweat	0	2000+ ml/hr
Water Gain		
Ingestion		
Fluids	1500-2000	2000+ ml/hr
Solids	500-600	1500 ml/hr
Body metabolism	250	1000 ml

From Wilkins RL, et al: *Egan's Fundamentals of Respiratory Care,* ed 8. St. Louis, Mosby, 2003.

2. Anion mean values (mEq/L):

HCO_3^-	27
Cl^-	103
Protein	16
Organic acids	6
PO_4^{-3}	2
SO_4^{-2}	1
Total	155

B. Plasma protein concentrations can be subdivided into:

	Mean values
Albumin	4.8 g/100 ml
Globulin	2.5 g/100 ml
Fibrinogen	300 mg/100 ml

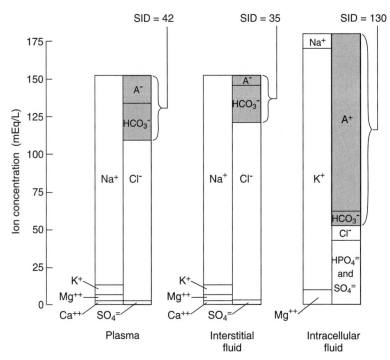

FIG. 14-1 Distribution of anions and cations in the plasma, interstitial fluid, and intracellular fluid. Strong ion difference (SID) represents the amounts of anions in the form of bicarbonate (HCO_3^-) and protein (A^-).

    C. The following neutral substances also are present in vascular fluid:

	Mean values
Glucose	90 mg/100 ml
Lipids	600 mg/100 ml

    D. Anion gap: The difference between the commonly measured anions and cations, reflecting the quantity of unmeasured anions:

$$\text{Anion gap} = [Na^+] + [K^+] - [Cl^-] + [HCO_3^-]$$
$$17 \text{ mEq/L} = [142 + 5] - [103 + 27]$$

        1. Normally the anion gap ranges from approximately 15 to 20 mEq/L.
        2. An increased anion gap is caused by a metabolic acidosis in which fixed acids accumulate in the body.
        3. An increased anion gap indicates an increase in unmeasured anions.
        4. However, a metabolic acidosis caused by HCO_3^- loss does not cause an increased anion gap because a HCO_3^- loss is associated with a Cl^- gain, maintaining electrical neutrality. This type of acidosis is referred to as a hyperchloremic acidosis.
        5. Causes of anion gap and nonanion gap metabolic acidosis are listed in Box 14-1.
        6. A decrease in the anion gap is caused by a metabolic alkalosis in which increased levels of base accumulate in the body (Box 14-2).

    F. Strong ion difference
        1. Another approach to defining electrolyte imbalances and, as a result, metabolic acid-base disturbances is by assessing the strong ion difference (SID).
        2. The SID represents the amount of anions necessary to balance the number of cations (primarily Na^+) to maintain electrical neutrality.

BOX 14-1

Causes of Anion Gap and Nonanion Gap Metabolic Acidosis

HIGH ANION GAP *Metabolically Produced Acid Gain* Lactic acidosis Ketoacidosis Renal failure (e.g., retained sulfuric acid) *Ingestion of Acids* Salicylate (aspirin) intoxication Methanol (formic acid) Ethylene glycol (oxalic acid)	**NORMAL ANION GAP (HYPERCHLOREMIC ACIDOSIS)** *Gastrointestinal Loss of HCO_3^-* Diarrhea Pancreatic fistula *Renal Tubular Loss: Failure to Reabsorb HCO_3^-* Renal tubular acidosis *Ingestion* Ammonium chloride Hyperalimentation intravenous nutrition

From Beachey W: *Respiratory Care Anatomy and Physiology: Foundations for Clinical Practice.* St. Louis, Mosby, 1998.

BOX 14-2

Causes of Metabolic Alkalosis (Increased Plasma HCO_3^-)

GASTROINTESTINAL LOSS OF HYDROGEN IONS Vomiting Nasogastric drainage *Renal* Diuretics (loss of chloride, potassium fluid volume)	Hypochloremia (increased H^+ secretion and HCO_3^- reabsorption) Hypokalemia (increased H^+ secretion and HCO_3^- reabsorption) Hypovolemia (increased H^+) **RETENTION OF BICARBONATE ION** $NaHCO_3$ infusion or ingestion

From Beachey W: *Respiratory Care Anatomy and Physiology: Foundations for Clinical Practice.* St. Louis, Mosby, 1998.

3. SID is regulated by the amount of renal reabsorption of Na^+: the greater the Na^+ reabsorption, the greater the SID, and the lesser the Na^+ reabsorption, the lesser the SID.
4. Protein is the other major component of the SID; however, unlike HCO_3^- it is not regulated with respect to maintenance of ion or acid-base balance.
5. Thus the SID is the amount of HCO_3^- and protein, the two major body buffers, needed to balance the cations.
6. As noted in Figure 14-1, the SID varies based on fluid compartment evaluated.
7. Because protein is not readily diffusible across the cell membrane, the intracellular SID is greater than the extracellular SID.
8. An increase in the SID is observed during metabolic alkalosis, and a decrease is seen during metabolic acidosis.
9. The normal SID in arterial blood is 40 to 44 mEq/L.

IV. **Composition of Extravascular (Interstitial) Fluid (see Figure 14-1)**
   A. The extravascular concentrations of most substances are about the same as their intravascular concentrations.
   B. The major exception is protein. Because protein is not freely diffusible across the capillary membrane, extravascular protein concentrations are less than one third intravascular concentrations.
   C. As with all other compartments, electrostatic balance is maintained.

V. **Composition of the Intracellular Compartment (see Figure 14-1)**
   A. Electrostatic balance is maintained within the intracellular space.
   B. However, the composition of anions and cations differs considerably from intravascular levels.

1. Cations, mean values (mEq/L):

Na$^+$	10
K$^+$	140
Ca^{+2}	0
Mg^{+2}	30
Total	180

2. Anions, mean values (mEq/L):

HCO$_3^-$	10
Cl$^-$	4
Protein	61
PO$_4^{-3}$	11
SO$_4^{-2}$	2
Other anions	92
Total	180

VI. **Movement Across Membranes**
   A. The following mechanisms are responsible for the movement of fluid and dissolved substances across membranes:
      1. Simple diffusion (see Chapter 2)
      2. Osmosis (see Chapter 2)
      3. Facilitated diffusion
      4. Active transport
   B. Facilitated diffusion (Figure 14-2) occurs from an area of high concentration of the diffusing substance to an area of low concentration. However, a carrier substance is necessary for movement to occur across the membrane.
      1. No energy is expended compared with active transport.
      2. Glucose moves across cell membranes by facilitated diffusion. Insulin allows a rapid attachment of glucose to the intramembrane carrier substance.
   C. Active transport is the movement of a substance from an area of low concentration to an area of high concentration (Figure 14-3).
      1. Movement is always uphill—low concentration to high concentration.
      2. Energy in the form of adenosine triphosphate (ATP) is necessary for transport to occur.
      3. The movement of many substances is controlled by active transport. Figure 14-3 depicts the most common active transport mechanism, the movement of Na$^+$ out of the cell and the movement of K$^+$ into the cell.

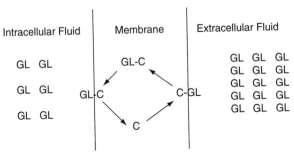

FIG. 14-2 Facilitated diffusion. Glucose (GL) reacts with a carrier (C) substance reversibly on the inside of the cell membrane allowing transport of the GL without the use of metabolic energy from outside to inside the cell.

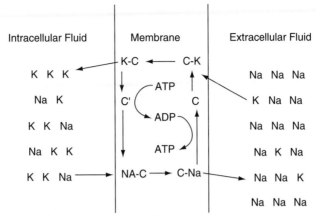

FIG. 14-3 Hypothetical scheme of active transport of sodium (Na^+) and potassium (K^+) across cellular membrane. (Energy in the form of ATP is used for each K^+ and Na^+ ion moved across the membrane.) *C,* Carrier substance; *ATP,* adenosine triphosphate; *ADP,* adenosine diphosphate.

VII. **Starling Law of Fluid Exchange**
  A. The Starling law of fluid exchange is the interrelationship among factors that determine the quantity and the direction of fluid movement across membranes.
  B. The relationship is expressed as:

$$J = k[(P_{cap} - P_{is}) - (\pi_{cap} - \pi_{is})]$$

  where J = net fluid movement; k = capillary membrane permeability; P_{cap} = capillary hydrostatic pressure; P_{is} = interstitial hydrostatic pressure; π_{cap} = plasma colloid osmotic pressure; and π_{is} = interstitial colloid osmotic pressure.
  C. Theoretically there are two pressures on each side of a capillary membrane.
    1. Hydrostatic pressure: Blood pressure or interstitial fluid pressure.
    2. Colloid osmotic pressure
      a. Colloid osmotic pressure is the osmotic pressure caused by nondiffusible protein.
      b. Because all dissolved substances except protein are readily diffusible, the effective osmotic pressure of either plasma or interstitial fluid is established by protein.
      c. The quantity of protein is approximately three times greater in the plasma than in the interstitial fluid.
  D. Capillary membrane permeability can be altered by many forms of physiologic stress, resulting in alterations in net fluid movement, given fixed hydrostatic and colloid osmotic pressures.
  E. The pressures across the *pulmonary* capillary membrane are depicted in Figure 14-4.
    1. Forces tending to move fluid *out* of the pulmonary capillary:

	Mean values (mm Hg)
Capillary hydrostatic pressure	7
Interstitial hydrostatic pressure (normally a negative pressure, thus forcing [pulling] fluid out of the capillary)	6
Interstitial colloid osmotic pressure	16
Total force moving fluid out of capillary	29

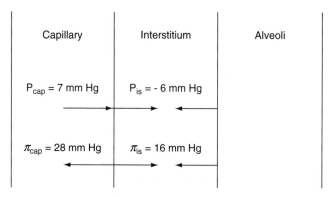

Pulmonary - Capillary Membrane

FIG. 14-4 Pressures affecting fluid exchange at the pulmonary capillaries. Arrows indicate direction of individual pressures causing fluid movement. P_{is}, Interstitial hydrostatic pressure; P_{cap}, capillary hydrostatic pressure; π_{is}, interstitial colloid osmotic pressure; π_{cap}, plasma colloid osmotic pressure.

2. Forces tending to *maintain fluid in* the pulmonary capillary:

	Mean values (mm Hg)
Plasma colloid osmotic pressure	28
Total force maintaining fluid inside the pulmonary capillaries	28

3. Net force causing fluid to leave pulmonary capillaries is approximately 1 mm Hg (29–28 mm Hg).
4. The amount of fluid leaving the capillary as a result of the 1-mm Hg pressure gradient depends on the permeability of the pulmonary capillary membrane.
5. The negative interstitial hydrostatic pressure not only assists in moving fluid out of pulmonary capillaries but also maintains the alveoli "dry." This force, along with the interstitial colloid osmotic pressure, moves fluid from the lung into the interstitial space.
6. The pulmonary interstitial colloid osmotic pressure is much higher than the systemic interstitial colloid osmotic pressure because the pulmonary capillaries are much more permeable than the systemic capillaries.
7. Any alteration in the pressures listed can result in increased fluid movement into the interstitium or the alveoli.
8. The most common causes of increased fluid movement are:
   a. Increased capillary hydrostatic pressure
      (1) Left heart failure
      (2) Fluid overload
   b. Increased capillary permeability: Any form of significant physiologic stress
      (1) Acute respiratory distress syndrome (ARDS)
      (2) Noxious gas inhalation
      (3) Pulmonary burns
      (4) Infection
   c. Decreased capillary colloid osmotic pressure
      (1) Hypermetabolic state
      (2) Starvation
      (3) Fluid overload
F. Forces affecting *systemic* capillary fluid movement, mean values (mm Hg; Figure 14-5).

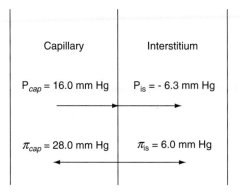

FIG. 14-5 Pressures affecting fluid exchange at the systemic capillaries. Arrows indicate direction of individual pressures causing fluid movement. P_{is}, Interstitial hydrostatic pressure; P_{cap}, capillary hydrostatic pressure; π_{is}, interstitial colloid osmotic pressure; π_{cap}, plasma colloid osmotic pressure.

1. Forces moving fluid *out* of the capillary are:

	Mean values (mm Hg)
Capillary hydrostatic pressure	16.0
Interstitial hydrostatic pressure (normally is negative pressure forcing [pulling] fluid out of the capillary)	6.3
Interstitial colloid osmotic pressure	6.0
Total force moving fluid out of the capillary	28.3

2. Forces moving fluid *into* the capillary are:

	Mean values (mm Hg)
Capillary colloid osmotic pressure	28
Total force moving fluid into the capillary	28

3. Net force causing fluid movement out of the capillary is approximately 0.3 mm Hg (28.3 – 28 mm Hg).
4. The amount of fluid leaving the capillary as a result of the 0.3-mm Hg pressure gradient depends on the permeability of the capillary membrane.
5. Any alteration in the pressures listed can cause fluid to move into the interstitium.
6. The most common causes of increased fluid movement are:
   a. Increased capillary hydrostatic pressure
      (1) Right ventricular failure
      (2) Fluid overload
   b. Increased capillary permeability: Any significant physiologic stress
      (1) Bacteremia
      (2) Septicemia
      (3) Trauma
   c. Decreased capillary colloid osmotic pressure
      (1) Hypermetabolic state
      (2) Starvation
      (3) Fluid overload

VIII. **Sodium**
   A. Normal serum sodium levels range from approximately 135 to 145 mEq/L, necessary to maintain extracellular fluid volume.

B. Serum Na$^+$ concentration is normally a reflection of extracellular fluid volume.

C. Approximately 70 to 100 mEq of Na$^+$ is excreted daily:

1. In feces and skin: 5 to 10 mEq
2. In sweat: 25 mEq
3. In urine: approximately 40 mEq

D. Hyponatremia (decreased serum Na$^+$ concentration) is present if serum [Na$^+$] level is <130 mEq/L.

1. Hyponatremia occurs in the presence of a decreased, increased, or normal extracellular fluid volume:
   a. Decreased extracellular fluid volume
      (1) Excessive Na$^+$ loss
         (a) Vomiting
         (b) Diarrhea
         (c) Excessive movement of fluid into the interstitial (third) space
      (2) Decreased Na$^+$ intake
   b. Normal extracellular fluid volume
      (1) Excessive antidiuretic hormone (ADH) secretion
      (2) Glucocorticoid deficiency, Addison's disease
      (3) Severe hypothyroidism
      (4) Fluid overload with normal renal function
   c. Increased extracellular fluid volume
      (1) Cardiac failure
      (2) Renal failure
      (3) Nephrotic syndrome
      (4) Hepatic insufficiency
      (5) Trauma
   c. Increased extracellular fluid volume
      (1) Congestive heart failure
      (2) Renal failure
      (3) Hepatic cirrhosis

2. The following clinical signs of hyponatremia are rare unless the [Na$^+$] level decreases <120 mEq/L:
   a. Headache
   b. Muscle cramps and weakness
   c. Thirst
   d. Nausea
   e. Agitation
   f. Anorexia
   g. Disorientation
   h. Apathy
   i. Lethargy

3. As the [Na$^+$] level decreases <110 mEq/L, drowsiness, progressing to coma, with convulsions occurs.

4. Management
   a. In the presence of a decreased extracellular fluid volume, intravenous (IV) replacement is begun immediately to reestablish Na$^+$ and fluid volume.
   b. In the presence of a normal extracellular fluid volume, management should focus on the underlying condition (i.e., diuretic therapy, excessive ADH production, and glucocorticoid deficiency).
   c. In the presence of an expanded extracellular fluid volume, the management should focus on the cause of the fluid overload.

E. Hypernatremia (increase in serum Na$^+$ concentration) always reflects a deficiency of water compared with total body solute volume ([Na$^+$] >145 mEq/L).

1. Etiology
   a. Water loss

    (1) Insensible loss
      (a) Increased sweating, fever, and exposure to high temperatures
      (b) Burns
      (c) Respiratory tract infections
    (2) Renal loss
      (a) Central diabetes insipidus
      (b) Nephrogenic diabetes insipidus
      (c) Osmotic diuresis
    (3) Hypothalamic disorders
      (a) Hypodipsia (decreased thirst)
      (b) Essential hypernatremia
   b. Sodium gain
    (1) Administration of hypertonic NaCl or $NaHCO_3$
    (2) Ingestion of Na^+
    (3) Primary hyperaldosteronism and Cushing's syndrome
  2. Clinical presentation
   a. Lethargy
   b. Muscle weakness
   c. Twitching
   d. Seizures
   e. Coma
   f. Death
  3. Because the brain adapts to the development of hypernatremia (hyperosmolal state) within 24 hours, the severity of symptoms is related to the degree and rate of development of hypernatremia.
  4. Management
   a. Focus is on managing the underlying problem and slowly returning Na^+ levels to normal by the administration of water.
   b. Rapid correction of hypernatremia with the administration of large quantities of water can result in cerebral edema, seizures, and death.

IX. Chloride

 A. Chloride balance is similar to Na^+ balance, necessary to maintain cellular electrostatic and fluid balance.
 B. Normal serum levels range from approximately 95 to 105 mEq/L.
 C. Hypochloremia (decreased serum Cl^- concentration <95 mEq/L) may be caused by:
  1. Increased secretion and loss of gastric fluids
  2. Increased renal excretion
  3. Aldosteronism
  4. Dilution
  5. Actual hyponatremia
  6. Bicarbonate ion retention
 D. Hyperchloremia (increased serum Cl^- concentration >105 mEq/L) may be caused by:
  1. Increased intake
  2. Decreased bicarbonate ion concentration
  3. Respiratory alkalosis
  4. Decreased renal excretion
  5. Dehydration
 E. Because of the exchange of Cl^- and HCO_3^- by the kidney, serum concentrations of these electrolytes are indirectly related. The pH of the urine and the plasma also change in the opposite direction as Cl^- levels change.
  1. Hypochloremia
   a. Increased serum HCO_3^-, alkalosis
   b. Decreased urine HCO_3^-, acidosis

    2. Hyperchloremia
       a. Decreased serum HCO_3^-, acidosis
       b. Increased urine HCO_3^-, alkalosis
  F. In chronic CO_2 retention with increased HCO_3^-, Cl^- is decreased.
  G. Because changes in $[Cl^-]$ closely mirror disturbances in $[Na^+]$ balance, symptoms of $[Cl^-]$ changes are similar to $[Na^+]$ changes.
  H. Management focuses on reversal of the underlying cause along with the administration of either NaCl or water, depending on the abnormality.

X. Potassium
  A. Normal serum K^+ concentrations are approximately 3.5 to 5.5 mEq/L, necessary to maintain normal cardiac and voluntary muscle function.
  B. Normal K^+ loss
    1. Via skin and feces: 15 to 30 mEq/L
    2. Via urine: 10 to 30 mEq/L
  C. Normal K^+ ingestion: 50 to 100 mEq
  D. Minimum required K^+ ingestion: 40 mEq
  E. Hypokalemia (decreased serum K^+ concentration <3.5 mEq/L)
    1. Causes
       a. Diuretic therapy
       b. Vomiting or nasogastric suction
       c. Malabsorption
       d. Laxative abuse
       e. Diarrhea
       f. Decreased intake
       g. Excessive output
       h. Hyperaldosteronism
       i. Steroid therapy
       j. Cirrhosis
       k. Liver failure
       l. Alkalosis
       m. Insulin-induced hypoglycemia
       n. Renal tubular acidosis
       o. Malnutrition
       p. Alcoholism
       q. Anorexia nervosa
       r. Licorice abuse
    2. Clinical signs and symptoms
       a. Metabolic alkalosis
       b. Acidic urine (because of exchange with H^+ as K^+ excretion decreases, H^+ excretion increases)
       c. Muscle weakness
       d. Fatigue
       e. Hypotension
       f. Confusion
       g. Cardiac arrhythmias (cardiac arrest)
       h. On electrocardiogram (ECG), flat or inverted T waves
       i. Loss of tendon reflexes
       j. Increased sensitivity to digitalis
    3. Management
       a. Management of underlying problem
       b. Administration of K^+
         (1) Essential if K^+ concentration is <3.0 mEq/L
         (2) May not be required if K^+ concentration is between 3.0 and 3.5 mEq/L

F. Hyperkalemia (increased serum K+ concentration >5.5 mEq/L)
1. Causes
   a. Increased intake
      (1) Iatrogenic, rapid IV administration
      (2) Excess oral intake
   b. Reduced excretion
      (1) Acute renal failure
      (2) Severe chronic renal failure
      (3) Sodium depletion
      (4) Steroid deficiency
      (5) Potassium-sparing diuretics
   c. Redistribution of K+, release from cells
      (1) Acidosis
      (2) Muscle injury catabolism
      (3) Leukemia chemotherapy
      (4) Hemolysis
      (5) Malignant hyperthermia
   d. Others
      (1) Thrombocytosis
      (2) Massive leukocytosis
      (3) Muscle exercise during venous occlusion
2. Clinical signs and symptoms
   a. Metabolic acidosis
   b. Alkaline urine
   c. Muscle weakness
   d. Occasional paralysis
   e. Listlessness
   f. Nausea, vomiting
   g. Occasional ileus
   h. Confusion
   i. Paresthesia
   j. Cardiac arrhythmias (cardiac arrest)
   k. On ECG, spiked T wave
3. Management
   a. Increased urinary excretion of K+ is essential (diuretic therapy).
   b. IV calcium chloride or calcium gluconate is given to antagonize the cardiotoxic effects of hyperkalemia.
   c. IV glucose and insulin are given to increase K+ uptake by cells.

XI. Calcium
A. Normal total serum Ca+2 concentrations are approximately 8.0 to 10 mg/dL, and normal ionized Ca+2 levels are 4.6 to 5.3 mg/dL, necessary to maintain normal cardiac and voluntary muscle function.
B. Approximately 50% of the calcium in the blood is bound to protein. The amount of Ca+2 bound to protein is affected by plasma pH.
   1. If plasma pH increases, more Ca+2 is bound to protein.
   2. If plasma pH decreases, less Ca+2 is bound to protein.
C. Hypocalcemia (decreased serum calcium concentration)
   1. Causes
      a. Hyperthyroidism
      b. Vitamin D deficiency
      c. Magnesium deficiency
      d. Renal failure
      e. Malnutrition
      f. Pancreatitis

g. Massive blood transfusion
h. Tumor lysis syndrome
2. Clinical signs and symptoms
   a. Impaired neuromuscular function
      (1) Paresthesia
      (2) Muscle cramps
      (3) Tetany
   b. Tingling, numbness
   c. Cardiac arrhythmias
3. Management of the underlying cause
   a. In acute hypocalcemia, IV calcium gluconate or calcium chloride can be administered.
   b. Adequate vitamin D ingestion must be ensured.

D. Hypercalcemia (increased serum Ca^{+2} concentration)
1. Causes
   a. Malignancy
   b. Primary hyperparathyroidism
   c. Acute renal failure
   d. Vitamin D intoxication
   e. Hyperthyroidism
   f. Increased absorption
   g. Sarcoidosis
   h. Multiple myeloma
   i. Paraproteinemia
2. Clinical signs and symptoms
   a. Tiredness, muscle weakness, and neuromuscular paralysis
   b. Cardiac arrhythmia
   c. Anorexia, nausea, and vomiting
   d. Weight loss
   e. Peptic ulcer, abdominal pain
3. Management
   a. Correction of dehydration and electrolyte imbalance
   b. Diuretic therapy to increase Ca^{+2} excretion
   c. Administration of phosphate to increase Ca^{+2} movement into bone
   d. Steroid therapy to reduce intestinal absorption of Ca^{+2}

XII. **Phosphate**
A. Normal serum PO_4^{-3} levels are 2.7 to 4.5 mg/dL, necessary for the normal production of ATP and muscle function.
B. Hypophosphatemia (decreased serum phosphate concentration <2.7 mg/dL)
1. Causes
   a. Primary hyperparathyroidism
   b. Alkalosis
   c. Low intake
   d. Chronic alcoholism
   e. Beriberi
   f. Septicemia
   g. Vitamin D deficiency
   h. Hemodialysis
   i. Glucose and insulin administration
   j. Reduced intake
   k. Steroid therapy
2. Clinical signs and symptoms
   a. Muscle weakness
   b. Paresthesia

        c. Rickets
        d. Impaired metabolism
        e. Seizures
        f. Reduced renal tubular bicarbonate reabsorption
        g. Impaired metabolism
        h. Coma

    3. Management
        a. Oral phosphate
        b. Intravenous K_2HPO_4

C. Hyperphosphatemia (increased serum phosphate concentration >4.5 mg/dL):
    1. Causes
        a. Hypoparathyroidism
        b. Vitamin D toxicity
        c. Renal failure
        d. High intake
        e. Acidosis
        f. Severe catabolic state
        g. Acromegaly
    2. Clinical signs and symptoms
        a. Ectopic calcification
        b. Secondary hyperparathyroidism
        c. Renal osteodystrophy
    3. Management
        a. Management of underlying cause
        b. Administration of aluminum hydroxide to decrease absorption
        c. Renal dialysis

XIII. Magnesium
  A. Normal serum Mg^{+2} concentration is 1.5 to 2.5 mEq/L, necessary for normal muscle function, voluntary and involuntary.
  B. Hypomagnesemia (decreased serum Mg^{+2} concentration <1.5 mEq/L)
    1. Causes
        a. Decreased intake
        b. Gastrointestinal disturbances
        c. Endocrine disturbances
        d. Renal disease
        e. Alcoholism
        f. Diabetic ketoacidosis
        g. Hypercalcemia
    2. Clinical signs and symptoms
        a. Muscle weakness
        b. Nausea and vomiting, abdominal pain
        c. Neuromuscular excitability, tetany, cramps, and paresthesia
        d. Central nervous system depression, irritability
        e. Tachycardia
    3. Management
        a. Management of underlying cause
        b. Administration of magnesium sulfate
  C. Hypermagnesemia (increased serum Mg^{+2} concentration)
    1. Causes
        a. Acute or chronic renal failure
        b. Eclampsia
        c. Adrenocortical insufficiency
        d. Metabolic acidosis
        e. Increased ingestion—magnesium-based laxatives

2. Clinical signs and symptoms
   a. Muscle weakness
   b. Loss of deep tendon reflexes
   c. Impaired autonomic nerve transmission
   d. Vasodilation
   e. Drowsiness
   f. Cardiac arrhythmia
3. Management
   a. Renal dialysis (if renal failure is present)
   b. Diuretic therapy

XIV. **Fluid Balance**
   A. The venous system is referred to as the *capacitance system* because it has the ability to store large quantities of blood.
   B. The storage capabilities of the venous system are depicted in Figure 14-6.
       1. Below minimum capacitance, large volume changes result in small pressure changes.
       2. Within the normal capacitance range, a volume change results in a small pressure change.
       3. Beyond the maximum capacitance level, a small volume change results in a large pressure change.
   C. Venous conductance is the ability of the venous system to conduct flow.
   D. Conductance is a reciprocal of resistance and is equal to flow divided by change in pressure.
   E. The greater the conductance, the greater the ability of the vessel to conduct flow.
   F. Either increasing driving pressure or increasing conductance increases venous return.
       1. Physiologically the body increases venotone to increase driving pressure, thus increasing venous return.
       2. Clinically increasing conductance is the most common method to increase venous return.
       3. Optimizing the vascular volume-to-vascular space relationship increases conductance.
       4. This is achieved by maintaining a vascular volume that moves the venous system to a capacitance level that is near its maximum capacitance.

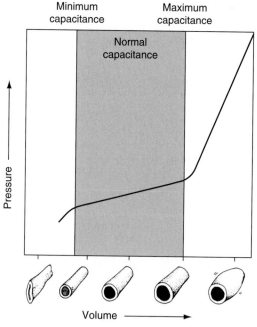

FIG. 14-6 Capacitance of the venous system.

G. Fluid administration (fluid challenge principle)
   1. This is an approach to fluid administration that results in optimization of the vascular volume-to-vascular space relationship.
   2. A general clinical and hemodynamic assessment of the patient is performed to establish baseline values. Specifically the pulmonary wedge pressure (PWP) or central venous pressure (CVP) is determined.
   3. Approximately 50 to 200 ml of fluid is rapidly administered. The volume used depends on the patient's clinical status.
   4. The patient is then assessed clinically for improvements in:
      a. Blood pressure
      b. Presence of crackles or wheezes
      c. Peripheral perfusion
      d. Urinary output
   5. The PWP or CVP is reassessed; if neither changes the challenge can be repeated. However, if they increase, careful reassessment of the cardiovascular system is required before additional fluid is administered.

BIBLIOGRAPHY

Beachey W: *Respiratory Care Anatomy and Physiology: Foundations for Clinical Practice*. St. Louis, Mosby, 1998.

Burton GG, Hodgkin JE, Ward JJ: *Respiratory Care: A Guide to Clinical Practice,* ed 4. Philadelphia, Lippincott, 1997.

Ellerbe S: *Fluid and Blood Component Therapy in the Critically Ill and Injured.* New York, Churchill Livingstone, 1981.

Guyton AC, Hall JE: *Textbook of Medical Physiology,* ed 10. Philadelphia, WB Saunders, 2000.

Hess D, MacIntyre N, Mishoe S, et al: *Respiratory Care: Principles and Practices.* St. Louis, Mosby, 2002.

Hicks GH: *Cardiopulmonary Anatomy and Physiology.* Philadelphia, WB Saunders, 2000.

Pieson DJ, Kacmarek RM: *Fundamentals of Respiratory Care.* New York, Churchill Livingstone, 1992.

Wilkins RL, Stoller JK, Scanlan CL: *Egan's Fundamentals of Respiratory Care,* ed 8. St. Louis, Mosby, 2003.

Chapter 15

Acid-Base Balance and Blood Gas Interpretation

I. **Electrolytes**
   A. An electrolyte is a substance that is capable of conducting an electrical current when placed into solution.
   B. When an electrolyte dissolves in solution, it dissociates, producing ions. For example, sodium chloride (NaCl) dissociates into sodium (Na^+) and chloride (Cl^-) ions.

$$NaCl \rightarrow Na^+ + Cl^- \tag{1}$$

   C. Strong electrolytes dissociate completely when dissolved in solution.
   D. Weak electrolytes only partially dissociate, with the majority of electrolytes remaining dissolved but undissociated.
   E. A weak acid electrolyte produces H^+ when dissolved.
   F. A weak basic electrolyte produces OH^- when dissolved.

II. **Law of Mass Action**
   A. The basic chemical and mathematical relationships involved in blood gas interpretation are based on the law of mass action (also referred to as the *law of electrolyte dissociation* or the *law of chemical equilibrium*).
   B. *The law of mass action* states that when a weak electrolyte is placed into solution, only a small percentage of it dissociates, and the majority remains undissociated. Determining the product of the molar concentrations of the dissociated species and dividing that by the molar concentration of the undissociated weak electrolyte yields a dissociation constant for that weak electrolyte. This constant is true for the particular electrolyte at the temperature at which it was originally determined.
   C. If the weak acid HA is placed into solution, it will reversibly dissociate to H^+ and A^- (the negative ion formed whenever H^+ dissociates from an acid):

$$HA \rightleftharpoons H^+ + A^- \tag{2}$$

   D. If 0.01 mol/L of HA were added to solution and 5% of HA dissociated, the following quantities of all three species would exist in solution:

HA 95% of 0.01, or 0.0095 mol/L
H^+ 5% of 0.01, or 0.0005 mol/L
A^- 5% of 0.01, or 0.0005 mol/L

Note: One H^+ and one A^- are formed as every HA molecule dissociates.

E. According to the law of mass action:

$$K = \frac{[H^+][A^-]}{[HA]} \qquad (3)$$

where K = the dissociation constant.

F. Inserting the molar concentrations of the individual species and calculating the dissociation constant yields the following:

$$0.0000263 = \frac{[0.0005][0.0005]}{[0.0095]}$$

Thus $K = 2.63 \times 10^{-5}$.

G. As explained in sections II and IV, the dissociation constant indicates the pH at which a buffer functions most efficiently.

H. The law of mass action applied to water is the basis for the pH scale.
1. Water (H_2O) dissociates into H^+ plus OH^-:

$$H_2O \rightleftharpoons H^+ + OH^- \qquad (4)$$

2. The molar concentration of H^+ and OH^- is 10^{-7} mol/L.
3. Because the concentration of the undissociated water is so large compared with the $[H^+]$ and $[OH^-]$, it is considered a constant:

$$\frac{[H^+][OH^-]}{K_{H_2O}} = K \qquad (5)$$

4. This relationship is frequently written as:

$$[H^+][OH^-] = K_w \qquad (6)$$

where K_w = the dissociation constant for H_2O.
5. The value of K_w is

$$[10^{-7}][10^{-7}] = 10^{-14}$$

6. Thus a neutral solution is one with 10^{-7} moles of H^+ per liter.
7. Because the H^+ concentration can vary from 10^{-1} to 10^{-14} in this relationship, the limits of the pH scale are defined.

$$pH \text{ is equal to } -\log[H^+] \qquad (7)$$

8. Therefore the pH scale goes from a pH of 1.0 ($[H^+] = 10^{-1}$ mol/L) to a pH of 14.0 ($[H^+] = 10^{-14}$ mol/L).
9. Remember the product of $[H^+]$ and $[OH^-]$ must equal 10^{-14}. As a result, as the $[H^+]$ increases, the $[OH^-]$ decreases and vice versa.

I. The law of mass action when applied to carbonic acid (H_2CO_3) dissolved in plasma at $37°$ C yields the following:
1. Carbonic acid (H_2CO_3) dissociates into $H^+ + HCO_3^-$ (bicarbonate ion):

$$H_2CO_3 \rightleftharpoons H^+ + HCO_3^- \qquad (8)$$

2. If the molar concentration of H^+ is multiplied by the molar concentration of HCO_3^-, and the answer is divided by the molar concentration of H_2CO_3, the dissociation constant for H_2CO_3 in plasma is calculated:

$$\frac{[H^+][HCO_3^-]}{[H_2CO_3]} = K \qquad (9)$$

3. K for the reaction 9 in blood is equal to 7.85×10^{-7}.

J.   The mathematical manipulation of the law of mass action results in the development of the Henderson-Hasselbalch equation, which is the basis for blood gas analysis.

III.   **Henderson-Hasselbalch Equation (Standard Buffer Equation)**
   A.   Derivation of the Henderson-Hasselbalch equation from equation 9:
      1.   Rearranging equation 9 and solving for [H⁺] results in the following:

$$[H^+] = \frac{K[H_2CO_3]}{[HCO_3^-]} \tag{10}$$

   2.   Taking the log to the base of 10 of each side of equation 10 yields the following:

$$\log [H^+] = \log K + \log \frac{[H_2CO_3]}{[HCO_3^-]} \tag{11}$$

   3.   Multiplying each side of equation 11 by −1 yields the following:

$$-\log [H^+] = -\log K - \log \frac{[H_2CO_3]}{[HCO_3^-]} \tag{12}$$

   4.   Rearranging $-\log \frac{[H_2CO_3]}{[HCO_3^-]}$ in equation 12 yields the following:

$$-\log [H_2CO_3]\,(-)\,-\log [HCO_3^-]$$
$$= -\log [H_2CO_3] + \log [HCO_3^-]$$
$$= +\log [HCO_3^-] - \log [H_2CO_3]$$
$$= +\log \frac{[HCO_3^-]}{[H_2CO_3]} \tag{13}$$

   5.   Inserting equation 13 in equation 12 yields the following:

$$-\log H^+ = -\log K + \log \frac{[HCO_3^-]}{[H_2CO_3]} \tag{14}$$

   6. $-\log H^+ = pH$ and $-\log K$ is termed the pK (refer to section IV). Equation 14 is rewritten as:

$$pH = pK + \log \frac{[HCO_3^-]}{[H_2CO_3]} \tag{15}$$

   7.   Equation 15 is the classic buffer equation (see section V) as applied to the $[HCO_3^-]/[H_2CO_3]$ buffer system.
   8.   A universal representation of the classic buffer equation as applied to a weak acid electrolyte is:

$$pH = pKa + \log \frac{[\text{Conjugate base}]}{[\text{Undissociated acid}]} \tag{16}$$

where pKa is the pK of a weak acid electrolyte.

   9.   If the derivation were carried out for a weak basic electrolyte, the standard equation would be:

$$pOH = pKb + \log \frac{[\text{Conjugate acid}]}{[\text{Undissociated base}]} \tag{17}$$

   10.   However, the types of buffer systems used in describing pulmonary physiology are all weak acid electrolytes.

IV.   **pK (−Log of the Dissociation Constant)**
   A.   This value represents the pH at which a buffer functions most efficiently.
   B.   When the pH of a solution equals the pK, 50% of the buffer exists in the form of the conjugate base, and 50% exists as the undissociated acid.

C. All buffers have a narrow pH range, identifying where they function most appropriately.
D. If the pH of a solution is above its pK, the solution generally will buffer acid more effectively than base.
E. If the pH of a solution is below its pK, the solution will buffer base more effectively than acid.
F. The farther away a solution's pH moves from its pK, the poorer its buffering capabilities.
G. If the pH of a buffered solution is outside the 1- to 1.5-pH range about the buffer's pK, the system's buffering capabilities are lost.

V. **Buffers**
   A. A buffer is a weak acidic or basic electrolyte that has the capability of determining the pH of a solution.
   B. Buffers are used to prevent significant changes in a solution pH.
   C. One should always choose a buffer whose pK is numerically near the pH of the solution to be buffered.
   D. Chemical functioning of buffers:
      1. If the buffer HA from section II is titrated into solution until the pH of the solution is equal to the pK of the buffer, an ideally buffered solution is established. The pK of this system is 4.58 ($-$log of 2.63×10^{-5}, see section II-F).
      2. After titration, the final concentrations of HA and A^- are equal to 0.01. Thus the classic buffer equation would be

$$pH = pK + \log \frac{[A^-]}{[HA]} \qquad (18)$$

   or

$$4.58 = 4.58 + \log \frac{0.01}{0.01}$$

   Note: The log of 0.01/0.01 is 0.
      3. If acid is added to this buffer, it reacts with the conjugate base (A^-) and forms more undissociated acid (HA):

$$A^- + H^+ \rightarrow HA \qquad (19)$$

   This should result in only a minimal change in the pH.
      a. If 0.001 mol/L of H^+ were added to the buffer, the H^+ would react with 0.001 mol/L of A^-:

$$A^- + H^+ \rightarrow HA \qquad (20)$$
$$0.001 + 0.001 \rightarrow 0.001$$

   Note: 100% efficiency is assumed.
      b. As a result, the concentration of A^- would decrease by 0.001, and the concentration of HA would increase by 0.001:

$$pH = 4.58 + \log \frac{0.01 - 0.001}{0.01 + 0.001} \text{ or } \frac{0.009}{0.011}$$

      c. The resulting pH of this solution would be 4.49, or a 0.09-pH unit change.
      d. By comparison, if 0.001 mol/L of H^+ were added to water with a pH of 7.0, the resulting pH would be approximately 2.99, more than a 4.0-pH unit change.
      4. If base is added to a buffer, it reacts with free H^+, allowing more HA to dissociate:

$$H^+ + OH^- \rightarrow H_2O \qquad (21)$$

causing the following:

$$HA \rightarrow H^+ + A^-$$ (22)

resulting in a minimal change in the pH.

a.   If 0.001 mol/L of OH⁻ were added to the buffer in equation 18, the OH⁻ would react with 0.001 mol/L of H⁺, causing 0.001 mol/L of A⁻ to be formed:

$$H^+ + OH^- \rightarrow H_2O$$
$$0.001 + 0.001 \rightarrow 0.001$$

causing the following:

$$HA \rightarrow H^+ + A^-$$
$$0.001 \rightarrow 0.001 + 0.001$$

b.   As a result, the concentration of HA decreases by 0.001, and the concentration of A⁻ increases by 0.001.

$$pH = 4.58 + \log \frac{0.01 + 0.001}{0.01 - 0.001} \text{ or } \frac{0.011}{0.009}$$

c.   The resulting pH of the solution would be 4.67, a 0.09-pH unit change.
d.   By comparison, if 0.001 mol/L of OH⁻ were added to water with a pH of 7.0, the resulting pH would be approximately 10.99, almost a 4.0-pH unit change.

VI.   The HCO_3^-/H_2CO_3 Buffer System

A.   The most important buffer system in the body is the HCO_3^-/H_2CO_3 system:

$$pH = pK + \log \frac{HCO_3^-}{H_2CO_3}$$ (23)

B.   The pK of this system is 6.1 ($K = 7.85 \times 10^{-7}$).
C.   Arterial $[HCO_3^-]$ is approximately 24 mEq/L.
D.   Arterial $[H_2CO_3]$ is approximately 1.2 mEq/L.
E.   Thus arterial pH is approximately 7.4:

$$7.4 = 6.1 + \log \frac{24 \text{ mEq/L}}{1.2 \text{ mEq/L}}$$

F.   The ratio of HCO_3^- to H_2CO_3 is 20:1:

$$\frac{HCO_3^-}{H_2CO_3} = \frac{24}{1.2} = \frac{20}{1}$$

G.   If this ratio increases (30:1), the arterial pH increases.
H.   If this ratio decreases (10:1), the arterial pH decreases.
I.   Clinically HCO_3^- and H_2CO_3 concentrations are extremely time consuming and costly to determine.
1.   Because $(P_{CO_2}) \times (0.0301)$ is equivalent to the H_2CO_3 concentration, this value can be substituted into equation 23 for H_2CO_3:

$$pH = 6.10 + \log \frac{[HCO_3^-]}{(P_{CO_2})(0.0301)}$$ (24)

2.   Clinically the pH of the blood is easily measured, as is the P_{CO_2}.
3. $[HCO_3^-]$ is always the calculated value when blood gas results are reported.
J.   In this buffer system $[HCO_3^-]$ is regulated and controlled by the kidney, and P_{CO_2} is regulated and controlled by the lung with the pH a result of $[HCO_3^-]$ and P_{CO_2}.

   K. The HCO_3^-/H_2CO_3 buffer system in blood is a poor chemical buffer.
1. This is true because of the pK (6.1) of the buffer in relation to the pH (7.4) of the arterial blood.
2. The pH of blood is outside the chemical buffering range of the HCO_3^-/H_2CO_3 system.
3. However, this system is considered an essential *physiologic* buffer (i.e., the lungs can control the excretion or retention of large quantities of acid in the form of CO_2).
4. The following reversible reaction illustrates the relationship:

$$CO_2 + H_2O \rightleftharpoons H_2CO_3 \rightleftharpoons H^+ + HCO_3^- \qquad (25)$$

5. If there is an increase in H^+, the reaction is shifted to the left, increasing plasma CO_2 levels, which are exhaled.
6. If there is a decrease in H^+, the reaction is shifted to the right, decreasing plasma CO_2 levels.
7. The effectiveness of HCO_3^- administration in the face of metabolic acidosis is based on equation 25 shifting to the left, allowing acid to be exhaled as CO_2. If ventilation cannot eliminate the increased CO_2 produced, the acidosis changes from metabolic to respiratory.

  VII. **Actual Versus Standard HCO_3^-**
    A. Actual HCO_3^-: Value calculated from actual, measured P_{CO_2} and pH of arterial blood.
1. Value normally given with arterial blood gas results.
2. Indicative of nonrespiratory acid-base imbalances.

    B. Standard HCO_3^-: Value calculated from measured pH and P_{CO_2} of venous blood after P_{CO_2} of blood has been equilibrated to 40 mm Hg.
1. Value usually reported with electrolyte studies by the clinical laboratory.
2. Indicative of a change in acid-base balance but not as precise when compared with arterial pH and P_{CO_2}.

    C. Arterial pH and P_{CO_2} most closely correlate with actual HCO_3^-.

 VIII. **Base Excess/Base Deficit**
    A. The total buffering capacity of the body can be broken down approximately as follows (Box 15-1):
1. Sixty percent by the HCO_3^-/H_2CO_3 system
2. Thirty percent by hemoglobin buffering system
3. Ten percent by all other blood buffers (e.g., phosphates, plasma proteins, and ammonia)

    B. Of the total body buffers, HCO_3^- and all proteins (including hemoglobin) are the most important.
    C. These two systems may be chemically depicted as follows:

$$CO_2 + H_2O \rightleftharpoons H_2CO_3 \rightleftharpoons HCO_3^- + H^+ \qquad (26)$$

$$H \, Prot \rightleftharpoons H^+ + Prot^- \qquad (27)$$

BOX 15-1

Primary Body Buffer Systems

Bicarbonate/carbonic acid*	HCO_3^-/H_2CO_3
Dibasic/monobasic phosphate	$HPO_4^{-2}/H_2PO_4^-$
Ammonia/ammonium ion	NH_3/NH_4^+
Hemoglobin/hemoglobin ion	Hb/HHb^+
Serum protein/protein ion	$Prot^-/HProt$

*Poor chemical buffer but essential physiologic buffer.

D. If a respiratory acidosis were to develop, the reaction shown in equation 26 would be driven to the right, causing an equal shift of the reaction shown in equation 27 to the left. As a result, the total amount of base in the body would remain unchanged.

E. If a respiratory alkalosis were to develop, the reaction shown in equation 26 would be driven to the left, causing an equal shift of the reaction shown in equation 27 to the right. As a result, the total amount of base in the body would remain unchanged.

F. The sum of $[HCO_3^-] + [Prot^-]$ is the buffer base (BB), which (as demonstrated in sections VIII-D and VIII-E) remains unchanged in all pure acute respiratory acid-base disturbances.

G. However, if metabolic acid is added to the body, the reactions shown in equations 26 and 27 would be driven to the left, and the quantity of BB would decrease; if metabolic base were added to the body, both reactions (26 and 27) would be driven to the right, and the quantity of BB would increase.

H. Base excess/base deficit (BE/BD) is defined as the actual BB minus the normal BB:

$$BE/BD = actual\ BB - normal\ BB \qquad (28)$$

I. In all pure acute respiratory acid-base disturbances, the BE/BD is normal. However, once compensation occurs, the BE/BD becomes positive or negative.

J. All metabolic acid-base disturbances are accompanied by a change in the BE/BD.

K. The BE/BD is the most reliable index of metabolic acid-base disorders.

L. The normal BE/BD is zero, with a range of ±2 mEq/L. The normal total BB is 54 mEq/L.

IX. **Normal Ranges for Blood Gases**
   A. *Absolute normals: Arterial blood* (mean population values):
      1. pH: 7.40
      2. P_{CO_2}: 40 mm Hg
      3. P_{O_2}: 100 mm Hg
      4. HCO_3^-: 24 mEq/L
      5. Base excess: 0
      6. Hemoglobin content: 14 g%
      7. Oxyhemoglobin saturation: 97.5%
      8. Oxygen content: 19.8 vol%
      9. Carboxyhemoglobin saturation: 0%
   B. *Normal ranges: Arterial blood* (±2 SDs from the population mean):
      1. pH: 7.35 to 7.45
      2. P_{CO_2}: 35 to 45 mm Hg
      3. P_{O_2}: 80 to 100 mm Hg
      4. HCO_3^-: 22 to 27 mEq/L
      5. Base excess: ±2 mEq/L
      6. Hemoglobin content: 12 to 15 g%
      7. Oxyhemoglobin saturation: ≥95%
      8. Oxygen content: >16 vol%
      9. Carboxyhemoglobin saturation: <2%
   C. *Absolute normals: venous blood* (mean population values):
      1. pH: 7.35
      2. P_{CO_2}: 46 mm Hg
      3. P_{O_2}: 40 mm Hg
      4. HCO_3^-: 27 mEq/L
      5. Oxyhemoglobin saturation: 75%
   D. *Normal range of neonatal arteriolized capillary blood*
      1. pH: 7.30 to 7.33
      2. P_{CO_2}: 40 to 45 mm Hg
      3. P_{O_2}: 35 to 40 mm Hg
      4. HCO_3^-: 18 to 20 mEq/L
      5. Oxyhemoglobin saturation: ≈75%

X. Mathematical Interrelationships Between pH, P_{CO_2}, and HCO_3^-

  A. If the constants and log relationship are eliminated in the HCO_3^-/H_2CO_3 buffer equation, the equation may be simplified to:

$$pH \approx \frac{HCO_3^-}{P_{CO_2}} \qquad (29)$$

  This demonstrates the mathematical interrelationship between these variables.

  B. Under all clinical circumstances the pH generally will be a result of the HCO_3^- and P_{CO_2} levels.

  C. In a pure respiratory abnormality where the HCO_3^- remains essentially constant, the P_{CO_2} and pH are indirectly related:

$$HCO_3^- \approx (pH)(P_{CO_2}) \qquad (30)$$

  D. In a pure metabolic abnormality where the P_{CO_2} remains essentially constant, the HCO_3^- and pH are directly related:

$$P_{CO_2} \approx \frac{HCO_3^-}{pH} \qquad (31)$$

  E. These interrelationships provide the basis for blood gas interpretation.

XI. Compensation for Primary Acid-Base Abnormalities

  A. Compensation involves the various mechanisms used by the body to normalize the pH after a primary acid-base abnormality. Compensation does not imply correction of the primary abnormalities.

  B. Compensation for primary respiratory acid-base imbalances is via the kidney (see Chapter 13).

  C. Compensation for primary metabolic acid-base abnormalities is via the respiratory system (see Chapter 6).

XII. Estimation of pH Changes Based Purely on P_{CO_2} Changes

  A. Because the pK of the HCO_3^-/H_2CO_3 system is 6.10 and the quantity of HCO_3^- is 20 times greater than the quantity of H_2CO_3, the body buffers acid more efficiently than base.

  B. If starting at a baseline pH of 7.40 and a P_{CO_2} of 40 mm Hg, for every 10-mm Hg P_{CO_2} increase there is an approximate 0.05-pH unit decrease:

   1. P_{CO_2} 50: pH 7.35: HCO_3^- 25
   2. P_{CO_2} 60: pH 7.30: HCO_3^- 26
   3. P_{CO_2} 70: pH 7.25: HCO_3^- 27
   4. P_{CO_2} 80: pH 7.20: HCO_3^- 28

   This relationship holds if *no* compensation by the kidney has occurred. The HCO_3^- increases as a result of a shifting of the components of the BB (see section VIII).

  C. If starting at a baseline pH of 7.40 and a P_{CO_2} of 40, for every 10-mm Hg P_{CO_2} decrease there is an approximate 0.10-pH unit increase:

   1. P_{CO_2} 35: pH 7.45: HCO_3^- 23
   2. P_{CO_2} 30: pH 7.50: HCO_3^- 22
   3. P_{CO_2} 25: pH 7.55: HCO_3^- 21
   4. P_{CO_2} 20: pH 7.60: HCO_3^- 20

   This relationship holds if no compensation by the kidney has occurred. The HCO_3^- decreases as a result of a shifting of the components of the BB (see section VIII).

XIII. Interpretation of Arterial Blood Gases

  A. Blood gas interpretation is performed in three steps:

   1. Interpretation of acid-base status
   2. Assessment of level of hypoxemia
   3. Assessment of tissue hypoxia

XIV. **Interpretation of Acid-Base Status**
   A. Table 15-1 lists ranges for interpretation of blood gases.
   B. The terminology used is uncompensated, partially compensated, and compensated.
   C. Approach to blood gas interpretation (see Table 15-1)
      1. Determine whether the pH is within the normal range
         a. If normal, the blood gas is normal or compensated.
         b. If it is outside the normal range, it is uncompensated or partially compensated.
      2. Determine whether the P_{CO_2} is normal or abnormal
         a. If the P_{CO_2} is normal and:
            (1) The pH is normal; then the blood gas is normal.
            (2) The pH is decreased; then an uncompensated metabolic acidosis exists.
            (3) The pH is increased; then an uncompensated metabolic alkalosis exists.
         b. If the P_{CO_2} is higher than normal and:
            (1) The pH is decreased and the HCO_3^- is normal; then an uncompensated respiratory acidosis exists.
            (2) The pH is decreased and the HCO_3^- is above normal; then a partially compensated respiratory acidosis exists.
            (3) The pH is between 7.35 and 7.40 and the HCO_3^- is elevated; then it is a compensated respiratory acidosis.
            (4) The pH is 7.40 to 7.45 and the HCO_3^- is elevated; then it *may be* a compensated metabolic alkalosis; however, this acid-base state is rare, and usually a compensated respiratory acidosis with a mild metabolic alkalosis exists.
            (5) The pH is increased with an elevated HCO_3^-; then a partially compensated metabolic alkalosis exists.

TABLE **15-1**

Blood Gas Interpretation

Status	pH	P_{CO_2}	HCO_3^-	Base Excess
Respiratory acidosis				
Uncompensated	↓ 7.35	↑ 45	Normal	Normal
Partially compensated	↓ 7.35	↑ 45	↑ 27	↑ +2
Compensated	7.35-7.45	↑ 45	↑ 27	↑ +2
Respiratory alkalosis				
Uncompensated	↑ 7.45	↓ 35	Normal	Normal
Partially compensated	↑ 7.45	↓ 35	↓ 22	↓ −2
Compensated	7.40-7.45	↓ 35	↓ 22	↓ −2
Metabolic acidosis				
Uncompensated	↓ 7.35	Normal	↓ 22	↓ −2
Partially compensated	↓ 7.35	↓ 35	↓ 22	↓ −2
Compensated	7.35-7.40	↓ 35	↓ 22	↓ −2
Metabolic alkalosis				
Uncompensated	↑ 7.45	Normal	↑ 27	↑ +2
Partially compensated*	↑ 7.45	↑ 45	↑ 27	↑ +2
Compensated*	7.40-7.45	↑ 45	↑ 27	↑ +2
Combined respiratory and metabolic acidosis	↓ 7.35	↑ 45	↓ 22	↓ −2
Combined respiratory and metabolic alkalosis	↑ 7.45	↓ 35	↑ 27	↑ −2

*Partially compensated or compensated metabolic alkalosis generally is rarely seen clinically because of the body's mechanism to prevent hypoventilation.

c. If the P_{CO_2} is lower than normal and:
  (1) The pH is increased and the HCO_3^- is normal; then an uncompensated respiratory alkalosis exists.
  (2) The pH is between 7.35 and 7.40 and the HCO_3^- is decreased; then a compensated metabolic acidosis exists.
  (3) The pH is between 7.40 and 7.45 and the HCO_3^- is decreased; then a compensated respiratory alkalosis exists.
  (4) The pH is increased and the HCO_3^- is decreased; then a partially compensated respiratory alkalosis exists.
  (5) The pH is decreased and the HCO_3^- is decreased; then a partially compensated metabolic acidosis exists.
d. Combined respiratory and metabolic acidosis or combined respiratory and metabolic alkalosis also can occur.
  (1) If the pH is markedly decreased, the P_{CO_2} is increased, and the HCO_3^- is decreased, then an uncompensated respiratory and metabolic acidosis exists.
  (2) If the pH is markedly increased, the P_{CO_2} is decreased, and the HCO_3^- is increased, then an uncompensated respiratory and metabolic alkalosis exists.
e. Figure 15-1 lists an algorithm for the interpretation of arterial blood gases.

XV. Assessment of Level of Hypoxemia
  A. For patients who are breathing room air and who are <60 years of age:
    1. Mild hypoxemia: Arterial P_{O_2} 70 to 79 mm Hg
    2. Moderate hypoxemia: Arterial P_{O_2} 50 to 69 mm Hg
    3. Severe hypoxemia: Arterial P_{O_2} <50 mm Hg

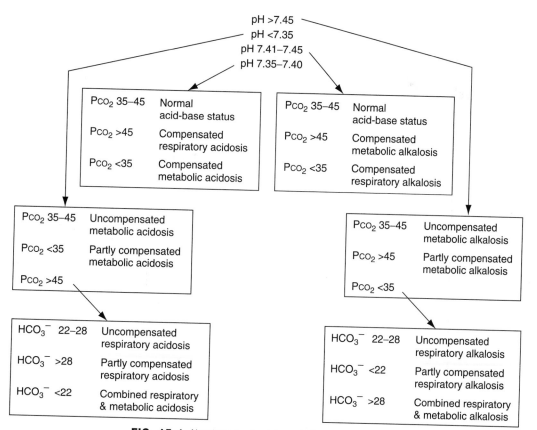

FIG. 15-1 Algorithm for the interpretation of blood gases.

B. For individuals >60 years of age, 1 mm Hg should be subtracted from the lower limits of mild and moderate hypoxemia for each year >60. At any age a PO_2 <40 mm Hg indicates severe hypoxemia, and a PO_2 <60 to 65 is always considered hypoxemic.

C. More precisely acceptable lower limits for PO_2 can be determined by the following (at sea level):
1. For patients in the supine position: $PO_2 = 103.5 - (0.42 \times age) \pm 4$ mm Hg.
2. For patients in the sitting position: $PO_2 = 104.2 - (0.27 \times age) \pm 3$ mm Hg.

D. Patients with F_IO_2 >0.21
1. Uncorrected hypoxemia: Arterial PO_2 less than room air acceptable limit.
2. Corrected hypoxemia: Arterial PO_2 between minimal acceptable room air limit and 100 mm Hg.
3. Excessively corrected hypoxemia: Arterial PO_2 >100 mm Hg.

XVI. **Assessment of Tissue Hypoxia**
A. At present there is no direct method to assess tissue hypoxia; it must be clinically assessed indirectly.
B. Normally adequate tissue oxygenation requires:
1. Normal volume of oxygen must be carried by arterial blood.
2. Acid-base status must be relatively normal.
3. Tissue perfusion must be adequate.
C. The likelihood of tissue hypoxia existing is increased in the presence of the following:
1. Severe hypoxemia
2. Metabolic acidosis
3. Decreased cardiac output or poor perfusion
D. If tissue hypoxia has occurred, blood lactate levels are increased.

XVII. **Acute Respiratory Failure**
A. A term used to define a circumstance where acute respiratory acidosis is associated with acute hypoxemia.
B. Acute respiratory failure requires:
1. pH < 7.35
2. $PaCO_2$ > 45 mm Hg
3. PaO_2 < 80 mm Hg

XVIII. **Acute Ventilatory Failure**
A. A term used to define a circumstance where acute respiratory acidosis is *not* associated with acute hypoxemia.
B. Acute ventilatory requires:
1. pH < 7.35
2. $PaCO_2$ > 45 mm Hg
3. PaO_2 normal limits

XIX. **Clinical Causes of Acid-Base Abnormalities**
A. Respiratory acidosis primary causes:
1. Cardiopulmonary disease, particularly end-stage chronic obstructive pulmonary disease (COPD) or chronic restrictive pulmonary disease.
a. COPD
b. Pneumonia
c. Fibrosis
d. Acute respiratory distress syndrome
e. Pulmonary edema
f. Others
2. Central nervous system depression by drugs, trauma, or lesion.
3. Obesity: Hyperventilation syndrome.

4. Neurologic or neuromuscular disease resulting in profound weakness of ventilatory muscles.
5. Fatigue after any acute pulmonary disease.
6. Chest wall restriction:
   a. Pneumothorax
   b. Pleural effusion
   c. Fibrothorax
   d. Kyphoscoliosis
B. Respiratory alkalosis: Primary causes:
   1. Hypoxemia: Its primary effect on the respiratory system is hyperventilation.
   2. Compensation for primary metabolic acidosis.
   3. Central nervous system stimulation by drugs, trauma, or lesion.
   4. Emotional disorders (e.g., pain, anxiety, or fear).
   5. Hepatic failure.
   6. High altitude.
   7. Mechanical ventilation.
   8. Septicemia, hypotension.
C. Metabolic acidosis
   1. Primary causes
      a. Lactic acidosis
         (1) In the absence of oxygen as final electron acceptor in the electron transport chain, aerobic metabolism is decreased.
         (2) An increase in anaerobic metabolism results, which increases formation of lactic acid, a nonvolatile organic acid.
         (3) If the oxygenation state of the patient is improved, lactic acidosis is reversed.
         (4) Normal lactate levels
             (a) 0.5 to 2.5 mmol/L
      b. Ketoacidosis
         (1) Primary causes
             (a) Uncontrolled diabetes mellitus
             (b) Starvation
             (c) High fat content in the diet for extended periods
             (d) Alcoholism
         (2) In all cases insufficient volumes of glucose enter the cell, resulting in an increase in metabolism of body fats.
         (3) The metabolic end products of fat metabolism are keto acids (e.g., acetone and β-hydroxybutyric acid).
         (4) The patient with diabetic acidosis is generally hyperventilating significantly, and his or her breath has a sweet, acetone odor.
         (5) The patient needs glucose and insulin.
      c. Renal failure (see Chapter 13)
         (1) May be caused by:
             (a) Renal tubular acidosis
             (b) Chronic pyelonephritis
             (c) Obstructive uropathy
         (2) Decreased renal function inhibits the body's primary mechanism for maintaining blood HCO_3^- levels and excretion of H^+.
         (3) Thus free $[H^+]$ increases and free $[HCO_3^-]$ decreases.
      d. Ingestion of base-depleting drugs or acids
         (1) Aspirin, salicylates
         (2) Methanol
         (3) Ethylene glycol
         (4) Paraldehyde
      e. Hypoaldosteronism

       f. Potassium-sparing diuretics

       g. Diarrhea

       h. Pancreatic or biliary fistulas, ureterosigmoidostomy

       i. Carbonic anhydrase inhibitors: acetazolamide

       j. Excessive intake of ammonium chloride, cationic anion acids

  D. Metabolic alkalosis

    1. Primary causes

       a. Hypokalemia (see Chapter 14)

       b. Hypochloremia (see Chapter 14)

       c. Gastric suction or vomiting

         (1) Because gastric contents are acidic (pH 1.0 to 2.0), excessive loss of gastric fluid results in alkalosis.

       d. Massive doses of steroids

         (1) Steroids increase reabsorption of Na^+ and accelerate excretion of H^+ and K^+.

       e. Diuretics

         (1) Diuretics cause an increase in the amount of K^+ excreted.

         (2) With excessive or uncontrolled use, hypokalemia may result.

       f. Ingestion of acid-depleting drugs or bases

         (1) $NaHCO_3$ (sodium bicarbonate)

       g. Primary aldosteronism

       h. Cushing's syndrome

XX. Mixed Venous Blood Gases

  A. $P\bar{v}o_2$, % $Hb\bar{v}o_2$, and $Cao_2 - C\bar{v}o_2$ levels are reflective of the adequacy of O_2 delivery to peripheral tissue.

  B. Alterations in these values may be caused by:

    1. Decreased O_2 content

    2. Decreased cardiac output (CO)

    3. Increased tissue metabolism

    4. Altered peripheral microcirculation (i.e., sepsis)

  C. All are predictive of alterations in CO if O_2 content, tissue metabolism, and peripheral distribution of CO are unaltered.

  D. A decrease in $P\bar{v}o_2$ and % $Hb\bar{v}o_2$ and an increase in $Cao_2 - C\bar{v}o_2$ are indicative of a decrease in CO relative to tissue demands and may be used as a reflection of cardiovascular reserve (Table 15-2).

    1. If CO decreases, the tissue must extract a greater quantity of O_2 per unit of blood.

    2. As a result $P\bar{v}o_2$ and % $Hb\bar{v}o_2$ must decrease, whereas the difference between arterial and venous O_2 contents ($Cao_2 - C\bar{v}o_2$) must increase.

  E. For maximum accuracy these values must be obtained from a pulmonary artery catheter. This is necessary because peripheral venous blood is reflective of only local events, whereas pulmonary artery values reflect means of all tissue beds.

  F. Many pulmonary artery catheters use oximetry to continuously monitor percentage of $Hb\bar{v}o_2$ or $P\bar{v}o_2$. Some believe the percentage of $Hb\bar{v}o_2$ or $P\bar{v}o_2$ is best used as an early indicator of a cardiovascular incident resulting in altered O_2 delivery.

TABLE 15-2

Mixed Venous Blood Gas Values During Various Levels of Cardiovascular Stress

Status	$Cao_2 - C\bar{v}o_2$ (vol%)		$P\bar{v}o_2$ (mm Hg)		% $Hb\bar{v}o_2$	
	Average	Range	Average	Range	Average	Range
Normal	5.0	3.4-6.0	40	37-43	75	70-76
Critically ill but stable	3.5	2.5-4.5	37	35-40	70	68-75
Critically ill with limited reserve	5.0	4.5-6.0	32	30-35	60	56-68
Cardiovascularly decompensated	>6.0	>6.0	<30	<30	<56	<56

XXI. Estimation of Base Excess/Base Deficit
    A. Determine the pH predicted by an acute change in the P_{CO_2}.
        1. For every 10-mm Hg P_{CO_2} increase, the pH decreases by 0.05.
        2. For every 10-mm Hg P_{CO_2} decrease, the pH increases by 0.10.
    B. Determine the difference between the actual and predicted pH.
        Example:
            Actual pH   7.50
            Predicted pH 7.35
            Difference   0.15
    C. Eliminate the decimal and multiply by 2/3 to obtain BE/BD in milliequivalents per liter.
        Example:
            ⅔ of 15 = 10 mEq/L
    D. If the actual pH is less than the predicted pH, this is a base deficit.
    E. If the actual pH is greater than the predicted pH, this is a base excess.
    F. This is an excess of 10 mEq/L of base in all extracellular fluid.

XXII. Calculation of Bicarbonate Administration
    A. Normally HCO_3^- is administered only in the case of severe metabolic acidosis.
    B. Severe metabolic acidosis is defined as a base deficit of at least 10 mEq/L and one of the following:
        1. A pH <7.20
        2. A pH between 7.20 and 7.25 with an unstable cardiovascular system.
    C. If the pH is >7.25, HCO_3^- is normally not administered, even if the base deficit is 10 mEq/L.
    D. Extracellular fluid volume in liters can be estimated by taking one fourth the body weight in kilograms.
    E. The total body deficit in base is determined by multiplying the extracellular fluid volume by the base deficit in milliequivalents per liter.
    F. One half of this estimated amount is normally administered.
        Example:
            Base deficit   15 mEq/L
            Weight   80 kg
            Extracellular fluid volume   80/4 = 20 L
            20 L × 15 mEq/L = 300 mEq total body deficit
            ½ of 300 mEq = 150 mEq administered

XXIII. Calculation of Ammonium Chloride (NH_3Cl) or Dilute Hydrochloric Acid (HCl) Administration
    A. In severe metabolic alkalosis, NH_3Cl or HCl can be administered to correct acute base excess.
    B. The same calculations outlined in Section XXII are used.

XXIV. Typical Blood Gas Contaminants
    A. Heparin
        1. Sodium heparin is commonly used to prevent coagulation of arterial blood to be used for blood gas analysis.
        2. Ammonium heparin may affect pH even in small quantities.
        3. Normal pH of sodium heparin is 6.0 to 7.0.
        4. Concentration used is 1000 units/ml.
        5. P_{CO_2} of sodium heparin is <2 mm Hg.
        6. P_{O_2} of sodium heparin is approximately 159 mm Hg.
        7. Normally 0.05 ml of heparin/ml of blood should be used for anticoagulation.
        8. If the concentration or volume of heparin used is above this level:
            a. The pH level of the blood may decrease or remain the same.
            b. The P_{CO_2} of the blood will decrease.

    c. The P_{O_2} may be altered, depending on the blood's original P_{O_2} in relation to heparin's P_{O_2}.

    d. The Hb_{O_2}% saturation may be altered, depending on the blood's original P_{O_2} and Hb_{O_2}% saturation.

    e. The Hb_{CO}% saturation will not be altered.

    f. Hemoglobin content will decrease.

    g. The HCO_3^- level will decrease.

    h. Base excess will decrease.

    i. Oxygen content may be altered.

  9. If insufficient heparin levels are used:

    a. Machine clotting is likely.

    b. Results are questionable.

 10. The problem of heparin contamination today is rare because most blood gas syringes come preheparinized and do not require the clinician to add fluid.

B. Saline and other intravenous solutions alter blood gas values in a manner similar to that of heparin except that the pH may also increase.

C. Air bubbles

  1. The pH level of the blood normally will increase.

  2. The P_{CO_2} of the blood normally will decrease.

  3. The P_{O_2} of the blood may be altered, depending on the blood's original P_{O_2} compared with atmospheric P_{O_2}.

  4. The Hb_{O_2}% saturation may be altered, depending on the blood's original P_{O_2} and Hb_{O_2}% saturation.

  5. The Hb_{CO}% saturation will be altered.

  6. Hemoglobin content is unaltered.

  7. The HCO_3^- level may decrease.

  8. Base excess may decrease.

  9. Oxygen content may be altered.

BIBLIOGRAPHY

Beachey W: *Respiratory Care Anatomy and Physiology: Foundations for Clinical Practice.* St. Louis, Mosby, 1998.

Burton GC, Hodgkin JE, Ward JJ: *Respiratory Care: A Guide to Clinical Practice,* ed 4. Philadelphia, JB Lippincott, 1997.

Cane RD, Shapiro BA: *Case Studies in Critical Care Medicine.* Chicago, Year Book Medical Publishers, 1985.

Comroe JH: *Physiology of Respiration,* ed 2. Chicago, Year Book Medical Publishers, 1974.

Davenport HW: *The ABC's of Acid-Base Chemistry,* ed 6. Chicago, University of Chicago Press, 1977.

Filey GF: *Acid-Base and Blood Gas Regulation.* Philadelphia, Lea & Febiger, 1972.

Guyton AC, Hall JE: *Textbook of Medical Physiology,* ed 10. Philadelphia, WB Saunders, 2000.

Hess D, MacIntyre N, Mishoe S, et al: *Respiratory Care: Principles and Practices.* St. Louis, Mosby, 2002.

Hicks GH: *Cardiopulmonary Anatomy and Physiology.* Philadelphia, WB Saunders, 2000.

Pierson DJ, Kacmarek RM: *Foundations of Respiratory Care.* New York, Churchill Livingstone Publishing, 1992.

Shapiro BA, Harrison RA, Cane R, et al: *Clinical Application of Blood Gases,* ed 4. Chicago, Year Book Medical Publishers, 1989.

Wilkins RL, Stoller JK, Scanlan CL: *Egan's Fundamentals of Respiratory Therapy,* ed 8. St. Louis, Mosby, 2003.

Chapter 16

Anatomy and Physiology of the Nervous System

I. **Structure of the Nerve Fiber**
   A. Each nerve fiber has three components: (Figure 16-1)
      1. Cell body or soma: The primary metabolic area of the nerve, site of initial synthesis of transmitter substances.
      2. Dendrite: The structures that carry impulses *to* the cell body. A single neuron may contain 10,000 dendrites.
      3. Axon: The structure that conducts impulses *away* from the cell body. Usually only one axon leaves a cell body; however, it may branch extensively.

II. **Classification of Neurons**
   A. Each neuron is classified by the direction of impulse transmission.
      1. Sensory (afferent) neurons: Transmit nerve impulses to the spinal cord or brain.
      2. Motor (efferent) neurons: Transmit nerve impulses from the brain or spinal cord to muscles or glands (effector organs).
      3. Interneurons (internuncial neurons): Conduct impulses from sensory to motor neurons entirely within the central nervous system (CNS).

III. **Nerve Cell Membrane Potential (Figure 16-2)**
   A. In the resting state, the inner surface of the cell membrane is negative compared with the positive outer surface. This sets up an electric potential across the cell membrane (normal polarity).
      1. Intracellular: The primary cation, potassium (K^+), is readily diffusible across the cell membrane.
      2. Extracellular: The primary cation, sodium (Na^+), is poorly diffusible across the cell membrane.
      3. High extracellular Na^+ (142 mEq/L) and low extracellular K^+ (5 mEq/L) levels, along with high intracellular K^+ (140 mEq/L) and low intracellular Na^+ (10 mEq/L) levels, are maintained in the resting state by the Na^+ pump (active transport).
      4. Active transport (Na^+ pump): The movement of Na^+ from the intracellular space to the extracellular space and the movement of K^+ from the extracellular space to the intracellular space. Adenosine triphosphate (ATP) provides the energy for the uphill transport of these ions.

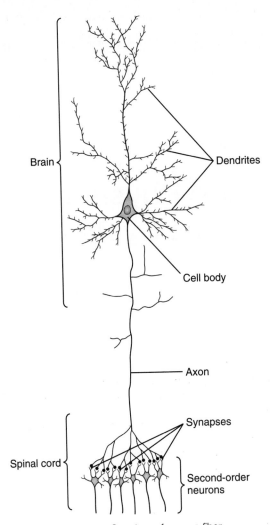

FIG. 16-1 Structure of a nerve fiber.

IV. Action Potential

A. For a nerve impulse to be transmitted, an alteration in the cell's resting membrane potential must be activated.

B. An action potential is a stimulus that is capable of significantly increasing the cell membrane's permeability to sodium.

C. The action potential is an all-or-nothing phenomenon (i.e., the stimulus must be strong enough to allow for a reversal in the membrane potential); Na^+ moves into the cells causing the intracellular side of the membrane to become positive. If the stimulus is not of sufficient strength, an action potential does not occur.

D. An action potential may be caused by:

1. Electric stimulation
2. Chemicals
3. Mechanical damage to the cell membrane
4. Heat or cold
5. Decreased serum calcium ion concentration $[Ca^{+2}]$, which increases the tendency for development of an action potential (low calcium tetany)

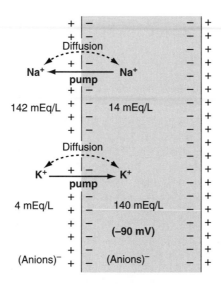

FIG. 16-2 Establishment of a resting membrane potential when the membrane potential is caused by diffusion of both sodium and potassium ions plus pumping of these ions by the Na+-K+ pump.

V. **Nerve Impulse Propagation (Figure 16-3)**
   A. The nerve impulse is a self-propagating wave of electric charge that travels along the surface of the neuron's membrane (i.e., the movement of the action potential along the cell membrane changing its charge). The nerve impulse travels in one direction only, from dendrite to cell body to axon.
   B. Depolarization: Stage 1 of the action potential, in which an impulse travels along the nerve fiber.
      1. Sodium ions rush to the inside of the cell membrane.
      2. A positive intracellular membrane charge is set up with a negative extracellular membrane charge.
      3. There is a complete reversal of the resting membrane potential.
   C. Repolarization: Stage 2 of the action potential, in which the membrane returns to the normal resting membrane potential.
      1. Immediately after the impulse passes a point on the membrane, the membrane's permeability to Na+ is again decreased.
      2. Na+ ions are actively removed from the cell by the Na pump.
      3. The resting membrane potential is reestablished.

VI. **Nerve Synapse**
   A. The nerve synapse (synaptic cleft) is the junction between one neuron and another neuron, muscle, or gland. It is an actual space between nerve fibers.
   B. Transmission of an impulse from the axon of one nerve to a dendrite, soma, or effector organ is a chemical process occurring across the synapse. The distance across the synapse is approximately 200 Å.
   C. Presynaptic terminals are located on the axon and contain vesicles that synthesize, store, and secrete a transmitter substance into the synapse. The transmitter substance stimulates the dendrite or soma of the next nerve, causing an action potential.
      1. Primary transmitter substances of the peripheral nervous system are:
         a. Acetylcholine
         b. Norepinephrine
   D. Postsynaptic terminals are located on dendrites, somas, or effector organs. After being stimulated, these terminals secrete a substance into the synapse to metabolize the transmitter substance.

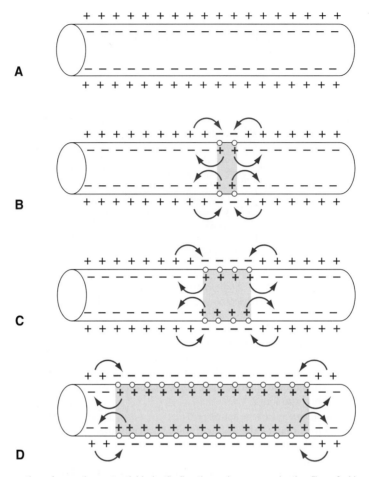

FIG. 16-3 Propagation of an action potential in both directions along a conductive fiber. **A,** Normal resting nerve fiber. **B,** Initial excitement—depolarization. **C** and **D,** Continuation of the action potential along the fiber.

E. Acetylcholine as the transmitter substance (Figure 16-4)
   1. Acetylcholine is synthesized in the terminal endings of cholinergic nerve fibers. After synthesis the acetylcholine is transported into the presynaptic vesicles where it is stored and released. It is formed from the reaction of acetyl coenzyme A with choline in the presence of choline acetyltransferase.
   2. Vesicles storing acetylcholine are formed in the cell body and migrate to the surface of the presynaptic terminal.
   3. When an action potential reaches the presynaptic terminal, acetylcholine is released into the synapse.
   4. The acetylcholine moves across the synapse and stimulates a receptor on the postsynaptic terminal.
   5. After stimulation the acetylcholine is released back into the synapse, and the postsynaptic terminal releases cholinesterase (acetylcholinesterase and acetylcholine esterase are terms synonymous with cholinesterase), which metabolizes acetylcholine, forming choline and acetate ion.
   6. The choline is reabsorbed into the presynaptic terminal and is available to form more acetylcholine.

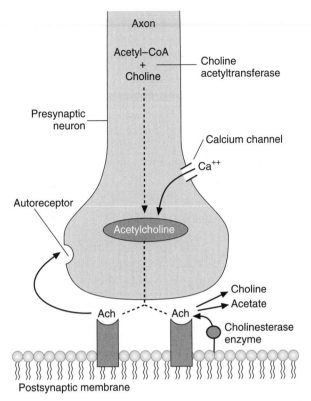

FIG. 16-4 Synthesis, storage, release, and inactivation of acetylcholine (see text).

F. Norepinephrine as the transmitter substance (Figure 16-5)
1. Norepinephrine is synthesized inside and outside the presynaptic vesicles, where it is stored and released.
2. The synthesis of norepinephrine proceeds as follows:
    (a) Tyrosine $\xrightarrow{\text{hydroxylation}}$ Dopa
    (b) Dopa $\xrightarrow{\text{decarboxylation}}$ Dopamine
    (c) Transport of dopamine into the vesicles
    (d) Dopamine $\xrightarrow{\text{hydroxylation}}$ Norepinephrine
3. Norepinephrine is released via a mechanism identical to acetylcholine (see section VI-E).
4. After stimulation norepinephrine has three possible immediate fates:
    a. Reabsorption into the presynaptic terminal (50% to 80% of secreted volume) for future secretion.
    b. Metabolism in adjoining tissue by catechol-O-methyl-transferase (COMT) or in the nerve ending by monoamine oxidase (MAO).
    c. Diffusion to surrounding tissues and eventually into the blood.
5. Complete metabolism of by-products formed in the synapse or norepinephrine entering the blood occurs in the liver via MAO and COMT.
6. In the adrenal medulla the formation of norepinephrine may proceed one step further to epinephrine by the process of methylation.
7. Duration of effect of norepinephrine in the synapse is only a few seconds. However, the norepinephrine and epinephrine released into the blood by the adrenal medulla remain active for up to several minutes.

VII. **Alteration of Nerve Impulse Transmission**
   A. Acidosis decreases transmission across the synapse.
   B. Alkalosis increases transmission across the synapse.

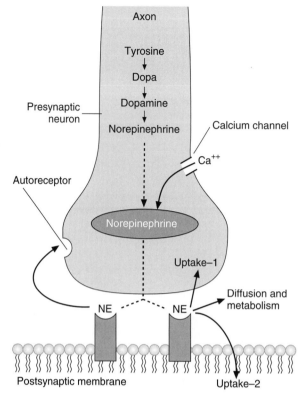

FIG. 16-5 Synthesis, storage, release, and inactivation of norepinephrine (see text).

VIII. **Neuromuscular Junction**
   A. This junction is the site of transmission of impulses from nerves to skeletal muscle fibers.
   B. The axon of the nerve branches at its end to form a structure called the motor endplate, which invaginates into muscle fiber but does not penetrate the muscle membrane.
   C. The motor endplate's terminal aspects are referred to as *sole feet*.
   D. Sole feet provide a large area of "contact" on the muscle surface. It is from the sole feet that the transmitter substance acetylcholine is secreted.
   E. After stimulation cholinesterase is secreted by the muscle fiber to metabolize the acetylcholine.

IX. **Reflex Arc or Reflex Action**
   A. The reflex arc is a functional process of the nervous system. Most neuromuscular and neuroglandular mechanisms are controlled by a reflex arc.
   B. The reflex arc consists of a series of neurons in which impulses are transmitted from a receptor to the CNS and then to a motor neuron to elicit a response.
   C. Most simple reflexes consist of an impulse from a sensory neuron being transmitted (normally in the spinal cord) to a motor neuron.
   D. Complex reflexes may involve many internuncial neurons.
   E. Reflex actions are involuntary, specific, predictable, and adaptive.

X. **Organization of the Nervous System**
   A. The nervous system is composed of the brain, spinal cord, ganglia (aggregations of nerve cell bodies), and nerves, which regulate and coordinate bodily activities.
   B. Divisions of the nervous system
      1. The CNS is composed of the brain and spinal cord, which acts as a switchboard, receiving and sending impulses to all areas of the body.

2. The peripheral nervous system is composed of neurons that enter and leave the CNS. The peripheral nervous system has two main divisions:
   a. Somatic nervous system, which is responsible for voluntary bodily functions.
   b. Autonomic nervous system (ANS), which is responsible for involuntary bodily functions.
C. Central nervous system
   1. The CNS is subdivided into the following structures:
      a. Cerebral cortex
      b. Diencephalon
         (1) Thalamus
         (2) Subthalamus
         (3) Hypothalamus
      c. Brain stem
         (1) Medulla
         (2) Pons
         (3) Midbrain
         (4) Cerebellum
      d. Spinal cord
   2. The cerebral cortex is primarily responsible for:
      a. All higher brain functions (e.g., memory, reasoning, sight, and hearing)
      b. Integration of all sensory stimuli
      c. Voluntary control of bodily activities
   3. The diencephalon is located between the hemispheres of the cerebral cortex and the brain stem containing the following structures:
      a. Thalamus
         (1) Primary relay station of the brain for:
            (a) Hearing
            (b) Touch
            (c) Pressure
            (d) Position
            (e) Pain
         (2) Site of action of many psychoactive drugs
      b. The subthalamus is responsible for the coordination of fine motor activity (extrapyramidal) along with the cerebellum.
      c. Hypothalamus
         (1) Responsible for many of the body's vegetative functions via the ANS and hormonal control.
            (a) Eating
            (b) Drinking
            (c) Sleeping
            (d) Temperature
            (e) Sexual behavior
            (f) Fluid and electrolyte balance
         (2) The hypothalamus assists in the modulation of emotion and behavior.
         (3) Many psychoactive drugs are active at the hypothalamus.
   4. The brain stem lies within the cranium and connects the diencephalon with the spinal cord. It contains the following structures:
      a. Medulla
         (1) The medulla contains control centers for the following:
            (a) Respiration (see Chapter 6)
            (b) Peripheral vasoconstriction
            (c) Gastrointestinal function
            (d) Sleeping
            (e) Walking

(2) The ascending reticular activating system (ARAS) travels through the medulla. The ARAS helps to modulate behavior.
   b. The pons contains two centers that effect respiration (see Chapter 6):
      (1) Apneustic center
      (2) Pneumotaxic center
   c. The midbrain acts as a relay station, controlling vision and hearing.
   d. The cerebellum coordinates fine motor activity along with the subthalamus.
5. Spinal cord
   a. Channels information from the brain to the periphery.
   b. Most reflexes are coordinated via the spinal cord.
D. Somatic nervous system (Figure 16-6)
   1. The somatic nervous system is responsible for all voluntary muscular activities.
   2. Contains sensory and motor neurons.
   3. Ganglia, a highly dense collection of nerve cell bodies, are located within the spinal cord.
E. Autonomic nervous system
   1. Contains only motor neurons (Figure 16-7).
   2. Input to the ANS is via the somatic nervous system that is coordinated by the CNS.
   3. Each nerve of the ANS has a ganglion, which is located outside of the spinal cord.
   4. The ANS is responsible for all involuntary bodily activities.
   5. It is subdivided into:
      a. Parasympathetic (craniosacral) nervous system (PNS)
      b. Sympathetic (thoracolumbar) nervous system (SNS)
   6. The two divisions are somewhat antagonistic.

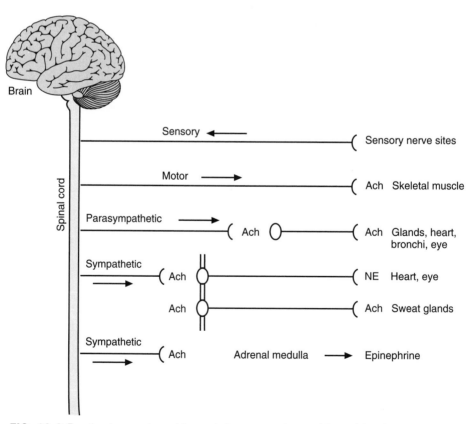

FIG. 16-6 Functional comparison of the central nervous system and the peripheral nervous system.

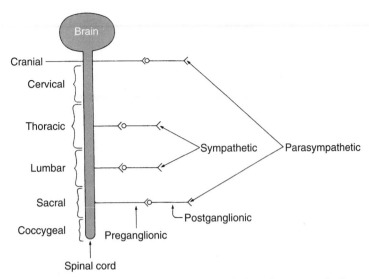

FIG. 16-7 Anatomic distribution of the nerve fibers of the sympathetic and parasympathetic nervous systems.

7. The ANS is activated and controlled primarily by the:
   a. Spinal cord
   b. Brain stem
   c. Hypothalamus
8. The ANS is activated secondarily by the:
   a. Cerebral cortex
   b. Visceral reflexes
9. SNS: Nerves of the SNS originate from the spinal cord at levels T-1 (thoracic) through L-2 (lumbar) (see Figure 16-7; Figure 16-8).
   a. Nerve fibers that transmit SNS impulses are either:
      (1) Preganglionic fibers
      (2) Postganglionic fibers
   b. The SNS fibers synapse primarily at ganglia located along the spinal cord. Here they form a chain of interconnecting ganglia referred to as the *sympathetic chain.*
   c. Some SNS fibers synapse at peripheral ganglia (celiac ganglion and hypogastric plexus), bypassing the sympathetic chain.
   d. Transmitter substances of the SNS:
      (1) Preganglionic fiber: Acetylcholine
      (2) Postganglionic fiber: Norepinephrine
      (3) Postganglionic fibers leading to the sweat glands, piloerector muscles of the hair, and some blood vessels have acetylcholine as a transmitter substance.
   e. Transmitter substance metabolism:
      (1) Acetylcholine: Metabolized by cholinesterase
      (2) Norepinephrine: Metabolized by MAO or COMT
10. PNS: Nerves of the PNS originate from sacral nerves 1 through 4 and cranial nerves III, VII, IX, and X. Eighty percent of all PNS impulses originate from *cranial nerve X* (*vagus nerve*) (see Figure 16-7; Figure 16-9).
    a. Nerve fibers that transmit PNS impulses are either:
       (1) Preganglionic fiber
       (2) Postganglionic fiber
    b. These fibers synapse at the ganglia of the PNS, which are located close to the organs they innervate.
    c. The transmitter substance for preganglionic and postganglionic fibers is acetylcholine (metabolized by cholinesterase) (Table 16-1).

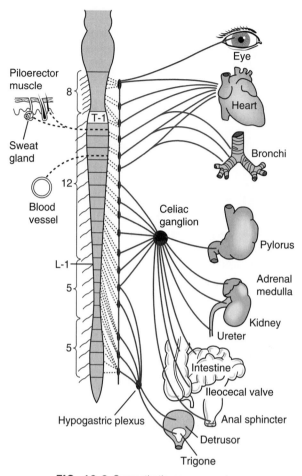

FIG. 16-8 Sympathetic nervous system.

F. Adrenal medulla: Secretes epinephrine (75% by volume) and norepinephrine (25% by volume) into the bloodstream, resulting in stimulation of the SNS.
    1. Innervation is via specific preganglionic fibers of the SNS.
    2. Adrenal secretions assist in maintaining normal tone of the SNS.
G. Effects of activation of the SNS and PNS:
    1. Adrenergic effect: An effect activated or transmitted by norepinephrine or epinephrine.
    2. Adrenergic receptor: A receptor stimulated by norepinephrine or epinephrine.
    3. Cholinergic effect: An effect activated or transmitted by acetylcholine.
    4. Cholinergic receptor: A receptor stimulated by acetylcholine.
    5. Table 16-2 lists the effects of the SNS and the PNS on various organs.
H. Adrenergic receptors:
    1. There are two major types of adrenergic receptors: *alpha* and *beta*. β receptors are divided into β_1 and β_2 receptors.
    2. Table 16-3 lists the responses elicited by activation of these receptors.
    3. Norepinephrine mainly excites α receptors but will excite β receptors but to a lesser extent.
    4. Epinephrine excites both types of receptors to an equal extent.
I. Cholinergic receptors
    1. There are two major types of cholinergic receptors: *muscarinic* and *nicotinic*.
    2. Muscarinic receptors are those receptors affected by muscarine, a poison produced by toadstools.

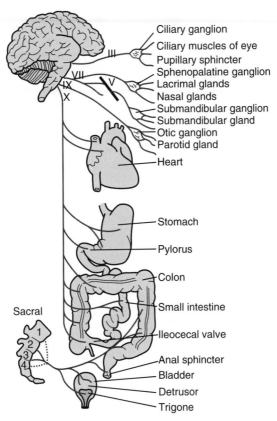

FIG. 16-9 Parasympathetic nervous system.

| TABLE **16-1** | | |

Comparison of the Structure of the Sympathetic Nervous System and the Parasympathetic Nervous System

Feature	SNS	PNS
Origin of nerve fibers from the CNS	T-1 to L-2	S-1 to S-4; cranial nerves III, VII, IX, X
Relative length		
Preganglionic fiber	Short	Long
Postganglionic fiber	Long	Short
Transmitter substance		
Preganglionic fiber	Acetylcholine	Acetylcholine
Postganglionic fiber	Norepinephrine	Acetylcholine
Transmitter substance metabolized by		
Preganglionic fiber	Cholinesterase	Cholinesterase
Postganglionic fiber	MAO and COMT	Cholinesterase

SNS, Sympathetic nervous system; *PNS*, parasympathetic nervous system; *CNS*, central nervous system; *MAO*, monoamine oxidase; *COMT*, catechol-*O*-methyl-transferase.

TABLE 16-2

Autonomic Effects on Various Organs of the Body

Organ	Effect of Sympathetic Stimulation	Effect of Parasympathetic Stimulation
Eye		
Pupil	Dilated	Constricted
Ciliary muscle	Slight relaxation (far vision)	Constricted (near vision)
Glands (nasal, lacrimal, parotid, submandibular, gastric, pancreatic)	Vasoconstriction and slight secretion	Stimulation of copious secretion
Sweat glands	Copious sweating (cholinergic)	Sweating on palms of hands
Apocrine glands	Thick, odoriferous secretion	None
Blood vessels	Most often constricted	Most often little or no effect
Heart		
Muscle	Increased rate	Slowed rate
	Increased force of concentration	Decreased force of contraction (especially at aria)
Coronaries	Dilated (β_2), constricted (α)	Dilated
Lungs		
Bronchi	Dilated	Constricted
Blood vessels	Mildly constricted	? Dilated
Gut		
Lumen	Decreased peristalsis and tone	Increased peristalsis and tone
Sphincter	Increased tone (most times)	Relaxed (most times)
Liver	Glucose released	Slight glycogen synthesis
Gallbladder and bile ducts	Relaxed	Contracted
Kidney	Decreased output and renin secretion	None
Bladder		
Detrusor	Relaxed (slight)	Contracted
Trigone	Contracted	Relaxed
Penis	Ejaculation	Erection
Systemic arterioles		
Abdominal viscera	Constricted	None
Muscle	Constricted (adrenergic α)	None
	Dilated (adrenergic β_2)	
	Dilated (cholinergic)	
Skin	Constricted	None
Blood		
Coagulation	Increased	None
Glucose	Increased	None
Lipids	Increased	None
Basal metabolism	Increased up to 100%	None
Adrenal medullary secretion	Increased	None
Mental activity	Increased	None
Piloerector muscles	Contracted	None
Skeletal muscle	Increased glycogenolysis	None
	Increased strength	
Fat cells	Lipolysis	None

From Guyton AC, Hall JE: *Textbook of Medical Physiology,* ed 10. Philadelphia, WB Saunders, 2000.

TABLE **16-3**		
Adrenergic Receptors and Responses		
Alpha	**Beta₁**	**Beta₂**
Vasoconstriction	Increased heart rate	Vasodilation
Iris dilation	Increased myocardial strength	Intestinal relaxation
Intestinal relaxation	Lipolysis	Uterus relaxation
Intestinal sphincter contraction		Bronchodilation
		Calorigenesis
Pilomotor contraction		Glycogenolysis
Bladder sphincter contraction		Bladder wall relaxation

From Guyton A, Hall J: *Textbook of Medical Physiology,* ed 10, Saunders, New York, 2001.

3. Nicotinic receptors are those receptors affected by nicotine.
4. Muscarinic receptors are on effector cells stimulated by the postganglionic fibers of the PNS and the postganglionic cholinergic fibers of the SNS.
5. Nicotinic receptors are found at the synapse between preganglionic and postganglionic fibers of SNS and PNS and at many nonautonomic nerve endings, specifically the neuromuscular junction.

BIBLIOGRAPHY

Beachey W: *Respiratory Care Anatomy and Physiology.* St. Louis, Mosby, 1998.

Goodman LS, Gilman A (eds): *The Pharmacological Basis of Therapeutics,* ed 8. New York, Macmillan Publishing, 1996.

Guyton AC, Hall JE: *Textbook of Medical Physiology,* ed 10. New York, WB Saunders, 2000.

Hicks GH: *Cardiopulmonary Anatomy and Physiology.* New York, WB Saunders, 2000.

Julian RM: *A Primer of Drug Action,* ed 3. San Francisco, WH Freeman & Co Publishers, 1981.

Rau JL: *Respiratory Care Pharmacology,* ed 6. St. Louis, Mosby, 2002.

Wilkins RL, Stoller JK, Scanlon CL: *Egan's Foundations of Respiratory Care,* ed 8. St. Louis, Mosby, 2003.

Chapter 17

Pharmacology

I. General Information
  A. Definitions
    1. Pharmacology: The study of the interaction of drugs with the organism.
    2. Drug: Any chemical compound that may be administered to or used in an individual to aid in the diagnosis, treatment, or prevention of disease, to relieve pain, or to control or improve any physiologic disorder or pathologic condition.
    3. LD_{50}: The dosage of a drug that would be lethal to 50% of a test population.
    4. ED_{50}: The dosage of a drug that would have therapeutic effects for 50% of a test population.
    5. Therapeutic index (TI): The numerical ratio of the LD_{50} to the ED_{50} (LD_{50}/ED_{50}). This ratio shows how close the lethal and therapeutic doses of a drug are for a test population. Low indices mean the therapeutic and lethal doses are similar and the drug has a high potential for overdose or toxic side effects (Figure 17-1).
    6. Side effect: Any physiologic response other than that for which the drug was administered.
  B. Pharmacologic nomenclature
    1. Chemical name: Name illustrative of chemical structural formula of the drug.
    2. Code name: An investigational designation, usually alphanumeric.
    3. Generic name: An assigned name given for clinical investigation of a promising chemical.
    4. Official name: Usually the generic name after the drug is accepted for general use.
    5. Trade, brand, or proprietary name: The name under which a particular manufacturer markets the drug.
    6. Example: Ipratropium bromide
      a. Code name: SCH 1000
      b. Chemical name: 8-Azoniabicyclo[3.2.1]octane, 3-(3-hydroxy-1-oxo-2-phenyl-propoxy)-8-methyl-8-(l-methyl-ethyl)-, bromide
      c. Official name: Ipratropium bromide
      d. Generic name: Ipratropium bromide
      e. Trade name: Atrovent (Boehringer-Ingelheim)
  C. Principles of drug action: There are three phases of drug action from initial dosing to pharmacologic effect. Each phase includes aspects of the pharmacology of the drug.
    1. Pharmaceutical phase: Administering the drug.
      a. Dosage forms: Tablet, capsule, liquid, powder, or ointment
      b. Route of administration (listed in order of speed in obtaining blood levels)
        (1) Intravenous (IV) injection
        (2) Via lung (aerosol)
        (3) Intramuscular (IM) injection
        (4) Subcutaneous (SC) injection
        (5) Sublingual and rectal absorption
        (6) Oral
        (7) Topical

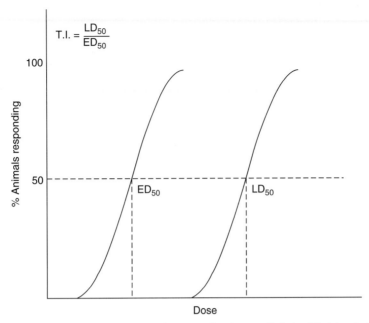

FIG. 17-1 Log-dose response curve demonstrating therapeutic index (TI) determination.

Note: Not all routes listed may be used to administer all drugs, and the speed of absorption by route may also vary.

2. Pharmacokinetic phase: The drug movement phase, including entry into or elimination from the body. This phase generally includes absorption, distribution, metabolism, and elimination of a drug. These factors determine onset of action, peak plasma drug level, and duration of drug action.

a. Absorption: Rate of absorption is determined by the specific physical and chemical characteristics of a drug.

  (1) The lung mucosa provides an excellent surface for absorption of inhaled drugs.

  (2) A substantial portion of an inhaled drug may be absorbed systemically in the mouth or proximal airways, thereby reducing its ability to affect the distal airways.

  (3) Only particles <3 μm in diameter are carried to the distal airways.

b. Distribution: Movement of the drug to an area of desired pharmacologic activity.

  (1) The primary mechanism for distribution is the circulatory system.

  (2) Topical administration for effect on skin or mucous membrane decreases the likelihood of further undesired distribution.

c. Metabolism: Inactivation of the drug by the body.

  (1) The primary organ for detoxification is the liver.

  (2) Secondary organs for detoxification are the kidneys and gastrointestinal (GI) tract.

  (3) The body's cells or plasma proteins may inactivate many drugs.

d. Excretion or clearance: Mechanism for elimination of the drug from the body.

  (1) Primary organ for excretion: Kidney

  (2) Secondary excretion sites

    (a) GI tract

    (b) Respiratory tract

    (c) All exocrine glands

3. Pharmacodynamic phase: Drug-receptor interaction

a. Drugs usually create their effect by stimulating or blocking a receptor.

      (1) An agonist is a drug that stimulates a receptor.

      (2) An antagonist is a drug that blocks a receptor.

   b. Drug-receptor types (Figure 17-2)

      (1) Ligand-gated channel receptors: These transmembrane receptors traverse the cell membrane, acting as a high-speed conduit for transfer of specific chemicals, often ions, into and out of the cell.

      (2) Tyrosine kinase linked receptor: Also a transmembrane receptor; binding of a drug to its extracellular receptor site enzymatically activates its intracellular end, acting as a tyrosine kinase. In this example, a phosphate group is added to (phosphorylates) the amino acid tyrosine in proteins that this receptor contacts, changing the protein to produce the clinical effect.

      (3) G protein-coupled receptors: Transmembrane receptors that act through an intermediary, the G protein, located within the cell membrane, bound to a molecule of guanosine diphosphate. In this example a drug-receptor binding stimulates the G protein to exchange a guanosine diphosphate molecule for a guanosine triphosphate molecule. Once phosphorylated, the G protein migrates to a separate protein target to create the end drug effect.

      (4) Steroid-receptor complex: Lipophilic steroid molecules readily pass through cell membranes and bind to receptors in the cell cytoplasm. Translocation of the steroid-receptor complex into the nucleus allows the complex to affect DNA transcription. The end effect of the drug occurs only after translation of new proteins from the affected DNA, making this a slow process.

   c. Drug-receptor interactions

      (1) Affinity: Tendency of a drug to combine with a matching receptor.

      (2) Potency: The activity of a drug per unit weight. A potent drug has a large biologic activity at a small unit dose (Figure 17-3).

      (3) Efficacy: The maximum effect produced by a drug regardless of dose (Figure 17-4).

      (4) Cumulation: A gradual increase in the body's total drug level that occurs when the administration rate of the drug is greater than the body's rate of removal.

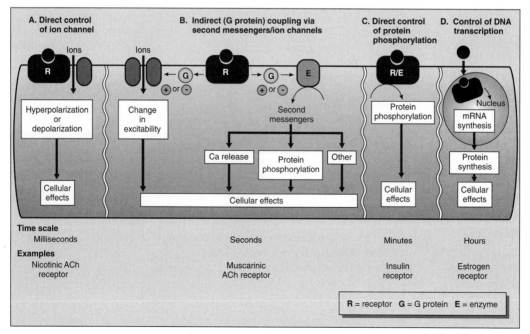

FIG. 17-2 Four classes of receptor-effector linkage.

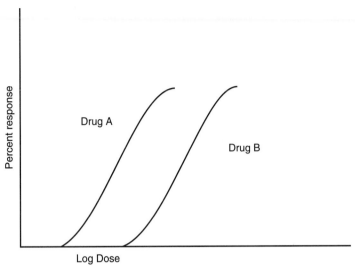

FIG. 17-3 Log-dose response curve comparing the potency of two drugs. The potency of drug A is greater than that of drug B.

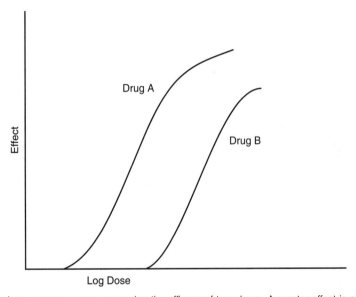

FIG. 17-4 Log-dose response curve comparing the efficacy of two drugs. A greater effect is caused by drug A than drug B. Drug A also is more potent than drug B.

        (5) Tolerance: The body's ability to increase its metabolism of a drug. Increasing amounts of the drug are required to produce the same effect.

        (6) Tachyphylaxis: The rapid development of tolerance.

  D. Drug interactions

    1. Additive: Two drugs, when given together, produce an effect equal to the sum of their individual effects.

    2. Potentiation: Potentiation occurs when a drug active at a specific receptor site is given with a drug inactive at that receptor site, and the resulting effect is greater than that of the active drug alone (1 + 0 = 3).

3. Synergism: Two drugs active at a receptor site, when given together, cause an effect greater than the sum of their individual effects (1 + 2 = 6).
4. Antagonist: This is a drug with affinity but no efficacy (i.e., it blocks an effect).
   a. Competitive: An antagonist whose effects are directly related to dosage. A competitive antagonist decreases potency but does not affect efficacy of the other drug.
   b. Noncompetitive: An antagonist whose effects are not dose related. Potency and efficacy of the other drug are decreased.
5. Agonist: This is a drug with affinity and efficacy (i.e., causes an effect).

E. The prescription: This is the written order for a drug composed of:
1. The patient's name, address, and the date.
2. Rx: "Take thou"; take and prepare the medication.
3. Inscription: Name and quantity of the drug.
4. Subscription: Directions (when applicable) to the pharmacist for compounding the drug.
5. Sig: Transcription, "write"; instructions to the patient for taking the drug.
6. Name of prescriber.

II. Administering Aerosolized Drugs (see Chapter 35)

A. Devices
1. Ultrasonic nebulizers (not recommended for bronchodilators)
2. Gas-powered small volume nebulizers
3. Metered dose inhaler (MDI), with or without extension (spacer) device

B. Particle size and deposition
1. Upper airway (above larynx): >5 μm
2. Central airways: 2 to 5 μm
3. Periphery: 1 to 2 μm

C. Basic protocol of administration
1. Gas-powered small reservoir nebulizers
   a. Fill volume: 2.5 to 4.0 ml
   b. Nebulizing flow: 6 to 8 L/min (viscous antibiotics, 12 L/min)
   c. Slow, deep inspirations with breath-hold
   d. Inspiratory nebulization only if possible
2. MDI
   a. Assemble, shake canister, and charge with one actuation.
   b. Hold 4 cm in front of open mouth or rest on mandibular teeth of open mouth.
   c. Exhale normally.
   d. Begin slow deep breath, and activate MDI.
   e. Inspire to total lung capacity, and hold breath at least 3 to 5 seconds.
   f. Exhale normally.
   g. Use of a spacer device is generally recommended.
3. General notes regarding administration
   a. Bronchodilators: Wait at least 1 minute, and then take a second puff.
   b. Corticosteroids: Take after bronchodilators, hyperextending the neck while inhaling; use a spacer; rinse mouth and throat after dosing.
   c. Dry powder inhalers: These require rapid inspiration with high flow rates (60 to 120 L/min) for dispersion.
   d. Spacers or extensions with MDIs reduce the need for coordination and oropharyngeal impaction.

III. Wetting Agents and Diluents

A. Isotonic solution: A solution equivalent to a 0.9% weight/volume (w/v) solution of NaCl. Isotonic solutions are used in respiratory therapy primarily in small-volume nebulizers to increase aerosol volume during drug delivery.
B. Hypertonic solution: A solution with a concentration >0.9% w/v solution of NaCl. Hypertonic solutions are used in respiratory therapy primarily for sputum induction.

C. Hypotonic solution: A solution with a concentration <0.9% w/v solution of NaCl. Hypotonic solutions are most commonly used in respiratory therapy in large-volume aerosol generators and seem to have less effect on increasing airway resistance than normal saline or water.

D. Distilled water: Used in respiratory therapy in all types of humidifiers.

IV. **Exogenous Surfactants**

A. Mode of action

1. Replace and replenish a deficient endogenous surfactant pool in neonatal respiratory distress syndrome (RDS).

2. Endogenous surfactant is normally recycled by reentering the type II alveolar cell as small vesicles. Exogenously administered surfactant can restore a depleted endogenous pool of surfactant, relieving RDS.

B. Composition of pulmonary surfactant

1. Surfactant, a complex mixture of lipids and proteins produced by type II alveolar cells, regulates the surface tension forces of the lipid alveolar lining (see Chapter 5).

   a. A film of liquid exists at the alveolar-air interface.

   b. As the alveolus is compressed during expiration, surfactant decreases surface tension, requiring less pressure and effort to reexpand the alveolus during the next inspiration.

2. Surfactant is composed of lipids (85% to 90%) and proteins (10% to 15%)

   a. Lipids

      (1) 85% to 90% of surfactant by weight.

      (2) 90% of lipids are phospholipids.

      (3) Phosphatidylcholine comprises 75% to 80% of the phospholipids.

      (4) Depalmitoylphosphatidylcholine (DPPC or lecithin) is the component predominantly responsible for decreasing alveolar surface tension.

   b. Proteins

      (1) 10% of surfactant by weight.

      (2) Only 20% of the proteins are surfactant-specific proteins; 80% are serum proteins.

      (3) The four surfactant-specific proteins are SP-A, SP-B, SP-C, and SP-D.

   c. The alveolar type II cell synthesizes all surfactant components.

C. Exogenous surfactant preparations

1. Colfosceril palmitate (Exosurf Neonatal)

   a. A protein-free, synthetic lyophilized powder reconstituted with 8 ml of preservative-free sterile water to form a milky white suspension.

   b. Colfosceril palmitate is depalmitoylphosphatidylcholine.

   c. Indications

      (1) Prophylactic therapy for infants with birth weight <1350 g.

      (2) Prophylactic therapy for infants with birth weight >1350 g and evidence of pulmonary immaturity and risk for RDS.

      (3) Rescue treatment of infants with RDS.

   d. Dosage

      (1) The first dose is 5 ml/kg, given as two divided doses.

      (2) A single vial of reconstituted Exosurf has a volume of 8 ml and can treat infants with birth weight up to 1600 g.

      (3) A second dose of 5 ml/kg is given 12 hours after the first.

      (4) A third dose, if necessary, is given 12 hours after the second dose.

   e. Administration

      (1) Instilled directly into the endotracheal tube (ETT) through a side-port adaptor that is Luer-Lok fitted to the ETT.

      (2) With the infant in the midline position, the first half dose is sequentially instilled in synchrony with the inspiratory phase of the ventilator.

      (3) The infant is then rotated to one side and ventilated for 30 seconds.

(4) Repositioned to midline, the infant is given the second half dose, then rotated to the opposite side, and ventilated for 30 seconds.

2. Beractant (Survanta)
   a. A natural bovine lung extract mixed with colfosceril palmitate (DPPC), palmitic acid, and tripalmitin.
   b. Contains surfactant proteins SP-B and SP-C but not SP-A.
   c. Indications
      (1) Used prophylactically for premature infants with birth weight <1250 g.
      (2) Used for infants with evidence of surfactant deficiency and risk of RDS.
      (3) Used for rescue treatment of infants with RDS.
   d. As Survanta, this surfactant preparation comes in an 8-ml solution suspended in 0.9% sodium chloride, having a concentration of 25 mg/ml. Thus one vial has 200 mg.
   e. Dosage
      (1) 100 mg/kg birth weight
      (2) If respiratory distress continues, a repeat dose can be given after 6 hours.
   f. Administration
      (1) To gently warm the refrigerated suspension, it should be set out at room temperature for 20 minutes.
      (2) Settling of the suspension should be countered by gentle agitation of the vial. The container should not be vigorously shaken.
      (3) The dose is given in four aliquots, instilled directly into the trachea through a 5-French catheter.
      (4) After each of the aliquots, the catheter is withdrawn, and the infant is ventilated and stabilized for at least 30 seconds.

3. Calfactant (Infasurf)
   a. An organic solvent extract of calf lung obtained by bronchoalveolar lavage.
   b. This surfactant preparation is a suspension containing SP-B and SP-C.
   c. Indications
      (1) Used prophylactically in infants <29 weeks gestational age.
      (2) Used for rescue of intubated premature infants aged <3 days who develop RDS.
   d. Dosage
      (1) 3 ml/kg birth weight
      (2) Repeat doses can be given 12 hours apart or as early as 6 hours for infants in continued distress.
      (3) Each 6-ml vial contains 210 mg phospholipids, enough to treat a 2-kg infant.
   e. Administration
      (1) Side-port adaptor
         (a) Two equal aliquots are given, one to each side while in the dependent position.
         (b) Instillation of small volumes is timed to coincide with the inspiratory phase of the ventilator.
      (2) Catheter
         (a) Four aliquots are given, each with the infant in a different position (prone, supine, left lateral, and right lateral)
         (b) The catheter is removed, and the infant is mechanically ventilated briefly between each instillation.

4. Poractant Alfa (Curosurf)
   a. A natural surfactant extracted from porcine lung, consisting of 99% phospholipids and 1% surfactant proteins SP-B and SP-C.
   b. Indications
      (1) Rescue or treatment of premature infants with RDS.
      (2) Used off-label for prophylaxis in RDS, acute respiratory distress syndrome (ARDS) from viral pneumonia, HIV-infected infants with *Pneumocystis*

carinii pneumonia, and management of ARDS after near drowning. Efficacy in all of these settings is controversial.

 c. Dosage
  (1) 2.5 ml/kg birth weight
  (2) Two subsequent doses of 1.25 ml/kg birth weight can be given in 12-hour intervals for continued distress.
  (3) Maximum recommended total dose is 5 ml/kg birth weight.
 d. Administration
  (1) Two equal aliquots are given through a 5-French catheter whose tip is positioned at the tip of the ETT.
  (2) Each aliquot is given to an alternate side, positioned dependently, stabilizing the infant by mechanically ventilating with 100% oxygen for at least 1 minute between doses.
  (3) Airway suctioning should be avoided for 1 hour after treatment, provided significant airway obstruction does not occur.

V. Mucolytics
 A. Mucomyst
  1. Trade name: Mucomyst
  2. Generic name: Acetylcysteine (N-acetyl-L-cysteine)
  3. Mechanism of action: Lyses disulfide bonds holding mucoproteins together, thus increasing fluidity of mucoid sputum.
  4. Concentration: 10% or 20% w/v solution
  5. Dosage
   a. Standard dosage: 4 ml of 10% w/v or 2 ml 20% w/v solution with 2 ml water or normal saline solution
   b. Maximum dosage: None specified
  6. Indications: Thick, retained mucoid or mucopurulent secretions
  7. Contraindications: Hypersensitivity
  8. Side effects and hazards
   a. Bronchospasm
   b. Excessive liquification of dried, retained secretions
   c. Stomatitis
   d. Hypersensitivity
   e. Nausea
   f. Rhinorrhea
  9. Comments
   a. Questionable efficacy when aerosolized.
    (1) Mucolytic activity well documented in vitro.
    (2) No data clearly demonstrate the clinical efficacy of aerosolized Mucomyst.
    (3) May be useful for direct bronchial instillation during bronchoscopy.
   b. Highly recommended that drug is administered in conjunction with bronchodilator.
   c. Should be refrigerated after opening.
   d. Foul smelling
   e. Should be administered in glass, plastic, or nontarnishable metal containers because it reacts with rubber, some plastics, and iron.
   f. Ineffective on predominantly purulent secretions.
   g. Supplied in 4-, 10-, and 30-ml vials.
   h. Should be administered after pretreatment with a bronchodilator.
 B. Dornase Alfa
  1. Trade name: Pulmozyme
  2. Generic name: Dornase alfa—originally *rh*DN*ase* (recombinant human DNase)
  3. Mechanism of action: A genetically engineered clone of human pancreatic DNase enzyme, it is a peptide proteolytic enzyme that can break down extracellular DNA and F-actin polymers from neutrophils found in purulent secretions.

4. Indication: Cystic fibrosis management to manage purulent mucoid secretions; more effective than Mucomyst in reducing the viscosity of sputum in cystic fibrosis.
5. Dosage
   a. 2.5 mg/ampule, 1 ampule daily via recommended nebulizer system (e.g., Hudson T Updraft II, Marquest II, or PARI LC Jet Plus).
   b. 3 to 5 ml of 5% to 10% w/v solution in 0.45% or 0.9% saline solution.
6. Contraindication: Hypersensitivity to dornase or other components of the drug preparation.
7. Side effects and hazards
   a. Unlike the earlier animal pancreatic dornase (Dornavac), dornase alfa does not cause antibody-mediated allergic reactions, such as bronchospasm.
   b. Pharyngitis and vocal alterations
   c. Laryngitis
   d. Conjunctivitis
   e. Rash
   f. Chest pain
   g. Less commonly a variety of respiratory symptoms (e.g., cough, dyspnea, rhinitis, and sinusitis), GI obstruction, hypoxia, and weight loss.

VI. **Mast Cell Stabilizers (Table 17-1)**
   A. Trade name: Intal
      1. Generic name: Cromolyn sodium
      2. Mechanism of action
         a. Inhibits release of histamine and leukotrienes during allergic, immunoglobulin (Ig) E-mediated responses of pulmonary mast cells.
         b. Suppresses response of mast cell to antigen-antibody reaction.
      3. Concentration: 20-mg capsules (powder) or 20 mg/2 ml H_2O ampules (liquid).
      4. Standard dosage: 20 mg three or four times daily.
      5. Maximum dosage: Same.
      6. Primary indications: Prophylactic maintenance for patients with severe bronchial asthma exercise-induced bronchospasm.
      7. Secondary indications: Result of the effect of cromolyn sodium on all mast cells.
         a. Allergic rhinitis
         b. Diarrhea in systemic mastocytosis
         c. Ulcers of the oral mucosa
         d. Nonspecific inflammatory bowel disease
      8. Contraindications: Hypersensitivity
      9. Side effects and hazards
         a. Local irritation
         b. Bronchospasm

TABLE **17-1**

Mast Cell Stabilizers

Drug	Brand Name	Formulation and Dosage
Cromolyn sodium	Intal	MDI: 800 µg/actuation Adults and children ≥5 yr: 2 inhalations QID SVN: 20 mg/ampule or 20 mg/vial
	Nasalcrom	Spray: 40 mg/ml (4%) Adults and children ≥6 yr: 1 spray each nostril 3-6 times daily every 4-6 hr
Nedocromil sodium	Tilade	MDI: 1.75 mg/actuation Adults and children ≥12 yr: 2 inhalations QID

MDI, Metered dose inhaler; *QID,* four times daily; *SVN,* small-volume nebulizer.
From Wilkins RL, et al: *Egan's Fundamentals of Respiratory Care,* ed 8. St. Louis, Mosby, 2003.

      c. Maculopapular rash

      d. Urticaria

      e. Cough

      f. Congestion

      g. Sneezing

      h. Epistaxis

    10. Comments

      a. Ineffective for acute asthmatic attack.

      b. Maximum effect seen after 4 weeks of continuous use.

      c. Sometimes effective in controlling exercise-induced asthma.

B. Trade name: Tilade

    1. Generic name: Nedocromil sodium

    2. Mechanism of action

      a. Inhibits most cell cytokine release

      b. Modulates the synthesis and release of proinflammatory cytokines

      c. Inhibits eosinophil chemotaxis and adhesion

    3. Concentration: 1.75 mg per MDI actuation (only preparation)

    4. Standard dosage: Two inhalations four times per day

    5. Maximum: Same

    6. Primary indication: Prophylactic therapy for the management of mild to moderate asthma.

    7. Contraindications: Hypersensitivity

    8. Side effects and hazards

      a. Unpleasant taste

      b. Headache

      c. Vomiting

      d. Dizziness

    9. Comments

      a. Not useful for acute asthmatic attack.

      b. As effective as cromolyn sodium.

      c. Dosed twice/day versus cromolyn sodium 4 times/day.

VII. Leukotriene Inhibitors (Antileukotrienes) (Table 17-2)

    A. Leukotriene characteristics

      1. Originally isolated from *leuko*cytes, leukotrienes have a carbon chain skeleton with three double bonds in series, a *triene*.

      2. Chemically they are lipid mediators of inflammation synthesized from arachidonic acid (AA).

TABLE 17-2

Leukotriene Inhibitors

Drug	Brand Name	Formulation and Dosage
Zafirlukast	Accolate	Tablets: 10 mg, 20 mg Adults and children >12 yr: 20 mg (1 tablet) BID, without food Children 5-11 yr: 10 mg BID
Montelukast	Singulair	Tablets: 10 mg, 5 mg, and 4 mg (cherry-flavored chewable) Adults and children >15 yr: 1 10-mg tablet each evening Children 6-14 yr: 1 5-mg chewable tablet each evening Children 2-5 yr: 1 4-mg chewable tablet each evening Children 12-23 mo: 4 mg oral granules each evening
Zileuton	Zyflo	Tablets: 600 mg Adults and children ≥12 yr: 1 600-mg tablet QID

BID, Twice daily; *QID,* four times daily.
From Wilkins RL, et al: *Egan's Fundamentals of Respiratory Care,* ed 8. St. Louis, Mosby, 2003.

   3. Potent bronchoconstrictors, they stimulate airway edema, mucus secretion, and recruitment of other inflammatory cells.
   4. They are particularly effective in controlling exercise-induced, aspirin-induced, and, less effectively, allergen-induced asthma.
B. Leukotriene production (Figure 17-5)
   1. In cell cytoplasm, phospholipase A_2 (PLA_2) moves to the cell nuclear membrane, where it hydrolyzes phospholipids to form free AA. AA binds to 5-lipoxygenase (5-LO)-activating protein (FLAP; AA-FLAP). 5-LO moves to the nuclear membrane and oxygenates AA of the AA-FLAP complex, resulting in 5-hydroperoxyeicosatetraenoic acid (HPETE). HPETE is converted to leukotriene A_4 (LTA_4), an unstable intermediate that is the source of all leukotrienes. LTA_4 is converted into leukotriene B_4 (LTB_4) or leukotriene C_4 (LTC_4), both of which move to the extracellular space. LTC_4, which structurally contains the amino acid cysteine, can be converted to leukotrienes D_4 and E_4 (LTD_4 and LTE_4). These three are known as the cysteinyl leukotrienes (CysLTs). The three CysLTs (LTC_4, LTD_4, and LTE_4) are the components previously known as slow reacting substance of anaphylaxis (SRS-A).
C. Leukotriene receptors
   1. Leukotrienes bind to leukotriene receptors to exert inflammatory effects.
      a. Increased bronchial hyperresponsiveness to other irritants such as histamine.
      b. Increased mucus secretion.
      c. Increased vascular permeability causing airway wall edema.
      d. Plasma exudation into airway lumen.
      e. Cumulative effect is increased secretion viscosity and possible airway occlusion often seen in asthma.

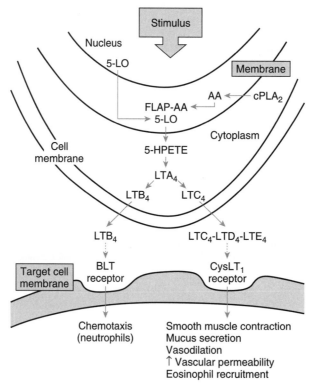

FIG. 17-5 A model of the synthesis of leukotrienes through the 5-lipoxygenase (5-LO) pathway and their effects on target cells. *AA*, Arachidonic acid; *BLT*, B leukotriene (LTB_4) receptor; *cPLA$_2$*, cytosolic phospholipase A_2; *CysLT$_1$*, cysteinyl leukotriene receptor; *FLAP*, 5-lipoxygenase-activating protein; *5-HPETE*, 5-hydroperoxyeicosatetraenoic acid; *LTA$_4$, LTB$_4$, LTC$_4$, LTD$_4$, LTE$_4$*, leukotrienes A_4, B_4, C_4, D_4, and E_4.

2. The CysLT$_1$ receptor, located on smooth muscle cells in the airway, mediates the proasthmatic action of the CysLTs.
   a. Stimulation of the CysLT$_1$ receptor causes bronchoconstriction.
   b. The CysLTs are more potent airway constrictors than histamine.
3. CysLT production
   a. The CysLTs are produced by eosinophils, mast cells, and macrophages, all of which are seen in the airways of persons with asthma.
   b. The CysLT$_2$ receptor subtype mediates constriction of vascular smooth muscle.
   c. Drugs that block the binding of leukotrienes to CysLT$_1$ have the generic suffix *-leukast.*
D. Zileuton (Zyflo)
   1. Characteristics
      a. Approved for use in early 1997.
      b. Orally active inhibitor of 5-LO, preventing catalysis of leukotrienes from AA.
      c. Indicated for prophylactic and long-term management of asthma in adults and children aged >12 years.
      d. Has no indication in an acute asthmatic attack.
   2. Dosage
      a. Available as a single tablet of 600 mg.
      b. One 600-mg tablet four times daily for total daily dose of 2400 mg.
   3. Pharmacokinetics
      a. Rapidly absorbed orally.
      b. 93% bound to plasma proteins.
      c. Half-life of 2.5 hours.
      d. Metabolized by cytochrome P450 enzymes in the liver.
      e. Eliminated in urine and feces.
   4. Precautions: Patients should be monitored for liver injury.
      a. Hepatic transaminase enzymes should be evaluated before initiation of treatment, monthly for the first 3 months, and every 2 to 3 months thereafter for the first year of treatment.
      b. With clinical signs of liver injury (e.g., right upper quadrant pain, nausea, fatigue, lethargy, pruritus, jaundice, or flulike symptoms), discontinue use.
   5. Hazards and side effects
      a. Headache, abdominal pain, loss of strength, and dyspepsia.
      b. Elevated liver function test values.
         (1) Hepatic transaminase enzymes should be monitored before and during treatment.
         (2) Liver function test values may return to normal either during or after treatment.
      c. Contraindicated in patients with acute liver disease or transaminase levels greater than three times normal.
      d. Zileuton interacts with theophylline and warfarin.
         (1) Can increase theophylline concentration.
         (2) Can increase prothrombin time when given with warfarin.
         (3) Dose adjustments of theophylline and warfarin may be needed.
E. Zafirlukast (Accolate)
   1. Characteristics
      a. Approved for use in the United States in 1996 as Accolate.
      b. Indicated for prophylaxis and long-term management of asthma in adults or children aged ≥12 years.
         (1) Inhibits asthma reactions induced by exercise, cold air, allergen, and aspirin.
         (2) Oral forms of the drug inhibit early- and late-phase asthma.
         (3) Oral form causes modest bronchodilation.
         (4) Inhaled form inhibits only the early response of asthma.
   2. Dosage
      a. 20-mg oral tablet taken twice daily.

    b. Should be taken 1 hour before or 2 hours after eating.

3. Mode of action

    a. Leukotriene receptor antagonist that blocks inflammatory effects of leukotrienes.

    b. Binds to the $CysLT_1$ receptors.

    c. Competitively inhibits leukotrienes LTC_4, LTD_4, and LTE_4, blocking inflammation.

4. Pharmacokinetics

    a. Rapidly absorbed orally, reaching peak plasma levels in 3 hours.

    b. Half-life approximately 10 hours.

    c. Metabolized in liver.

    d. 10% excreted in urine, remainder in feces.

    e. Administration of zafirlukast with food reduces mean bioavailability by 40%.

5. Hazards and side effects

    a. Headache, infection (primarily respiratory), nausea, diarrhea, and generalized and abdominal pain.

    b. Liver disease will increase drug plasma levels.

    c. Doses >40 mg daily can cause elevations in serum liver enzymes.

    d. Instances of hepatitis and hyperbilirubinemia reported in patients receiving 40 mg/day for 100 days.

F. Montelukast (Singulair)

  1. Characteristics

    a. Approved for use in February 1998.

    b. Orally active leukotriene receptor antagonist.

    c. Indicated for prophylaxis and long-term management of asthma.

      (1) Has no bronchodilatory effect in short-term asthma treatment.

      (2) Approved for use in pediatric patients (children aged ≥2 years).

      (3) Efficacious in management of mild to moderate asthma and exercise-induced bronchial constriction.

      (4) Exhibits improved asthma control in children aged 6 to 14 years and in adults and adolescents aged >15 years.

  2. Dosage

    a. Supplied in 10-mg oral tablet or 4-mg and 5-mg chewable cherry-flavored tablets.

    b. Adults and adolescents aged >15 years: one 10-mg tablet daily, taken in the evening.

    c. Pediatric patients aged 6 to 14 years: one 5-mg chewable tablet daily, taken in the evening.

    d. Pediatric patients aged 2 to 5 years: one 4-mg chewable tablet daily, taken in the evening.

  3. Mode of action

    a. Competitive antagonist for the CysLTs LTC_4, LTD_4, and LTE_4.

    b. Binds to the $CysLT_1$ receptor subtype, preventing leukotriene receptor stimulation in airway smooth muscle and secretory gland cells.

    c. Shown to inhibit early- and late-phase asthmatic bronchoconstriction.

  4. Pharmacokinetics

    a. Rapidly absorbed orally.

      (1) A 10-mg dose reaches peak plasma concentration in 3 to 4 hours.

      (2) A 10-mg dose has mean bioavailability of 64%, not influenced by intake of food.

    b. A 5-mg fasting dose had slightly higher concentrations than when taken with food.

    c. A 4-mg tablet reached peak plasma concentrations in 2 hours.

    d. Mean plasma life in adults: 2.7 to 5.5 hours.

    e. Metabolized in liver and excreted via bile.

    f. Mild to moderate liver disease will increase plasma levels.

  5. Hazards and side effects

    a. Adverse effects (e.g., diarrhea, laryngitis, pharyngitis, nausea, otitis, sinusitis, and viral infection) occurred in approximately 2% of users.

    b. Liver enzymes were not elevated.

VIII. **Aerosolized Antimicrobial Agents**
  A. Class features
    1. Aerosolized delivery achieves high drug concentration in lung tissue.
    2. Antibiotics effective against particular organisms, such as *Pseudomonas*; have poor lung bioavailability when taken orally.
  B. Precautions
    1. Nebulization of antibiotics should occur in contained rooms to prevent escape of the drug and possible development of resistant organisms within the local environment.
    2. Caregivers should be protected to prevent development of sensitivity reactions or resistance to antibiotics.
    3. Antibiotic solutions vary in viscosity from the aqueous solutions for which disposable nebulizers were designed.
      a. Nebulizer-compressor systems should be tested for adequate delivery of antibiotics.
      b. Higher nebulizer flow rates may be necessary.
  C. Tobramycin
    1. Characteristics
      a. An aminoglycoside used for management of *Pseudomonas aeruginosa*, a pathogen often associated with chronic infection of cystic fibrosis patients.
      b. Tobramycin solution for inhalation (TOBI) is a preservative-free preparation that may reduce the risk of adverse effects.
      c. TOBI should be administered in the PARI LC Plus nebulizer to ensure adequate drug output and particle size.
    2. Side effects
      a. Ototoxicity
      b. Nephrotoxicity
      c. Side effects minimized when taken by aerosol.
    3. Contraindicated in patients with hypersensitivity to aminoglycosides.
    4. Dose: 300 mg twice daily in repeated cycles of 28 days on drug, followed by 28 days off drug.
    5. Delivery
      a. Extubated patients: Via Pari nebulizer and Pulmo-Aide compressor.
      b. Intubated patients: Via conventional small-volume nebulizer in-line with ventilator circuit, using additional expiratory circuit limb filter.
  D. Colistimethate (Coly-Mycin, Colistin)
    1. Characteristics
      a. A polypeptide antibiotic used in aerosol form for management of *Pseudomonas* pneumonia.
      b. Most often used for immunocompromised patients or patients with cystic fibrosis.
    2. Contraindicated in patients with known hypersensitivity to the drug.
    3. Dose: 150 mg (4 ml) twice daily.
    4. Delivery
      a. Extubated patients: Via Pari nebulizer.
      b. Intubated patients: Via conventional small-volume nebulizer in-line with ventilator circuit, using additional expiratory circuit limb filter.
  E. Amphotericin B
    1. Characteristics: An antifungal agent given prophylactically to prevent fungal pneumonia in immunocompromised patients.
    2. Contraindicated in patients with known hypersensitivity to the drug.
    3. Dose
      a. Usual dose: 10 mg twice daily.
      b. A vial with 50 mg powder is reconstituted in 10 ml sterile water for inhalation, creating a concentration of 5 mg/ml.
        (1) One dose is 2 ml.

          (2) The remaining solution, when refrigerated, is good for 24 hours after being mixed.

          (3) Because amphotericin B is a colloid, mixing the powder with saline will cause precipitation.

    4. Delivery

        a. Extubated patients: Via Pari nebulizer.

        b. Intubated patients

          (1) Using a small-volume nebulizer, dilute the 2-ml dose (5 mg/ml) with 2 ml water for a final solution of 4 ml.

          (2) Use additional ventilator expiratory limb filter to prevent drug interference with exhalation valve or flow sensor.

        c. Amphotericin B, incompatible with most drugs, should not be mixed with other drugs in the nebulizer.

        d. Side effects and hazards

          (1) Bronchospasm and cough may occur; pretreat with a bronchodilator.

          (2) Nausea and vomiting.

F. Gentamicin

    1. Characteristics

        a. An aminoglycoside antibiotic aerosolized to manage pulmonary gram-negative infections.

G. Pentamidine (Pentam-300)

    1. Characteristics

        a. An antiprotozoal agent used for prophylaxis of *P. carinii* pneumonia, often seen in immunocompromised patients.

        b. Has been replaced by trimethoprim-sulfamethoxazole (TMP/SMX) for treatment (IV) and prophylaxis (nebulized) in patients allergic to sulfa drugs.

    2. Dose

        a. 300 mg for prophylactic use.

        b. Up to 600 mg for active *P. carinii* pneumonia.

    3. Delivery

        a. Administer with a Respirgard II nebulizer.

        b. Patient should be in a negative pressure room.

        c. Staff should use a tuberculin mask when in the room during treatment.

        d. Pretreat patient with bronchodilator if bronchospasm is encountered.

    4. Side effects and hazards

        a. Hypotension

        b. Dyspnea

        c. Nausea and vomiting

        d. Pancreatitis

        e. Hyperglycemia or hypoglycemia

H. Ribavirin

    1. Characteristics

        a. An antiviral agent used for the management of respiratory syncytial virus (RSV) infection.

        b. Delivered by small particle aerosol generator (SPAG), a specialized nebulizer and drying chamber system.

          (1) Sticky consistency of the drug particles may create problems during nebulization.

          (2) ETTs may become partially or completely obstructed.

          (3) Function of mechanical ventilator circuitry or valves may be compromised by particle buildup.

    2. Side effects

        a. Skin rash

        b. Eyelid erythema

        c. Conjunctivitis

I. Table 17-3 lists commonly used antibacterial agents with their mechanisms of action, spectra of activity, and toxicities.

J. Table 17-4 lists commonly used antifungal agents and antituberculous agents with their mechanisms of action, spectra of activity, and toxicities.

IX. **Adrenergic Bronchodilators (β-Adrenergic Agonists): General Considerations (Table 17-5)**
   A. Features
      1. The most widely prescribed class of bronchodilator.
      2. Indicated to relieve airflow obstruction in diseases such as asthma, acute and chronic bronchitis, emphysema, bronchiectasis, and cystic fibrosis.
      3. Divided into two main categories by the 1997 National Asthma Education and Prevention Program Expert Panel II guidelines.
         a. "Rescue" agents: Short-acting β_2 agonists indicated for relief of acute airflow obstruction.
         b. "Controller" agents: Long-acting drugs used for maintenance bronchodilation and relief of nocturnal symptoms.
   B. General classification
      1. α-Receptor stimulation: Causes vasoconstriction and increased blood pressure (vasopressor effect).
      2. β_1-Receptor stimulation: Causes increased heart rate and myocontractility (increased chronotropic and inotropic effects).
      3. β_2-Receptor stimulation: Relaxes bronchial smooth muscle, stimulates mucociliary activity, and has some inhibitory action on inflammatory mediator release.
   C. Mechanism of action for β_2-receptor-mediated relaxation of airway smooth muscle (Figure 17-6)
   D. Specific adrenergic bronchodilators (see Table 17-5)
   E. Ultra-short-acting catecholamines
      1. Features
         a. All are catecholamines that lack β_2 specificity, commonly resulting in tachycardia and increased blood pressure.
         b. All have a short duration of action because they are metabolized by the enzyme catechol-O-methyl-transferase.
      2. Epinephrine
         a. Used as a bronchodilator since the start of the 20th century.
         b. Stimulates α-adrenergic and β-adrenergic receptors.
         c. Racemic epinephrine is often used for its vasoconstrictive action in management of stridor associated with laryngeal edema and croup.
      3. Ephedrine
         a. Widely used for management of asthma until the 1970s.
         b. Possesses long-acting stimulant effects and was sold over-the-counter as a central nervous stimulant in the 1970s.
         c. Removed from over-the-counter sales in the 1980s because of its abuse as a stimulant and because it was used as a precursor in the synthesis of amphetamine.
      4. Isoproterenol
         a. Developed in the 1940s.
         b. First bronchodilator with only β agonist effects.
         c. Causes bronchodilation by relaxing bronchial smooth muscle but also relaxed vascular smooth muscle, causing decreased peripheral vascular resistance and lower blood pressure.
         d. Stimulation of β_1 receptors could cause increased heart rate and contractility.
         e. Rarely used today.
   F. Short-acting noncatecholamines
      1. Features
         a. Longer-acting β_2-specific drugs, with duration of action of 4 to 6 hours.

TABLE 17-3

Common Antibacterial Antibiotics, Mechanisms, Spectra of Activity, and Toxicities

Class	Examples	Mechanism of Action	Spectrum of Activity	Toxicity
Penicillins	Penicillin, amoxicillin, amoxicillin-clavulanate (Augmentin), piperacillin, ticarcillin	Cleave bonds contained in peptidoglycan cell wall, disrupting bacterial structural integrity	G+/G–, and anaerobic activities increasing with successive generations	Hypersensitivity, GI intolerance, hepatitis with prolonged use
Cephalosporins	Cefazolin (Ancef), cephalexin (Keflex), ceftriaxone (Rocephin), ceftazidime	Same as penicillins	Same as penicillins	Rare cytopenias
Carbapenems	Imipenem	Same as penicillins	Broad G+, G–, anaerobic coverage	Seizure, GI intolerance, occasional cytopenias
Monobactams	Aztreonam	Same as penicillins	Broad G+, G–, anaerobic coverage	Similar to penicillins
Aminoglycosides	Gentamicin, tobramycin (TOBI)	Antiribosomal: interfere with translation of proteins from mRNA by binding the bacterial ribosome 30S subunit, bacteriocidal	G–	Nephrotoxicity, ototoxicity, rare paralysis; levels requiring monitoring
Tetracyclines	Tetracycline, doxycycline, minocycline	Antiribosomal; bind the 30S subunit; bacteriocidal at high concentrations	G+, atypicals	Tooth and bone defects, phototoxicity, GI intolerance, benign intracranial hypertension, mild hepatitis
Sulfonamides	Trimethoprim/sulfamethoxazole (TMP/SMX, Bactrim, Septra)	Block metabolic pathway for folate production	G+, G–, *Pneumocystis carinii*	Hypersensitivity, possible trigger of hemolysis in G6PD deficiency
Fluoroquinolones	Ciprofloxacin, levofloxacin, gatifloxacin	Inhibit DNA gyrase, interfere with DNA synthesis	G–, G+, atypicals	Cartilage erosion in animals; not administered to children, except those with cystic fibrosis
Macrolides	Erythromycin, clarithromycin (Biaxin), azithromycin (Zithromax)	Antiribosomal: bind 50S subunit; bacteriostatic	G+, some G–; good atypical coverage, including *Legionella* species	GI intolerance
Others	Vancomycin	Inhibits cell wall synthesis	G+, including MRSA; *Enterococcus* species	Hypotension and rash with infusion, ototoxicity
	Metronidazole		Anaerobes	Ethanol intolerance, seizures, peripheral neuropathy
	Chloramphenicol	Antiribosomal: binds 50S subunit	G+, many G–, anaerobes, rickettsiae	Aplastic anemia; used only when strongly indicated
	Clindamycin	Antiribosomal: bacteriocidal at high concentrations	G+ and anaerobes	*Clostridium difficile* colitis

G+, Gram-positive bacteria; G–, gram-negative bacteria; GI, gastrointestinal; DNA, deoxyribonucleic acid; MRSA, methicillin-resistant *Staphylococcus aureus*.
From Hess DR, et al: *Respiratory Care: Principles and Practices*. Philadelphia, WB Saunders, 2002.

TABLE 17-4

Common Antibiotics, Mechanisms, Spectra of Activity, and Toxicities

Class	Examples	Mechanism of Action	Spectrum of Activity	Toxicity
Antifungals				
Imidazoles	Fluconazole, itraconazole	Inhibit ergosterol production	*Aspergillus, Blastomyces,* and *Histoplasma* species, onychomycosis	ECG QT prolongation when given with cisapride, hepatotoxicity
Polyenes	Amphotericin B	Disrupt ergosterol-based cell membrane	All; preferred for severe infections	Fever, rigors, hypotension with infusion, nephrotoxicity, hypersensitivity, cytopenias
Antivirals	Acyclovir, famciclovir, valacyclovir	Guanosine analogues incorporated into DNA, blocking further DNA synthesis; interfered with DNA synthesis	HSV, VZV, CMV	Headache, nausea
	Amantadine, rimantadine	Block attachment of virus and/or release of viral nucleic acid into host cell	Influenza A	Reversible neurotoxicity
	Ganciclovir	Guanine analogue incorporated into DNA, blocking further DNA synthesis; interferes with DNA synthesis	CMV	Cytopenias, impaired male fertility
	Foscarnet	Pyrophosphate analogue blocking DNA synthesis by interfering with DNA polymerase	HSV, VZV, CMV, EBV	Nephrotoxicity in most patients, electrolyte abnormalities, seizures, anemia
	Ribavirin	Unknown	RSV	Possible clogging of ventilator valves, severe bronchospasm, rash
Antituberculous	Rifampin	Inhibits DNA polymerase	G+, G−, MTB	Flulike syndrome, hepatotoxicity
	Isoniazid (INH)	Unknown	MTB	Hepatotoxicity, neurotoxicity, hypersensitivity
	Ethambutol (EMB)	Inhibits protein synthesis?	MTB	Optic neuritis
	Pyrazinamide (PZA)	Unknown	MTB	Hepatotoxicity, hyperuricemia, hypersensitivity
	Streptomycin	Antiribosomal; binds with 30S subunit; bacteriocidal	MTB, G−	Hepatotoxicity, ototoxicity, Neurotoxicity

ECG, Electrocardiographic; *HSV,* herpes simplex virus; *VZV,* varicella-zoster virus; *CMV,* cytomegalovirus; *EBV,* Epstein-Barr virus; *MTB, Mycobacterium tuberculosis; RSV,* respiratory syncytial virus.
From Hess DR, et al: *Respiratory Care: Principles and Practice.* Philadelphia, WB Saunders, 2002.

TABLE 17-5

Inhaled Adrenergic Bronchodilator Agents Currently Available in the United States

Drug	Brand Name	Receptor Preference	Adult Dosage	Time Course (Onset, Peak, Duration)
Epinephrine	Adrenalin Cl	(α, β)	SVN: 1% solution (1:100), 0.25-0.5 ml (2.5-5.0 mg) QID; MDI: 0.2 mg/puff; 2 puffs as ordered or needed	3-5 min, 5-20 min, 1-3 hr
Racemic epinephrine	MicroNefrin, AsthmaNefrin, various	(α, β)	SVN: 2.25% solution, 0.25-0.5 ml (5.63-11.25 mg) QID	3-5 min, 5-20 min, 0.5-2 hr
Isoproterenol	Isuprel, Isuprel Mistometer	(β)	SVN: 0.5% solution (1:200), 0.25-0.5 ml (1.25-2.5 mg) QID, MDI; 103 µg/puff QID	2-5 min, 5-30 min, 0.5-2 hr
Isoetharine	Isoetharine HCl	(β_2)	SVN: 1% solution, 0.25-0.5 ml (2.5-5.0 mg) QID	1-6 min, 15-60 min
Terbutaline	Brethaire	(β_2)	MDI: 200 µg/puff, 2 puffs every 4-6 hr; TABS: 2.5 or 5 mg, 5 mg every 6 hr; INJ: 1 mg/mL, 0.25 mg SC	5-30 min, 30-60 min, 3-6 hr
Metaproterenol	Alupent	(β_2)	SVN: 5% solution, 0.3 ml (15 mg), TID, QID; MDI: 650 µg/puff, 2-3 puffs TID, QID; TABS: 10 or 20 mg, 20 mg TID, QID; SYRUP: 10 mg/5 ml, 2 tsp TID, QID	1-5 min, 60 min, 2-6 hr
Albuterol	Proventil, Proventil HFA, Ventolin	(β_2)	SVN: 0.5% solution, 0.5 ml (2.5 mg) TID, QID; MDI: 90 µg/puff, 2 puffs TID, QID; TABS: 2 mg, 4 mg TID, QID; SYRUP: 2 mg/5 ml, 1-2 tsp TID, QID	15 min, 30-60 min
Bitolterol	Tornalate	(β_2)	SVN: 0.31 mg and 0.2% solution, 1.25 ml (2.5 mg) BID-QID; MDI: 370 µg/puff, 2 puffs every 8 hr	3-4 min, 30-60 min, 5-8 hr
Pirbuterol	Maxair	(β_2)	MDI: 200 µg/puff, 2 puffs every 4-6 hr	5 min, 30 min, 5 hr
Levalbuterol	Xopenex	(β_2)	SVN: 0.31 mg and 0.63 mg/3 ml TID or 1.25 mg/3 ml TID	15 min, 30-60 min, 5-8 hr
Salmeterol	Serevent	(β_2)	MDI: 25 µg/puff, 2 puffs BID; DPI: 50 µg/blister BID	20 min, 3-5 min, 12 hr
Formoterol	Foradil	(β_2)	DPI: 12 µg/inhalation BID	5 min, 30-60 min, 12 hr

SVN, Small-volume nebulizer; *QID,* four times daily; *MDI,* metered dose inhaler; *TABS,* tablets; *INJ,* injection; *SC,* subcutaneous; *TID,* three times daily; *BID,* twice daily.
From Wilkins RL, et al: *Egan's Fundamentals of Respiratory Care,* ed 8. St. Louis, Mosby, 2003.

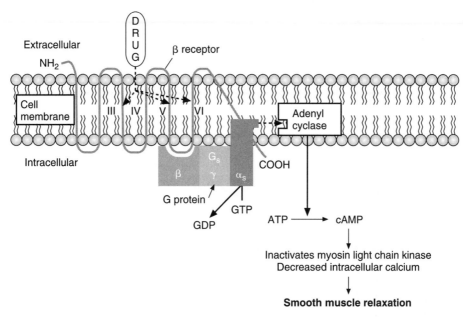

FIG. 17-6 Mode of action by which a β agonist stimulates the G protein-linked β receptor, causing smooth muscle relaxation. Adrenergic agonists such as albuterol or epinephrine attach to β receptors, which are polypeptide chains traversing the cell membrane seven times. This causes activation of the stimulatory G protein, designated G_S, linked to the receptor. When stimulated, the receptor undergoes a conformational change, and the α subunit of the G protein attaches to adenyl cyclase. Activation of adenyl cyclase by the G_S protein increases synthesis of the second messenger, cyclic adenosine monophosphate (cAMP). This ultimately causes smooth muscle relaxation and bronchodilation.

      b. Better suited to maintenance therapy than catecholamines.

      c. Modest duration of action results in loss of bronchodilatation overnight.

  2. Albuterol

      a. A rapid-acting β agonist primarily used for symptomatic relief of bronchospasm.

      b. The most commonly prescribed pulmonary medication in the United States, with few side effects.

  3. Levalbuterol

      a. The R-enantiomer of albuterol, a single isomer β_2-selective agonist.

      b. The R-enantiomer form causes most of the bronchodilatory effect on airways.

      c. Levalbuterol binds with greater affinity to receptor sites, providing effective bronchodilation at lower doses than albuterol.

      d. Clinically often used at half the dosage of albuterol.

      e. Laboratory evidence indicates that a 0.63-mg dose produces a forced expiratory volume in one sec change equivalent to a 2.5-mg dose of albuterol.

  4. Bitolerol

      a. Similar to albuterol but has a slightly longer duration of action.

      b. Bitolerol is a prodrug that is metabolized to the active form colterol, a catecholamine.

      c. The gradual hydrolysis of the prodrug creates the sustained release effect.

G. Long-acting adrenergic bronchodilators

  1. Features

      a. Long-acting β_2 agonists with slower onset of action.

      b. Indicated for maintenance bronchodilation and control of nocturnal symptoms in asthma or other obstructive diseases.

      c. Often combined with antiinflammatory agents for control of airway inflammation and bronchospasm.

2. Salmeterol
   a. The first long-acting adrenergic bronchodilator in the United States.
   b. Duration of action: 12 hours.
   c. Onset of action is >20 minutes, with peak effect in 3 to 5 hours, making it poorly suited for relief of acute airflow obstruction or bronchospasm.
3. Formoterol
   a. β_2-Specific drug approved for use in United States in 2001.
   b. Duration of action: 12 hours.
   c. Long duration of action because of the lipophilic nature of its long side chain structure.
   d. Onset of action and peak effect similar to albuterol.

H. General therapeutic uses of sympathomimetics
   1. Management of generalized bronchoconstriction
   2. Management of mucosal congestion
   3. Management of allergic disorders
   4. Control of hemorrhage
   5. Management of hypotension
   6. Cardiac stimulation
   7. Management of heart block
   8. Treatment of central nervous system (CNS) disorders

I. Contraindications
   1. Hyperthyroidism
   2. Hypertension
   3. Tachycardia

J. Side effects and hazards
   1. Palpitations
   2. Tachycardia
   3. Hypertension
   4. Restlessness
   5. Fear
   6. Anxiety
   7. Tension
   8. Tremor
   9. Weakness
   10. Dizziness
   11. Pallor

K. Comments
   1. Tolerance is frequently observed (tachyphylaxis).
   2. Synergistic effects may be seen.

X. **Anticholinergic Bronchodilators (Table 17-6)**
   A. Features
      1. Blocks cholinergic-induced bronchoconstriction.
         a. Indicated for maintenance management of chronic obstructive pulmonary disease (COPD).
         b. As effective as the β agonists for COPD patients but less effective for those with asthma.
      2. Mode of action: Competitive antagonist for acetylcholine at muscarinic receptors on airway smooth muscle (antimuscarinic agents) (Figure 17-7).
   B. Atropine
      1. A tertiary ammonium compound long known to have bronchodilatory action.
      2. Multiple undesirable side effects rendered it obsolete as a bronchodilator once ipratropium was developed in the 1980s.
   C. Ipratropium bromide
      1. The primary anticholinergic agent used for management of airway obstructive conditions.

TABLE 17-6

Inhaled Anticholinergic Bronchodilator Agents*

Drug	Brand Name	Adult Dosage	Time Course (Onset, Peak, Duration)
Ipratropium bromide	Atrovent	MDI: 18 µg/puff, 2 puffs QID; SVN: 0.02% solution (0.2 mg/ml), 500 µg TID, QID; Nasal spray: 0.03%, 0.06%; 2 sprays per nostril 2 to 4 times daily (dosage varies)	Onset: 15 min, peak: 1-2 hr, duration: 4-6 hr
Ipratropium bromide and albuterol	Combivent	MDI: ipratropium 18 µg/puff and albuterol 90 µg/puff, 2 puffs QID	Onset: 15 min, peak: 1-2 hr, duration: 4-6 hr
	DuoNeb	SVN: ipratropium 0.5 mg and albuterol 3.0 mg (equal to 2.5 mg albuterol base)	
Oxitropium bromide†		MDI: 100 µg/puff, 2 puffs BID, TID	Onset: 15 min, peak: 1-2 hr, duration: 8 hr
Tiotropium bromide‡	Spiriva	DPI: 18 µg/inhalation, 1 inhalation daily	Onset: 30 min, peak: 3 hr, duration: 24 hr

*Ipratropium bromide is the only agent currently approved for use in the United States as an inhaled bronchodilator. A holding chamber is recommended with MDI administration to prevent accidental eye exposure.
†Available outside the United States.
‡Investigational.
MDI, Metered dose inhaler; *SVN*, small-volume nebulizer; *QID*, four times daily; *TID*, three times daily; *BID*, twice daily; *DPI*, dry powder inhaler.
From Wilkins RL et al: *Egan's Fundamentals of Respiratory Care*, ed 8. St. Louis, Mosby, 2003.

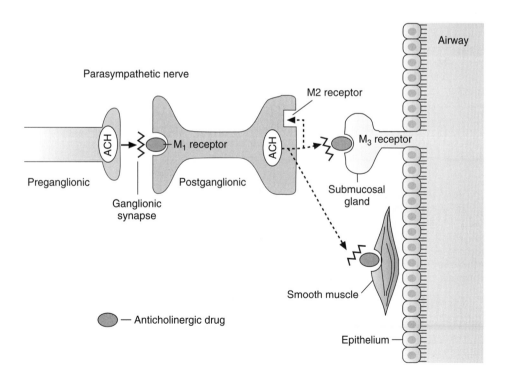

FIG. 17-7 Mode of action of anticholinergic agents in blocking muscarinic receptors in the airway to inhibit cholinergic-induced bronchoconstriction.

2. Ipratropium's quaternary ammonium structure allows it to carry a positive charge, thus inhibiting its diffusion across cell membranes.
   a. This feature restricts ipratropium's distribution, limiting side effects.
   b. By not being able to cross the blood-brain barrier, absorption to the CNS is also limited.
3. Half-life of 3 hours requires dosing every 4 to 6 hours.
4. Also available in a metered dose inhaler formulation combined with albuterol (Combivent).
5. Given only by inhalation because it is poorly absorbed through the oral mucosa.
6. Does not have the secretion drying effects of atropine or glycopyrrolate.

D. Tiotropium bromide (Spiriva): Structurally similar to ipratropium but selective for muscarinic receptors M_1 and M_3.
   1. Tiotropium can confer bronchodilation for up to 24 hours in COPD patients.
   2. Has a slower onset than ipratropium but after onset maintains a higher level of baseline bronchodilation.
   3. Not yet approved for use in the United States.

E. Oxitropium bromide: A derivative of scopolamine used outside the United States as an aerosolized anticholinergic bronchodilator for management of COPD.

TABLE 17-7

Corticosteroids Available by Aerosol for Oral Inhalation

Drug	Brand Name	Formulation and Dosage
Beclomethasone dipropionate	OVAR	MDI: 40 µg/puff and 80 µg/puff Adults ≥12 yr: 40-80 µg BID* or 40-160 µg BID[†] Children 5-11 yr: 40 µg BID*[†]
Triamcinolone acetonide	Azmacort	MDI: 100 µg/puff Adults: 2 puffs TID or QID Children: 1-2 puffs TID or QID
Flunisolide	AeroBid, AeroBid-M	MDI: 250 mg/puff Adults: 2 puffs BID Children: 2 puffs BID
Fluticasone propionate	Flovent	MDI: 44 µg/puff, 110 µg/puff, 220 µg/puff Adults ≥12 yr: 88 µg BID,* 88-220 µg BID,[†] 880 µg BID[‡]
	Flovent Rotadisk	DPI: 50 µg, 100 µg, 250 µg Adults: 100 µg BID,* 100-250 µg BID,[†] 1000 µg BID[‡] Children 4-11 yr: 50 µg BID
Budesonide	Pulmicort Tubuhaler	DPI: 200 µg/actuation Adults: 200-400 µg BID,* 200-400 µg BID,[†] 400-800 µg BID[‡] Children ≥6 yr: 200 µg BID
	Pulmicort Respules	SVN: 0.25 mg/2 ml, 0.5 mg/2 ml Children 1-8 yr: 0.5 mg total dose given daily or BID in divided doses*[†]; 1 mg given as 0.5 mg BID or daily[‡]
Fluticasone propionate/ salmeterol	Advair Diskus	DPI: 100 µg fluticasone/50 µg salmeterol, 250 µg fluticasone/50 µg salmeterol, or 500 µg fluticasone/50 µg salmeterol Adults and children >12 yr: 100 µg fluticasone/50 µg salmeterol 1 inhalation BID about 12 hr apart (starting dose if not currently on inhaled corticosteroids); maximum recommended dose is 500 µg fluticasone/50 µg salmeterol BID

*Recommended starting dose if on bronchodilators alone.
[†]Recommended starting dose if on inhaled corticosteroids previously.
[‡]Recommended starting dose if on oral corticosteroids previously.
MDI, Metered dose inhaler; *BID,* twice daily; *TID,* three times daily; *QID,* four times daily; *DPI,* dry powder inhaler; *SVN,* small-volume nebulizer.
From Wilkins RL, et al: *Egan's Fundamentals of Respiratory Care,* ed 8. St. Louis, Mosby, 2003.

XI. Inhaled Corticosteroids (Table 17-7)
  A. Features
   1. Development of inhaled corticosteroids allowed control of airway inflammation without the side effects associated with systemic steroid use. Direct delivery to the lungs reduced systemic absorption and allowed long-term steroid use with minimal side effects.
   2. Continuous treatment by inhaled corticosteroids has become standard maintenance therapy for those with moderate and severe asthma and is indicated for short-term use in exacerbations of asthma.
     a. In exacerbations of asthma, the underlying poorly controlled inflammation should be managed by an increase in corticosteroids.
       (1) Exacerbations of asthma are usually preceded by a period of increasing bronchial inflammation.
       (2) The inflammatory process is often treated with a 5- to 20-day course of oral corticosteroids, initially dosed at 20 to 40 mg prednisone daily.
     b. The antiinflammatory effects of steroids may take hours to develop. Therefore, serious asthmatic attacks should be managed with a short-acting bronchodilator to prevent acute respiratory failure.
   3. All corticosteroids used for management of asthma are glucocorticoids.
  B. Mode of action
   1. Glucocorticoids are lipid-soluble drugs that exert effects on intracellular receptors (Figure 17-8).

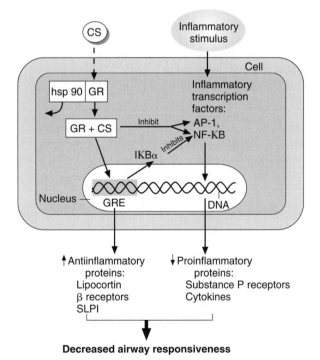

FIG. 17-8 Mode of action of corticosteroids. Corticosteroids (CS) diffuse into the cell and bind to a glucocorticoid receptor (GR). When the steroid binds to the GR, a protein, hsp 90, dissociates from the GR, and the steroid-GR complex moves into the cell nucleus. The drug-receptor complex binds to glucocorticoid response elements (GREs) of the nuclear DNA to up-regulate transcription of antiinflammatory substances such as lipocortin, a protein that inhibits the generation of the arachidonic acid cascade by phospholipase A_2. There is evidence that steroids also up-regulate inhibitors of factors in the cell, such as nuclear factor-κB (NF-κB), which can cause transcription of inflammatory substances. There may be direct inhibition of factors such as NF-κB to further limit the inflammatory process.

    2. Full antiinflammatory effects do not occur for hours to days after beginning treatment, making them unsuitable for use as a rescue drug.

C. Specific inhaled corticosteroids: New synthetic hydrocortisone analogues have high antiinflammatory action with few systemic side effects.

    1. Dexamethasone
        a. The first corticosteroid developed for inhalation.
        b. Its high level of systemic absorption rendered it obsolete once other inhaled corticosteroids were developed.

    2. Beclomethasone dipropionate (Vanceril, Beclovent, QVAR)
        a. The second inhaled corticosteroid available in the United States, after the Decadron (dexamethasone) Respihaler, which is no longer available.
        b. A medium potency inhaled corticosteroid that is rapidly metabolized in the GI tract, preventing its use in an oral form.
        c. Available in MDI formulation as Vanceril and Beclovent.
        d. Reformulated with a hydrofluoroalkane propellant MDI in 40-μg and 80-μg strength as QVAR.
        e. Available for nasal inhalation as Vancenase and Beconase to manage inflammation of the nasopharynx and sinuses.

    3. Triamcinolone acetonide (Azmacort)
        a. Low systemic absorption because of its nonpolar and water-insoluble nature.
        b. Less topically active than beclomethasone.
        c. Its low potency and short duration of action require high initial doses (12 to 16 inhalations/day) for those with severe asthma.
        d. Marketed with a built-in spacer.

    4. Flunisolide (Aerobid)
        a. Also a low potency agent, similar in potency to triamcinolone, but with a longer duration of action.
        b. Reaches peak plasma level between 2 and 60 minutes after inhalation.
        c. The plasma half-life is approximately 1.8 hours.
        d. Poor taste complicates its regular use in pediatric patients.

    5. Budesonide
        a. A high potency agent with a potency greater than beclomethasone, triamcinolone, or flunisolide but less potent than fluticasone.
        b. Delivered by Pulmicort Turbuhaler, a breath-activated MDI.
        c. Peak plasma concentrations occur between 15 and 45 minutes after inhalation.
        d. Plasma half-life is 2 hours.

    6. Fluticasone propionate (Flovent, Flonase)
        a. The highest potency inhaled glucocorticoid agent, available in MDI form.
            (1) MDI strengths: 44 μg, 110 μg, and 220 μg.
            (2) Each actuation releases 50 μg, 125 μg, or 250 μg from the MDI valve, resulting in 44 μg, 110 μg, and 220 μg exiting the mouthpiece.
        b. Available for nasal inhalation as Flonase.

    7. Fluticasone propionate/salmeterol (Advair)
        a. A combination of fluticasone and salmeterol, a long-acting β_2 agonist.
        b. Glucocorticoids and β-adrenergic agonists have beneficial complementary interactions.
            (1) Steroids increase upregulation of β receptors.
            (2) Development of tolerance to β-adrenergic agonists is suppressed by steroid use.
            (3) Salmeterol initiates an antiinflammatory effect in vascular cells, even in the absence of glucocorticoids, by promoting binding of the glucocorticoid receptor to the response element of the cell's DNA.

XII. Sympathomimetics Used for Their Effects on the Cardiovascular System
    A. Norepinephrine
        1. Trade name: Levophed, Noradrenalin

2. Generic name: Norepinephrine
3. Effects: Vasoconstriction and cardiac stimulation
    a. α: Strong vasoconstriction
    b. β_1: Weak
    c. β_2: None
    d. Increases myocardial oxygen consumption, which may result in tissue hypoxia and ischemic injury, particularly when used in high doses.
4. Indications: Hypotension
5. Administration: IV only

B. Dopamine HCl
1. Trade name: Intropin, Dopastat
2. Generic name: Dopamine HCl
3. Action:
    a. A precursor of norepinephrine; stimulates dopaminergic, β_1-adrenergic, and α-adrenergic receptors in a dose-dependent fashion.
    b. Also stimulates the release of norepinephrine.
4. Effects: Dose dependent
    a. Low dosages (1 to 2 µg/kg/min)
        (1) Stimulates dopaminergic receptors, increasing cerebral, renal, and mesenteric vasodilation.
        (2) Increases venous tone because of β-adrenergic stimulation.
        (3) Urine output may increase, but heart rate and blood pressure are usually unchanged.
        (4) May cause a mild increase in cardiac output because of vasodilation.
    b. Moderate dosages (2 to 10 µg/kg/min)
        (1) Stimulates β_1-and α-adrenergic receptors.
        (2) β_1-adrenergic stimulation increases cardiac output, partially antagonizing α-adrenergic-mediated vasoconstriction.
        (3) Substantial increases in venous tone and central venous pressures occur at doses >2.5 µg/kg/min.
        (4) Resultant effect is enhanced cardiac output with a modest increase in systemic vascular resistance.
    c. High dosages: Systemic vasoconstriction
        (1) α-Adrenergic effects predominate at doses >10 µg/kg/min, resulting in renal, mesenteric, and peripheral arterial and venous vasoconstriction.
        (2) Hemodynamic effects similar to norepinephrine occur at doses >20 µg/kg/min.
    d. Dopamine increases myocardial work without compensatory increases in coronary blood flow, leading to an imbalance between oxygen supply and demand that may create myocardial ischemia.
5. Indications
    a. Hypotension
    b. Shock
    c. Renal failure
    d. Myocardial infarction
    e. Other hemodynamic problems
6. Administration: IV only in appropriate dilution of nonalkaline solutions.
7. Side effects and hazards
    a. Widening QRS interval
    b. Angina
    c. Conduction disturbances
    d. Tachycardia

C. Dobutamine: A synthetic sympathomimetic catecholamine.
1. Trade name: Dobutrex
2. Generic: Dobutamine

3. Action: Potent inotrope; stimulates β_1- and α-adrenergic myocardial receptors.
   a. Mild vasodilator because of dual effects of stimulating α-adrenergic peripheral receptors but antagonistically stimulating more potent β_2-adrenergic receptors.
   b. Increases cardiac output and decreases peripheral vascular resistance.
      (1) Increases renal and mesenteric blood flow by increasing cardiac output.
      (2) At conventional doses (2 to 20 µg/kg/min), less apt to induce tachycardia than Isuprel or dopamine.
      (3) Net hemodynamic effects are similar to dopamine combined with a vasodilator such as nitroprusside.
   c. Does not increase myocardial oxygen demand by inducing norepinephrine release, as occurs with dopamine.
4. Indications:
   a. Congestive heart failure (CHF)
   b. Hemodynamic abnormalities
5. Administration: IV only
6. Side effects and hazards
   a. Premature ventricular contractions
   b. Anginal pain
   c. Ischemic injury
7. Comments
   a. Has inotropic selectivity (less increase in heart rate than other drugs).
   b. Decreases systemic vascular resistance.
   c. No increase in pulmonary or systemic blood pressure noted with administration.

XIII. **Noncatecholamines Affecting the Sympathetic Nervous System**
   A. Ephedrine
      1. Trade name: Ephedrine
      2. Generic name: Ephedrine
      3. Mechanism of action: Causes release of epinephrine and norepinephrine stored throughout the body.
      4. Effects (lasting up to 6 hours)
         a. Bronchodilation
         b. Mild cardiac stimulation
         c. Peripheral vasoconstriction
         d. Mild CNS stimulation
      5. Indications
         a. Nonemergency allergic reactions
         b. Chronic asthma
         c. Nasal congestion
      6. Administration: Oral, IM, or SC
   B. Methylxanthines (primarily theophylline)
      1. Trade name: Aminophylline
      2. Generic name: Theophylline
      3. Role: Traditionally used for treatment of patients with asthma and COPD; its current clinical role has been reduced to second- or third-line agents.
         a. Role in asthma
            (1) Methylxanthines are not indicated for acute exacerbations of asthma. Theophylline has a relatively weak bronchodilating effect when compared with β agonists.
            (2) Sustained-release theophylline has been used as a long-term controller drug for management of asthma.
            (3) Low-dose inhaled corticosteroids or cromolyn-like agents are preferred to theophylline for management of stable asthma.
            (4) Antileukotrienes are more therapeutic and have fewer side effects than theophylline.

   b. Role in COPD
      (1) Theophylline is considered effective for COPD but recommended as an alternative to inhaled bronchodilators because of potential toxicity.
      (2) For acute exacerbations of COPD, IV theophylline is recommended only after β_2 agonists or anticholinergic bronchodilators fail.
4. Mechanism of action unknown
   a. Formerly thought that theophylline inhibited the enzyme phosphodiesterase, which led to increased intracellular cyclic adenosine monophosphate (cAMP), that causes relaxation of bronchial smooth muscle.
   b. At clinical dosage levels in humans, theophylline is a poor inhibitor of cAMP-specific phosphodiesterase, invalidating the aforementioned explanation.
   c. Theophylline is a weak and nonselective inhibitor of cAMP-specific phosphodiesterase.
   d. Currently there is no definitive explanation for the bronchodilatory effects of theophylline.
5. Effects
   a. Mild bronchodilation
   b. Cardiac stimulation
   c. Coronary artery dilation
   d. Skeletal muscle stimulation
   e. Diuresis
   f. CNS stimulation
   g. Increased ventilatory drive
6. Indications
   a. Acute and chronic asthma
   b. Abnormal respiratory patterns (e.g., Cheyne-Stokes)
   c. Apnea of prematurity (neonates)
      (1) Methylxanthines, primarily theophylline, were formerly considered first-line agents to stimulate breathing in apnea of prematurity.
      (2) Caffeine citrate has become the respiratory stimulant of choice for this role.
7. Dosage
   a. It is difficult to determine therapeutic doses of theophylline because people metabolize theophylline at different rates.
   b. The recommended therapeutic range for management of asthma is 5 to 15 µg/ml.
   c. For COPD, the American Thoracic Society (2001) recommends a therapeutic range of 10 to 12 µg/ml.
8. Side effects (normally noted if therapeutic level is exceeded)
   a. GI irritation
   b. Headache
   c. Hyperactivity
   d. Dizziness
   e. Nausea
   f. Palpitation
   g. Chest pain
   h. Cardiac arrhythmias
   i. Seizures
9. Administration: Oral, IM, IV, or by suppository

XIV. **Parasympathomimetics (Cholinergic Agents)**
   A. Action: Enhance effects of parasympathetic nervous system (Figure 17-9).
      1. In the parasympathetic nervous system, the neurotransmitter acetylcholine conducts nerve impulses across synapses.
         a. A nerve impulse (action potential) arriving at the presynaptic neuron site causes the release of calcium.
         b. Calcium affects the release of acetylcholine at the end of the nerve fiber.

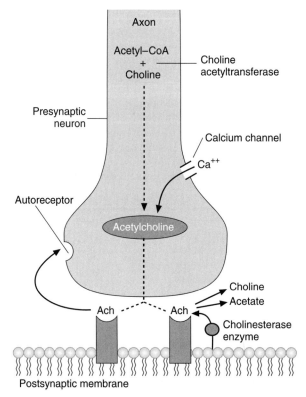

FIG. 17-9 Cholinergic nerve transmission mediated by the neurotransmitter acetylcholine (Ach). Cholinesterase enzymes terminate the action of the neurotransmitter: attachment of Ach to presynaptic autoreceptors inhibits further neurotransmitter release.

  c. Acetylcholine attaches to receptors on the postsynaptic membrane, creating an effect at the tissue or organ site.
 2. Acetylcholinesterase in the synapse enzymatically cleaves acetylcholine, terminating the effect at the receptor site.
 B. Classification of effects
 1. *Muscarinic*: Affects parasympathetic postganglionic fibers, thus stimulating only the parasympathetic nervous system.
 2. *Nicotinic*: Affects acetylcholine receptors at autonomic ganglia and skeletal neuromuscular junctions where acetylcholine is the transmitter substance, thus stimulating sites outside the parasympathetic nervous system.
   a. Voluntary muscle
   b. Sympathetic nervous system
   c. CNS
   d. Adrenal medulla
 C. Cholinergic agents
 1. Direct acting: Mimic acetylcholine, thereby binding to muscarinic or nicotinic receptors directly.
 2. Indirect acting:
   a. Inhibits cholinesterase, creating an excess of acetylcholine at the parasympathetic nerve endings (muscarinic) or neuromuscular junction (nicotinic).
   b. The excess acetylcholine attaches to receptor sites, stimulating the cholinergic response.
   c. Therapeutic uses
    (1) Paralytic ileus
    (2) Atony of urinary bladder

(3) Glaucoma
(4) Myasthenia gravis
(5) Atropine intoxication
(6) Reversal of nondepolarizing neuromuscular-blocking agents

D. Exemplary drugs
   1. Physostigmine: Stimulates muscarinic receptors in the iris and ciliary muscle of the eye, causing constriction of the pupil and thickening of the lens.
   2. Pyridostigmine (Mestinon)
   3. Neostigmine increases acetylcholine at the neuromuscular junction, reversing neuromuscular blockade caused by paralytics such as pancuronium.
   4. Edrophonium (Tensilon)
      a. Short acting (5 to 15 minutes), thereby useful as a diagnostic agent.
      b. Tensilon test
         (1) Inhibition of cholinesterase creates an excess of acetylcholine, causing receptor fatigue, leading to muscle weakness.
         (2) If Tensilon is given and muscle strength is improved, insufficient cholinergic agents are present.
         (3) If Tensilon is given and muscle strength is not improved, excess anticholinergic agents may be present.

E. Side effects associated with excessive stimulation of parasympathetic nervous system
   1. GI disorders
   2. Cardiovascular problems
   3. Excessive secretion by exocrine glands (e.g., mucous and salivary)

XV. **Parasympatholytics (Anticholinergic Agents)**
   A. Action: Inhibition of parasympathetic nervous system.
   B. Mechanism of action:
      1. Blocks acetylcholine receptors (cholinergic antagonists) by competitive inhibition of acetylcholine at muscarinic sites only.
      2. Parasympatholytic agents are solely antimuscarinic because of being limited to parasympathetic terminal fiber sites.
   C. Therapeutic uses
      1. CNS disorders
      2. Preanesthesia medication
      3. Ophthalmologic (pupil dilation)
      4. Upper airway allergies
      5. GI disorders
      6. Genitourinary tract disorders
      7. Common cold
      8. Over-the-counter sleeping pills
      9. Motion sickness, nausea, and vomiting
      10. Cardiovascular problems
      11. Used with parasympathomimetics for reversal of neuromuscular-blocking agents
      12. Bronchodilation
   D. Side effects
      1. Dry mouth
      2. Blurred vision
      3. Urinary retention
      4. Lightheadedness
      5. Fatigue
      6. Tachycardia
   E. Representative parasympatholytic drugs
      1. Atropine, *Atropa belladonna*
         a. A competitive antagonist of acetylcholine at muscarinic receptor sites.
         b. Nonspecific for muscarinic receptor subtypes (blocks M_1, M_2, and M_3).

      c. Structurally a tertiary ammonium compound that carries no electrical charge, allowing it to be easily absorbed, creating the possibility of many side effects.

      d. Blocks parasympathetic component of smooth muscle tone, causing relaxation of bronchial smooth muscle. Since the development of ipratropium, no longer used as a bronchodilator.

      e. Blocks vagal component of cardiac innervation, increasing heart rate.

      f. Decreases mucous gland secretions, creating "dry mouth" because salivary gland secretions are reduced.

      g. Decreases smooth muscle tone, mobility, and acid secretion within the GI tract.

      h. Reduces smooth muscle tone of the bladder, causing urinary retention.

      i. Reduces perspiration by blocking acetylcholine receptors of sweat glands.

  2. Ipratropium bromide (Atrovent, see Section X, Anticholinergic bronchodilators)

  3. Glycopyrrolate (Robinul)

      a. A derivative of atropine that is also not well absorbed across cell membranes, leading to fewer side effects than atropine.

      b. Used during reversal of neuromuscular blockade as an antimuscarinic agent with few CNS side effects.

      c. Not approved for inhalation but has been used IV as a less expensive alternative to Atrovent.

      d. Onset of action: 15 to 30 minutes

      e. Peak effect: 0.5 to 1.0 hour

      f. Duration of action: Approximately 6 hours

  4. Scopolamine hydrobromide (Hyoscine)

      a. A tertiary ammonium compound similar in structure to atropine.

      b. Can produce drowsiness or amnesia.

      c. Can reduce motion sickness through its antimuscarinic effects on the vestibular system of the ear.

  5. Anticholinergics

      a. Parkinson's disease

        (1) Procyclidine (Kemadrin)

        (2) Trihexyphenidyl (e.g., Aphen, Artane)

        (3) Benztropine (Cogentin)

        (4) Biperiden (Akineton)

        (5) Ethopropazine (Pardisol)

        (6) Orphenadrine (Disipal)

        (7) Diphenhydramine (Benadryl and other formulations)

      b. Antispasmodic

        (1) L-Hyoscyamine (Anaspaz)

        (2) Clidinium (Quarzan)

XVI. Sympatholytics (Adrenergic-Blocking Agents)

  A. Action: Inhibition of the sympathetic nervous system.

  B. α-Receptor subtypes: α receptors are divided into α_1 and α_2 subtypes based on location and variation in pharmacologic response.

    1. α-Receptor subtypes in peripheral nerves

      a. α_1 Receptors are located on postsynaptic sites (e.g., vascular smooth muscle), where stimulation results in vasoconstriction.

      b. α_2 Receptors are found in presynaptic sites.

        (1) Stimulation of presynaptic α_2 receptors inhibits further neurotransmitter release, leading to vasodilation.

        (2) Peripheral α_2 receptors thereby autoregulate neurotransmitter release, forming a negative feedback control of the neurotransmitter.

    2. α-Receptor subtypes in the CNS

      a. α_2 Receptors are located in postsynaptic sites of the CNS.

      b. α_2 Receptor agonists decrease blood pressure by decreasing sympathetic release from the CNS.

C. α-Receptor blockade

    1. α-Receptor antagonists may produce opposite effects based on whether they affect α_1- or α_2-receptor subtypes.

    2. Example:

        a. Prazosin prevents vasoconstriction (decreases blood pressure) via blockade of α_1-excitatory receptors.

        b. Yohimbine prevents vasodilation (increases blood pressure) via blockade of α_2-inhibitory receptors.

    3. α_1-Adrenergic antagonists

        a. Selectively block postsynaptic α_1 receptors, causing arterial and venous dilation, reducing peripheral vascular resistance.

          (1) Decrease preload and afterload.

          (2) Can cause tachycardia, orthostatic hypotension, palpitations, syncope, and headaches, particularly on initial dosage.

        b. Examples:

          (1) Doxazosin (Cardura)

          (2) Prazosin (Minipress)

          (3) Terazosin (Hytrin)

    4. α_2-Adrenergic antagonist

        a. Representative drug: Yohimbine

        b. Acts within the CNS at postsynaptic α_2 receptor sites.

        c. Blocks brain stem α_2-inhibitory receptors, increasing sympathetic stimulation from the CNS, preventing vasodilation.

D. β-Adrenergic blocking agents

    1. Mechanism of action: Competitive inhibition at β_1- and β_2-adrenergic receptor sites.

    2. Effects

        a. Reduced heart rate

        b. Reduced blood pressure

        c. Reduced myocardial oxygen consumption

    3. Therapeutic uses

        a. Hypertension

          (1) Blockade of myocardial β receptors decreases rate and contractility, reducing cardiac output.

          (2) Blocks β receptors on renal juxtaglomerular cells, inhibiting renin production, resulting in decreased angiotensin II concentration.

          (3) Blockade of CNS β receptors decreases sympathetic tone.

          (4) Decreases norepinephrine production via blockade of peripheral β receptors.

        b. Cardiac arrhythmias: Slows A-V nodal conduction, helping prevent atrial fibrillation, atrial flutter, and paroxysmal supraventricular tachycardia (PSVT).

        c. Angina pectoris

        d. Migraine prophylaxis

        e. Glaucoma

    4. Side effects and hazards

        a. CHF and associated pulmonary edema

        b. Hypotension

        c. Bronchospasm

          (1) Exacerbation of stable asthma or COPD may occur with use of β blockade.

          (2) β_1-selective drugs (e.g., atenolol and metoprolol) have fewer pulmonary side effects at low doses but are less β_1 specific at higher doses.

        d. Contraindicated in patients with bradycardia or significant A-V block.

    5. Representative drugs

        a. Propranolol (Inderal): Nonselective blockade of β_1 and β_2 receptors, thus potentially affecting cardiac and pulmonary systems.

    b. Metoprolol (Lopressor): β_1 selective at low doses.

    c. Atenolol (Tenormin): β_1 selective at low doses.

    d. Timolol (Bleocardin, Timolide)

    e. Nadolol (Corgard)

    f. Pindolol (Visken): Possesses intrinsic sympathomimetic activity, decreasing the intensity of its β blockade.

    g. Acebutolol (Sectral)

  E. α- and β-adrenergic blockers: labetalol (Normodyne, Trandate) and carvedilol (Coreg)

XVII. Advanced Cardiac Life Support Medications

  A. Antiarrhythmic agents

    1. Amiodarone: A complex drug with effects on sodium, potassium, and calcium channels and has α- and β-adrenergic blocking effects.

      a. Has broad atrial and ventricular antiarrhythmic effects and lesser negative inotropic effects.

      b. Alters accessory conductive pathways, thus effective in controlling rapid ventricular rate in supraventricular tachycardia (SVT).

      c. Dose:

        (1) 150 mg over 10 minutes, followed by infusion of 1 mg/min for 6 hours, then 0.5 mg/min continuous infusion.

        (2) Recurrent arrhythmias treated with a repeated 150-mg infusion up to a maximum daily dose of 2 g.

        (3) In pulseless ventricular tachycardia or ventricular fibrillation, give a 300-mg rapid infusion diluted with 20 to 30 ml saline.

    2. Lidocaine

      a. A primary agent for management of wide complex tachycardia. Suppresses ventricular arrhythmias associated with acute myocardial ischemia and infarction (AMI).

        (1) Its antiventricular arrhythmic use in AMI reduces the incidence of ventricular fibrillation but does not decrease mortality rate.

        (2) Routine prophylactic use in patients with AMI is not recommended.

      b. Appropriate as a second-line agent for controlling hemodynamically stable ventricular tachycardia.

      c. Useful for controlling hemodynamically compromising premature ventricular contractions.

      d. Not indicated for management of supraventricular tachycardia.

      e. Cardiac arrest dose:

        (1) 1.0 to 1.5 mg/kg IV bolus

        (2) For refractory ventricular tachycardia/ventricular fibrillation, an additional bolus of 0.5 to 0.75 is given over 3 to 5 minutes.

        (3) Maximum cumulative dose should not exceed 3 mg/kg.

    3. Procainamide

      a. Effective for management of supraventricular arrhythmias and ventricular tachycardia.

      b. Alters conduction across an accessory pathway, thus effective in breaking SVT.

      c. Has vasodilatory and negative inotropic effects that may lead to hypotension.

    4. Adenosine: An endogenous purine nucleoside that depresses sinus and A-V node conduction.

      a. Used to manage narrow complex tachycardia, narrow complex SVT, and wide complex tachycardia that is supraventricular in origin.

      b. Produces a short-lived pharmacologic conductive block at the A-V node.

      c. Initial dose: 6 mg bolus over 1 to 3 seconds followed by 20-ml saline flush.

      d. A repeat dose of 12 mg may be given twice if no response is obtained.

      e. Half-life of adenosine is <5 seconds.

    5. Atropine (also see section XVI, E, Anticholinergic Agents)

    a. Reverses cholinergic-mediated bradycardia, decreased systemic vascular resistance, and decreased blood pressure.

    b. Recommended dose:

       (1) For asystole and pulseless electrical activity: 1.0 mg IV, repeated in 3 to 5 minutes.

       (2) For bradycardia: 0.5 to 1.0 g IV every 3 to 5 minutes to a maximum of 0.04 mg/kg.

    c. Well absorbed through the tracheal route of administration.

    d. Should be used carefully for AMI; excessive increases in heart rate may worsen ischemia or increase a zone of infarction.

    e. Contraindicated in type II A-V block and third-degree block with new wide QRS complexes.

6. β-Adrenergic blockers (also see Section XVII, D, Sympatholytics)

    a. Indicated for all patients with AMI and high-risk unstable angina.

    b. Atenolol, metoprolol, and propranolol significantly reduce ventricular fibrillation in post-MI patients who did not receive fibrinolytic agents.

    c. Esmolol: A short-acting (half-life, 2 to 9 minutes) β_1-selective β blocker used for management of SVTs.

    d. Side effects of β blockade: Bradycardia, A-V conduction delay, and hypotension.

    e. Contraindicated in second- or third-degree heart block, severe CHF, and lung disease associated with severe bronchospasm.

7. Verapamil and diltiazem: Calcium channel blockers

    a. Action: Slows conduction and increases refractoriness within the A-V node by blocking calcium channels.

       (1) Can terminate A-V nodal reentry arrhythmias.

       (2) Can control ventricular response rate in patients with atrial fibrillation, atrial flutter, or multifocal atrial tachycardia (MAT).

       (3) May decrease myocardial contractility, thus may worsen CHF in patients with severe left ventricular dysfunction.

    b. Verapamil initial dose: 2.5 to 5 mg IV given over 2 minutes. Repeated doses of 5 to 10 mg may be given every 15 to 30 minutes. Maximum cumulative dose: 20 mg.

       (1) Indicated only for narrow complex PSVT or supraventricular arrhythmias.

       (2) Contraindicated in patients with impaired left ventricular function or CHF.

    c. Diltiazem initial dose: 0.25 mg/kg, followed by a second dose of 0.35 mg/kg.

       (1) Produces less myocardial depression than verapamil.

       (2) Can be used as a maintenance infusion to control the ventricular rate in atrial fibrillation or atrial flutter.

8. Dopamine (also see Section XII, B, Sympathomimetics utilized for their effects on the cardiovascular system.)

    a. An endogenous catecholamine with dopaminergic, α- and β-adrenergic agonist activity.

    b. Currently the preferred catecholamine for bradycardia in which atropine is contraindicated or ineffective.

    c. Exhibits dose-dependent effects.

9. Magnesium

    a. A deficiency of magnesium can be associated with ventricular arrhythmias.

    b. Considered the hallmark therapy for ventricular dysrhythmia, even in the absence of magnesium deficiency.

    c. Dose: 1 to 2 g magnesium sulfate, diluted in 100 ml D_5W, given over 1 to 2 minutes.

10. Sotalol

    a. A nonselective β blocker approved for ventricular and supraventricular arrhythmias.

    b. Prolongs action potential and increases refractoriness of cardiac tissue.

    c. Dose: Given IV, 1 to 1.5 mg/kg at a rate of 10 mg/min.

      d. Its slow infusion rate renders it impractical during cardiopulmonary resuscitation (CPR) or for emergent hypotensive crises.

B. Agents for optimizing cardiac output and blood pressure

  1. Vasopressin: The endogenous antidiuretic hormone, acts as a nonadrenergic peripheral vasoconstrictor when given in unnaturally high doses.

    a. Directly stimulates smooth muscle vasopressin V_1 receptors.

    b. Does not vasodilate skeletal muscle vessels or increase myocardial oxygen consumption during CPR because it has no β-adrenergic activity.

      (1) During CPR, vasopressin causes peripheral vasoconstriction in skeletal muscle, skin, intestine, and fat, with less constriction of coronary and renal vasculature, but vasodilates the cerebral vasculature.

      (2) Repeated doses of vasopressin are more effective than epinephrine to maintain coronary perfusion pressure.

    c. Half-life in animal models is 10 to 20 minutes (much longer than epinephrine).

    d. Used as a continuous infusion to increase vascular tone and support hemodynamics in septic shock and sepsis syndrome (systemic inflammatory response syndrome).

  2. Epinephrine: An endogenous catecholamine synthesized in the adrenal medulla.

    a. Has potent α and β effects.

    b. Increases myocardial oxygen demand but may not increase perfusion enough to prevent myocardial hypoxia.

    c. Traditionally has been the first-line pressor and cardiac stimulant in CPR but is currently being supplanted by vasopressin.

    d. Recommended dose: 1 mg IV push every 3 to 5 minutes.

  3. Norepinephrine (see Section XII, A, Sympathomimetics utilized for their effects on the cardiovascular system)

  4. Dopamine (see Section XII , B, Sympathomimetics utilized for their effects on the cardiovascular system)

  5. Dobutamine (see Section XII , C, Sympathomimetics utilized for their effects on the cardiovascular system)

  6. Amrinone and milrinone (phosphodiesterase inhibitors)

    a. Positive inotropic agents that selectively inhibit cAMP phosphodiesterase, the enzyme that hydrolyzes cAMP.

      (1) Elevated cAMP increases intracellular calcium, enhancing myocardial contractility.

      (2) Elevated cAMP causes vasodilation of arterial smooth muscle, which may result in hypotension.

      (3) Phosphodiesterase inhibitors are an alternative to dobutamine-induced tachycardia.

    b. Have a more significant effect on preload than catecholamines.

    c. Hemodynamic effects are similar to dobutamine.

    d. Indicated in severe heart failure or cardiogenic shock that is unresponsive to standard treatment.

    e. Amrinone may worsen myocardial ischemia or increase ventricular ectopy.

  7. Calcium

    a. Important in myocardial contractility and impulse generation.

    b. In cardiac arrest administration of calcium has demonstrated no benefit.

    c. If hyperkalemia, hypocalcemia, or calcium channel blocker toxicity exists, administration of calcium may be helpful.

    d. Dose

      (1) Calcium chloride: 10% solution dosed at 2 to 4 mg/kg, repeated at 10-minute intervals as necessary.

      (2) Calcium gluconate: 5 to 8 ml

  8. Digitalis

    a. Slows atrioventricular node conduction, thereby decreases the ventricular rate in atrial fibrillation or flutter.

    b. Effectively controls ventricular response rate in patients with chronic atrial fibrillation.

        (1) Less effective in patients with paroxysmal atrial fibrillation.

        (2) Not effective for rate control in CHF, hyperthyroidism, or during exercise (high adrenergic states).

    c. Calcium channel blockers or β-adrenergic blockers should be used for initial ventricular rate control in atrial fibrillation.

    d. Digitalis toxic-to-therapeutic ratio is narrow, particularly during hypokalemia.

    e. Digitalis toxicity can cause cardiac arrest or ventricular arrhythmias.

9. Nitroglycerin

    a. A potent venodilator, vasodilates coronary vessels and collaterals, decreasing end-diastolic pressure and myocardial oxygen demand.

        (1) Primarily a venodilator.

        (2) At high doses can effect arterial dilation.

    b. Indicated in AMI, angina, hypertension, and acute heart failure.

    c. Nitroglycerin effects depend on intravascular volume status.

        (1) In hypovolemic states, vasodilation increases the risk of hypotension.

        (2) Further hypotension may reduce coronary blood flow and increase myocardial ischemia.

    d. Delivered by sublingual tablets for relief of acute angina.

        (1) Each nitroglycerin tablet contains 0.3 to 0.4 mg.

        (2) Provides immediate onset of action with duration of action approximately 30 minutes.

        (3) Tablets should be repeated every 5 minutes until angina is relieved.

        (4) If symptoms are not relieved after a maximum of three doses within 15 minutes, emergency care should be summoned.

    e. Adverse reactions may include palpitations, hypotension, dizziness, tachycardia, and headache.

10. Sodium nitroprusside

    a. A potent peripheral vasodilator for management of severe heart failure and acute hypertensive crises.

    b. Venodilation reduces preload, potentially relieving pulmonary congestion and reducing left ventricular pressure and volume.

    c. Higher doses cause arterial dilation, decreasing arterial resistance to flow (afterload).

        (1) Decreased afterload increases systolic ejection, reducing left ventricular distention.

        (2) Myocardial oxygen consumption is reduced by more efficient myocardial contractility.

    d. Nitroprusside affects the pulmonary system by dilating pulmonary arteries, reversing hypoxic pulmonary vasoconstriction, thereby increasing intrapulmonary shunt, resulting in decreased Pao_2.

    e. Dose

        (1) Usual range: 0.1 to 5.0 μg/kg/min

        (2) Prepared by adding 50 or 100 mg to 250 ml of D_5W or saline.

        (3) Photosensitive; therefore, tubing and solution should be wrapped by opaque material.

    f. Side effects

        (1) Hypotension

        (2) Potential for cyanide toxicity

            (a) Metabolically catabolized to cyanide and thiocyanate.

            (b) Cyanide toxicity can be detected by the development of a metabolic acidosis.

XVIII. Steroids

    A. Adrenocorticotropic hormone (ACTH) and adrenocorticosteroids

        1. ACTH (corticotropin) is produced and released from the adenohypophysis (anterior pituitary).

        2. Physiology of steroid regulation

            a. Release of ACTH into the blood causes the adrenal cortex to release steroids into the bloodstream.

            b. Release of ACTH is affected directly by corticotropin-releasing factor (CRF), which is secreted by the hypothalamus.

            c. Blood level of CRF is indirectly affected by blood steroid levels.

            d. Thus there is a cyclic relation between ACTH, CRF, and steroid levels.

            e. An increase in steroid level causes a decrease in CRF levels, which causes a decrease in ACTH levels. This results in a decrease in steroid levels, which causes an increase in CRF levels, and so forth, thus maintaining a normal equilibrium.

        3. Actions

            a. Stimulate glucose formation (i.e., increase blood glucose levels).

            b. Decrease glucose utilization.

            c. Promote storage of glucose in liver.

            d. Regulate rate of synthesis of proteins.

            e. Control distribution of body fat.

            f. Regulate lipid metabolism.

            g. Regulate reabsorption of sodium ions from kidney tubules.

            h. Increase urinary excretion of potassium and hydrogen.

            i. Maintain normal function of skeletal muscles.

            j. Increase hemoglobin and red blood cell content of blood.

            k. Maintain normal lymphoid tissue.

            l. Prevent or suppress inflammatory responses caused by hypersensitivity.

        4. Mechanisms of action

            a. Modification of cell function protein production and direct stimulation of tissue receptor sites to inhibit the complex mechanisms of inflammation.

            b. Allergic disorders: Has a catabolic effect on lymphoid tissue.

            c. Edema: Decreases capillary permeability by an unknown mechanism.

        5. Therapeutic uses

            a. Allergic asthma

            b. Acute and chronic adrenal insufficiency

            c. Suppression of immune response in organ transplant patients

            d. Congenital adrenal hyperplasia

            e. Adrenal insufficiency secondary to anterior pituitary insufficiency

            f. Arthritis

            g. Rheumatic carditis

            h. Osteoarthritis

            i. Acute inflammatory diseases

        6. Side effects

            a. Aerosol administration

                (1) Upper airway fungal infections

                (2) Hoarseness

                (3) Coughing

                (4) Dry mouth

                (5) Adrenal insufficiency after transfer from systemic steroids

            b. Systemic administration

                (1) Cushing's disease

                    (a) Moon face

                    (b) Hirsutism

                    (c) Muscle wasting

                    (d) Variable hypernatremia

                    (e) Hypokalemia

          (2)   Hypertension
          (3)   Aggravation of diabetes mellitus (hyperglycemia)
          (4)   Necrotizing arteritis in rheumatoid patients
          (5)   Aggravation of peptic ulcer
          (6)   Psychotic manifestations (mood changes)
          (7)   Adrenal atrophy
          (8)   Obesity
          (9)   Growth suppression
        (10)   Thinning of skin
        (11)   Muscle wasting
        (12)   Osteoporosis
        (13)   Immunosuppression

    7. Representative aerosolized drugs (see Section XI, Inhaled Corticosteroids)
    8. Representative systemic drugs
        a. Cortisone
        b. Hydrocortisone
        c. Prednisone
        d. Prednisolone
        e. Methylprednisolone
        f. Betamethasone

XIX. Neuromuscular-Blocking Agents

    A. Major action: Interruption of transmission of nerve impulse at skeletal neuromuscular junction, resulting in paralysis.

    B. Categories
        1. Nondepolarizing agents
            a. Mechanism of action: Competitive inhibition of acetylcholine at muscle post-synaptic receptor sites. The muscle tissue itself remains sensitive to external stimulation.
            b. Effects
               (1)   Nondepolarizing agents act by competitive inhibition, thus their effects are dose related.
               (2)   Maximal effects are attained in 2 to 10 minutes and persist for 30 to 60 minutes.
               (3)   Hypotension as a result of histamine release is seen occasionally with *d*-tubocurarine.
               (4)   Bradycardia occasionally is seen with pancuronium.
               (5)   Cholinesterase-inhibiting agents (e.g., neostigmine) may reverse effects of this group of drugs.
            c. Representative drugs

Representative drugs	Duration (minutes)
(1) Tubocurarine (*d*-tubocurarine)	>35
(2) Pancuronium (Pavulon)	>35
(3) Metocurine (Metubine)	>35
(4) Atracurium (Tracrium)	20-35
(5) Vecuronium (Norcuron)	20-35
(6) *cis*-Atracurium	20-35

            d. Neuromuscular-blocking agents commonly used in the intensive care unit (ICU) (Table 17-8)
        2. Depolarizing agents
            a. Mechanism of action
               (1)   They cause persistent depolarization of the postjunctional membrane by competitively binding at acetylcholine receptor sites, rendering them incapable of repolarization.
               (2)   As this wave of depolarization proceeds, a rippling of voluntary muscles occurs (muscle fasciculation), usually from the head downward. Because

---

	TABLE **17-8**			

Neuromuscular Blocking Agents Commonly Used in the Intensive Care Unit

	Pancuronium	Vecuronium	Tubocurarine	*Cis*-Atracurium
Intubation dose	0.08-0.1 mg/kg	0.1-0.2 mg/kg	0.5-0.6 mg/kg	0.15-0.2 mg/kg
Infusion dose	1 μg/kg/min	1 μg/kg/min	0.08-0.12 mg/kg/hr	2 μg/kg/min
Cost	Low	High	Low	Moderate

these agents are chemically similar to acetylcholine, they cause continual stimulation of the motor endplate.
   (3) This continual stimulation does not allow time for repolarization; therefore, the muscle develops a flaccid paralysis.
   (4) There are no drugs known that reverse depolarizing agents. With time depolarizing agents are metabolized by acetylcholinesterase.
   b. The muscle fiber itself is still sensitive to external stimulation.
   (1) Effects are seen in approximately 30 to 40 seconds and persist 3 to 5 minutes.
   (2) Effects are not reversible.
   c. Representative drugs   Duration (minutes)
   (1) Succinylcholine (Anectine)   10-15
   (2) Decamethonium (Syncurine)   20-35
        (a) Available in Europe
        (b) Not metabolized by acetylcholinesterase.
        (c) Requires hepatic and renal function for elimination.

XX. **Narcotics and Analgesics**
   A. Primary use (narcotics): Analgesia and relief of severe pain.
   B. Mechanism of action: Unclear, but these drugs affect neurotransmission at specific CNS sites, affect autonomic nervous system transmission, and cause some histamine release.
   C. General pharmacologic effects
      1. Analgesic
         a. Alters the perception of pain.
         b. Interferes with the continuance of pain impulses in the spinal cord.
         c. Alters the body's response to the pain stimulus.
         d. May elevate the pain threshold.
      2. Euphoric: Seen at therapeutic dosages.
      3. Hypnotic: With increasing dosages, more subjective CNS depression.
      4. Metabolic: Transient hyperglycemia.
      5. Endocrine: Stimulates the release of antidiuretic hormone.
      6. Pupil size: Miosis
      7. GI tract: Constipation because of decreased overall activity.
      8. Nausea and vomiting: Direct stimulation of medullary control center.
      9. Cardiovascular system
         a. If patient is well oxygenated and in normal acid-base balance, there are no significant effects.
         b. Cardiac arrhythmias may be seen with acid-base abnormalities.
         c. Hypotension may result because of direct effect on venous smooth muscle and release of histamine.
      10. Respiratory system
         a. Direct depression of medullary respiratory center response to CO_2 changes.
         b. Significant decrease in respiratory rate, tidal volume, and minute volume is seen with large dosages.
      11. Cough reflex: Decreased as a result of direct depression of medullary cough center.

D. Therapeutic uses
   1. Analgesia
   2. Cough control
   3. Emetic
   4. Antidiarrheic
   5. Pulmonary edema
   6. Control of patients on ventilators
E. Representative drugs
   1. High potency
      a. Morphine (generic and trade)
      b. Oxymorphone (Numorphan)
      c. Heroin
      d. Fentanyl
      e. Methadone (Dolophine)
      f. Hydromorphone
   2. Intermediate potency
      a. Meperidine (Demerol)
      b. Oxycodone (Percodan)
   3. Low potency
      a. Codeine (generic and trade)
      b. Diphenoxylate (Lomotil)
F. Nonnarcotic analgesics and antiinflammatory agents: All have analgesic properties and are normally used for mild or chronic pain.
   1. Salicylates
      a. Aspirin (acetylsalicylic acid)
      b. Methyl salicylate
   2. Aniline derivatives
      a. Phenacetin
      b. Acetaminophen (Tempra, Tylenol)
   3. Pyrazole derivatives
      a. Phenylbutazone (Butazolidin)
      b. Oxyphenbutazone (Oxalid)
   4. Central-acting agents
      a. Methotrimeprazine (Levoprome)
   5. Nonsteroidal antiinflammatory drugs (NSAIDs)
      a. Indomethacin (Indocin)
      b. Ibuprofen (Motrin)
      c. Ketoprofen (Orudis)
      d. Fenoprofen (Nalfon)
   6. Narcotics commonly used in the ICU (Table 17-9)

XXI. **Narcotic Antagonists**
A. Sole use: To reverse effects of narcotics.
B. Mechanism of action: Competitive displacement of agonist from receptor site.
C. Partial antagonists
   1. Cause narcotic-like effects in absence of a narcotic.
   2. Cause increased respiratory depression if administered in a nonnarcotic overdose (e.g., barbiturates).
   3. Representative drugs
      a. Nalorphine (Nalline)
      b. Levallorphan (Lorfan)
D. Pure antagonists: Have only narcotic antagonist properties.
   1. Will not increase respiratory depression in a nonnarcotic overdose.
   2. Representative drug: Naloxone (Narcan)

	Morphine	Fentanyl	Hydromorphone
TABLE **17-9** *Narcotics Commonly Used in the Intensive Care Unit*			
Onset of action	Rapid	Rapid	Rapid
Intermittent dose	0.01-0.15 mg/kg	0.35-1.5 µg/kg	10-30 µg/kg
Infusion dose	0.07-0.5 mg/kg/hr	0.7-1.0 µg/kg/hr	7-15 µg/kg/hr
Cost	Low	Moderate	Moderate

E. Duration of effect
   1. Forty-five to 60 minutes *(careful monitoring of overdosed patient must be maintained).*
   2. Narcotic's effect may significantly outlast that of the narcotic antagonist.

XXII. **Sedatives and Hypnotics**
  A. Solid or liquid substances that cause a longer generalized depression of the CNS than do anesthetic gases.
  B. Mechanism of action: Selective depression of ascending reticular activating system at either the cellular or synaptic level, resulting in loss of consciousness.
  C. Physiologic effects
    1. Behavioral changes caused by increased dosages
      a. Sedation: Generalized decreased responsiveness
      b. Disinhibition: Impaired judgment and loss of self-control
      c. Relief of anxiety
      d. Ataxia and nystagmus
      e. Sleep (hypnosis)
      f. Anesthesia
    2. Electroencephalographic pattern changes consistent with generalized CNS depression
    3. Poor analgesia
    4. Anticonvulsant: Phenobarbital the most effective
    5. Withdrawal state with repeated long-term use and abrupt discontinuance
    6. Habit forming
    7. Voluntary muscle relaxation from spinal cord depression
    8. Depression of respiratory medullary center with larger doses
    9. Profound vasomotor depression and shock with larger doses
   10. No direct effect on myocardium
  D. Therapeutic uses
    1. Sleep induction
    2. Relief of anxiety (sedation)
    3. Management of neurotic anxiety
    4. Relief of depression
    5. Voluntary muscle relaxation
    6. Anticonvulsant
  E. Side effects
    1. Drowsiness
    2. Impaired performance and judgment
    3. Hangover
    4. Drug abuse
    5. Withdrawal state
    6. Overdose
  F. Contraindications
    1. Hypothyroidism
    2. Hypoadrenalism
  G. Types
    1. Barbiturates

a. Ultra-short-acting: Anesthetic agents
    (1) Hexobarbital (Sombucaps)
    (2) Thiopental (Pentothal)
b. Short-acting: Primarily for sleep induction
    (1) Pentobarbital (Nembutal)
    (2) Secobarbital (Seconal)
c. Intermediate-acting: Relief of anxiety
    (1) Amobarbital (Amytal)
    (2) Aprobarbital (Alurate)
d. Long-acting: Anticonvulsant
    (1) Phenobarbital (generic and trade)
    (2) Mephobarbital (Mebaral)
2. Nonbarbiturate sedatives: Hypnotics
    a. Short-acting
        (1) Methaqualone (Quaalude)
        (2) Paraldehyde (generic and trade)
        (3) Chloral hydrate (generic and trade)
        (4) Flurazepam (Dalmane)
    b. Intermediate-acting
        (1) Meprobamate (Miltown, Equanil)
        (2) Glutethimide (Doriden)
        (3) Diazepam (Valium)
    c. Long-acting: Chlordiazepoxide (Librium)
3. Other antianxiety agents
    a. Lorazepam (Ativan)
    b. Midazolam (Versed)
    c. Propofol (Diprivan)
    d. Haloperidol (Haldol)
4. Agents commonly used in the ICU (Table 17-10)

XXIII. **Diuretics and Antihypertensive Agents**
    A. Functional renal unit: The nephron (Figure 17-10)
        1. Approximately 20% of blood entering the glomerulus is filtered, forming a cell-free ultrafiltrate within the glomerulus.
        2. Flowing through the nephrons, >99% of the ultrafiltrate is reabsorbed.
        3. Diuretic drugs alter the reabsorption of water within the nephron system.
    B. Electrolyte balance within the nephron
        1. Sodium
            a. 80% of sodium in the ultrafiltrate is reabsorbed in the proximal tubule.
            b. 20% is absorbed in the distal tubule.

TABLE 17-10

Sedatives Commonly Used in the Intensive Care Unit

	Lorazepam (Ativan)	Midazolam (Versed)	Diazepam (Valium)	Haloperidol (Haldol)	Propofol (Diprivan)
Onset of action	5-20 min	2-5 min	2-5 min	3-20 min	1-2 min
Intermittent dose	0.02-0.06 mg/kg every 2-6 hr	0.02-0.08 mg/kg every 0.5-2 hr	0.03-0.01 mg/kg every 0.5-6 hr	0.03-0.15 mg/kg every 0.5-6 hr	—
Infusion rate	0.01-0.10 mg/kg/hr	0.04-0.20 mg/kg/hr	—	0.04-0.15 mg/kg/hr	5-80 µg/kg/min
Cost	Low	High	Low	Low	High

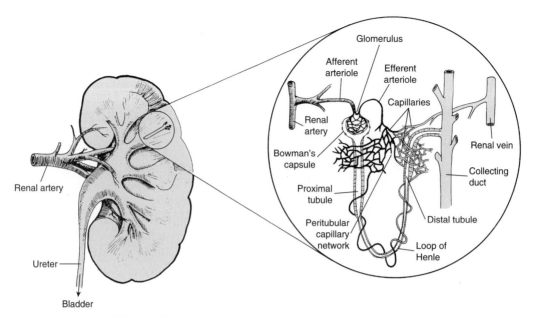

FIG. 17-10 Basic structure of the kidney, with detail of the nephron.

2. Potassium
    a. Nearly all ultrafiltrate potassium is reabsorbed in the proximal tubules.
    b. Small amounts of potassium are secreted by the distal tubule.
3. Chloride and bicarbonate are reabsorbed passively in proximal and distal tubules.
4. Water reabsorption occurs passively, following osmotic gradients created by electrolytes, primarily sodium. Drugs that decrease sodium reabsorption decrease reabsorption of water.
C. Classes of diuretics (Figure 17-11)
    1. Osmotic diuretics: Interfere with water reabsorption in the descending loop of Henle and in the proximal tubule.
        a. Once filtered into the nephron, osmotic diuretics stay within the tubule lumen and prevent the reabsorption of sodium.
        b. Increased sodium and (because of preservation of electrical neutrality within the tubule) chloride delivered to the distal tubule promote an exchange of sodium for potassium, increasing potassium elimination.
        c. Mannitol: The preferred osmotic diuretic because of its low toxicity and short half-life.
    2. Carbonic anhydrase inhibitors: Prevent reabsorption of sodium and bicarbonate ions in the proximal tubule.
        a. Carbonic anhydrase enzymatically hydrates bicarbonate, which can then be reabsorbed.
        b. Sodium is reabsorbed with bicarbonate to preserve electrical neutrality.
        c. Carbonic anhydrase inhibitors thus increase the excretion of sodium and bicarbonate, resulting in a metabolic acidemia.
        d. Because carbonic anhydrase inhibitors act only on the proximal tubule, sodium can be reabsorbed in the ascending limb of the loop of Henle and in the distal tubule. Thus carbonic anhydrase inhibitors are weak diuretics.
    3. Loop diuretics: Inhibit absorption of chloride ions in the ascending loop of Henle (sodium and water passively follow the chloride).
        a. Loop diuretics produce an acute vasodilatory effect that may be caused by the renal release of vasodilating prostaglandins.

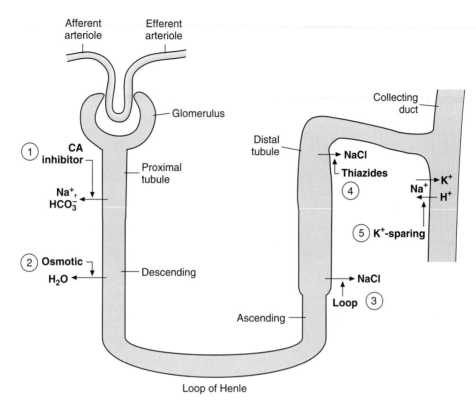

FIG. 17-11 The nephron, from glomerulus to collecting duct, showing the various sites of action for the diuretic groups. CA, Carbonic anhydrase.

(1) This acute vasodilatory effect can decrease pulmonary capillary wedge pressure and systemic vascular resistance.

(2) Before any diuresis, this short-term effect aids patients with CHF or pulmonary edema.

b. Examples

(1) Furosemide

(2) Bumetanide

(3) Torsemide

4. Thiazide diuretics

a. Block sodium and chloride ion reabsorption in the distal tubule.

b. Because only 5% of sodium is reabsorbed in the distal tubule, thiazide diuretics are much less potent than loop diuretics.

5. Potassium-sparing diuretics block sodium reabsorption in the distal tubule and collecting duct.

a. Normally sodium is exchanged for potassium and hydrogen in the distal tubule. Blockade of this exchange results in preservation of potassium, hence the term potassium-sparing diuretics.

b. As a class they are weak diuretics.

D. Complications of diuresis

1. Hypokalemia

a. Normally 80% of sodium is absorbed in the proximal tubule. In the distal convoluted tubule, most of the remaining 20% of sodium in the ultrafiltrate is reabsorbed by exchange of Na^+ for K^+ ions.

b. Diuretics that increase the concentration of sodium at the distal convoluted tubule promote increased exchange of Na^+ for K^+, which may create hypokalemia.

2. Acid-base alterations
   a. Volume depletion because of diuretic use may result in hypokalemia and hypochloremia. As K^+ and Cl^- are excreted, HCO_3^- is retained, creating a metabolic alkalosis.
   b. Repletion of K^+ or Cl^- corrects the alkalosis by allowing excretion of HCO_3^-.
3. Hyperglycemia has been associated with the use of loop and thiazide diuretics. The mechanism is not clear.

BIBLIOGRAPHY

American Medical Association: *AMA Drug Evaluations Annual.* Chicago, American Medical Association, 1992.

American Thoracic Society, 2001.

Arky R: *Physician's Desk Reference,* ed 51. Montvale, NJ, Medical Economics, 1999.

Cummins RO: *Advanced Cardiac Life Support.* Dallas, American Heart Association, 1977.

Global Initiative for Chronic Obstructive Lung Disease (GOLD) Workshop Report: National Heart, Lung, and Blood Institute, Bethesda, Md, World Health Organization, 2001.

Guidelines 2000 for Cardiopulmonary Resuscitation and Emergency Cardiovascular Care: An International Consensus on Science. *Resuscitation* 46:1-447, 2000.

Hess DH, MacIntyre N, Mishoe S, et al: *Respiratory Care: Principles and Practices.* Philadelphia, WB Saunders, 2002.

Jacobi J, Fraser GL, Coursin DB, et al: Clinical practice guidelines for the sustained use of sedatives and analgesics in the critically ill. *Crit Care Med* 30:119-141, 2002.

Murray MJ, Cowen J, DeBlock H, et al: Clinical practice guidelines for sustained neuromuscular blockage in the adult critically ill patient. *Crit Care Med* 30:142-156, 2002.

Rau JL: *Respiratory Care Pharmacology,* ed 6. St. Louis, Mosby, 2002.

Stiell IG, Hebert PC, Wells GA, et al: Vasopressin versus epinephrine for inhospital cardiac arrest: a randomized controlled trial. *Lancet* 358:105-109, 2001.

Truitt T, Witko J, Halpern M: Levalbuterol compared to racemic albuterol. *Chest* 123:128-135, 2003.

Wenzel V, Krismer AC, Arntz HR, et al: A comparison of vasopressin and epinephrine for out-of-hospital cardiopulmonary resuscitation. *N Engl J Med* 350:105-113, 2004.

Wilkins RL, Stoller JK, Scanlon CL, et al: *Egan's Fundamentals of Respiratory Care,* ed 8. St. Louis, Mosby, 2003.

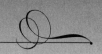

Chapter 18

Clinical Assessment of the Cardiopulmonary System

I. Clinical Assessment of the Cardiopulmonary System Requires a Number of Specific Steps.
   A. Review of the patient's chart:
      1. Present illness
      2. General and medical history
      3. Personal habits and lifestyle
      4. Occupational and environmental history
   B. Interview of the patient: Medical history:
      1. Patient identification
      2. Chief complaint
      3. History of present illness
      4. Medical history
      5. Family history
      6. Personal habits and lifestyle
      7. Occupational and environmental history
      8. Review of system
   C. Physical examination:
      1. Inspection
      2. Palpation
      3. Percussion
      4. Auscultation

II. Chart Review
   A. Before entering a patient's room his or her chart should be reviewed completely.
   B. This review should identify the reason for the patient's admission and the type of therapy he or she is to receive.
   C. An initial review of the chart helps to outline areas where the clinician would ask the patient questions and to help focus the physical examination.
   D. This initial review also frequently provides insights into the patient's history, his or her family history, and social and environmental issues that may affect his or her disease.

III. The Patient Interview: Medical History
   A. The interview provides unique information because it is the patients' prospective on their illness.

   B. The interview is designed to accomplish three related goals:
     1. Establish a rapport between patient and clinician.
     2. Obtain essential diagnostic information.
     3. Monitor changes in the patient's symptoms and response to therapy.
   C. Effective patient interviewing requires that the clinician pay attention to a number of professional issues as listed in Box 18-1.
   D. Questions during the interview can be structured in a number of different ways depending on the type of response the clinician desires. Table 18-1 lists a number of different types of questions.
   E. Occupational or environmental exposures are a key aspect of a patient interview. Table 18-2 lists a number of common exposures associated with pulmonary disease.
   F. Symptoms expressed as a concern by patients should be explored in detail. Box 18-2 lists specific questions that should be asked regarding a specific symptom.
   G. All interviews of patients receiving respiratory care should focus on the following symptoms and signs.
     1. Cough
       a. The most common symptom of cardiopulmonary disease.
       b. Is it dry or loose, productive or nonproductive?
       c. A dry nonproductive cough is typical of congestive heart failure (CHF) or pulmonary fibrosis.

BOX 18-1

Guidelines for Effective Patient Interviewing

1. Project a sense of undivided interest in the patient:
   - Provide for privacy and do not permit interruptions.
   - Review records and prepare materials before entering the room.
   - Listen and observe carefully.
   - Be attentive and respond to the patient's priorities, concerns, feelings, and comfort.
2. Establish your professional role during the introduction.
   - Dress and groom professionally.
   - Enter the room with a smile and unhurried manner.
   - Make immediate eye contact.
   - If the patient is well enough, introduce yourself with a firm handshake.
   - State your role and the purpose of your visit, and define the patient's involvement in the interaction.
3. Show your respect for the patient's beliefs, attitudes, and rights:
   - Be sure the patient is appropriately covered.
   - Position yourself so that eye contact is comfortable for the patient. (Ideally, patients should be sitting up, with their eye level at or slightly above yours).
   - Avoid standing at the foot of the bed or with your hand on the door because this may send the nonverbal message that you do not have time for the patient.

- Ask the patient's permission before moving any personal items or making adjustments in the room.
- Remember that the patient's dialog with you and his or her medical records are confidential.
- Be honest; never guess at an answer or provide information that you do not know. Do not provide information beyond your scope of practice; providing new information to the patient is the privilege and responsibility of the attending physician.
- Make no moral judgments about the patient; set your values for patient care according to the patient's values, beliefs, and priorities.
- Expect the patient to have an emotional response to illness and the health care environment.
- Listen, then clarify and teach, but never argue.
- Adjust the time, length, and content of the interview to your patient's needs.

4. Use a relaxed, conversational style:
   - Ask questions and make statements that communicate empathy.
   - Encourage the patient to express his or her concerns.
   - Expect and accept some periods of silence.
   - Close even the briefest interview by asking whether there is anything the patient needs or wants to discuss.
   - Tell the patient when you will return.

From Wilkins RL et al: *Egan's Fundamentals of Respiratory Care*, ed 8. St. Louis, Mosby, 2003.

TABLE **18-1**

Types of Questions in Taking a Medical History

Question Type	Description	Comments	Examples
Open-ended	Broad, general question about patient's symptom or illness	Allows patients to give history spontaneously without bias or influence from interviewer; patients direct discussion to whatever they want to cover first; can provide greatest amount of information; should generally be used first in interview	"Tell me about your shortness of breath." "What brings you to the clinic today?"
Focused	Interviewer defines area of inquiry more than in open-ended question or statement	Directs discussion into more specific area but still gives patients latitude in answering	"What treatment have you had for this condition in the past?" "What are the physical requirements of your job?"
Closed-ended	More specific question, which can generally be answered yes or no or by giving objective data such as dates, names, or numbers	Best way to obtain specific data but limits scope of information by restricting patients to individual items requested	"Have you ever had tuberculosis?" "How may puffs from your inhaler do you use in a given day?"
Compound	Two or more separate questions asked at once, without giving patients chance to respond to them individually	May confuse patients; prevents patients from giving answers to all components; induces patients to focus on last question in series; should not be used	"Tell me about yourself—how old are you, where do you live, and what do you do for a living?" "Have you ever smoked cigarettes, used drugs, worked with asbestos, or been exposed to tuberculosis?"
Leading	Interviewer phrases questions so as to lead patient in a particular direction in answering	Reflects interviewer's bias; tends to produce inaccurate, unreliable answer; should not be used	"You're feeling better today, aren't you?" "You've never used drugs, have you?"

From Pierson DJ, Kacmarek RM: *Foundations of Respiratory Care.* New York, Churchill Livingstone, 1992.

    d. A loose, productive cough is often associated with bronchitis and asthma.
    e. The most common cause of acute cough is viral infection.
    f. Chronic coughing is associated with asthma, postnasal drip, chronic bronchitis, and gastroesophageal reflux.
  2. Sputum production
    a. Sputum containing pus is purulent.
    b. Purulent sputum is thick, colored, and sticky.
    c. Clear and thick sputum is mucoid.
    d. Recent changes in the quantity, color, or viscosity of sputum are often signs of infection.
  3. Hemoptysis
    a. Defined as coughing up blood or blood-streaked sputum.

TABLE **18-2**

TABLE **18-2**

Common Occupational or Environmental Exposures Associated with Pulmonary Disease

Occupation or Activity	Exposure	Disease
Asbestos mining/milling/ manufacture; pipe fitting; shipbuilding/ship fitting; insulation, construction, demolition, living with someone employed in any of the above	Asbestos	Lung cancer, asbestosis, malignant mesothelioma, nonmalignant inflammatory pleural effusion
Hard-rock mining, quarrying, stone cutting, abrasive industries, foundry work, sandblasting	Crystalline quartz (silica)	Silicosis
Coal mining	Coal dust	Coal workers' pneumoconiosis
Farming, grain handling	Grain dust	Chronic bronchitis, chronic obstructive pulmonary disease
Farming, animal attendants	Moldy hay (spores of thermophilic actinomycetes [fungus])	Hypersensitivity pneumonitis (farmer's lung)
Cotton/flax/hemp workers, textile industry	Cotton dust	Byssinosis
Pigeon breeding, bird handling	Proteins derived from parakeets, budgerigars, pigeons, chickens, turkeys (avian droppings or feathers)	Hypersensitivity pneumonitis (e.g., pigeon-breeders' lung), bird-fanciers' lung
Woodworking, lumber industry	Wood dust, *Alternaria* (fungus),Western red cedar, oak, others	Hypersensitivity pneumonitis, woodworker's lung, occupational asthma

From Pierson DJ, Kacmarek RM: *Foundations of Respiratory Care.* New York, Churchill Livingstone, 1992.

BOX 18-2

What, Where, When, and How: Ten Questions to Ask a Patient About a Pain or Other Symptom

1. What does it feel like?
   Have the patient use own words in describing the character of the symptoms (e.g., dyspnea or pain).
2. Where is it?
   If the symptom is a pain, ask the patient to localize it as precisely as possible.
3. Where else does it go?
   Inquire about radiation of the pain to other parts of the body.
4. How bad is it?
   If possible, have the patient quantitate the symptom (e.g., by using a hypothetical scale of 1 of 10, with 10 being the worst discomfort ever experienced).
5. How long does it last?
   Again quantitate as much as possible. Does the pain come and go or is it constant? Is it always the same?

6. When does it occur?
   Ask about associations with time of day, physical activity, body position, emotion or stress, and any relationship to eating or drinking.
7. What brings it on or makes it worse?
   What would the patient do who wanted to bring on the pain or make it worse?
8. What relieves it or makes it better?
   Ask about any medication or activity that the patient has noted improves the symptom.
9. How does it affect you?
   What activities are prevented or limited by the symptom? Quantitate if possible. Ask the patient to compare present limitations with past performance or present capabilities with those of peers.
10. What else is associated with it?
    Inquire about other phenomena (e.g., fever, diaphoresis, dyspnea) that occur with the symptom in question.

From Pierson DJ, Kacmarek RM: *Foundations of Respiratory Care.* New York, Churchill Livingstone, 1992.

    b. Hematemesis is vomiting of blood, blood from the gastrointestinal tract.

    c. Massive hemoptysis is >300 ml.

    d. Nonmassive hemoptysis is seen in tuberculosis, lung cancer, and pulmonary embolism.

    e. Blood-streaked sputum is often associated with infection.

    f. Massive hemoptysis is seen in lung abscess, bronchiectasis, and trauma.

4. Pedal edema

    a. Swelling of lower extremities

    b. Normally associated with heart failure, usually right-sided failure.

    c. May be severe enough to result in "pitting" when compressed.

5. Jugular vein distention

    a. With the head of the bed elevated 45 degrees, venous distention >3 to 4 cm above the sternal angle is abnormal.

    b. Associated with right-sided heart failure.

6. Dyspnea

    a. Patient-perceived shortness of breath.

    b. Occurs when the patient's sense of the work of breathing exceeds that associated with the effort performed.

    c. Orthopnea is dyspnea in the supine or lying position and is associated with heart failure.

    d. Platypnea is dyspnea in the upright position seen in patients with right to left intracardiac shunts associated with congenital cardiac disease and venous to arterial shunts in the lung related to severe lung disease or chronic liver disease. Orthodeoxia is oxygen desaturation in the upright position.

7. Chest pain

    a. Chest pain is usually classified as pleuritic or nonpleuritic.

    b. Pleuritic chest pain is usually located laterally and posteriorly, worsens with a deep breath, and is described as sharp and stabbing.

    c. Pleuritic pain is associated with inflammation of the pleura as a result of pneumonia or pulmonary embolism.

    d. Nonpleuritic chest pain is located in the center of the chest and may radiate to the shoulder or back. It is not affected by breathing and is described as a dull ache or pressure.

    e. The most common cause of nonpleuritic chest pain is angina, which is associated with coronary artery disease.

    f. Nonpleuritic chest pain is also associated with gastroesophageal reflex, esophageal spasm, chest wall pain (costochondritis), and gallbladder disease.

8. Cyanosis

    a. A bluish discoloration of the skin and mucous membrane caused by the presence of at least 5 g of deoxygenated hemoglobin.

    b. May be either peripheral or central.

    c. Typically seen in association with hypoxemia in the absence of anemia.

9. Clubbing

    a. Diffuse bulbous enlargement of terminal phalanges of the fingers and toes.

    b. Occurs as a result of a buildup of fibroelastic soft tissue in the nail bed.

    c. Clubbing is usually asymptomatic and of an unknown mechanism.

    d. Normally seen in:

        (1) Lung cancer

        (2) Bronchiectasis

        (3) Cystic fibrosis

        (4) Lung abscess

        (5) Empyema

        (6) Interstitial lung disease

        (7) Cyanotic congenital heart disease

    10. Stridor
       a. A harsh, high-pitched sound, normally during inspiration.
       b. Associated with partial upper airway obstruction.
    11. Wheezing
       a. A high-pitched musical sound produced when a patient breathes.
       b. Occurs as a result of lower airway narrowing.
       c. May occur during any portion of the respiratory cycle.
    12. Level of consciousness
       a. Is the patient oriented to person, place, and time?
       b. Box 18-3 lists the terms with their definition of various levels of consciousness.
       c. If the patient is falling asleep during the interview, his or her CO_2 level may be elevated.

IV. Vital Signs
  A. Temperature: An indicator of metabolic rate.
    1. Normal temperature
       a. Oral: 97.0 to 99.5° F or 36.5 to 37.5° C.
       b. Axillary: 96.7 to 98.5° F or 35.9 to 36.9° C.
       c. Rectal: 98.7 to 100.5° F or 37.1 to 38.1° C.
       d. Ear: Essentially the same as rectal if measured correctly.
    2. Hyperthermia (fever): In the hospitalized patient it is normally indicative of infection, which is usually bacterial but may be viral.
       a. Fever increases overall metabolic rate:
          (1) For every 1° C increase in body temperature, O_2 consumption and CO_2 production increase by 10%.
          (2) Fever combined with hypoxemia may result in poor tissue oxygenation.
    3. Hypothermia is rare in hospitalized patients but may be a result of:
       a. Severe head injury affecting the hypothalamus
       b. Hypothyroidism

BOX 18-3

Levels of Consciousness

Confused
The patient:
- Exhibits slight decrease of consciousness
- Has slow mental responses
- Has decreased or dulled perception
- Has incoherent thoughts

Delirous
The patient:
- Is easily agitated
- Is irritable
- Exhibits hallucinations

Lethargic
The patient:
- Is sleepy
- Arouses easily
- Responds appropriately when aroused

Obtunded
The patient:
- Awakens only with difficulty
- Responds appropriately when aroused

Stuporous
The patient:
- Does not awaken completely
- Has decreased mental and physical activity
- Responds to pain and exhibits deep tendon reflexes
- Responds slowly to verbal stimuli

Comatose
The patient:
- Is unconscious
- Does not respond to stimuli
- Does not move voluntarily
- Exhibits possible signs of upper motor neuron dysfunction, such as Babinski's reflex or hyperreflexia
- Loses reflexes with deep or prolonged coma

From Wilkins RL et al: *Egan's Fundamentals of Respiratory Care*, ed 8. St. Louis, Mosby, 2003.

        c.   Exposure to cold (emergency room)
   4. Hypothermia decreases O_2 consumption and CO_2 production.
        a.   Shivering during hypothermia generates heat and consumes energy.
        b.   Peripheral vasoconstriction minimizes heat loss secondary to convection.
B. Pulse: A general reflection of pump capabilities of the heart.
   1. Heart rate in adults is normally 60 to 100 beats/min.
        a.   Heart rates >100 beats/min (tachycardia) may be a reflection of the following:
            (1) Fear
            (2) Anxiety
            (3) Low blood pressure
            (4) Anemia
            (5) Fever
            (6) Hypoxemia
            (7) Response to certain medications (e.g., sympathomimetics)
        b.   Heart rates <60 beats/min (bradycardia):
            (1) Are much less common than tachycardia.
            (2) May be a response of a diseased myocardium to severe stress.
            (3) May be a response to certain medications.
                (a) Parasympathomimetics (e.g., atropine)
                (b) β_1 Blockers (e.g., propranolol [Inderal])
                (c) Digitalis
   2. Rhythm: A regular rhythm should be noted. Irregular rhythm may indicate:
        a.   Premature ventricular contractions
        b.   Premature atrial contractions
        c.   Heart blocks
   3. Strength: The force of the beat should be easily noted.
        a.   A weak, thready pulse is normally associated with hypotension.
        b.   A strong bounding pulse may be associated with hypertension.
        c.   Pulsus paradoxus or paradoxical pulse: A decrease in pulse strength during spontaneous inhalation; frequently a result of changes in auto-positive end-expiratory pressure levels during inspiration and expiration.
        d.   Pulsus alternans: An alternating succession of strong and weak pulses, suggestive of left-sided heart failure.
C. Blood pressure: The force exerted by the arterial pressure against the wall of the artery.
   1. Systolic pressure is normally 95 to 139 mm Hg (between 130 and 139 mm Hg currently referred to as prehypertension) in the adult.
   2. Diastolic pressure is normally 60 to 89 mm Hg in the adult.
   3. Pulse pressure is the difference between the systolic and diastolic pressure, normally 35 to 40 mm Hg. If it is <25 to 30 mm Hg, the peripheral pulse is difficult to palpate. This pressure provides the gradient for peripheral perfusion.
   4. Hypertension is a pressure ≥140/90 mm Hg and may be reflective of:
        a.   Hypoxemia
        b.   Increased intracranial pressure
        c.   CHF (right sided)
        d.   Fluid overload
        e.   A response to medication (e.g., sympathomimetics)
   5. Prehypertension, a systolic pressure of 130 to 140 mm Hg, is now considered a precursor to hypertension and requires a change in lifestyle and in some cases treatment.
   6. Hypotension is a pressure <95/60 mm Hg and may be reflective of:
        a.   Fluid depletion
        b.   CHF (left sided)
        c.   Peripheral vasodilation (sepsis)
        d.   A response to medication (e.g., vasodilators)
        e.   Positive pressure ventilation
        f.   Positive end-expiratory pressure

D. Respiratory rate
   1. Normal adult respiratory rate is 12 to 18 breaths/min.
   2. Tachypnea rates >18 breaths/min may be a result of:
      a. Hypoxemia
      b. Fever
      c. Metabolic acidosis
      d. Fear
      e. Anxiety
      f. Interstitial alveolar edema stimulating type J receptors
   3. Bradypnea rates <12 breaths/min may be a result of:
      a. Hypothermia
      b. Head trauma
      c. Narcotic overdose
      d. Sedative overdose

V. **Physical Assessment of the Chest**
   A. Chest assessment includes the following (sequentially performed as listed):
      1. Inspection
      2. Palpation
      3. Percussion
      4. Auscultation
   B. Inspection is the observation of the patient's chest configuration and pattern of breathing. During inspection, the following should be evaluated:
      1. Position
         a. Is the patient sitting comfortably, or does he or she require support to ventilate?
         b. The position assumed provides information about the patient's use of accessory muscles of ventilation or the presence of pain.
            (1) Use of accessory muscles results in positioning to support their use (i.e., sitting with elbows on bedside table, leaning forward).
            (2) If pain is present, the point of pain will be favored, and a position to minimize movement of the affected area is assumed.
      2. Chest configuration
         a. Anteroposterior to lateral diameter ratio is normally 1:2. If the patient is barrel-chested, the ratio approaches 1:1, a common finding in patients with chronic obstructive pulmonary disease (COPD).
         b. Bony deformities of the thorax
            (1) Kyphosis: Posterior curvature of the thoracic vertebral column.
            (2) Scoliosis: Lateral curvature of the spinal column.
            (3) Kyphoscoliosis: Combination of kyphosis and scoliosis.
            (4) Pectus carinatum: Protrusion of the sternum anteriorly.
            (5) Pectus excavatum: Depression of the sternum.
            (6) Any thoracic deformity may result in restriction of ventilation.
      3. Ventilatory pattern
         a. Sequence of normal lung expansion
            (1) Abdominal protrusion
            (2) Lateral costal expansion
            (3) Upper chest expansion
            (4) Abnormal sequencing may be a result of underlying lung disease or an increase in cardiopulmonary stress.
               (a) Paradoxical breathing: Abdomen retracted during inspiration, usually indicative of fatigue of the diaphragm.
               (b) Respiratory alternans: The periodic change from a normal ventilatory pattern to a paradoxical pattern, indicative of impending or early fatigue of the diaphragm.
         b. Uniform bilateral chest expansion

(1) The chest cage should move equally bilaterally.
(2) Splinting of an area of the chest may be a result of:
    (a) Pain
    (b) Pneumonia
    (c) Atelectasis
    (d) Pleural effusion
    (e) Pneumothorax

c. Use of accessory muscles of ventilation
(1) Normal inspiration requires only contraction of the diaphragm and external intercostals.
(2) Exhalation is passive.
(3) Use of accessory muscles is an indication of increased work of breathing (see Section VI).

d. Acute cardiopulmonary stress normally results in an increased ventilatory rate.

e. Patients with chronic obstructive lung disease may have a decreased ventilatory rate, whereas patients with chronic restrictive lung disease may have an increased ventilatory rate.

f. Pursed lipped breathing is indicative of chronic airway obstruction.

g. Inspiratory/expiratory ratios should be about 1:2.

h. The presence of audible wheezes, crackles, or rhonchi is indicative of secretions or bronchospasm.

C. Palpation is the touching of the chest to evaluate movement and underlying lung function.
1. Symmetric movement of the thoracic cage.
2. Tone of ventilatory muscles.
3. Presence of consolidation, pneumothorax, atelectasis, or pleural effusion. These may cause a shift in the mediastinum. Palpation of the trachea at the suprasternal notch identifies shifting.
   a. Pneumothorax shifts the trachea and lungs away from the area of the pneumothorax.
   b. Consolidation and atelectasis shifts the trachea and lungs toward the affected area.
   c. Unilateral pleural effusion shifts the trachea and lungs away from the effusion. A bilateral effusion may not affect position.
4. Fremitus: The vibration produced over the thoracic cage by the conduction of sound waves.
   a. Evaluation of fremitus is performed bilaterally to compare the tactile vibrations between sides of the chest.
   b. Normally fremitus is equal throughout all lung fields; however, it may be increased over the apex of the right lung.
   c. Fremitus is increased if lung density is increased (e.g., pneumonia or consolidation).
   d. Fremitus is decreased if atelectasis from obstruction is present or if fluid or air accumulates in the pleural space.
   e. A generalized or diffuse decrease in fremitus is noted in those with COPD and muscular or obese chest walls.
5. Subcutaneous emphysema: If it is present, an air leak has allowed gas to enter the tissue.

D. Percussion is the production of audible and tactile vibrations over the chest by tapping the chest wall (Figure 18-1).
1. If lung tissue is normal, percussion produces a moderately low-pitched sound.
2. The presence of increased air in the thoracic cavity produces a lower-pitched, more muffled drumlike sound, frequently referred to as *hyperresonance*.
3. Decreased air in the thoracic cavity, consolidation, atelectasis, or a pleural effusion causes the percussion note to be higher pitched but dull or flat.
4. Percussion should be performed over all lung fields following a specific pattern as illustrated in Figure 18-2.

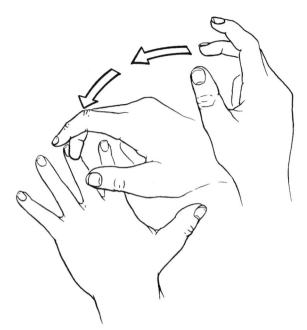

FIG. 18-1 Chest percussion technique.

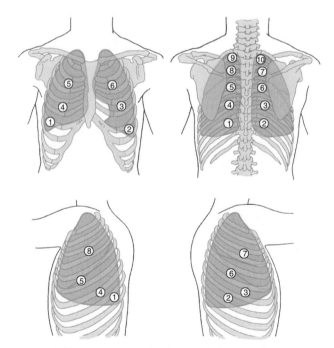

FIG. 18-2 Sequencing for auscultation technique.

E. Auscultation is the evaluation of breath sounds with a stethoscope (see Figure 18-2).
   1. Normal breath sounds (Figure 18-3)
      a. Over the trachea, the sound is loud with a tubular quality, referred to as *bronchial* or *tracheal breath sounds*.
      b. Auscultation of the parenchyma reveals a soft muffled sound referred to as *vesicular breath sounds*. These are usually heard during inspiration but only minimally during exhalation.

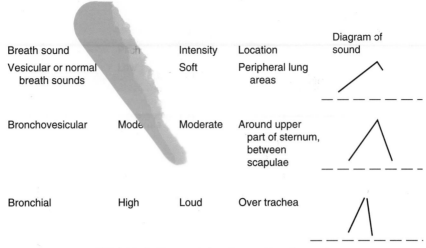

Breath sound		Intensity	Location	Diagram of sound
Vesicular or normal breath sounds		Soft	Peripheral lung areas	
Bronchovesicular	Mode	Moderate	Around upper part of sternum, between scapulae	
Bronchial	High	Loud	Over trachea	

FIG. 18-3 Characteristics of normal breath sounds.

    c. The sound heard over the airways is termed *bronchovesicular*. It is softer than bronchial breath sounds and lower in pitch, being heard during inspiration and expiration.

  2. Adventitious or abnormal breath sounds (Tables 18-3 and 18-4)

    a. *Crackles (rales)*: A discontinuous sound (<20 msec) that is perceived as a wet, crackling, bubbling sound associated with gas moving through liquid. Normally they are heard during:

      (1) Pulmonary edema

      (2) CHF

      (3) The opening of collapsed airways during inspiration

      (4) In the presence of excessive secretions

    b. *Rhonchi*: A continuous sound (>25 msec) that is low in pitch and normally indicative of secretions in large airways. In patients who can successfully mobilize their own secretions, rhonchi clear with coughing.

    c. *Wheezes*: A continuous sound (>25 msec) that is high pitched and normally indicative of bronchospasm or mucosal edema in medium to larger airways. Wheezes do not clear with coughing.

    d. *Pleural friction rub*: A creaking or grating sound as a result of inflamed pleural surfaces rubbing together during breathing.

VI. Work of Breathing

  A. During normal breathing the muscles of ventilation consume 5% to 10% of the total oxygen consumed to perform the work of breathing.

  B. The effort required to perform the work of breathing depends on the following:

    1. Airway resistance (increased; increases work)

    2. Compliance (decreased; increases work)

TABLE 18-3

Recommended Terminology for Lung Sounds Versus Terminology in Other Publications

Recommended Term	Classification	Terms Used in Other Publications
Crackles	Discontinuous	Rales
		Crepitations
Wheezes	High-pitched, continuous	Sibilant rales
		Musical rales
		Sibilant rhonchi
	Low-pitched, continuous	Rhonchi
		Sonorous rales

From Wilkins RL, Krier SJ, Sheldon RL: *Clinical Assessment in Respiratory Care,* ed 4. St. Louis, Mosby, 2000.

TABLE **18-4**			

Application of Adventitious Lung Sounds

Lung Sounds	Possible Mechanism	Characteristics	Causes
Wheezes	Rapid airflow through obstructed airways caused by bronchospasm, mucosal edema	High-pitched most often occur during exhalation	Asthma, congestive heart failure, bronchitis
Stridor	Rapid airflow through obstructed airway caused by inflammation	High pitched, often occurs during inhalation	Croup, epiglottitis, bronchitis
Crackles			
Inspiratory and expiratory	Excess airway secretions moving with airflow	Coarse and often clear with cough	Bronchitis, respiratory infections
Early inspiratory	Sudden opening of proximal bronchi	Scanty, transmitted to mouth, not affected by cough	Bronchitis, emphysema, asthma
Late inspiratory	Sudden opening of peripheral airways	Diffuse, fine, occur initially in the dependent regions	Atelectasis, pneumonia, pulmonary edema, fibrosis

From Wilkins RL, Krider SJ, Sheldon RL: *Clinical Assessment in Respiratory Care,* ed 4. St. Louis, Mosby, 2000.

    3. Respiratory rate (increased; increases work)
    4. Tidal volume (increase and decrease may increase work)
    5. Use of accessory muscles (increases work)
    6. Ventilatory pattern (abnormal patterns increase work)
  C. Normally the ventilatory pattern a patient assumes is that which requires the least work.
    1. Figure 18-4, *A,* relates the components of the work of breathing to the respiratory rate and tidal volume.
    2. Resistance work refers to the amount of work necessary to overcome nonelastic resistance to ventilation. If nonelastic resistance were the only force opposing ventilation, the ideal ventilatory pattern would be a slow rate and a large tidal volume.
    3. Elastic work refers to the amount of work necessary to overcome elastic resistance. If elastic resistance were the only force opposing ventilation, a rapid ventilatory rate with a small tidal volume would be ideal.
    4. Total work refers to actual work expended with varying ventilatory rates and tidal volumes. Note the ideal rate is approximately 12 to 18 breaths/min with an ideal tidal volume of approximately 6 ml/kg predicted body weight.
    5. Figure 18-4, *B,* illustrates the effect an increase in elastic work has on ventilatory pattern.
      a. Because elastic resistance to ventilation has increased, the least amount of work is accomplished at a high ventilatory rate and a small tidal volume.
      b. With most acute pulmonary diseases there is an increase in elastic work; therefore, ventilatory rates increase and tidal volumes decrease.
    6. If resistance work were increased, the total work curve in Figure 18-4, *A,* would shift to the left.
      a. The ideal respiratory pattern would produce a slow rate with large tidal volumes. This pattern minimizes the effect of the increased resistance.
      b. This would be the ideal ventilatory pattern for patients in asthmatic attacks. However, fear and anxiety frequently result in the opposite pattern (fast and shallow) being assumed.
    7. Refer to Chapter 5 for quantification of work of breathing.

 VII. Ventilatory Reserve
  A. Ventilatory reserve is the ability of the organism to respond to increased levels of cardiopulmonary stress.

A

Normal Compliance

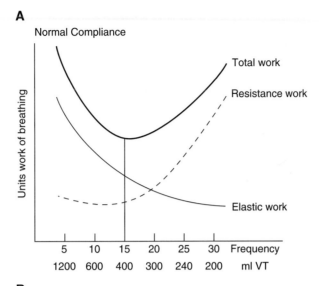

B

Decreased Compliance

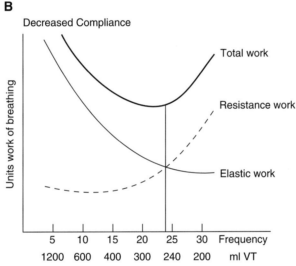

FIG. 18-4 A, Graphic representation of total work of breathing when minute ventilation is unchanged but ventilatory pattern (tidal volume and frequency) is varied. Note that for any minute ventilation there is a ventilatory pattern that requires minimal work. Total work is the summation of resistance work (nonelastic resistance) and elastic work (elastic resistance). **B,** If elastic work is increased, the pattern of ventilation at which the minute volume can be achieved with minimal work is dramatically altered. Work of breathing is a major factor determining ventilatory pattern.

    B. During normal breathing, the efficiency of the ventilatory muscles is poor. Approximately 90% of the oxygen consumed to perform the work of breathing is lost as heat.

    C. The efficiency of the ventilatory muscles is further reduced with chronic pulmonary disease and with an increased minute ventilation.

    D. Figure 18-5, *A*, depicts the relationship between minute volume and percentage of oxygen consumed for breathing in patients without chronic pulmonary disease (solid line) and patients with chronic pulmonary disease (dotted line).

        1. The percentage of oxygen consumed for breathing markedly increases as minute volume increases.

        2. In patients with chronic pulmonary disease the percentage of oxygen consumed for breathing at basal level is already increased (20%). With increased minute volume there

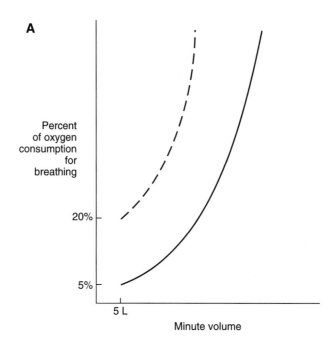

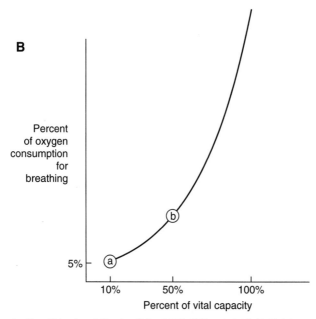

FIG. 18-5 A, The work of breathing in relation to vital capacity (VC; see text). **B,** Point *a* represents a tidal volume (V_T) of 500 ml with a VC of 5 L; point *b* represents a V_T of 500 ml with a VC of 1 L.

is a tremendous increase in oxygen consumption. These patients have markedly lower reserves than patients without chronic pulmonary disease.

E. Figure 18-5, *B*, illustrates the relationship between percentage of oxygen consumed for breathing and the percentage of the vital capacity (VC) that is the tidal volume.

1. As the tidal volume becomes a greater percentage of the VC, the amount of oxygen consumed for breathing increases.

2. When the tidal volume is 50% of the VC, limited ventilatory reserves exist, and the likelihood of sustained spontaneous ventilation is questionable.

VIII. Vital Capacity/Maximum Inspiratory Pressure

A. A normal VC is approximately 70 to 90 ml/kg of ideal body weight.

B. VCs are frequently used as an estimate of the patient's ventilatory reserve.

C. If the VC is >15 ml/kg of ideal body weight, it is assumed that the individual has the capability to respond to increased levels of cardiopulmonary stress.

D. However, if the VC is <10 ml/kg, prolonged sustained spontaneous ventilation is questionable. This individual has virtually no reserves.

E. At VCs between 10 and 15 ml/kg, reserves are marginal, and appropriate monitoring should be instituted.

F. Maximum inspiratory pressure (MIP) is also a parameter used to assess ventilatory reserves.

G. If the MIP is more negative than −30 cm H_2O in a 20-second period and the patient has normal lungs and is recovering from anesthesia, neuromuscular or neurologic disease, or an overdose, sustained spontaneous ventilation is probable.

H. In patients with chronic pulmonary disease or acute respiratory failure associated with multiorgan system failure, the use of a −30 cm H_2O range for MIP becomes less reliable.

   1. In this population, MIP or VC values provide a daily guide to ventilatory muscle capability but are unreliable as a specific indicator of spontaneous ventilatory capability.

   2. The measurement of MIP before and after weaning trials provides information on the development of exhaustion. A lower value after a weaning trial compared with initial values indicates exhaustion and an inability to continue spontaneous breathing.

I. During the measurement of MIP, the diaphragm must be at its resting level for maximum performance. Thus the greater the length of the diaphragmatic muscle fibers (smaller lung volume), the greater their contractile force.

   1. In the intensive care unit, evaluation of MIP is difficult if a one-way valve system is not used (Figure 18-6).

   2. The use of a one-way valve allows the patient to exhale after each attempted inspiration, resulting in a lower lung volume and greater force generation.

   3. Normally inspiratory occlusion is maintained for 20 seconds unless adverse reaction occurs.

      a. Cardiac arrhythmias

      b. Tachycardia, bradycardia

      c. Arterial desaturation

   4. MIP generally should be measured only in patients with stable cardiopulmonary status who can withstand the stress.

IX. Rapid Shallow Breathing Index

A. Normally the relationship between respiratory rate and tidal volume in liters is approximately 20 to 60 in the average adult.

B. This relationship has been used to determine whether a patient is ready to be discontinued from ventilatory support.

C. In critically ill patients a rapid shallow breathing index (RSBI) <105 indicates a high probability of being able to breathe unassisted.

D. An RSBI ≥105 indicates ventilatory support is still required.

E. It is critical that the RSBI be determined the same way it was studied if it is to be maximally predictive.

   1. Patient is disconnected from the ventilator.

   2. Allowed to breathe room air unsupported.

   3. Respiratory rate is counted for a full minute.

   4. Tidal volume is measured with a pneumotachograph and mask or mouthpiece for a full minute and the average determined.

   5. Respiratory rate is then divided by average tidal volume expressed in liters.

X. Assessment of Peripheral Perfusion

A. Adequacy of peripheral perfusion can be estimated by:

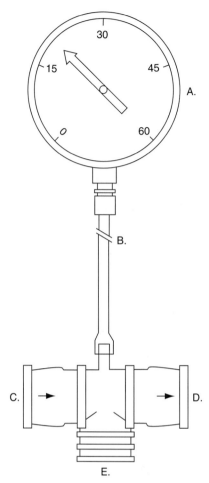

FIG. 18-6 Technical setup for performance of maximum inspiratory pressure measurement. **A,** Pressure manometer. **B,** Connecting tubing. **C,** One-way valve. **D,** One way-valve. **E,** Patient connection of Briggs T piece.

      1. Sensorium
      2. Urinary output
      3. Capillary refill
      4. Skin turgor
      5. Cyanosis
      6. Peripheral pulses
      7. Skin temperature
    B. Sensorium
      1. Confusion, agitation, and disorientation are all signs of cerebral hypoxia that can be caused by decreased oxygen carriage or decreased cerebral perfusion.
      2. Somnolence and drowsiness are signs of increased arterial P_{CO_2} levels.
    C. Urinary output
      1. Normal urinary output is approximately 40 to 60 ml/hr.
      2. Decreased urinary output is frequently a sign of decreased peripheral perfusion.
    D. Capillary refill decreases as peripheral perfusion decreases.
    E. Skin turgor also decreases as peripheral perfusion decreases.
    F. Cyanosis
    G. Thready, faint, or distant peripheral pulses are noted as peripheral perfusion decreases.

  XI. **Physical Signs Associated with Common Abnormal Pulmonary Pathology (Table 18-5)**

TABLE 18-5

Physical Signs of Pulmonary Abnormalities

Abnormality	Initial Impression	Inspection	Palpation	Percussion	Auscultation	Possible Causes
Acute airway obstruction	Appears acutely ill	Use of accessory muscles	Reduced expansion	Increased resonance	Expiratory wheezing	Asthma, bronchitis
Chronic airway obstruction	Appears chronically ill	Increased anteroposterior diameter, use of accessory muscles	Reduced expansion	Increased resonance	Diffuse reduction in breath sounds, early inspiratory crackles	Chronic bronchitis, emphysema
Consolidation	May appear acutely ill	Inspiratory lag	Increased fremitus	Dull note	Bronchial breath sounds, crackles	Pneumonia, tumor
Pneumothorax	May appear acutely ill	Unilateral expansion	Decreased fremitus	Increased resonance	Absent breath sounds	Rib fracture, open wound
Pleural effusion	May appear acutely ill	Unilateral expansion	Absent fremitus	Dull note	Absent breath sounds	Congestive heart failure
Left bronchial obstruction	Appears acutely ill	Unilateral expansion	Absent fremitus	Dull note	Absent breath sounds	Mucous plug
Diffuse interstitial fibrosis	Often normal	Rapid shallow breathing	Often normal, increased fremitus	Slight decrease in resonance	Late inspiratory crackles	Chronic exposure to inorganic dust
Acute upper airway obstruction	Appears acutely ill	Labored breathing	Often normal	Often normal	Inspiratory/expiratory stridor	Epiglottitis, croup, foreign body aspiration

From Wilkins RL, Krider SJ, Sheldon RL: *Clinical Assessment in Respiratory Care*, ed 4. St. Louis, Mosby, 2000.

XII. Laboratory Assessment in Cardiopulmonary Disease

    A. Hematology

        1. Complete red blood cell count (CBC)

            a. Red blood cell (RBC) count (normal levels)

                (1) Men: 4.8 to $6.0 \times 10^6/mm^3$

                (2) Women: 4.1 to $5.1 \times 10^6/mm^3$

            b. Hemoglobin (normal levels)

                (1) Men: 13 to 16 g/dl or g%

                (2) Women: 12 to 14 g/dl or g%

            c. Hematocrit (normal levels)

                (1) Men: 40% to 54%

                (2) Women: 37% to 47%

            d. White blood cell (WBC) count: 5,000 to $10,000/mm^3$

            e. Differential of WBCs

                (1) Neutrophils: 50% to 75%

                    (a) Segmented neutrophils: 90% to 100% of total neutrophils

                    (b) Bands: 0% to 10% of total neutrophils

                (2) Eosinophils: 2% to 4%

                (3) Basophils: <0.5%

                (4) Lymphocytes: 20% to 40%

                (5) Monocytes: 3% to 8%

            f. Platelet count: 200,000 to $350,000/mm^3$

        2. Anemia: A below-normal quantity of hemoglobin, RBC count, or hematocrit and greatly decreases oxygen-carrying capacity. It may be a result of:

            a. Hemorrhage (bleeding)

            b. Deficiency in cell formation

            c. Abnormal cell formation

        3. Polycythemia: An increase in hemoglobin, RBC count, or hematocrit. It may result from:

            a. Chronic hypoxemia

            b. Altered production by bone marrow

        4. Abnormalities in WBC count and their differential are a result of infection, allergic reaction, or leukemia.

            a. An increase in overall WBC count (i.e., leukocytosis) is normally noted in bacterial infections.

            b. A decrease in overall WBC count (i.e., leukopenia) is normally noted in leukemia, radiation therapy, and chemotherapy.

            c. Neutrophilia (increased neutrophils): A common response to stress and the body's first response to:

                (1) Bacterial infection

                (2) Inflammation

            d. A *leftward shift* of the neutrophils: Increased levels of bands (immature neutrophils) as a result of stress. The greater the stress, the greater the percent bands.

            e. Eosinophilia: An increase in the number of eosinophils, usually a result of:

                (1) Allergic reaction

                (2) Parasitic infection

            f. Lymphocytosis: An increase in the number of lymphocytes, usually a result of a viral infection.

            g. Monocytosis: An increase in the number of monocytes, usually a result of:

                (1) Chronic infections

                (2) Malignancies

            h. Basophilia: An increase in the number of basophiles usually seen in:

                (1) Leukemia

                (2) Other myeloproliferative disorders

(a) Polycythemia vera

(b) Essential thrombocythemia

(c) Myelofibrosis

5. Platelet count

   a. Platelets are necessary for normal coagulation of blood. If the platelet count is low, small skin hemorrhages are noted:

   (1) Petechiae

   (2) Ecchymoses

   (3) Oozing from mucosal surfaces

   b. Platelet counts are reduced by:

   (1) Various drug therapies

   (2) Bone marrow diseases

   (3) Idiopathic thrombocytopenic purpura (ITP)

   (4) Disseminating intravascular coagulation (DIC)

   c. An increase in platelets may be a result of:

   (1) Stress

   (2) Bone marrow disease

   d. Increased platelet levels increase the likelihood of thrombosis (blood clots).

B. Coagulation studies

1. Four distinct tests generally are used to evaluate the tendency of blood to clot.

   a. Bleeding time

   b. Platelet count (see Section XII-A.5)

   c. Activated partial thromboplastin time (APTT)

   d. Prothrombin time (PT)

2. Bleeding time: Evaluates the ability of small skin vessels to constrict and evaluates the function of platelets. Normal time is up to 6 minutes.

3. APTT: Evaluates the amount of time it takes plasma to form a fibrin clot once the body's intrinsic clotting pathways are activated. Normal time is 32 to 51 seconds.

4. PT: Evaluates the amount of time it takes extrinsic blood factors to form a clot once activated. Normal PT is 12 to 15 seconds.

5. All times are lengthened during hemophilia.

6. APTT: Monitored during heparin therapy.

7. PT: Monitored during warfarin sodium (Coumadin) therapy.

C. Electrolytes (see Chapter 14)

D. Blood urea nitrogen and creatinine levels and urinalysis (see Chapter 13).

BIBLIOGRAPHY

Barnes T: *Respiratory Care Practice.* Chicago, Year Book Medical Publishers, 1988.

Beachey W: *Respiratory Care Anatomy and Physiology: Foundations for Clinical Practice.* St. Louis, Mosby, 1998.

Burton GG, Hodgkin JE, Ward JJ: *Respiratory Care: A Guide to Clinical Practice,* ed 4. Philadelphia, JB Lippincott, 1997.

Hess D, MacIntyre N, Mishoe S, et al: *Respiratory Care: Principles and Practice.* St. Louis, Mosby, 2002.

Hicks GH: *Cardiopulmonary Anatomy and Physiology.* Philadelphia, WB Saunders, 2000.

Kacmarek RM, Chapman M, Palazzo P, et al: Comparison of two techniques for the determination of maximal inspiratory pressure (MIP) in mechanically ventilated patients. *Respir Care* 34:868-878, 1989.

Pierson DJ, Kacmarek RM: *Foundations of Respiratory Care.* New York, Churchill Livingstone, 1992.

Shapiro BA, Harrison RA, Kacmarek RM, et al: *Clinical Application of Respiratory Care,* ed 4. Chicago, Year Book Medical Publishers, 1990.

Wilkins RL, Sheldon RL, Krider SJ: *Clinical Assessment in Respiratory Care.* St. Louis, Mosby, 1985.

Wilkins RL, Stoller JK, Scanlan CL: *Egan's Fundamentals of Respiratory Care,* ed 8. St. Louis, Mosby, 2003.

Chapter 19

Pulmonary Function Testing

Pulmonary function tests (PFTs) provide measurements of airway function and mechanics, lung volumes, gas exchange, and cardiopulmonary exercise tolerance.

I. **Lung Volumes and Capacities**
   A. The gas in the respiratory system is divided into four lung volumes and four lung capacities.
      1. Lung volumes (Figure 19-1)
         a. Residual volume (RV): Volume of gas remaining in the lung after a maximal exhalation.
         b. Expiratory reserve volume (ERV): Volume of gas that can be exhaled after a normal exhalation.
         c. Tidal volume (V_T or TV): Volume of gas inspired during a normal inspiration.
         d. Inspiratory reserve volume (IRV): Volume of gas that can be inspired after a normal inspiration.
      2. Lung capacities are composed of two or more lung volumes.
         a. Total lung capacity (TLC): Volume of gas contained in the lung at maximum inspiration (RV + ERV + V_T + IRV).
         b. Inspiratory capacity (IC): Maximum volume of gas that can be inhaled after a normal exhalation (V_T + IRV).
         c. Vital capacity (VC): Maximum volume of gas that can be exhaled after a maximal inspiration (ERV + V_T + IRV).
         d. Functional residual capacity (FRC): Volume of gas that remains in the lung after a normal exhalation (RV + ERV).
   B. Normal lung volumes and capacities for a healthy young male with 1.7 m^2 body surface area (165 lb, 6 ft tall, 25 years old) are:
      1. TLC: 6.00 L
      2. VC: 4.80 L, approximately 80% of TLC
      3. IC: 3.60 L, approximately 60% of TLC
      4. FRC: 2.40 L, approximately 40% of TLC
      5. RV: 1.20 L, approximately 20% of TLC
      6. ERV: 1.20 L, approximately 20% of TLC
      7. V_T: 0.5 L, approximately 6.3 ml/kg of ideal body weight (10% of TLC)
      8. IRV: 3.1 L, approximately 50% to 55% of TLC
   C. All lung volumes and capacities depicted in Figure 19-1 can be measured by direct spirometry except:
      1. RV
      2. FRC
      3. TLC

II. **Spirometry Refers to Simple, Widely Used Tests That Measure VC and Its Subdivisions (Adapted from AARC Clinical Practice Guidelines)**
   A. Slow VC measurement (see Figure 19-1)

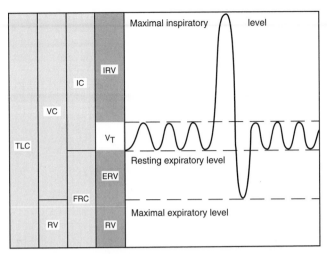

FIG. 19-1 Lung volumes and capacities. Diagrammatic representation of various lung compartments based on a typical spirogram. *TLC,* Total lung capacity; *VC,* vital capacity; *RV,* residual volume; *FRC,* functional residual capacity; *IC,* inspiratory capacity; V_T, tidal volume; *IRV,* inspiratory reserve volume; *ERV,* expiratory reserve volume. Shaded areas indicate relationships between the subdivisions and relative sizes as compared with the TLC. The resting expiratory level should be noted because it remains more stable than other identifiable points during repeated measurements and therefore is used as a starting point for FRC determinations.

1. The subject breathes normally for several breaths, followed by a maximal inspiration and a maximal exhalation.
2. The resting expiratory level must be stable to obtain valid test results.
3. Large TVs or an irregular pattern will result in inaccurate measurements of IC and ERV. These values are used to calculate RV and TLC.

  B. Forced vital capacity (FVC) and its subdivisions are the most widely used PFTs. The graphic representation of this simple maneuver provides information for the determination of many useful variables or calculations.

1. The subject breathes normally for several breaths, then inspires maximally and exhales as forcefully and fully as possible.
2. FVC and VC should be within 200 ml of each other in healthy patients.
3. Decreased FVC is a nonspecific finding; any disorder that affects the elasticity of the lungs can decrease FVC.
   a. With severe airway obstruction, such as emphysema, or small airway collapse, gas is trapped in the alveoli, reducing FVC.
   b. Restrictive lung diseases, such as pulmonary fibrosis or pneumonia, can reduce FVC.
4. FEV_1 is the forced expiratory volume that can be exhaled in 1 second.
   a. FEV_T for other time intervals (T) can easily be determined from the FVC curve.
   b. FEV_1 is reported as volume, although it is essentially a measurement of flow (volume/time).
   c. A decrease in FEV_1 indicates obstructive changes in small airways.
   d. Large airway obstruction from a tumor or a foreign body causes a decrease in FEV_1, which continues through the entire FVC.
5. $FEV_T\%$ is the ratio of the FEV for any given time interval (T) to the FVC (Figure 19-2).
   a. The percentage of the FVC that can be expired in 1 second, or $FEV_1\%$, is calculated below:

$$FEV_1\% = \frac{FEV_1}{FVC} \times 100 \qquad (1)$$

   b. $FEV_1\%$ tends to decrease with age, as the elasticity of the lung decreases.
   c. Normal values for young adults

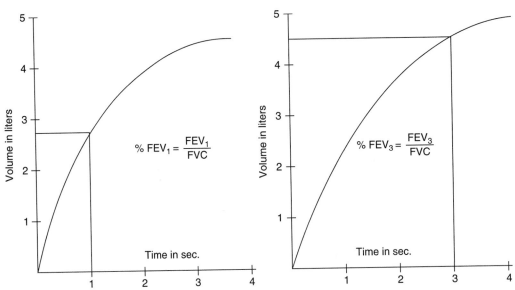

FIG. 19-2 Method to determine $FEV_1\%$ and $FEV_3\%$. See text for details.

        (1) $FEV_{0.5}\%$ is equal to 50% to 60% of the FVC.
        (2) $FEV_1\%$ is equal to 75% to 85% of the FVC.
        (3) $FEV_3\%$ is equal to 95% to 100% of the FVC.
   d.   A decrease in $FEV_1\%$ is the most important indicator of obstructive disease.
   e. $FEV_1\%$ is increased or normal with restrictive disease.
  6. $FEF_{25\%-75\%}$ is the average expiratory flow rate of the middle 50% of the FVC (Figure 19-3).
    a.   Reflects flow from medium and small airways.
    b.   Smoking causes changes in flow from medium airways before there is evidence of obstruction in small airways.
    c.   To evaluate $FEF_{25\%-75\%}$
        (1)   Determine the points on the FVC curve at which 25% and 75% of the volume is exhaled.
        (2) $FEF_{25\%-75\%}$ in L/sec is equal to the slope of the line connecting these two points.
  7. $FEF_{200-1200}$ is the average expiratory flow rate between the first 200 ml and 1200 ml of exhaled volume during an FVC maneuver (see Figure 19-3).
    a.   Reflects flow from large airways.
    b.   To evaluate $FEF_{200-1200}$
        (1)   Determine the points on the FVC curve at which 200 ml and 1200 ml are exhaled.
        (2) $FEF_{200-1200}$ in L/sec is equal to the slope of the line connecting these two points.
  8. The $FEF_{200-1200}$ value in L/sec is multiplied by 60 to convert it to L/min.
  9. Diagnosis of obstructive disease using PFT results
    a. $FEF_{25\%-75\%}$ for young, healthy adults is 4 to 5 L/sec, but results vary considerably.
    b.   FVC, FEV_1, and $FEV_1\%$ should be considered together to determine the presence and severity of an obstructive disorder.
    c.   Other measurements, such as $FEF_{25\%-75\%}$, are useful to confirm the diagnosis but should not be used as a primary indicator.
 C. Maximum voluntary ventilation (MVV)
   1. Calculates the maximum volume of gas that a patient can ventilate in 1 minute.
   2. The patient is directed to breathe rapidly and deeply for 12 to 15 seconds.

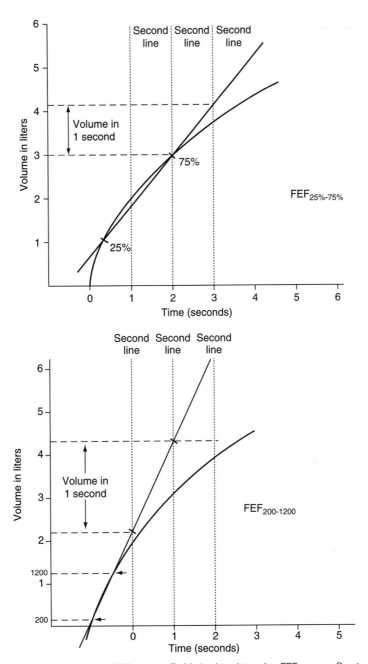

FIG. 19-3 A, Method to determine FEF$_{25\%-75\%}$. **B,** Method to determine FEF$_{200-1200}$. See text for details.

3. The total volume inspired or expired during the testing interval is measured.
4. The volume is extrapolated to 1 minute. For example, if the patient breathed 40 L in 15 seconds:

$$\text{MVV} = 40 \text{ L/15 sec} \times 60 \text{ sec/min} = 160 \text{ L/min} \qquad (2)$$

5. MVV must be corrected to body temperature and pressure saturated (BTPS).
6. Normal MVV for young healthy men is 150 to 200 L/min; slightly lower values are normal for women.

7. Decreased values indicate increased airway resistance or obstruction, decreased lung or thoracic compliance, or ventilatory muscle weakness.

D. Peak expiratory flow (PEF) rate
   1. The highest expiratory flow rate occurs during the early part of exhalation.
   2. When PEF is reported with other spirometry values, it is expressed as L/sec. When it is performed alone using a peak flowmeter, it is expressed as L/min.
   3. Peak flows normally are equal to 400 to 600 L/min for young, healthy men and 300 to 500 L/min for young, healthy women.
   4. Decreased peak flows indicate airway obstruction in large airways.

E. Flow-volume (F-V) curves (Figure 19-4)
   1. An F-V loop graphically depicts flow rate plotted against volume change during an FVC maneuver.
   2. To perform this maneuver, the patient maximally inspires, followed by a single forced exhaled vital capacity (FEVC) and forced inspired vital capacity (FIVC).
   3. A tidal F-V loop superimposed on a VC loop allows easy determination of many flow and volume variables.

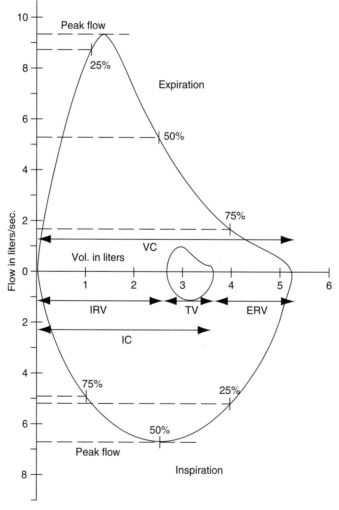

FIG. 19-4 Normal flow-volume loop with superimposed tidal volume (TV) loop. All normal spirometry values plus peak inspiratory and expiratory flows along with flow at 25%, 50%, and 75% of inspiration and expiration may be determined.

4. Computer-generated graphics allow easy manipulation and comparison of F-V loops.
   a. Most computerized spirometers indicate time increments on the curve so that FEV_1 can be read from the loop.
   b. Successive F-V loops can be superimposed on each other to demonstrate reproducibility or response to bronchodilators (Figure 19-5).
   c. Superimposed loops may show decreasing flows with successive efforts. FVC maneuvers can induce bronchospasm in patients with reactive airways.
   d. Some pulmonary disorders can be identified from specific, reproducible changes in the shape of the F-V loop (Figure19-6).
   e. Normal or predicted loops can be easily compared with suspected abnormal loops.

III. **Useful Guidelines for Spirometry Equipment and for Evaluating and Reporting Test Results**
   A. The American Thoracic Society sets standards for spirometry equipment.
      1. Volume measurement range of 0.5 to 8 L.
      2. Flow measuring range of 0 to 14 L/sec.
      3. Capable of accumulating volume for 15 seconds.
      4. The maximum acceptable error for volume measurements is ±3% or ±0.050 L, whichever is greater.
      5. Resistance and backpressure must be <1.5 cm H_2O/L/sec over the standard flow range.
   B. Criteria to evaluate accuracy of spirometry results
      1. Spirometry measurements depend on patient effort. Practitioners should be careful to ensure reproducibility before test values are reported.
      2. Evaluation of the volume-time tracing
         a. The curve should be smooth and show at least 6 seconds of forced effort.
         b. A plateau lasting at least 1 second should be evident. There should be <30 ml of volume change during the plateau.
         c. The test can be acceptable when the FVC maneuver is stopped at <6 seconds for a clinical reason, such as excessive coughing or dizziness.

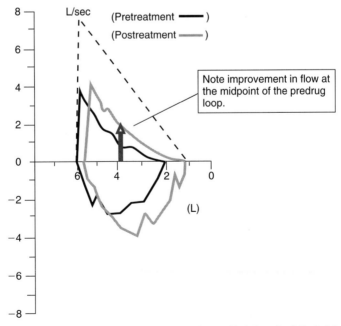

FIG. 19-5 Bronchodilator response—isovolume flow-volume loops. Each loop is plotted at the absolute lung volume at which it was measured. The increase in $FEF_{50\%}$ accurately describes the degree of bronchodilator response.

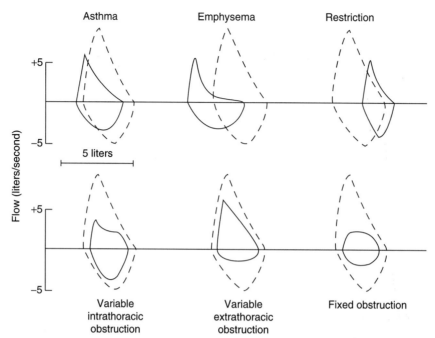

FIG. 19-6 Normal and abnormal flow-volume loops. Six curves are shown plotting flow in L/sec against the forced vital capacity (FVC). In each example the expected curve is shown by the dashed lines, whereas the curve illustrating the particular disease pattern is superimposed. In patients who have asthma and emphysema, the portion of the expiratory curve from the peak flow to residual volume (RV) is characteristically concave. The total lung capacity (TLC) and RV points are displaced toward higher lung volumes (to the left of the expected curves in this diagram). These patterns indicate hyperinflation and/or air trapping. In restrictive patterns the shape of the loop is preserved, but the FVC is decreased. The TLC and RV are displaced toward lower lung volume (to the right of the expected curves). The bottom three examples depict types of large airway obstruction. Variable intrathoracic obstruction shows reduced flows on expiration despite near-normal flows on inspiration, resulting from flow limitation in the large airways during a forced expiration. Variable extrathoracic obstruction shows an opposite pattern. Inspiratory flow is reduced, whereas expiratory flow is relatively normal. Fixed large airway obstruction is characterized by equally reduced inspiratory and expiratory flows. Comparison of the $FEF_{50\%}$ with the $FIF_{50\%}$ may be helpful to differentiate large airway obstructive processes. Because the magnitude of inspiratory flow is effort dependent, low inspiratory flows should be carefully evaluated.

    d.   Patients with severe airway obstruction may continue to exhale at low flow rates for >15 seconds. Stopping the maneuver at 15 seconds will not significantly change the results.

  3. Evaluation of the start-of-test

    a.   The beginning of the maneuver should be abrupt and distinct.

    b.   Time zero should be calculated by back extrapolation of each FVC curve (i.e., a straight line drawn through the steepest part of the curve is extended until it intersects the x-axis. The point of intersection is time zero.)

    c.   The volume exhaled at the back-extrapolated time zero should be <5% of the FVC or <0.150 L, whichever is greater (Figure 19-7).

  4. Reproducibility

    a.   A minimum of three acceptable maneuvers should be recorded.

    b.   A maximum of eight attempts should be performed to show reproducible efforts.

    c.   If two acceptable maneuvers cannot be recorded after eight attempts, the test should not be reported.

    d.   The largest and second largest FVC and FEV_1 measurements from acceptable curves should be within 200 ml. A maximum of 5% difference has also been used as the reproducibility criterion.

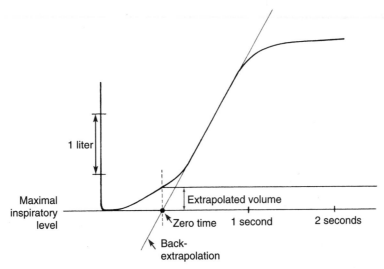

FIG. 19-7 Back-extrapolation of a volume-time spirogram. Back-extrapolation is a method to correct measurements made from a spirogram that does not show a sharp deflection from the maximal inspiratory level. This occurs when a patient does not begin forced exhalation rapidly enough or hesitates at the start of test. A straight line drawn through the steepest part of a volume-time tracing is extended to cross the volume baseline (maximum inspiration). The point of intersection is the back-extrapolated time zero. Timed volumes, such as FEV_1, are measured from this point rather than from the initial deflection from the baseline or from the point of maximal flow. The perpendicular distance from maximal inspiration to the volume-time tracing at time zero defines the back-extrapolated volume. To accurately determine FEV_1, the back-extrapolated volume should be <5% of the forced vital capacity (FVC) or <150 ml, whichever is greater. FVC efforts with larger extrapolated volumes should be considered unacceptable. These measurements are commonly performed using a computer.

C. Reporting of spirometry results
1. Lung volumes are always corrected to BTPS.
2. The largest FVC and FEV_1 from acceptable curves are reported even if the two values are from different curves.
3. Flows that depend on the FVC are taken from the single best maneuver.
4. The maneuver with the largest sum of FVC and FEV_1 is considered the best effort.

IV. **Tests Used to Measure Lung Volumes and Gas Distribution (Adapted from the AARC Clinical Practice Guidelines)**
A. Volumes of gas and lung capacities that can be exhaled from the lung (i.e., VT, VC, IRV, ERV, and IC) can be measured directly with spirometry.
B. Lung volumes and capacities that cannot be exhaled (i.e., FRC, TLC, and RV) are determined using indirect methods.
C. The FRC value is measured using indirect methods and used to calculate TLC and RV.
D. Computed tomography (CT) scans and magnetic resonance imaging (MRI) provide a direct view of gas distribution in the lungs and can be used to determine FRC, TLC, and RV.
E. The multiple-breath nitrogen washout study uses an open circuit method to determine FRC (Figure 19-8).
1. Because nitrogen makes up approximately 80% of FRC when the subject is breathing room air, the volume of nitrogen in the total exhaled gas will equal approximately 80% of the FRC.
2. The patient breathes 100% oxygen through a valve-mouthpiece system for 7 minutes or until the alveolar concentration of nitrogen decreases to approximately 1%.
3. Measurements are started at end expiration.
4. A rapid response nitrogen (N_2) analyzer and a spirometer measure breath-by-breath N_2 concentration and exhaled volume. Values are summed to provide the total volume of N_2 washed out.

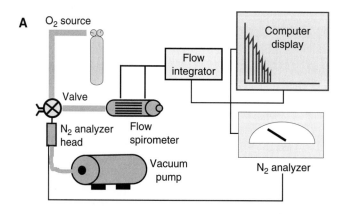

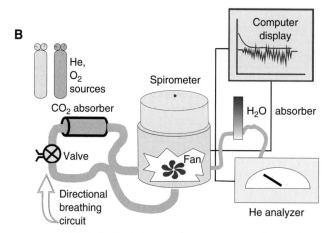

FIG. 19-8 Open- and closed-circuit functional residual capacity (FRC) systems. **A,** Open-circuit equipment used for N_2 washout determination of FRC. The subject inspires O_2 from a regulated source and exhales past a rapidly responding N_2 analyzer into a pneumotachometer. Flow and gas concentration are integrated and displayed on a computer screen. FRC is calculated from the total volume of N_2 exhaled and the change in alveolar N_2 from the beginning to the end of the test (see text). **B,** Closed-circuit equipment used for He dilution FRC determination includes a volume-based spirometer with an He analyzer, CO_2 absorber, and a directional breathing circuit. A fan or blower promotes gas mixing within the rebreathing system. A breathing valve near the mouth allows the subject to be "switched in" to the system after He has been added and the system volume determined. The O_2 source allows the addition of O_2 during the test to replenish that taken up by the subject and to maintain a constant system volume. The CO_2 absorber permits rebreathing without accumulation of CO_2. A chemical absorber removes water vapor before the He analyzer samples the gas. Tidal breathing and the He dilution curve are displayed on the computer.

5. Corrections must be made for the 30 to 40 ml of N_2 that are washed out of the blood and tissue during each minute of the test.
6. FRC is calculated using the equations below.

$$\text{FRC} = \text{FeN}_{2\ \text{final}} \times \text{Exhaled volume} - \frac{N_{2\ \text{tissue}}}{\text{FeN}_{2\ \text{alveolar 1}} - \text{FeN}_{2\ \text{alveolar 2}}} \qquad (3)$$

where: $N_{2\text{tissue}}$ = volume of N_2 washed out in blood and tissue (35 ml/min); $\text{FeN}_{2\ \text{final}}$ = fraction of N_2 in the total exhaled volume; $\text{FeN}_{2\ \text{alveolar 1}}$ = fraction of N_2 in alveolar gas at the beginning of the test; and $\text{FeN}_{2\ \text{alveolar 2}}$ = fraction of N_2 in alveolar gas at the end of the test

7. ERV obtained from a slow VC maneuver is used to calculate RV and TLC

$$RV = FRC - ERV$$
$$TLC = VC + RV$$

8. The washout time should be reported with the results because the pattern of and the time required for N_2 washout are used as indices of distribution of ventilation.

F. The multiple-breath helium dilution study uses a closed circuit method to determine FRC (Figure 19-9).

1. Because helium (He) is metabolically inert, a known volume of He may be distributed throughout the lung and the circuit without absorption of a significant volume.

2. A spirometer is filled with a known volume of air. He is added until a concentration of approximately 10% is reached. The exact concentration and volume of He in the system are measured and recorded before the test.

3. The patient breathes through a valve-mouthpiece connected to a rebreathing system containing a CO_2 absorber. Oxygen is added to maintain an F_IO_2 of approximately 0.21.

4. The valve is opened at end-expiration, and the test continues for up to 7 minutes or until a stable He concentration is reached.

5. At the completion of the test, the concentration of He in the system is measured.

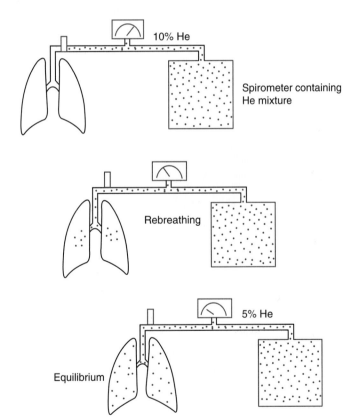

10% He

Spirometer containing He mixture

Rebreathing

5% He

Equilibrium

FIG. 19-9 Closed-circuit (He dilution) determination of functional residual capacity (FRC). At the beginning of the test the subject's lungs contain no He *(top)*. The subject then rebreathes a mixture of He and air or O_2 from a secondary system *(middle)*. He is diluted until equilibrium is reached. The volume of He initially present and its concentration are known, and the volume of the rebreathing system can be calculated. At the end of the test the same volume of He has been diluted in the rebreathing system and the lungs *(bottom)*. FRC is derived from the change in He concentration and the known system volume. The patient must be switched from breathing air to the He mixture at the end-expiratory level for accurate measurement of FRC. Residual volume (RV) is derived by subtracting the expiratory reserve volume (ERV).

6. FRC is calculated using the equations below.

$$FRC = \frac{(\% \, He_{initial} - \% \, He_{final})}{\% \, He_{final}} \times system \ volume \qquad (4)$$

where: $\% \, He_{initial}$ = He concentration in the system at start of test and $\% \, He_{final}$ = He concentration at end of test

$$System \ volume = \frac{volume \ of \ He \ added}{initial \ He \ concentration} \qquad (5)$$

7. A correction factor of 100 ml is sometimes subtracted from the calculated FRC to account for the small amount of He that is absorbed into the blood during the test.
G. Advantages and disadvantages are similar for He dilution and N_2 washout techniques.
   1. Both tests are essentially independent of patient effort. Normal tidal breathing and an adequate seal on the mouthpiece are the only requirements.
   2. Any leak in the system will result in the addition of room air to the sample, resulting in overestimation of volume. Leaks are easily detectable on graphic tracings by a spike in N_2 concentration or unexpected change in He concentration (Figure 19-10).
   3. Accuracy depends on even distribution ventilation of all areas of the lung. Patients with obstructive lung disease have poorly ventilated lung units that require a lengthy time to wash out N_2 or mix He, resulting in underestimation of volumes.
   4. Both tests are considered reliable, reproducible, and simple for patient and therapist.

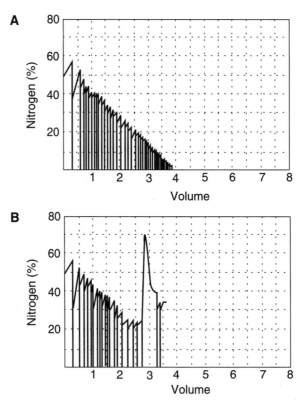

FIG. 19-10 Open-circuit N_2 washout tracings. **A,** A computer-generated recording of an N_2 washout test in a healthy subject. The tracings show a continuous decrease in end-tidal N_2 concentration with successive breaths. The test is continued until the N_2 concentration decreases to <1%. **B,** A similar plot of N_2 washout from a healthy subject, but in this instance a leak develops during the test. Leaks may occur if the patient does not maintain a tight seal at the mouthpiece. Leaks are usually easy to detect because room air enters the system and indicates an abrupt increase in N_2 concentration.

H. Body plethysmography (Figure 19-11) (adapted from the AARC Clinical Practice Guidelines)

1. This test calculates the total thoracic gas volume (V_{TG}), including gas trapped distal to completely obstructed airways or located in the abdomen or intestines.
2. The patient is placed in the plethysmograph or body box and breathes through a mouthpiece with a shutter valve that, when closed, obstructs airflow. Airway pressure at the mouth is measured using a pressure transducer attached to the mouthpiece.
3. During testing, the patient breathes gas from within the box.
4. The patient pants at a frequency of 1 to 2 breaths/sec while pressures at the mouth and within the box are measured simultaneously.
5. At FRC level the shutter is briefly closed to create an obstruction of the airway, and pressures are again measured. Changes in lung volume are reflected by changes in box pressure.
6. Mouth pressure theoretically equals alveolar pressure when the shutter occludes the airway. Occlusion of the shutter results in no airflow, allowing the two pressures to equilibrate. Esophageal pressure measurements obtained from an esophageal balloon are sometimes used instead of airway pressure.
7. The total volume of the plethysmograph is known, and the volume of gas displaced by the patient can be calculated. The volume of gas in the box surrounding the patient is determined by subtracting the volume the patient occupies from the volume of the box.

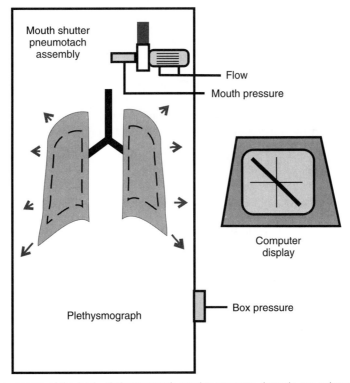

Mouth shutter
pneumotach
assembly

Flow

Mouth pressure

Computer
display

Plethysmograph

Box pressure

FIG. 19-11 Components of the body plethysmograph used to measure thoracic gas volume (V_{TG}). Boyle's law states that the volume varies inversely with the pressure if the temperature is held constant. A pressure-type plethysmograph, with pressure transducers for measurements of box pressure and mouth (alveolar) pressure is shown. The mouth shutter momentarily occludes the airway so that alveolar pressure can be estimated. The subject pants gently against the closed shutter. Gas in the lungs is alternately compressed and decompressed. Changes in lung volume are reflected by changes in box pressure. These changes are displayed as a sloping line on a computer display. When the original pressure (P), the new pressure (P′), and the new volume (V′ or V + ΔV) are known, the original volume (V or V_{TG}) can be computed from Boyle's law.

8. Boyle's law relating pressure to volume is used in the following calculations:

$$P_1V_1 = P_2V_2 \tag{6}$$

where: P_1 = original pressure inside the box (atmospheric pressure) or 760 mm; V_1 = original volume in the box – the volume occupied by patient (determined using body surface area); P_2 = pressure in the box as a result of expansion of the thorax (760.2 mm Hg); and V_2 = final volume in the box

$$(760 \text{ mm Hg})(1000 \text{ L}) = (760.2 \text{ mm Hg})(V_2)$$

$$V_2 = \frac{(760 \text{ mm Hg})(1000 \text{ L})}{760.2 \text{ mm Hg}}$$

$$V_2 = 999.737 \text{ L}$$

9. The difference between V_1 and V_2 is equal to the decreased volume in the plethysmograph after chest expansion. Because this is a sealed system, the change in volume in the plethysmograph is equal to the change in the volume in the patient's thorax. The change in volume is calculated below.

$$V_1 - V_2 = \Delta V \tag{7}$$
$$1000 \text{ L} - 999.737 \text{ L} = 0.263 \text{ L}$$

10. As the patient pants against an obstruction and the volume in the thorax increases, the pressure in the thorax decreases.
Again using Boyle's law:

$$P_1V_1 = P_2V_2 \tag{8}$$

where: P_1 = proximal airway pressure at resting FRC levels (760 mm Hg); V_1 = volume of FRC (unknown); P_2 = pressure in airway after inspiring against an occlusion; in this example: 700 mm Hg; and V_2 = volume in thorax is equal to the original volume (V_1) + ΔV calculated in equation 7.

$$(P_1)(V_1) = (P_2)(V_1 + \Delta V) \tag{9}$$
$$(760 \text{ mm Hg})(V_1) = (700 \text{ mm Hg})(V_1 + 0.263 \text{ L})$$
$$(760 \text{ mm Hg})(V_1) = (700 \text{ mm Hg})(V_1) + (700 \text{ mm Hg})(0.263 \text{ L})$$
$$(760 \text{ mm Hg})(V_1) = (700 \text{ mm Hg})(V_1) + 181.1 \text{ mm Hg} \bullet \text{L}$$
$$(60 \text{ mm Hg})(V_1) = 184.1 \text{ mm Hg} \bullet \text{L}$$
$$V_1 = 3.07 \text{ L}$$

where V_1 is the volume of gas in the thorax (V_{TG})

11. Tidal breathing is first measured to determine end-expiration.
12. The shutter automatically closes while the patient pants.
13. Electrical shutter valves and computerized systems eliminate the need to occlude the airway precisely at end-expiration.
14. Patients usually pant at a level slightly above FRC. The computer will add or subtract the change in volume from the volume before panting began to more accurately determine FRC.
15. Mouth and box pressure measurements are plotted continuously on the computer display. The slope of the resulting line is equal to change in alveolar pressure/change in alveolar volume and can be substituted into the above equations.
16. Advantages and disadvantages
   a. Patient effort and understanding of the procedure are essential. Some patients cannot tolerate the plethysmograph because of claustrophobia.

b. V_{TG} measures all gas in the thorax, including that trapped distal to collapsed airways. In diseases causing uneven distribution of ventilation and air trapping, FRC measurements are higher than those obtained by He dilution or N_2 washout but may be more accurate.

c. However, if those tests are continued for >7 minutes, the accuracy of the results will be closer to those measured using the plethysmograph.

d. V_{TG} measurement is considered quick, precise, and reproducible.

I. The single-breath nitrogen washout study (SB N_2) is used to measure distribution of ventilation and closing volume (Figure 19-12).

   1. Closing volume (CV) is the portion of a slow VC that can be exhaled after the most gravity-dependent airways start to collapse.

   2. Normally during a maximal exhalation, peripheral bronchioles collapse as lung volume approaches RV. In many disease states, an increased volume of gas is present in the lungs when these bronchioles begin to collapse.

   3. During a maximal inspiration from RV, gas is distributed in the lungs in a predictable pattern because of differences in transpulmonary pressure between the apices and bases caused by gravity and lung position.

      a. Initially gas moves into the conducting airways and begins to fill the apices.

      b. Before the apices are filled, gas begins to fill the lung bases.

      c. Toward the end of inspiration, the bases and apices fill.

      d. Alveoli in the apices are described as slow alveoli because they fill first and empty last.

      e. Alveoli in the bases are described as fast alveoli because they fill last and empty first.

   4. The apparatus used for SB N_2 testing is similar to that used for the open-circuit FRC test.

   5. The patient exhales to RV level and maximally inspires from a reservoir containing 100% O_2. The patient then exhales slowly and evenly to RV at a flow rate of 0.3 to 0.5 L/sec.

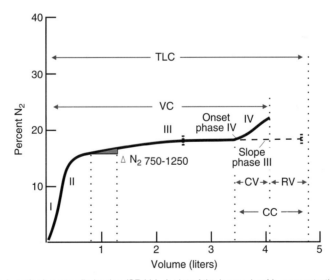

FIG. 19-12 Single-breath nitrogen elimination (SB N_2). A plot of the increasing N_2 concentration on expiration after a single vital capacity breath of 100% O_2. The curve is divided into four phases. Phase I is the extreme beginning of the expiration when only O_2 is being exhaled. Phase II shows an abrupt increase in N_2 concentration as mixed bronchial and alveolar air is expired. Phase III is the alveolar gas plateau, and N_2 concentration changes slowly as long as ventilation is uniformly distributed. Phase IV is an abrupt increase in N_2 concentration as basal airways close and a larger proportion of gas comes from the N_2-rich lung apices. Several useful parameters are derived from the SB N_2 tracing. The $\Delta N_{2\ 750-1250}$ and slope of Phase III are indices of the evenness of ventilation distribution. Closing volume (CV) can be read directly from the onset of Phase IV until residual volume (RV) is reached; vital capacity (VC) can also be read directly.

6. The N_2 concentration is plotted against the exhaled volume, and the resulting graph is divided into four distinct phases.
   a. Phase 1: Gas from the conducting airways (anatomic deadspace) is exhaled first. The gas is 100% O_2, with N_2 concentration near zero.
   b. Phase 2: A mixture of bronchial and alveolar gas next is exhaled, and N_2 concentration increases sharply.
   c. Phase 3: Gas from the alveoli then is exhaled. N_2 concentration increases slowly during this phase, resulting in a plateau on the graph.
   d. Phase 4: Bronchioles in the lung bases close, and gas from the apices is exhaled. This causes a sharp increase in N_2 concentration and indicates the closing volume.
7. CV is expressed as a percentage of the VC.
   a. In young, healthy adults, CV is equal to approximately 10% of VC.
   b. An increase in CV is considered normal as people age. A normal CV for a 60-year-old person may be 40%.
   c. Increases in CV appear to be an early indicator of small airway obstruction.
8. Closing capacity (CC) is a term used to express the percentage of the TLC that the CV + the RV represents. Normally in young, healthy adults CC is approximately 30%, but it varies widely between individuals.
9. Delta percent nitrogen ($\Delta\%N_2$) is an expression used to indicate the change in nitrogen concentration between the first 750 ml and 1250 ml exhaled.
   a. In healthy, young adults $\Delta\%N_2 \leq 1.5\%$ and for older adults, up to 3%.
   b. As the $\Delta\%N_2$ increases, it indicates uneven distribution of ventilation.
   c. Patients with severe emphysema can have a $\Delta\%N_2 > 10\%$.
10. Clinical applications
    a. Initially used to establish small airway disease because values are increased in most smokers and values are normal in most nonsmokers.
    b. Not useful to determine whether patients with small airway disease will develop clinically detectable airflow obstruction.
    c. Primarily used for epidemiologic purposes.
    d. Clinical usefulness remains controversial.

V. **Diffusion Studies (Adapted from the AARC Clinical Practice Guidelines)**
   A. Diffusion studies are used to assess the ability of the lungs to exchange gas across the alveolar-capillary membrane.
   B. Carbon monoxide (CO) is used because of its strong affinity for hemoglobin. The primary factor limiting its diffusion is the status of the alveolar-capillary membrane.
   C. Normally there is no CO in pulmonary capillary blood; therefore, the partial pressure of CO (P_{ACO}) in the alveoli creates a pressure gradient that drives CO uptake.
   D. All methods are based on the following equation:

$$D_{LCO} = \frac{\dot{V}CO}{P_{ACO} - P_{CCO}} \tag{10}$$

where: D_{LCO} is in ml/min/mm Hg CO; $\dot{V}$ CO = pulmonary capillary uptake of CO in ml/min at standard temperature and pressure dry (STPD); P_{ACO} = mean alveolar partial pressure of CO; and P_{CCO} = mean capillary partial pressure of CO, assumed to be zero
   E. Two approaches to the measurement of CO uptake from the lung, or CO diffusing capacity (D_{LCO}), have been developed.
      1. The single-breath method is the most commonly used method.
         a. The patient maximally inspires from a mixture of gases containing 0.3% CO with 10% He balance air, followed by a 10-second breath-hold.
         b. The patient exhales, and after a volume approximating that of the anatomic deadspace is exhaled a sample is collected. This sample is analyzed to determine the concentrations of CO and He in exhaled alveolar gas.
         c. The change in He concentration reflects dilution and is used to calculate the initial P_{CCO} before any CO is diffused into the blood.

2. The steady-state method
   a. During steady-state determinations, the subject breathes a fixed concentration of CO until a steady state is established (a constant value for exhaled CO).
   b. D_{LCO} then is calculated from the difference between inhaled and exhaled CO.
   c. There are a number of testing methods for steady-state determinations; none are used as widely as the single-breath method.

F. Test results
   1. Normal resting D_{LCO} for the average young man is 25 ml/min/mm Hg CO.
   2. Women have slightly lower normal values, correlating with smaller lung volumes.
   3. D_{LCO} increases as much as two to three times during exercise.
   4. D_{LCO} is often decreased in those with restrictive lung diseases resulting from pulmonary fibrosis.

VI. **Bronchial Provocation Tests**
   A. Uses of bronchial provocation tests
      1. To assess patients with normal PFTs and symptoms of bronchospasm.
      2. To quantify severity of asthma and assess changes in airway reactivity.
      3. Screening of those who may be at risk from or to document the effects of environmental or occupational exposure to toxins.
   B. Patients must be asymptomatic at baseline.
   C. Bronchodilators and antihistamines must be withheld before the test. Inhaled corticosteroids should not be withheld (Table 19-1).
   D. Appropriate emergency equipment and monitoring devices should be readily available.
   E. Baseline spirometry tests are measured before the challenge and compared with serial spirometry measurements taken at specified time intervals after the challenge.
   F. Methacholine challenge (adapted from the AARC Clinical Practice Guidelines)
      1. Baseline FEV_1 measurements are made before the administration of the aerosolized drug and after each successive dose is administered.
      2. The first dose of methacholine administered is 0.025 mg/ml. The dose used for each subsequent administration is determined using a predetermined dosing schedule. Dosing schedules commonly specify doubling the dose each time, up to a maximum of 25 mg/ml (Box 19-1).
      3. The methacholine concentration that causes a 20% decrease in the FEV_1 from baseline is referred to as the provocative dose or $PD_{20\%}$.
      4. The test is stopped once $PD_{20\%}$ is reached.
      5. Normal, healthy subjects have a $PD_{20\%}$ that is greater than the maximum dose used for testing. These individuals do not show a 20% decrease in FEV_1 during a methacholine challenge.
      6. A $PD_{20\%}$ of ≤8 mg/ml is common in patients with hyperreactive airways.

TABLE 19-1

Drugs That Should and Should Not Be Withheld Before Bronchial Challenge

Short-acting β-adrenergic agents (oral or inhaled)	12 hr
Long-acting β-adrenergic agents (oral or inhaled)	48 hr
Anticholinergic aerosols	12 hr
Sustained-action theophylline preparations	48 hr
Cromolyn sodium and related preparations	48 hr
Leukotriene inhibitors	24 hr
Antihistamines	48 hr
Corticosteroids, inhaled or oral	Subjects should be challenged while taking a normal dose
Antihistamines	72-96 hr
H_1-receptor antagonists	48 hr
Caffeine-containing drinks (e.g., cola, coffee)	6 hr
β-Blocking agents	May increase the response

BOX 19-1
Methacholine Challenge Dosing Schedule

0.075 mg/ml
0.150 mg/ml
0.310 mg/ml
0.620 mg/ml
1.25 mg/ml
2.50 mg/ml
5.00 mg/ml
10.0 mg/ml
25.0 mg/ml

G. Histamine challenge
 1. Histamine produces bronchoconstriction using a different pathway from methacholine.
 2. Histamine has side effects such as flushing and headache, but recovery of baseline function is faster than with methacholine, and it is thought to be less cumulative in its effects.
 3. A protocol of increasing dosages of histamine phosphate is followed until the $PD_{20\%}$ is determined, similar to the procedure used in the methacholine challenge.
H. Eucapnic hyperventilation
 1. Bronchospasm can be induced in individuals with hyperreactive airways.
    a. By the loss of heat and water from the upper airways.
    b. By breathing cold, dry air.
 2. In both testing methods the patient breathes at a high level of ventilation (at or approaching MVV) for a specified number of minutes.
 3. During hyperventilation carbon dioxide is mixed with inspired air to prevent respiratory alkalosis.
 4. After hyperventilation spirometry values are measured at specific intervals and are compared with those measured at baseline.
 5. The test is considered negative if there is no decrease in FEV_1 within 20 minutes after hyperventilation.
I. Exercise challenge
 1. Exercise-induced asthma (EIA)
    a. Characterized by bronchospasm that occurs during or just after vigorous exercise.
    b. Related to heat and water loss from the upper airway caused by high levels of ventilation required during exertion.
 2. Evaluation of EIA is useful in certain situations:
    a. Patients with exertional shortness of breath but with normal pulmonary function.
    b. Patients with asthma symptoms whose results were negative when they performed other bronchial provocation tests.
    c. To assess effectiveness of therapy in patients with known EIA.
    d. Screening of patients with asthma before taking part in athletics.
 3. The patient's electrocardiograph (ECG) and blood pressure must be continuously monitored during testing.
 4. The patient uses either a treadmill or cycle ergometer and exercises for 6 to 8 minutes at 60% to 85% of the individual's predicted maximum heart rate.
 5. After exercise spirometry measurements are taken at intervals and compared with the individual's baseline.
 6. As with hyperventilation testing if there is no decrease in FEV_1 within 20 minutes, the test is considered negative.
 7. Most of the time EIA causes bronchospasm after, rather than during, exercise, unless the testing is continued for a longer period.

VII. Ventilatory Response Tests

    A. In healthy, normal individuals CO_2 is the primary stimulus to breathe, and O_2 is a secondary stimulus.

    B. Control of breathing and the drive to breathe can be altered in many disease states. These tests may be of value for patients with the following disorders:

        1. Myxedema

        2. Obesity-hypoventilation syndrome

        3. Obstructive sleep apnea

        4. Idiopathic hypoventilation

    C. Occlusion pressure

        1. The $P_{0.1}$ is the amount of negative pressure generated at the mouth in the first 100 msec of inspiration against an occluded airway.

        2. The $P_{0.1}$ correlates with changes in minute ventilation and changes in hypercapnia or hypoxemia.

        3. Because there is no airflow during measurement, $P_{0.1}$ eliminates interference from mechanical abnormalities of the lung, such as decreased compliance or increased resistance.

        4. $P_{0.1}$ is a reflection of the neural output from the medullary centers in the brain that determine frequency and depth of breathing.

        5. Normal $P_{0.1}$ is 1.5 to 5 cm H_2O.

        6. An increased $P_{0.1}$ indicates a reduced drive to breathe.

    D. Ventilatory response to CO_2 can be quantified by measuring changes in minute ventilation ($\dot{V}_E$) that result when the subject breathes low concentrations of CO_2.

        1. Testing is performed under normoxic conditions (PaO_2 >90 mm Hg).

        2. The measurement is expressed as L/min/mm Hg PCO_2.

        3. Open-circuit method

            a. The patient breathes concentrations of CO_2 (1% to 7%) through a demand valve or reservoir until equilibrium is reached.

            b. $PETCO_2$, $PaCO_2$, $P_{0.1}$, and $\dot{V}_E$ are measured at each concentration.

        4. Closed-circuit or rebreathing method

            a. The patient breathes a gas containing 95% O_2 and 5% CO_2 from a one-way circuit for 4 minutes or until $PETCO_2$ is >9% (Figure 19-13).

            b. Changes in $\dot{V}_E$ are plotted against $PETCO_2$ to form a response curve.

        5. Normal individuals exhibit a linear increase in $\dot{V}_E$ of approximately 3 L/min/mm Hg PCO_2, with a range of responses from 1 to 6 L/min/mm Hg PCO_2.

        6. It is unclear why some individuals with obstructive disease develop a reduced response to CO_2 and others do not.

    E. Ventilatory response to O_2 can be quantified by measuring changes in $\dot{V}_E$ that result when the subject breathes several concentrations of oxygen.

        1. Testing is performed under isocapneic conditions ($PaCO_2$ = 40 mm Hg).

        2. Open-circuit method (step test)

            a. The patient breathes gas containing 12% to 20% oxygen, with CO_2 added to maintain a constant $PaCO_2$.

            b. When a steady state is reached, PaO_2, $\dot{V}_E$, and $P_{0.1}$ are measured.

            c. The procedure is repeated at lower oxygen concentrations to create a response curve.

            d. Continuous monitoring of $PETCO_2$ and SpO_2 is required.

        3. Closed-circuit method (progressive hypoxemia)

            a. The patient breathes from a one-way circuit containing a CO_2 scrubber and an adjustable blower.

            b. To maintain isocapnia, CO_2 can be added or the blower can be adjusted to direct some of the circuit gas into the scrubber.

            c. As O_2 is gradually consumed, the F_IO_2 in the circuit decreases.

            d. Measurements of $\dot{V}_E$, $P_{0.1}$, and SpO_2 or PaO_2 are recorded.

        4. In normal subjects, if PaO_2 is in the range of 40 to 60 mm Hg, ventilatory response appears to increase exponentially, but there is a wide range of responses among individuals.

        5. Hypoxic response increases if hypercapnia is present and decreases with hypocapnia.

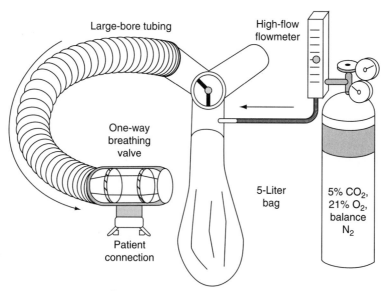

FIG. 19-13 Breathing circuit for eucapnic voluntary hyperventilation (EVH). A gas containing 5% CO_2, 21% O_2, and balance N_2 is directed through a precision high-flow flowmeter to a reservoir bag. Flow is adjusted to a target ventilation level, such as 30 times the subject's FEV_1. The subject then breathes from the bag via a one-way valve with large-bore tubing. The subject is coached to increase ventilation so as to keep the bag partially deflated. The test is continued for a predetermined interval, usually 6 minutes.

Labels in figure:
- Large-bore tubing
- High-flow flowmeter
- One-way breathing valve
- 5-Liter bag
- 5% CO_2, 21% O_2, balance N_2
- Patient connection

VIII. **Pulmonary Response to Exercise (Adapted from the AARC Clinical Practice Guidelines)**

   A. Pulmonary exercise testing can be used for the following purposes:
   1. To evaluate work capacity and to provide rehabilitative, vocational, or recreational direction.
   2. To demonstrate oxygen desaturation and determine appropriate supplemental O_2 therapy.
   3. To determine whether exercise limitation is caused by pulmonary or cardiovascular insufficiency.

   B. A variety of protocols can be used for exercise testing.
   1. Timed walk (usually 6 or 12 minutes)
      a. Distance and number of stops necessary are recorded during a walk lasting a specified time interval.
      b. Used as an evaluation for rehabilitation programs.
      c. This is a steady-state test and is simple to perform.
   2. Master step test
      a. The number of stairs climbed, the time, and number of rest periods are recorded.
      b. Either constant or variable step height is combined with increasing step rates.
   3. Progressive multistage or incremental tests
      a. These tests examine the effects of increasing workload, but a steady state is not necessarily achieved.
      b. The incline of the treadmill or resistance to pedaling is increased at predetermined intervals.

   C. Direct measurements made during exercise
   1. Work output
   2. Exercise time
   3. Minute ventilation
   4. Respiratory rate
   5. SpO_2
   6. ECG

7. Oxygen consumption
8. Carbon dioxide production
9. Arterial blood gases

D. Derived values from basic data
   1. Anaerobic threshold is that point during exercise when the oxygen demand exceeds oxygen delivery.
      a. Lactic acid increases.
      b. Carbon dioxide production markedly increases.
      c. Minute ventilation markedly increases.
      d. Oxygen consumption rate of increase is not altered.
   2. Respiratory exchange ratio (R):

$$R = \frac{CO_2 \text{ production}}{O_2 \text{ consumption}} \qquad (11)$$

   3. Oxygen pulse is the O_2 consumption divided by the heart rate.

E. Cardiac versus pulmonary limitation to exercise
   1. In cardiac diseases MVV is rarely reached, whereas with respiratory disease it is exceeded.
   2. The anaerobic threshold is rarely reached in respiratory disease but is usually exceeded in cardiac disease.
   3. Pulse and oxygen saturation decrease in respiratory and cardiac disease but more so with cardiac disease.

IX. **Reference Values in Pulmonary Function Measurements**
   A. Variation in pulmonary function measurements occurs naturally in healthy individuals and is important when comparing measured and reference values.
   B. Physical characteristics influence pulmonary function.
      1. Age: Lung volumes and capacities decrease as a person ages.
      2. Gender: Females generally have smaller body proportions than males and therefore smaller lung volumes and capacities.
      3. Body position (standing versus sitting): Lung volumes and capacities are smaller in subjects tested in the sitting position because excursion of the diaphragm is limited.
      4. Race or ethnic background: Differences in lung volumes and capacities among races are well documented and exist mainly because of differences in stature and body proportions. There is no single factor that accounts for these differences.
      5. Weight or body surface area: Again differences are related to body proportions, and lung volumes and capacities increase in larger subjects.
   C. The quality of instruction and the patient's ability to follow instructions influence test results and often result in variation in individuals, especially for spirometry testing.
   D. Most pulmonary function measurements regress or vary in a predictable way in relation to certain physical factors.
   E. Reference or predicted values are derived from statistical analysis of the pulmonary function of a group of normal subjects with:
      1. No individual or familial history of lung disease.
      2. Minimal exposure to risk factors such as smoking or environmental pollution.
   F. Published reference values such as tables, nomograms, and regression equations are available.
   G. Computerized testing equipment is used to apply reference values to values measured in patients.
   H. All lung volumes and capacities are expressed at BTPS. Measured values at atmospheric temperature and pressure saturated (ATPS) must be converted to BTPS using Charles' law (see Chapter 2).
   I. There are several methods that can be used to determine the lower limits of normal.
      1. The confidence limit method uses a normal bell-shaped distribution to define 95% confidence limits. Values that fall outside 2 SDs from the mean reference value are considered abnormal.

2. The fifth percentile method is used to determine the percentage of the reference value above which 95% of the healthy population falls.

3. The confidence limit and the fifth percentile methods give similar results for variables with normal distributions.

4. The fifth percentile method does not require a normal distribution.

5. Some PFT laboratories use a fixed percentage (e.g., ±20%) to determine the lower limit of normal for all values.

J. Considerations when choosing reference values for an individual PFT laboratory

1. Type of equipment used in the reference study: Does it comply with the recommendations of the American Thoracic Society?

2. Methodologies: Were procedures used in the reference study similar to those used in the laboratory, particularly for spirometry, lung volumes, and D_{LCO}?

3. Sample populations: Age ranges in the reference study should be noted. Did the study determine regressions for individual ethnic groups? Were smokers or other potentially unhealthy subjects used as normal control subjects?

4. Statistical data: Are lower limits of normal defined? Are data such as SD and confidence intervals presented so that limits can be calculated?

5. Conditions of the study: Was the study performed at a similar altitude and environmental conditions?

6. Published reference equations: Are values generated in the study similar to other published references?

BIBLIOGRAPHY

American Association for Respiratory Care: Clinical practice guidelines: body plethysmography. *Respir Care* 46:506-513, 2001.

American Association for Respiratory Care: Clinical practice guidelines: exercise testing for evaluation of hypoxemia and/or desaturation: 2001 revision & update. *Respir Care* 46:514-522, 2001.

American Association for Respiratory Care: Clinical practice guideline: methacholine challenge testing: 2001 revision & update. *Respir Care* 46:523-530, 2001.

American Association for Respiratory Care: Clinical practice guideline: single-breath carbon monoxide diffusing capacity, 1999 update. *Respir Care* 44:539-546, 1999.

American Association for Respiratory Care: Clinical practice guideline: spirometry, 1996 update. *Respir Care* 41:629-636, 1996.

American Association for Respiratory Care: Clinical practice guideline: static lung volumes: 2001 revision & update. *Respir Care* 46:531-539, 2001.

(The above resources can also be found on the Internet at *www.aarc.org*.)

ACSM: Roitman JL (ed): *Resource Manual for Guidelines for Exercise Testing and Prescription*, ed 4. Philadelphia, Lippincott, 2001.

Beauchamp RK: Pulmonary function testing procedures. In Barnes TA (ed): *Respiratory Care Practice*. Chicago, Year Book Medical Publishers, 1988.

Cairo JM, Pilbeam SP: *Mosby's Respiratory Care Equipment*, ed. 7. St. Louis, Mosby, 2003.

Cherniack RN: *Pulmonary Function Testing*, ed 2. Philadelphia, WB Saunders, 1992.

Clausen JL (ed): *Pulmonary Function Testing Guidelines and Controversies: Equipment, Methods, and Normal Values*. New York, Grune & Stratton, 1982.

Forster RE: *The Lung: Clinical Physiology and Pulmonary Function Tests*, ed 3. St. Louis, Mosby, 1988.

Ruppel G: *Manual of Pulmonary Function Testing*, ed 8. St. Louis, Mosby, 2003.

West JB: *Pulmonary Physiology and Pathophysiology: An Integrated, Case-Based Approach*. Baltimore, Lippincott Williams & Wilkins, 2001.

Wilkins RL, Stoller JK: *Egan's Fundamentals of Respiratory Care*, ed 8. St. Louis, Mosby, 2003.

Wilson AF (ed): *Pulmonary Function Testing Indications and Interpretations*. New York, Grune & Stratton, 1985.

U.S. Department of Labor, Occupational Safety and Health Administration contains information about personnel and testing standards for pulmonary functions testing involved with various environmental exposures. Available at: www.osha.gov.

Chapter 20

Obstructive Pulmonary Disease and General Management Principles

I. **General Comments**

   A. The acronym for chronic obstructive pulmonary disease (COPD) is applied to patients with long-term chronic obstructive pulmonary disease, who show persistent airway obstruction, normally manifested by decreased expiratory flow rates. The airflow obstruction may be associated with airway hyperactivity and may be partially reversible.

   B. Prevalence

     1. COPD is the fourth leading cause of death in the United States, preceded by cerebrovascular disease, cancer, and heart disease.

     2. In 2000, the World Health Organization estimated that 2.74 million deaths worldwide were attributed to COPD.

     3. Between 1985 and 1995, the number of physician visits for COPD in the United States increased from 9.3 million to 16 million.

     4. Approximately 14 million people in the United States have been diagnosed with COPD, and this number has increased by 42% since 1982.

     5. There seems to be a greater incidence of COPD in men than in women; however, the percentage of women with COPD is steadily increasing.

     6. On autopsy, some degree of emphysema appears in a large percentage of the population.

     7. Emphysema is the second leading cause of disability, arteriosclerotic heart disease being first.

   C. General causes of COPD

     1. Smoking: Of all risk factors, smoking shows the highest correlation with COPD; however, individual response to short-term and long-term exposure varies considerably from individual to individual. The reasons for this variation in response are not well understood. Smoking:

       a. Inhibits ciliary function.

       b. Causes bronchospasm.

       c. Affects macrophage activity.

       d. Causes disruption of the alveolar septal wall and capillary endothelium.

     2. Pollution: Particulate and gaseous.

     3. Passive smoking: Evidence indicates the passive inspiration of smoke from the environment increases the risk of COPD. Passive smoking exposes the individual to the same toxic substance, although in lower concentration than the active smoker.

     4. Occupational exposure to dusts and fumes.

     5. Infection, which may cause decreased pulmonary clearance, resulting in an increased incidence of recurrent infection.

6. Heredity
   a. α_1-Antitrypsin deficiency, which results in emphysematous changes measurable in the third and fourth decades (see Section II, Emphysema).
   b. Cystic fibrosis (see Chapter 29).
   c. Asthma (see Section VI, Asthma).
7. Allergies (e.g., chronic asthma), which can lead to permanent pulmonary changes.
8. Socioeconomic status: Higher incidence has been demonstrated in low socioeconomic groups.
9. Alcohol ingestion, although no direct link has been demonstrated. Alcohol ingestion:
   a. Decreases ciliary function.
   b. Decreases alveolar macrophage function.
   c. Decreases surfactant production.
   d. Alters antibacterial defenses of the lung.
10. Aging, which causes natural degenerative changes in the respiratory tract resembling emphysematous changes.

D. Physical appearance of patient
   1. *Barrel-chested*: A result of increased air trapping
      a. Increase in anteroposterior diameter
      b. Increase proportional to increase in functional residual capacity (FRC)
   2. *Clubbing* (pulmonary hypertrophic osteopathy): Bulbous enlargement of terminal portion of the digits, altering the cuticular angle, may be present if there have been frequent pulmonary infections.
   3. *Cyanosis*: A result of hypoxemia coupled with secondary polycythemia
   4. Decreased and adventitious breath sounds
   5. Often a hyperresonant chest
   6. Ventilatory pattern
      a. Increased use of accessory muscles
      b. Paradoxical movement of the abdomen frequently observed
      c. Prolonged expiratory time
      d. Active exhalation
      e. Pursed-lip breathing
   7. Malnourished, secondary to loss of appetite (anorexia)
   8. Anxious
   9. General muscle atrophy
   10. May be edematous with jugular vein distention if congestive heart failure (CHF) present
E. General pulmonary function changes (Table 20-1)
   1. Pulmonary compliance is frequently increased.
   2. Airway resistance increases as a result of mucosal edema and bronchiolar wall weakening.
   3. Prolonged expiratory times when numbers 1 and 2 are present.
   4. Increased FRC.

TABLE 20-1

Changes in Pulmonary Function Associated with Obstructive and Restrictive Lung Disease

Pulmonary Function Study	Obstructive Disease	Restrictive Disease
TLC	Normal or increased	Decreased
VC	Normal or decreased	Decreased
FRC	Increased	Normal or decreased
RV	Increased	Normal or decreased
RV/TLC ratio	Increased	Normal
FEV$_1$%	Decreased	Normal
MMEFR$_{25\%-75\%}$	Decreased	Normal or decreased

TLC, Total lung capacity; *VC*, vital capacity; *FRC*, functional residual capacity; *RV*, residual volume; *FEV$_1$%*, percentage of forced vital capacity in 1 second; *MMEFR$_{25\%-75\%}$*, maximum midexpiratory flow rate between 25% and 75%.

5. Increased residual volume (RV).
6. Increased RV/total lung capacity (TLC) ratio.
7. Increased or normal TLC.
8. Decreased or normal vital capacity (VC).
9. Decreased or normal inspiratory capacity (IC) and inspiratory reserve volume (IRV) secondary to increased FRC.
10. Increased expiratory reserve volume (ERV).
11. Decreased expiratory flow studies: $FEV_1\%$, $FEV_3\%$, maximum midexpiratory flow rate between 25% and 75% ($MMEFR_{25\%-75\%}$), forced expiratory flow determined between the first 200 ml and 1200 ml of exhaled volume ($FEF_{200-1200}$), and maximum voluntary ventilation (MVV). The level of reduction is associated with severity of disease (Figure 20-1).

F. General radiographic findings (Figure 20-2)
1. Increased anteroposterior diameter
2. Flattened hemidiaphragms
3. Hyperinflation
4. Pulmonary vascular engorgement with increased vascular markings
5. Increased retrosternal airspace
6. Normal or increased heart shadow
7. Normal or thin elongated mediastinum
8. Hypertranslucency
9. Possible peripheral bullae or blebs
10. In severe cases or end-stage disease, frequently right ventricular hypertrophy and CHF

G. Dyspnea
1. In all patients dyspnea on exertion is one of the first noticeable symptoms.
2. As the disease process progresses, dyspnea becomes apparent even at rest.
3. Dyspnea normally increases as the work of breathing progressively increases.
4. The percentage of the oxygen consumed to ventilate is increased, severely limiting the patient's level of physical exertion as the disease progresses.

H. Ventilatory drive and COPD
1. The ventilatory drive of COPD patients may vary considerably.
2. Some continue to increase their ventilatory efforts as the disease progresses, despite increases in work of breathing.

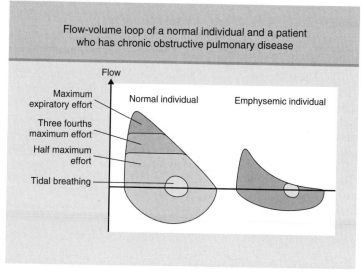

FIG. 20-1 Flow-volume loop of a normal individual and a patient with chronic obstructive pulmonary disease (COPD). Patients who have COPD may reach airflow limitation even during tidal breathing.

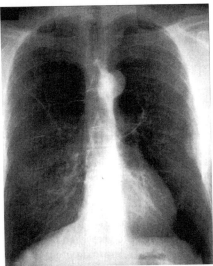

FIG. 20-2 Radiograph of a patient with chronic obstructive pulmonary disease. Note the hyperinflated lungs and decrease in pulmonary markings.

    a. These patients possess normal or increased ventilatory drives. In the past these patients were referred to as "pink puffers."

    b. This group usually does not become carbon dioxide retainers, despite continual disease progression.

    c. As a result administration of high F_IO_2 does not depress ventilation. Normal carbon dioxide responsiveness continues until there is complete failure of ventilatory muscles.

    d. These patients present in acute distress, with normal or decreased PCO_2 levels.

    e. The level of PCO_2 rapidly increases when failure overwhelms ventilatory capabilities (Figure 20-3).

  3. Conversely, many COPD patients have marked alterations in ventilatory drive.

    a. Their sensitivity to oxygen frequently is increased, and carbon dioxide is reduced.

    b. This group in the past was referred to as "blue bloaters."

    c. They experience progressive increases to baseline PCO_2 levels as their disease progresses.

    d. At presentation with an acute exacerbation of the disease, markedly elevated PCO_2 levels may be noted. Blood gas interpretation is usually acute respiratory acidosis superimposed on chronic respiratory acidosis with severe hypoxemia.

    e. These patients are classified as individuals who *will not* breathe during failure, whereas those with normal drives *simply cannot breathe* at the time of failure.

  I. General pattern of arterial blood gas changes demonstrated by carbon dioxide retainers as their disease progresses from mild to severe:

    1. Because of the pathophysiology of COPD, ventilation/perfusion inequalities develop.

    2. Mismatching of ventilation and blood flow results in hypoxemia. It should be noted that hypoxemia normally is the first measured blood gas abnormality.

    3. Hypoxemia becomes increasingly worse as the disease process progresses, resulting in stimulation of peripheral chemoreceptors.

    4. Stimulation of peripheral chemoreceptors may result in hyperventilation, the body's attempt to correct hypoxemia.

    5. If hyperventilation persists, the kidneys compensate for the acid-base imbalance. Blood gas analysis reveals compensated respiratory alkalosis (chronic alveolar hyperventilation) with hypoxemia.

    6. Hyperventilation continues until oxygen consumption by the patient's respiratory musculature exceeds the benefits received by hyperventilation.

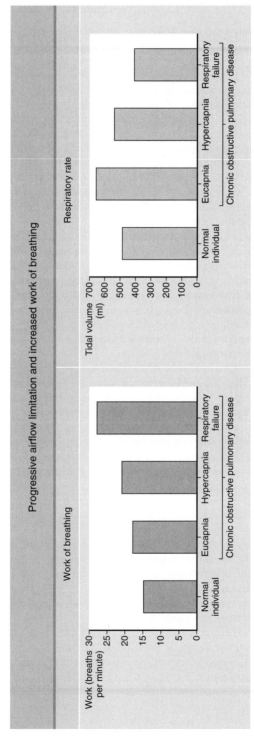

FIG. 20-3 With progression of airflow limitation, work of breathing increases. To provide the increased oxygen demanded by the breathing pump, tidal volume increases in eucapnic patients, begins to decrease as the response decreases with hypercapnia, and decreases below the normal value in patients with respiratory failure. Respiratory rate increases as patients progress from eucapnia to hypercapnia, and it reaches the highest value in patients in respiratory failure.

7. The percentage of total oxygen consumption used for ventilation becomes greatly increased because the efficiency of the respiratory system is greatly reduced by disease and increased accessory muscle use.

8. The body can no longer maintain the level of alveolar ventilation necessary to maintain adequate oxygen tensions without severely compromising oxygen delivery to other organs.

9. Because of the depressed ventilatory drive of the individual and the high cost of breathing, carbon dioxide is allowed to increase in an attempt to conserve energy.

10. This results in further progression of the hypoxemia.

11. The total oxygen reservoir may be decreased even further.

12. This is counterbalanced to a degree by a reduction in oxygen consumption by the respiratory muscles, a decrease in the patient's overall level of activity, and secondary polycythemia.

13. Alveolar ventilation continues to decrease. This is evidenced by increasing carbon dioxide levels and further development of hypoxemia.

14. With time the patient begins to retain carbon dioxide. Blood gases at this time reveal compensated respiratory acidosis with moderate to severe hypoxemia.

15. It is at this point when carbon dioxide starts to be retained that the patient's primary stimulus to breathe may become oxygen.

16. If oxygen were administered in sufficient amounts, the hypoxic stimulus to breathe could be reduced, potentially to the point of apnea in a few select patients.
    a. This is an unusual occurrence.
    b. Most patients who are CO_2 retainers do not function on a hypoxic drive.
    c. However, care should always be exercised when administering oxygen, but oxygen should not be withheld from a hypoxemic patient because of fear of further hypoventilation.

17. The disease continues to progress with increasing levels of carbon dioxide retention and more severe hypoxemia.

18. The disease process becomes end stage and terminal. The patient's level of physical activity is severely limited, and he or she is reduced to a pulmonary cripple (Figure 20-4).

J. Cor pulmonale
1. Cor pulmonale denotes right ventricular hypertrophy secondary to abnormalities of lung structure and function. CHF may or may not be present.
2. It is a frequent sequel to chronic bronchitis and cystic fibrosis.
3. Pathogenesis
   a. Developing pulmonary disease results in increasing hypoxemia, which causes constriction of the pulmonary arterioles.
   b. Constriction causes pulmonary hypertension. The decreased size of the capillary bed seen with advancing pulmonary disease also contributes to development of pulmonary hypertension.
   c. Pulmonary hypertension causes the right side of the heart to work harder. With time, right ventricular hypertrophy develops.
   d. Pulmonary hypertension, if not controlled, precipitates the development of right ventricular failure.
   e. This results in peripheral edema because of increased resistance to venous return and decreased right ventricular function.
   f. Failure of the right side of the heart is more frequently seen in association with pulmonary disease than is left-sided heart failure.
   g. However, over time the patient with right-sided heart failure can also develop left-sided heart failure.

II. **Emphysema**
A. Emphysema is characterized by enlargement of air spaces distal to terminal bronchioles, with loss of elastic tissue and destruction of alveolar septal walls.
B. Etiology
1. Smoking (high correlation with emphysema)

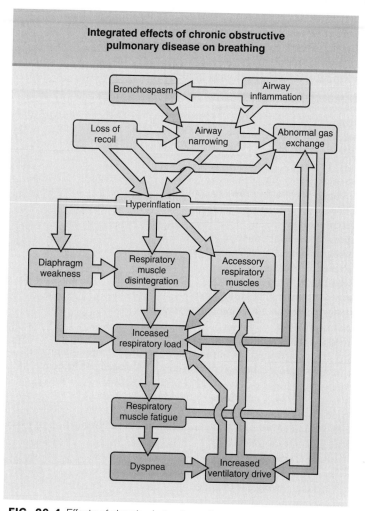

FIG. 20-4 Effects of chronic obstructive pulmonary disease on breathing.

2. High correlation with long-term air pollution.
3. Occupational hazards, dust, fumes, and similar factors
4. Heredity
   a. Patients may have α_1-antitrypsin deficiency, a lack of the enzyme that metabolizes trypsin, a digestive enzyme.
   b. If the trypsin is not metabolized, it will cause destruction of normal pulmonary tissue.
C. Types
   1. Centrilobular
      a. Destructive changes occur primarily in the respiratory bronchioles.
      b. Incidence is much higher in men than women.
      c. Primary lesions appear in the upper lobes.
      d. There is a high correlation with centrilobular emphysema and smoking; frequently it is a sequel to chronic bronchitis.
      e. It rarely occurs in nonsmokers.
   2. Panlobular
      a. Changes at alveolar level where destruction of septa predominates.
      b. Effects seemingly generalized in distribution.
      c. Seen with α_1-antitrypsin deficiency and the natural aging process.

3. Bullous
    a. Destructive changes at the alveolar and respiratory bronchiolar level.
    b. Prominent bleb and bullae formation.
D. Clinical manifestations
    1. Shortness of breath, developing gradually
    2. Nonproductive cough
    3. Frequent respiratory infections
    4. Cyanosis
    5. Barrel-chested appearance
    6. Hyperresonant chest
    7. Polycythemia
    8. Use of accessory muscles
    9. Clubbing, when infections are common
    10. Anorexia
    11. Muscle atrophy
    12. Suprasternal retractions
E. Chest radiography findings (Figure 20-5)
    1. Flattened hemidiaphragms
    2. Hypertranslucency
    3. Increased retrosternal air space
    4. Attenuated peripheral pulmonary vasculature
    5. Small heart
    6. Elongated cardiac silhouette
F. Pulmonary function studies (as outlined in Section I, General Comments)
G. Management (as outlined in Section V, General Management Principles in COPD)

III. Bronchitis
A. Acute bronchitis
    1. Acute inflammation of tracheobronchial tree with production of excessive mucus.
    2. Clinical manifestations
        a. Mucosal edema
        b. Increased sputum production
        c. Hacking paroxysms of cough
        d. Raw, burning substernal pain
    3. Causes
        a. Infectious: Viral, bacterial, or fungal
        b. Allergic
        c. Chemical, smoke, irritant gases, and similar factors

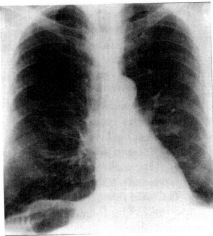

FIG. 20-5 Posteroanterior chest radiograph of a patient with emphysema.

4. Treatment: Usually by administration of antibiotics, expectorants, aerosol therapy, and occasionally antitussives.
5. Normally a self-limiting process without serious complications or residual effects.

B. Chronic bronchitis
1. Chronic cough with excessive sputum production of unknown specific etiology for 3 months per year for 2 or more successive years
2. Caused by frequent acute episodes of bronchitis, which may result from:
   a. Smoking (by far the leading cause)
   b. Air pollution
   c. Chronic infections
3. Clinical manifestations
   a. Onset normally insidious, with patient rarely aware of its development
   b. Steps in development
      (1) Smoker's cough, followed by a
      (2) Morning cough, leading to
      (3) Continual cough, especially during cold weather and exacerbations
   c. Sputum
      (1) Normally sputum production increases slowly until there is continual abnormal production.
      (2) Sputum is usually thick, gray, and mucoid until chronic infections develop, then turning mucopurulent.
4. Pathophysiology
   a. Mucosal glands
      (1) Size increases in relation to wall thickness; normally gland size is approximately one third of the height of the bronchial walls.
      (2) In chronic bronchitis, gland size is approximately two thirds of the height of the bronchial walls.
      (3) The number of mucus-secreting glands increases.
   b. Submucosal gland hypertrophy
   c. Increased population of goblet cells replacing ciliated columnar cells (epithelial metaplasia)
   d. Mucosal edema
   e. Smooth muscle hypertrophy
   f. All the above collectively result in:
      (1) Diminished airway lumen
      (2) Secretion accumulation
      (3) Submucosal infiltration
      (4) General increase in sputum production
      (5) Loss of ciliated cells
      (6) Sputum production in nonciliated airways
      (7) Impaired clearance mechanism
5. Chest radiography findings
   a. Early in the disease, radiographic changes are not significant, especially if the disease is associated only with larger airways.
   b. If the disease has moved to the periphery, hyperinflation with flattened hemidiaphragms may be noticed.
   c. Peripheral pulmonary vasculature may be prominent.
   d. Cardiac shadow is enlarged.
   e. There is pulmonary vascular engorgement.
   f. Chest radiography is usually of little use in establishing diagnosis.
   g. A positive patient history usually is the best diagnostic tool.
6. Pulmonary function studies
   a. In early stages all pulmonary function studies may be normal, except for slight decreases in expiratory flow rates.
   b. As the disease process progresses, pulmonary function results are consistent with those presented in Section I, General Comments.

    7. Treatment
        a. Most important: Removal of patient from irritants.
        b. Aerosol and bronchodilator therapy if there is a reversible component to airflow obstruction.
        c. Antibiotics if indicated for bacterial infection.
        d. Treatment regimen fairly consistent with that outlined in Section V, General Management Principles in COPD.

IV. Bronchiectasis
    A. Permanent abnormal dilation and distortion of bronchi and/or bronchioles
    B. Classification: There are three types of bronchiectasis (Figure 20-6).
        1. Cylindrical (tubular)
            a. Bronchial walls are dilated, with regular outlines.
            b. It is the least severe type because bronchiectatic areas drain fairly well.
        2. Fusiform (cystic)
            a. Bronchial walls have large, irregularly shaped distortions with bulbous ends.
            b. Evidence of bronchitis or bronchiolitis often is present.
        3. Saccular
            a. There is complete destruction of bronchial walls.
            b. Normal bronchial tissue is replaced by fibrous tissue.
            c. It is the most severe type and has poorest prognosis.
    C. Etiology
        1. Despite controversy, probable contributing factors are as follows:
            a. Recurrent infection, gram-negative infections being prominent
            b. Complete airway obstruction
            c. Atelectasis
            d. Congenital abnormalities
    D. Pathophysiology
        1. Loss of cilia
        2. Inflammatory infiltration
        3. Sloughing of mucosa with ulceration and possible abscess formation
        4. Adjacent and distal lung tissue generally has reduced volume with patchy scarring and consolidation, all believed to be secondary to the obstruction of the bronchi.
    E. Diagnosis
        1. The bronchogram is the only absolute diagnostic tool.
        2. Bronchoscopy may afford direct visualization of bronchiectatic lesions.
        3. Chest radiography findings (see Section IV-G, Chest Radiographic Findings)
        4. Sputum examination (see Section IV-F, Clinical Manifestations)

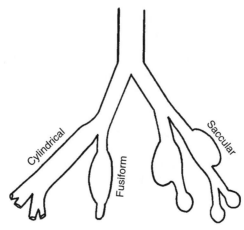

FIG. 20-6 Various morphologic types of bronchiectasis.

F. Clinical manifestations
1. Chronic loose cough, often exacerbated by change of position
2. Clubbing of fingers
3. Recurrent infections
4. Increased sputum production of a characteristic three-layer nature on standing
   a. Top layer: Thin, frothy
   b. Middle layer: Turbid, mucopurulent
   c. Bottom layer: Opaque, mucopurulent to purulent with mucous plugs (Dittrich's plugs), sometimes foul smelling
5. Hemoptysis (common)
6. Severe ventilation/perfusion abnormalities
7. Halitosis

G. Chest radiography findings
1. Usually normal unless disease is advanced and associated with other types of COPD
2. May show multiple cysts with associated fluid level
3. May show cor pulmonale

H. Pulmonary function studies
1. Cylindric type may show no changes or decreases in expiratory flow rates.
2. The saccular or cystic types show decreased flow rates, especially if associated with bronchitis, emphysema, or cystic fibrosis.

I. Management
1. Aggressive bronchial hygiene with aerosol therapy, including bronchodilators if airflow obstruction is present.
2. Appropriate antibiotic therapy
3. Possible lung resection if lesions are localized

V. **General Management Principles in COPD**
According to the Global Initiative for Chronic Obstructive Lung Disease, management of COPD consists of the following:

A. Overall management of COPD
1. Prevent disease progression
2. Relieve symptoms
3. Improve exercise tolerance
4. Improve health status
5. Prevent and treat complications
6. Reduce mortality

B. Stable COPD
1. Smoking cessation
   a. Regardless of level of disability, cessation of smoking is beneficial.
   b. Progress of disease is reduced if smoking stopped.
   c. However, no treatment can reverse or stop disease progression.
2. Vaccination
   a. Influenza virus is recommended.
   b. Pneumococcal vaccination is controversial.
3. Bronchodilators
   a. Response to bronchodilator therapy with pulmonary function studies generally should be demonstrated ($\geq 15\%$ increase in baseline FEV_1 is considered positive).
   b. However, many believe bronchodilator therapy should be administered regardless of demonstrated response.
   c. Long-acting β agonists taken twice daily may be preferable.
   d. Some patients respond to anticholinergics (atropine-like drugs) better than β agonists because of altered autonomic receptor distribution with age (see Chapter 17).
      (1) Atropine
      (2) Ipratropium bromide (Atrovent)
      (3) Glycopyrrolate (Robinul)

    e. A combination of β agonist and anticholinergic therapy may be helpful and is available in metered dose inhaler (MDI) form (Combivent).

4. Corticosteroids
   a. Corticosteroids are used primarily to reduce mucosal edema.
   b. Aerosolized approaches are generally desired over systemic because of side effects of the systemic route; however, neither has been shown to have a significant effect.
   c. Aerosolized corticosteroids commonly used are:
      (1) Beclomethasone (Becotide, Vanceril)
      (2) Flunisolide (AeroBid)
      (3) Triamcinolone (Azmacort)
      (4) Fluticasone (Flovent)

5. Antibiotics
   a. Some recommend low-dose long-term antibiotic therapy for those with persistent and frequently reoccurring pulmonary infections.
   b. Agents frequently used are:
      (1) Ampicillin
      (2) Trimethoprim-sulfamethoxazole (Bactrim, Septra)
      (3) Tetracycline
      (4) Erythromycin
      (5) Chloramphenicol
      (6) Azithromycin (Zithromax)

6. Oxygen therapy (see Chapter 34)
7. Mechanical ventilation (see Chapter 21)
8. Nocturnal nasal continuous positive airway pressure (CPAP) therapy (see Chapter 32)
9. Improvement of patient's exercise tolerance by general graded body toning and stamina-developing exercises
10. Maintenance of cardiovascular status by management of CHF
11. Avoidance of exposure to all types of airway irritants
12. Proper education and psychological and sociologic support

C. Acute exacerbation of COPD
   1. Acute exacerbations may be associated with a number of specific concomitant problems (Table 20-2).
   2. Oxygen therapy: F_1O_2 generally is titrated to maintain Po_2 in the 60 mm Hg range. No need exists to increase Po_2 to the 90 mm Hg range.
   3. Antibiotic therapy: Acute exacerbations are commonly associated with pneumonia. Appropriate therapy should begin immediately.
   4. Bronchodilator therapy should be started immediately.
      a. Aminophylline: Use of aminophylline has declined over the past several years. The exact mechanism of action is not clear. It had previously been thought to increase cellular levels of cyclic adenosine monophosphate; however, this is not the case. Possible mechanisms of action likely include increased intracellular calcium transport, adenosine antagonism, and inhibition of prostaglandin E_2.
         (1) Loading dose: 5 to 6 mg/kg intravenously
         (2) Maintenance dose: 0.5 to 0.6 mg/kg/hr intravenously
      b. Aerosolized β_2 agonists
      c. Anticholinergics
      d. A combination of a through c may be used.
   5. Adequate hydration
      a. With some, appropriate systemic hydration markedly increases the mobility of secretions because many patients are dehydrated, increasing viscosity of pulmonary secretions.
   6. Corticosteroid therapy
      a. Use of aerosolized steroids at home is common.
      b. During acute exacerbation systemic steroids may be helpful for some patients. Therapy consists of 0.5 mg/kg of methylprednisone given intravenously every 6 hours and may be abruptly withdrawn after 72 hours of treatment.

TABLE 20-2

Comorbid Conditions That Present as Exacerbations of COPD

Condition	Common Clinical Symptoms	Diagnostic Laboratory Tests	Treatment
Acute bronchitis	Productive cough, increased dyspnea, substernal discomfort, purulent sputum	Leukocytosis, sputum, Wright stain, and Gram stain	Antibiotics, systemic and airway hydration
Pneumonia	Fever, productive cough, pleuritic chest pain	As above, plus chest radiograph and blood cultures	As above; if toxic or in impending respiratory failure, hospitalization
Asthmatic bronchoconstriction	Increased cough, dyspnea, wheeze	Increased blood and sputum eosinophil count, elevated IgE in bronchial asthma	Corticosteroids, avoidance of causative agent if possible, desensitization when indicated sodium cromolyn
Medication errors and noncompliance, tobacco smoke exposure, industrial smoke and fume exposure, failure to comply with exercise conditioning regimen	Progressive dyspnea "worsening"	Persistent eosinophilia, nontherapeutic serum theophylline levels, presence of carboxyhemoglobin, work history	Patient and family education, use of intelligent caregivers, job modification, closer work with pulmonary rehabilitation team
Malnutrition or weight gain	Weakness, weight loss or gain	Weight, characteristic blood chemistry and hematologic abnormalities	Nutrition, counseling dietary supplementation as indicated
Pneumothorax	Acute dyspnea, chest pain, syncope	Chest radiograph	Hospitalization for thoracotomy tube to suction
Acute myocardial infarction and/or CHF	Increasing dyspnea, may not have typical anginal chest pain	ECG, chest radiograph (may not be typical), cardiac enzymes	Hospitalization for cardiovascular monitoring
Pulmonary embolism and infarction	Acute dyspnea, hemoptysis (in infarction)	Chest radiograph, ventilation/perfusion lung scan (may be difficult to interpret), pulmonary angiogram	Anticoagulation or thrombolysis
Bronchogenic carcinoma	Weight loss recurrent pneumonia, hemoptysis, chest pain	Chest radiograph, computed tomography scan, cytology, bronchoscopy	Thoracotomy and resection (if possible), radiation, chemotherapy

COPD, Chronic obstructive pulmonary disease; *Ig*, immunoglobulin; *CHF*, congestive heart failure; *ECG*, electrocardiography.
From Burton GG: Exacerbations of chronic obstructive pulmonary disease: pharmacologic management. In Kacmarek RM, Stoller JK (eds). *Current Respiratory Care.* Toronto, BC Decker, 1988.

7. Diuretic therapy
   a. Many COPD patients also have CHF.
   b. Appropriate diuretic therapy to normalize fluid balance is indicated.
8. Nutritional support
   a. Many COPD patients demonstrate chronic nutritional deficiencies.
   b. Preceding admission, nutritional maintenance decreases as respiratory symptoms progress.
   c. See Chapter 24 for details.
9. Bronchial hygiene techniques, although controversial, are often used (see Chapter 36).
D. Ventilatory management in acute exacerbations of COPD
   1. Indication for ventilatory support varies among experts but generally should be associated with reversibility of the event responsible for failure. Unless the state before the acute exacerbation can be reestablished, the likelihood of chronic ventilatory support is highly probable.
   2. General principles: The goal of ventilator management for these patients generally is to provide rest for fatigued ventilatory muscles while minimizing the potential for ventilator-induced lung injury (see Chapter 21).
   3. Before intubation and mechanical ventilation a trial of noninvasive ventilation should be attempted. Patients experiencing acute exacerbation of COPD are the patients most likely to have a favorable response to this intervention.

VI. **Asthma**
   A. Asthma, according to the American Thoracic Society, is "characterized by an increased responsiveness of the trachea and bronchi to various stimuli and is manifested by widespread narrowing of the airways that changes in severity either spontaneously or as the result of treatment."
   B. Categories
      1. *Allergic*: Implies that asthma is a result of an antigen-antibody reaction on mast cells of the respiratory tract. This reaction causes release of histamine, bradykinins, eosinophilic chemotactic factor of anaphylaxis, and slow-reacting substance of anaphylaxis. These substances then elicit the clinical responses associated with an asthmatic attack and cause high serum immunoglobulin (Ig) E levels along with sputum and serum eosinophilia.
      2. *Idiopathic*: Implies that asthma is a result of an imbalance of the autonomic nervous system (i.e., the response of β- and α-adrenergic sites and cholinergic sites of the autonomic nervous system is not properly coordinated).
      3. *Nonspecific*: Implies that the origin of asthmatic reactions is unknown. The asthmatic attack may follow viral infection, emotional changes, or exercise.
   C. Etiology
      1. The complete causes generally are unknown, but heredity plays a significant role. Allergies and environmental factors also are frequently implicated.
      2. If the disease develops between ages 5 through 15 years, it usually has an allergic basis.
      3. If onset is after age 30 years, the disease normally is considered nonspecific.
      4. Incidence: The actual incidence of asthma is difficult to determine. It is based on diagnosis, which varies because of several factors, including the definition used and access to health care.
         a. Worldwide the incidence of asthma in children is believed to be approximately 2% to 5% but has been reported to be as high as 34%.
         b. Approximately 1% of the adult population has asthma.
         c. Often at the onset of adolescence, the disease begins to disappear.
   D. Diagnosis
      1. Diagnosis depends on skin testing for antibodies and on the patient's and the patient's family history.
      2. In allergic asthma, antibody IgE serum levels are approximately six times that of normal.
      3. In idiopathic asthma, patients show an abnormal response to drug therapy: decreased β-sympathetic response and increased α-sympathetic response.
      4. In nonspecific asthma, frequent presenting symptoms are nasal polyps and aspirin intolerance.
      5. Eosinophilia of sputum and blood are common.

E. Pathophysiology
   1. Thickening of subepithelial membranes
   2. Hypertrophy of mucous glands
   3. Eosinophilic infiltrates common in sputum and serum
   4. Decrease in number of pulmonary mast cells
   5. Mucosal edema and bronchoconstriction
   6. Increased production of thick viscid secretions
F. Clinical manifestations
   1. Severe respiratory distress
   2. Rapid, shallow respiratory pattern
   3. Wheezing that is often audible without a stethoscope
   4. Weak cough
   5. Tachycardia and hypertension
   6. Sometimes diaphoresis
   7. Possibly cyanosis
   8. Barrel-chested appearance with hyperresonance
   9. Anxiety
   10. Intercostal, substernal, and subcostal retractions
   11. Paradoxical chest movement
   12. Accessory muscle usage
   13. Shortness of breath
   14. Prolonged expiratory time
G. Chest radiography findings
   1. During an attack a classic hyperinflation pattern is seen.
   2. Between attacks the chest radiographic findings may be normal.
H. Pulmonary function studies
   1. During an attack expiratory flow rates and VC are reduced. Bronchodilator therapy during pulmonary function testing often results in a significant improvement in test results (Figure 20-7).

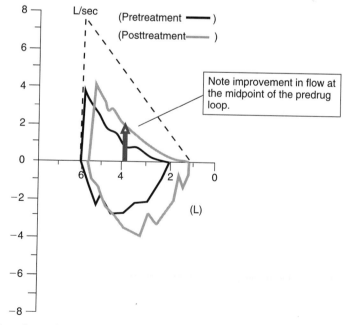

FIG. 20-7 Isovolume flow-volume loops. Each loop is plotted at the absolute lung volume at which it was measured. The increase in $FEF_{50\%}$ accurately describes the degree of bronchodilator response.

2. Between attacks pulmonary function studies may be normal or show decreased expiratory flow rates.

I. Exacerbating factors: One of the hallmarks of asthma is that it varies in severity and resolves either spontaneously or with treatment. Between attacks the patient may have little or no evidence of disease. Exacerbating factors or "triggers" result in acute onset and may include the following:

1. Infection
2. Allergens (e.g., grass, tree pollen, pets, house dust, and mites)
3. Air pollution
4. Exercise
5. Occupation (e.g., environment and sensitizing agents)
6. Drugs
7. Premenstrual and menstrual periods
8. Physical and emotional stress

J. Status asthmaticus
1. Status asthmaticus is a sustained asthmatic attack that does not respond to conventional therapy.
2. Severe hypoxemia is normally present.
3. May result in:
   a. Lactic acidosis
   b. Respiratory failure
   c. Mechanical ventilation
   d. Death

K. Management of stable asthma: The National Institutes of Health, Heart, Lung, and Blood recommend a stepwise approach based on classification of the severity of the patient's disease to maintain control of asthma with the least amount of medication and hence minimal risk of side effects.

1. Classification of asthma severity (Table 20-3)
   a. Severe persistent
      (1) Continual symptoms
      (2) Limited physical activity
      (3) Frequent exacerbations
   b. Moderate persistent
      (1) Daily symptoms
      (2) Daily use of short-acting inhaled β_2 agonist
      (3) Exacerbations after activity
      (4) Exacerbations ≥ 2 times a week; may last days
   c. Mild persistent
      (1) Symptoms >2 times a week but <1 time a day
      (2) Exacerbations may affect activity.
   d. Mild intermittent
      (1) Symptoms ≤ 2 times a day
      (2) Asymptomatic and normal peak flow between exacerbations
      (3) Exacerbations brief (from a few hours to a few days); intensity may vary.

2. Stepwise approach to managing asthma includes long-term control, quick relief, and education and is based on the following goals (Table 20-4):
   a. Preventing chronic and troublesome symptoms (e.g., coughing or breathlessness in the night, in the early morning, or after exertion).
   b. Maintaining (near) "normal" pulmonary function.
   c. Maintaining normal activity levels (including exercise and physical activity).
   d. Preventing recurrent exacerbations of asthma and minimizing the need for emergency department visits or hospitalizations.
   e. Providing optimal pharmacotherapy with minimal or no adverse effects.
   f. Meeting patients' and families' expectations of and satisfaction with asthma care.

TABLE **20-3**

Goals of Treatment and Classification of Asthma Severity

Goals of Asthma Treatment
- Prevent chronic and troublesome symptoms (e.g., coughing or breathlessness in the night, in the early morning, or after exertion)
- Maintain (near) "normal" pulmonary function
- Maintain normal activity levels (including exercise and other physical activity)
- Prevent recurrent exacerbations of asthma and minimize the need for emergency department visits or hospitalizations
- Provide optimal pharmacotherapy with minimal or no adverse effects
- Meet patients' and families' expectations of and satisfaction with asthma care

CLASSIFY SEVERITY OF ASTHMA

	Clinical Features Before Treatment*		
	Symptoms†	**Nighttime Symptoms**	**Lung Function**
Step 4 (severe persistent)	• Continual symptoms • Limited physical activity • Frequent exacerbations	Frequent	• FEV_1 or PEF ≤60% predicted • PEF variability >30%
Step 3 (moderate persistent)	• Daily symptoms • Daily use of inhaled short-acting β_2-agonist • Exacerbations affect activity • Exacerbations ≥2 times a week; may last days	>1 time a week	• FEV_1 or PEF >60%–<80% predicted • PEF variability >30%
Step 2 (mild persistent)	• Symptoms >2 times a week but <1 time a day • Exacerbations may affect activity	>2 times a month	• FEV_1 or PEF ≥80% predicted PEF variability 20–30%
Step 1 (mild intermittent)	• Symptoms ≤2 times a week • Asymptomatic and normal PEF between exacerbations • Exacerbations brief (from a few hours to a few days); intensity may vary	≤2 times a month	• FEV_1 or PEF ≥80% predicted • PEF variability <20%

*The presence of one of the features of severity is sufficient to place a patient in that category. An individual should be assigned to the most severe grade in which any feature occurs. The characteristics noted in this figure are general and may overlap because asthma is highly variable. Furthermore, an individual's classification may change over time.

†Patients at any level of severity can have mild, moderate, or severe exacerbations. Some patients with intermittent asthma experience severe and life-threatening exacerbations separated by long periods of normal lung function and no symptoms.

From National Institutes for Health: *Guidelines for the Diagnosis and Management of Asthma* Publication Number 97–4051, 1997).

3. Key recommendations for long-term asthma management:
    a. Persistent asthma is most effectively controlled with daily long-term control medication, specifically, antiinflammatory therapy.
    b. A stepwise approach to pharmacologic therapy is recommended to gain and maintain control of asthma.
        (1) The amount and frequency of medication are dictated by asthma severity and directed toward suppression of airway inflammation.
        (2) Therapy should be initiated at a higher level than the patient's step of severity at the onset to establish prompt control and then stepped down.
        (3) Continual monitoring is essential to ensure that asthma control is achieved.
        (4) Step-down therapy is essential to identify the minimal medication necessary to maintain control.

TABLE **20-4**

Stepwise Approach for Managing Asthma in Adults and Children Over 5 Years of Age[*]

	Long-Term Control	Quick Relief	Education
Step 4 (severe persistent)	Daily medications: ■ **Antiinflammatory: inhaled corticosteroid (high dose)** AND ■ Long-acting bronchodilator: either long-acting inhaled β_2-agonist, sustained-release theophylline, or long-acting β_2-agonist tablets AND ■ Corticosteroid tablets or syrup long term (make repeat attempts to reduce systemic steroids and maintain control with high-dose inhaled steroids)	■ Short-acting bronchodilator: **inhaled β_2-agonists as needed for symptoms** ■ Intensity of treatment will depend on severity of exacerbation ■ Use of short-acting inhaled β_2-agonists on a daily basis, or increasing use, indicates the need for additional long-term-control therapy	Steps 2 and 3 actions plus: ■ Refer to individual education/counseling
Step 3 (moderate persistent)	Daily medication: ■ Either **Antiinflammatory: inhaled corticosteroid (medium dose)** OR Inhaled corticosteroid (low-medium dose) and add a long-acting bronchodilator, especially for nighttime symptoms; either **long-acting inhaled β_2-agonist,** sustained-release theophylline, or long-acting β_2-agonist tablets ■ If needed Antiinflammatory: inhaled corticosteroids (medium-high dose) AND Long-acting bronchodilator, especially for nighttime symptoms; either long-acting inhaled β_2-agonist sustained-release theophylline, or long-acting β_2-agonist tablets	■ Short-acting bronchodilator: **inhaled β_2-agonists as needed for symptoms** ■ Intensity of treatment will depend on severity of exacerbation ■ Use of short-acting inhaled β_2-agonists on a daily basis, or increasing use, indicates the need for additional long-term-control therapy	Step 1 actions plus: ■ Teach self-monitoring ■ Refer to group education if available ■ Review and update self-management plan
Step 2 (mild persistent)	One daily medication: ■ Antiinflammatory: either **inhaled corticosteroid** (low doses) or **cromolyn or nedocromil** (children usually begin with a trial of cromolyn or nedocromil)	■ Short-acting bronchodilator: **inhaled β_2-agonists as needed for symptoms** ■ Intensity of treatment will depend on severity of exacerbation	Step 1 actions plus: ■ Teach self-monitoring ■ Refer to group education if available ■ Review and update self-management plan

TABLE 20-4

Stepwise Approach for Managing Asthma in Adults and Children Over 5 Years of Age[*]*—cont'd*

	Long-Term Control	Quick Relief	Education
	▪ Sustained-release theophylline to serum concentration of 5–15 mcg/ml is an alternative, but not preferred, therapy Zafirlukast or zileuton may also be considered for patients ≥12 years of age, although their position in therapy is not fully established	▪ Use of short-acting inhaled β_2-agonists on a daily basis, or increasing use, indicates the need for additional long-term-control therapy	
Step 1 (mild intermittent)	▪ No daily medication needed	▪ Short-acting bronchodilator: inhaled β_2-agonists as needed for symptoms ▪ Intensity of treatment will depend on severity of exacerbation ▪ Use of short-acting inhaled β_2-agonists more than 2 times a week may indicate the need to initiate long-term-control therapy	▪ Teach basic facts about asthma ▪ Teach inhaler/spacer/ holding chamber technique ▪ Discuss roles of medications ▪ Develop self-management plan ▪ Develop action plan for when and how to take rescue actions, especially for patients with a history of severe exacerbations ▪ Discuss appropriate environmental control measures to avoid exposure to known allergens and irritants

↓ Step down
Review treatment every 1 to 6 months; a gradual stepwise reduction in treatment may be possible

↑ Step up
If control is not maintained, consider step up. First, review patient medication technique, adherence, and environmental control (avoidance of allergens or other factors that contribute to asthma severity)

NOTE:
▪ The stepwise approach presents general guidelines to assist clinical decision-making; it is not intended to be a specific prescription. Asthma is highly variable; clinicians should tailor specific medication plans to the needs and circumstances of individual patients.
▪ Gain control as quickly as possible; then decrease treatment to the least medication necessary to maintain control. Gaining control may be accomplished by either starting treatment at the step most appropriate to the initial severity of the condition or starting at a higher level of therapy (e.g., a course of systemic corticosteroids or higher dose of inhaled corticosteroids).
▪ A rescue course of systemic corticosteroids may be needed at any time and at any step.
▪ Some patients with intermittent asthma experience severe and life-threatening exacerbations separated by long periods of normal lung function and no symptoms. This may be especially common with exacerbations provoked by respiratory infections. A short course of systemic corticosteroids is recommended.
▪ At each step, patients should control their environment to avoid or control factors that make their asthma worse (e.g., allergens, irritants); this requires specific diagnosis and education.
▪ Referral to an asthma specialist for consultation or co-management is *recommended* if there are difficulties achieving or maintaining control of asthma or if the patient requires step 4 care. Referral may be *considered* if the patient requires step 3 care.
[*]Preferred treatments are in bold print.
From National Institutes for Health: *Guidelines for the Diagnosis and Management of Asthma* Publication Number 97-4051, 1997.

c. Regular follow-up visits (at 1- to 6-month intervals) are essential to ensure that control is maintained and the appropriate step down in therapy is considered.
d. Therapeutic strategies should be considered in concert with clinical-patient partnership strategies; education of patients is essential to achieve optimal pharmacologic therapy.

    e. At each step patients should be advised to avoid or control allergens, irritants, or other factors that make the patient's asthma worse.

    f. Referral to an asthma specialist for consultation or co-treatment of the patient is recommended if there are difficulties achieving or maintaining control of asthma or if the patient requires step 4 care. Referral may be considered if the patient requires step 3 care. For infants and young children referral is recommended if the patient requires step 3 or step 4 care and should be considered if the patient requires step 2 care.

4. Other steps to be taken by the patient for the management of asthma:

    a. Avoid irritants and allergens.

    b. Avoid occupational and environmental triggers.

    c. Perform daily monitoring of peak flow to serve as an early warning sign of an impending onset.

       (1) Peak flow monitoring should be done at the same time each day, preferably in the morning.

       (2) A daily log should be kept to determine the patient's normal range.

       (3) A decrease in peak flow should be reported to the patient's physician.

5. Pharmacologic treatment: Pharmacologic treatment is divided into two categories. Drugs that are used to manage asthma are called relievers, whereas those that are used to prevent asthma attacks are referred to as controllers (see Chapter 17).

    a. Controllers:

       (1) Inhaled corticosteroids

          (a) Beclomethasone dipropionate

          (b) Budesonide

          (c) Flunisolide

          (d) Fluticasone

          (e) Triamcinolone acetonide

       (2) Systemic corticosteroids

          (a) Methylprednisone

          (b) Prednisone

       (3) Cromolyn

       (4) Nedocromil

       (5) Long-acting β agonists

          (a) Salmeterol

          (b) Sustained-release albuterol tablet

       (6) Methylxanthines

          (a) Theophylline

       (7) Leukotriene modifiers

          (a) Zafirlukast

          (b) Zileuton

    b. Relievers

       (1) Short-acting inhaled β agonists

          (a) Albuterol

          (b) Pirbuterol

          (c) Terbutaline

          (d) Bitolterol

       (2) Anticholinergics

          (a) Ipratropium

       (3) Systemic corticosteroids

          (a) Methylprednisone

          (b) Prednisone

6. Immunotherapy is used against identified antigens. Immunotherapy can be expected to:

    a. Increase serum and/or secretory IgG and IgA levels that block IgE capacity to bind to mast cells.

    b. Decrease IgE levels.

    c. Decrease mast cell sensitivity.

L. Management of acute exacerbation and status asthmaticus
  1. Pharmacologic management centers on relief of airway obstruction.
    a. Inhaled β_2-adrenergic agents
    b. Aminophylline
    c. Anticholinergic agents
    d. Corticosteroids (normally do not demonstrate efficacy until 6 to 8 hours after administration)
    e. Management generally is similar to stable asthma, except dosages and frequencies are increased, and more invasive routes of administration are chosen.
  2. Systemic hydration demonstrates variable results depending on the length of time the asthmatic attack has been in progress before admission and the level of dehydration.
  3. The use of airway clearance techniques, expectorants, and mucolytic agents during the acute phase is questionable.
  4. Oxygen therapy should be administered liberally by cannula or simple mask if hypoxemia is present. A cannula is normally much better tolerated than a mask.
  5. Heliox: The administration of a helium oxygen mixture is a useful adjunct to reducing the work of breathing and oxygen consumption. Patients who fail to respond to the conventional approach outlined previously may have a favorable response to inhaled heliox and thus be spared intubation and mechanical ventilation.
    a. Heliox has a lower density than air or oxygen.
    b. This results in less resistance in areas where flow is turbulent.
    c. Lower resistance to gas flow results in decreased work of breathing, improved ventilation, and reduced oxygen consumption.

M. Ventilatory management of status asthmaticus: Intubation and mechanical ventilation generally are difficult for patients with asthma and if possible should be avoided through the aggressive use of more conservative therapies (see Chapter 21).
  1. Indications for mechanical ventilation
    a. Acute ventilatory failure with a P_{CO_2} >50 mm Hg is an indication for ventilation.
      (1) If P_{CO_2} level is >50 mm Hg, ventilatory muscle fatigue may have occurred.
      (2) Airflow obstruction may be nearly complete.
    b. Normally persons with asthma are relatively healthy before an acute attack; thus they can be expected to hyperventilate in the presence of hypoxemia.
    c. If the severity of the attack persists or increases despite treatment, that is, if
      (1) Hypoxemia persists.
      (2) Peak flow decreases.
      (3) FEV_1 decreases.
      (4) Abnormal breath sounds increase.
      (5) Aeration decreases.
      (6) P_{CO_2} will begin to increase because of exhaustion.
    d. Once P_{CO_2} returns to normal (40 to 45 mm Hg) with persistent symptomatology failure is imminent in the presence of a continued acute asthma.
    e. Intubation and mechanical ventilation should be immediately instituted to prevent further clinical deterioration.
      (1) Positive end-expiratory pressure (PEEP) generally is contraindicated in asthma because it may increase air trapping.
      (2) However, in mechanically ventilated patients demonstrating auto-PEEP, low levels of PEEP ($\leq$5 cm H_2O) may reduce air trapping and improve ventilation (see Chapter 40).
  2. If bronchospasm persists, some recommend the use of gaseous anesthetic agents that are potent bronchodilators. However, intravenous anesthetics also have potent bronchodilator effects.
    a. Ether
    b. Halothane
    c. Enflurane
    d. Isoflurane

3. Once the acute attack is resolved, ventilator discontinuance should progress rapidly.
4. Many persons with asthma respond adversely (i.e., increase in bronchospasm) to an artificial airway when sedation has been reversed. Once it has been established that spontaneous ventilation is feasible, rapidly extubate.

BIBLIOGRAPHY

Albert RK, Spiro SG, Jett JR: *Comprehensive Respiratory Medicine*. London, Mosby, 2001.

Burton GG: Exacerbations of chronic obstructive pulmonary disease: Pharmacologic management. In Kacmarek RM, Stoller JK (eds): *Current Respiratory Care*. Toronto, BC Decker, 1988.

Cherniack RM, Cherniack L: *Respiration in Health and Disease*, ed 3. Philadelphia, WB Saunders, 1983.

Fanta CH: Acute exacerbations of asthma and status asthmaticus: Pharmacologic management. In Kacmarek RM, Stoller JK (eds): *Current Respiratory Care*. Toronto, BC Decker, 1988.

Farzan S: *A Concise Handbook of Respiratory Diseases*, ed 3. Norwalk, CT, Appleton and Lange, 1992.

Hess DR, MacIntyre NR, Mishoe SC, Galvin WF, Adams AB, Saposnick AB: *Respiratory Care Principles and Practices*. Philadelphia, WB Saunders, 2002.

Marcy TW, Matthay RA: Stable asthma. In Kacmarek RM, Stoller JK (eds): *Current Respiratory Care*. Toronto, BC Decker, 1988.

National Institutes of Health: *Global Initiatives for Chronic Obstructive Lung Disease*. Bethesda, MD, National Institutes of Health, 2001, publication number 2710.

National Institutes for Health: *Guidelines for the Diagnosis and Management of Asthma*. Bethesda, MD, National Institutes of Health, 1997, publication number 97-4051.

Pare JAP, Fraser RG: *Synopsis of Diseases of the Chest*. Philadelphia, WB Saunders, 1983.

Petty TL: *Intensive and Rehabilitative Respiratory Care*, ed 3. Philadelphia, Lea & Febiger, 1982.

Pierson DJ: Exacerbation of chronic bronchitis and emphysema: Ventilatory management. In Kacmarek RM, Stoller JK (eds): *Current Respiratory Care*. Toronto, BC Decker, 1988.

Pierson DJ, Kacmarek RM: *Foundations of Respiratory Care*. New York, Churchill Livingstone, 1992.

Ruppel GL: *Manual of Pulmonary Function Testing*, ed 8. St. Louis, Mosby, 2003.

Shapiro BA, Harrison RA, Kacmarek RM, et al: *Clinical Application of Respiratory Care*, ed 3. Chicago, Year Book Medical Publishers, 1985.

Tisi GM: *Pulmonary Physiology in Clinical Medicine*, ed 2. Baltimore, Williams & Wilkins, 1983.

Whitcomb ME: *The Lung: Normal and Diseased*. St. Louis, Mosby, 1982.

Wilkins RL, Stoller JK, Scanlan CL: *Egan's Fundamentals of Respiratory Care*, ed 8. St. Louis, Mosby, 2003.

Chapter 21

Obstructive Pulmonary Disease and Ventilatory Management

I. Obstructive Pulmonary Diseases Are Characterized by Airflow Limitation

II. Specific Diseases in This Category Include:
   A. Emphysema
   B. Chronic bronchitis
   C. Asthma
   D. Bronchitis
   E. Cystic fibrosis
   F. Bronchiectasis

III. In Obstructive Pulmonary Disease Airflow Limitation Results from:
   A. Inflammation
   B. Airway hyperactivity
   C. Secretions
   D. Loss of structural integrity of the lung

IV. All of the Above Lead to:
   A. Air trapping
   B. Increased work of breathing
   C. Ventilatory muscle dysfunction
   D. These are the major concerns affecting the approach and ease of providing ventilatory support to patients with obstructive pulmonary disease.

V. Air Trapping (see Chapter 40) (Figure 21-1)
   A. The trapping of gas at end-exhalation in the lung parenchyma.
   B. This results in an increase in the functional residual capacity and an alteration in the end-expiratory position of the diaphragm.
   C. Air trapping results in the development of auto-positive end-expiratory pressure (PEEP).
   D. The level of auto-PEEP is determined by the tidal volume, respiratory system compliance, airway resistance, and expiratory time:

   $$\text{auto-PEEP} = \frac{V_T}{[(C) \times (e^{K_E/T_E} - 1)]} \tag{1}$$

   where $K_E = 1/R_E \times C$, e is the base of the natural logarithm, T_E is expiratory time, R_E is expiratory airways resistance, and C is respiratory system compliance.
   E. In obstructive lung disease auto-PEEP develops because of:

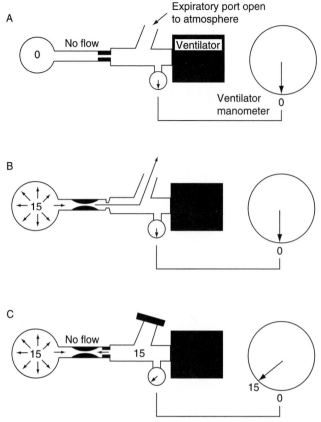

FIG. 21-1 Relationship between alveolar, central airway, and ventilator circuit pressure under **(A)** normal conditions and in the presence of severe dynamic airway obstruction, **(B)** with expiratory port open, and **(C)** with expiratory port occluded. Auto-positive end-expiratory pressure (PEEP) level is identified by creating an end-expiratory hold, allowing alveolar, central airway, and ventilator circuit pressure to equilibrate. Note that during equilibration auto-PEEP level can be read on the system manometer.

1. Increased compliance: All diseases except asthma
2. Increased airway resistance: All diseases but especially asthma

F. With most obstructive diseases there is instability of the small airways. As a result these airways dilate during inspiration but narrow during expiration.

G. This is referred to as dynamic airway obstruction.

H. In most obstructive lung disease it is the combination of dynamic airway obstruction and increased respiratory system compliance that accounts for the development of auto-PEEP.
1. Auto-PEEP caused by this mechanism is usually not increased by the addition of applied PEEP until the applied PEEP level is ≥80% of the auto-PEEP level.
2. To trigger an assisted breath the patient must first decompress the auto-PEEP.
3. Appling PEEP in the presence of dynamic airway obstruction (see Figure 21-1) decreases the pressure threshold needed to trigger the ventilator.

I. In asthma the limitation of airway flow is a result of increased fixed airway resistance caused by bronchospasm and edema.
1. In this setting auto-PEEP level is not beneficially affected by the application of PEEP.
2. For patients with asthma the application of PEEP usually does not offset the auto-PEEP as in dynamic airway obstruction. For those with asthma applied PEEP is normally additive to auto-PEEP.

J. Beyond altered lung mechanics, minute ventilation has the greatest overall effect on the level of air trapping and auto-PEEP.

1. The greater the minute ventilation, the greater the auto-PEEP.
2. The lower the minute ventilation, the lower the auto-PEEP.

K. Refer to Chapter 40 for a full discussion on identification of auto-PEEP level.
   1. As noted in Figure 21-2 for spontaneously breathing patients triggering the ventilator, auto-PEEP is most commonly observed by a difference in the patients' ventilatory rate and the ventilator response rate.
   2. If the patient's rate is higher than the ventilator response rate it is almost ensured that the cause is auto-PEEP.
   3. To offset the effect of auto-PEEP on patient triggering (in dynamic airway obstruction) PEEP should be slowly applied in 1- to 2-cm H_2O steps until every patient effort triggers the ventilator.
   4. In some patients this may require applied PEEP as high as 15 cm H_2O.

VI. Increased Work of Breathing

   A. The biggest adverse impact of auto-PEEP for patients with obstructive lung disease is an increase in work of breathing.
   B. As discussed previously if a patient must decompress the auto-PEEP level to inspire, work of breathing increases. For example:

• Airway pressure =	0.0 cm H_2O
• Auto-PEEP level =	10.0 cm H_2O
• Pressure gradient needed to cause flow into the airway	10.0 cm H_2O
• Normal transpulmonary pressure during breathing	3.0 cm H_2O
• Total pressure gradient to breath in the presence of 10.0 cm H_2O auto-PEEP	13.0 cm H_2O

   C. In patients with severe obstructive lung disease with air trapping and auto-PEEP, the diaphragm is flattened. This prevents its contraction from increasing the anterior-posterior diameter of the thorax and laterally expanding the lower rib cage. This frequently results in paradoxical breathing:
   1. Anterior abdominal wall moves inward.
   2. Lateral rib cage moves inward.
   3. Expansion of the upper chest wall.

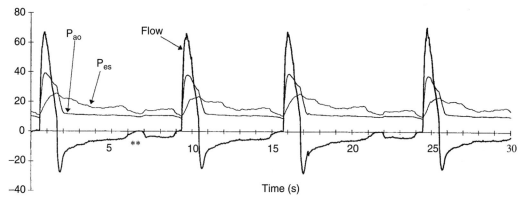

FIG. 21-2 Esophageal pressure (P_{es}), airway opening pressure (P_{ao}), and flow at the tracheostomy in a patient with dysynchrony on volume-cycled (assist/control) mode. The units are cm H_2O for the pressure tracing and L/min for flow. The patient's inspiratory efforts are identified by the negative P_{es} swings. The positive end-expiratory pressure is set at 0. P_{ao} appropriately decreases to 0 during expiration, demonstrating little circuit or valve resistance. Dysynchrony is evident with one triggered breath every three to four efforts. Prolonged expiratory flow is caused by airflow limitation. P_{es} swings have little effect in retarding the expiratory flow and even less effect on P_{ao}, depending on the phase of expiration.

VII. **The Overall Indications for Ventilation in Patients With Chronic Pulmonary Disease Are:**
   A. Acute or chronic ventilatory failure
   B. Unloading work of breathing
   C. Resting ventilatory muscles
   D. Improving bronchial hygiene

VIII. **Noninvasive Positive Pressure Ventilation**
   For all patients with obstructive pulmonary disease requiring ventilatory support, except those with asthma, noninvasive positive pressure ventilation (NPPV) should be the first ventilatory option (see Chapter 43).
   A. The data clearly indicate that the use of NPPV in these patients results in:
      1. A decreased need for intubation
      2. Decreased length of mechanical ventilation
      3. Decreased length of intensive care unit (ICU) stay
      4. Decreased rate of nosocomial pneumonia and other infections
      5. Decreased cost of care
      6. Improved mortality
   B. NPPV should be applied with a ventilator that allows assessment of patient-ventilator synchrony; waveforms should be available (Box 21-1).
   C. Initially an oronasal mask should be used.
   D. Mode of ventilation should be pressure support or pressure assist/control (B_IPAP).
   E. Peak airway pressure should not exceed 20 cm H_2O to avoid gastric distention.
   F. PEEP should be set to minimize the effort to trigger inspiration as a result of auto-PEEP: approximately 3 to 10 cm H_2O.
   G. Ventilatory pressures do not need to be elevated; for most patients a ventilating pressure (pressure support level) of 8 to 12 cm H_2O is adequate to produce an appropriate VT.
   H. VT should only be approximately 4 to 8 ml/kg predicted body weight; excessive VT increases dysynchrony.
   I. Respiratory rate should be up to the patient. Back-up rate should be set at approximately 8 to 10 breaths/min.
   J. Inspiratory time should be equal to the patient's neuroinspiratory time, usually 0.6 to 1.0 second.

IX. **Invasive Ventilation of Obstructive Lung Disease (Box 21-2)**
   A. Because of respiratory muscle dysfunction and increased work of breathing, assist/control and pressure support are the modes of choice.
   B. Volume or pressure targeting can be used, but pressure ventilation is preferred because it better ensures that gas delivery matches ventilatory demand.
   C. VT is targeted or set at approximately 8 to 10 ml/kg provided plateau pressure is ≤25 cm H_2O.
   D. If plateau pressure is >25 cm H_2O, tidal volume should be approximately 6 to 8 ml/kg predicted body weight (PBW).
      PBW (kg) males = 50 + 0.91 (height in cm, 152)
      PBW (kg) females = 45.5 + 0.91 (height in cm, 152)

BOX 21-1

Initial Setting of Ventilator During NPPV in Acute Respiratory Failure

Ventilator: Provides waveforms of airway pressure and flow
Mode: Pressure support or pressure assist/control (B_IPAP)
Mask: Oronasal
Peak airway pressure: 20 cm H_2O maximum
PEEP: 3 to 10 cm H_2O
Ventilating pressure: 8 to 12 cm H_2O
Inspiratory time: ≤0.6 to 1.0 second
Tidal volume: Approximately 6 to 8 ml/kg
Respiratory rate: Patient determined

BOX 21-2

Initial Ventilator Setting During Invasive Ventilation of Patients With Obstructive Pulmonary Disease

Ventilator: Any ICU ventilator ideally with waveforms, airway pressure, and flow displayed.
Mode: Pressure assist/control, pressure support, or volume assist control.
Tidal volume: Targeted or set 8 to 10 ml/kg PBW if plateau pressure ≤25 cm H_2O, approximately 6 ml/kg PBW if plateau pressure between 26 and 30 cm H_2O.
Plateau pressure: Ideally <25 cm H_2O, absolutely should be <30 cm H_2O.
PEEP: 5 to 10 cm H_2O
F_IO_2: ≤0.50 to maintain PaO_2 55 to 75 mm Hg
Rate: Patient set with back-up rate 10 to 16 breaths/min
I:E: ≤1:3
Inspiratory time: 0.6 to 1.0 second
Flow waveform: Decelerating in volume A/C
Peak flow: ≥80 L/min in volume A/C

   E. PEEP is set to offset the effects of auto-PEEP and ensure all patient inspiratory efforts trigger an assisted breath, usually 5 to 10 cm H_2O.
   F. Inspiratory time should be equal to the patient's neuroinspiratory time. The more stressed the patient, the shorter the inspiratory time, usually 0.6 to 1.0 second.
   G. The inspiration-to-expiration (I:E) ratio is not set, but it should be as low as tolerated. The expiratory time should be lengthy to avoid air trapping, usually ≤1:3.
   H. The flow waveform in volume ventilation should be decelerating with a peak flow ≥60 liters per minute (LPM) to ensure that initial gas delivery will meet the patient's inspiratory demand.
   I. F_IO_2 is set to ensure PaO_2 is between approximately 55 and 75 mm Hg. This usually requires an F_IO_2 ≤0.5.
   J. Respiratory rate is usually patient determined. However, many of these patients, after minor sedation, allow the ventilator to control rate. A back-up rate of 10 to 16 breaths/min generally maintains adequate ventilation.
   K. Adequate ventilation is a $PaCO_2$ equal to preventilation baseline, which may be 60 to 80 mm Hg. The key here is to maintain the pH at baseline values usually ≥7.30.
   L. Patients with bronchitis, emphysema, and cystic fibrosis are generally ventilated the same way as patients with chronic obstructive pulmonary disease (COPD).

  X. **Ventilatory Management of Asthma (Box 21-3)**
   A. All patients with severe asthma requiring ventilatory support develop air trapping and auto-PEEP.
   B. The air trapping occurs because of increased fixed airway resistance as a result of bronchospasm and edema. The accumulation of a large amount of secretions also causes a ball-valve obstruction, increasing air trapping.

BOX 21-3

Ventilatory Management of Severe Asthma

Ventilator: Provides waveforms of airway pressure and flow.
Mode: Initially VA/C but once ventilation can be achieved with a peak PA/C level of 30 cm H_2O, PA/C can be used.
V_T: 4 to 8 ml/kg predicted body weight, level to maintain plateau pressure <30 cm H_2O.
Rate: 8 to 16 breaths/min, lowest rate minimizing auto-PEEP, patient dependent.
Flow waveform: Decelerating
Inspiratory time: 1 to 1.5 seconds
Peak flow: Sufficient to ensure V_T delivery in set inspiratory time >60 LPM
F_IO_2: Sufficient to maintain PaO_2 >60 mm Hg
PEEP: 0 to 5 cm H_2O should not increase plateau pressure when applied.

C. This high level of auto-PEEP coupled with an increased drive to breathe results in large intrathoracic pressure swings producing marked pulsus paradoxus.

D. Mechanical ventilation is indicated when the asthmatic patient can no longer maintain adequate gas exchange.
1. This point is difficult to determine.
2. Because most patients are young, they can work to maintain a $PaCO_2$ $\leq$40 mm Hg until they are exhausted.
3. But once exhausted their $PaCO_2$ can increase rapidly.
4. As a result once $PaCO_2$ increases to >45 to 50 mm Hg and acidosis begins to develop, ventilatory support is indicated.

E. Heliox: For many patients the administration of heliox (see Chapter 34) can markedly reduce the effort to breathe.
1. Unfortunately this does not occur for all patients.
2. At this time there is no method to determine who can be successfully treated with heliox and who cannot.

F. NPPV has been used for some patients with severe asthma.
1. We have not found NPPV useful.
2. Patients alert and oriented and not sedated with severe asthma have a difficult time tolerating a tight-fitting mask.

G. Two major concerns exist when initially ventilating a patient with severe asthma.
1. Auto-PEEP
2. Adequate driving pressure to deliver a VT

H. Patients with asthma requiring intubation are markedly difficult to ventilate because of high airway resistance.
1. Large driving pressures are needed to move airflow past the obstruction.
2. Initially the only mode that can ventilate these patients is volume assist/control (VA/C).
3. In VA/C a high driving pressure can be achieved, but because of a low VT, plateau pressures can still be maintained at <30 cm H_2O.
4. Peak pressure may need to be 60 to 80 cm H_2O to deliver a VT of 4 ml/kg PBW in a 1.5-second inspiratory time and still maintain a plateau pressure of <30 cm H_2O.
5. Although a high peak pressure is not desirable, there is no evidence that it causes lung injury because it only represents the pressure driving gas to the obstruction, not the pressure affecting the peripheral lung.
6. Plateau pressure represents the peak alveolar distending pressure, which has been associated with marked alveolar damage.
7. Once reversal of some of the acute obstruction occurs, the mode can be charged to pressure assist/control (PA/C).
8. With PA/C peak pressure should be kept $\leq$30 cm H_2O because with PA/C peak pressure is essentially equal to peak alveolar distending pressure.
9. The change from VA/C to PA/C should only occur when a peak pressure of $\leq$30 cm H_2O in PA/C can deliver the desired tidal volume.

I. Most patients with severe asthma require heavy sedation, and some patients also need paralysis to effectively provide mechanical ventilation.
1. During the initial phase of ventilation in those with severe asthma, spontaneously breathing patients fight the ventilator.
2. After initial stabilization, the least sedation that ensures adequate ventilation is indicated.

J. As already stated VT is set low, 4 to 8 ml/kg PBW.

K. The actual VT setting depends on the plateau pressure, which should be $\leq$30 cm H_2O.

L. Inspiratory time: For patients with severe asthma, time is needed to allow gas to enter the lung past obstructions. Inspiratory times ideally should be approximately 1 to 1.5 seconds. With shorter times effective ventilation may not be possible.

M. Auto-PEEP is a major problem and more difficult to manage than in patients with COPD.
1. As illustrated in Figure 21-3 auto-PEEP cannot be effectively measured in those with severe asthma.

End-expiratory airway occlusion

Measured AP = 5 cm H$_2$O

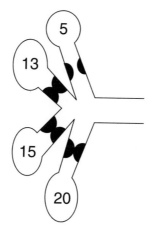

FIG. 21-3 A hypothetical model to explain underestimation of end-expiratory alveolar pressure using measured auto-positive end-expiratory pressure (auto-PEEP) in patients with severe asthma. Alveolar pressure (cm H$_2$O) in four different lung units is shown. At end-expiration, only the upper lung unit is communicating with the central airway, causing the airway occlusion pressure (measured auto-PEEP) to be much lower than end-expiratory alveolar pressure in the other hyperinflated but noncommunicating lung units.

    2. Obstruction is fixed and near complete in some airways; as a result at end exhalation some airways are completely obstructed, preventing communication of pressure with central airways.

    3. As a result the auto-PEEP behind these obstructed areas is not included in the measurement of auto-PEEP.

    4. This has been referred to as occult auto-PEEP.

    5. When the measured auto-PEEP level is 8 cm H$_2$O, the actual auto-PEEP level may be 15 cm H$_2$O.

    6. For patients with severe asthma it is better to monitor plateau pressure change as a reflection of changing auto-PEEP than auto-PEEP itself.

       a. If an increase in rate increases plateau pressure, auto-PEEP increased.

       b. If a decrease in rate decreases plateau pressure, auto-PEEP decreased.

N. Ideal respiratory rate for a given patient may vary widely in those with severe asthma.

    1. It is difficult to identity a specific rate that results in the best ventilation and least auto-PEEP for all patients.

    2. In some a low rate with a higher V$_T$ results in the least auto-PEEP and best P$_{CO_2}$.

    3. In others a higher rate with a smaller V$_T$ results in the least auto-PEEP and best P$_{CO_2}$.

    4. Ideal rates across patients can vary between approximately 8 and 20 breaths/min.

O. Applied PEEP in most patients with severe asthma does increase the level of total PEEP (auto-PEEP + applied PEEP).

    1. As a result, >5 cm H$_2$O applied PEEP is not recommended.

    2. If 5 cm H$_2$O applied PEEP increases the plateau pressure it should be removed.

    3. However, there are some asthmatic patients that do respond similarly to COPD patients. The application of applied PEEP decreases the measured auto-PEEP, but these are rare patients.

P. Permissive hypercapnia: The first patients to experience permissive hypercapnia were asthmatic patients.

    1. Because these are usually young otherwise healthy patients they frequently can tolerate a pH <7.20, sometimes a pH of 7.00.

2. The dilemma is which is more detrimental: the acidosis caused by the hypercapnia or the high plateau pressure needed to better ventilate.
3. If the patient's hemodynamic status tolerates the acidosis, plateau pressure should not be increased to correct it.

Q. F_IO_2 is adjusted to maintain the PaO_2 >60 mm Hg.

R. There are some data that indicate ventilating patients with heliox mixtures decreases plateau pressure and improves $PaCO_2$.
1. This is poorly defined in the literature, but we have observed improvement in select patients.
2. Heliox concentration should be at least 50% helium.
3. If the patient cannot tolerate ≤50% oxygen, heliox is not indicated.
4. Few ventilators function properly with heliox because of its density. Internal monitoring systems cannot accurately determine volume.
5. This prevents some ventilators from functioning properly.
6. If heliox is used, careful monitoring of plateau pressure is essential.
7. The readout of VT will always be incorrect, underestimating the delivered VT.

XI. **Use of New Modes of Ventilation (see Chapter 39)**
   A. There are no data to indicate that the newer modes of ventilation improve outcome in patients with either COPD or asthma.
   B. Especially with asthma, patients are usually sedated to apnea, with VA/C and PA/C the modes of choice.
   C. For COPD patients assisted ventilation is common, but again none of the new modes has demonstrated any benefit.
   D. However, many COPD patients are ventilated in pressure support. Adjustment of *rise time* and *expiratory cycling criteria* is helpful to improve patient-ventilator synchrony.
      1. Rise time: Adjusts the slope of the pressure rise at the onset of pressure support (Figure 21-4).
      2. The greater the patient's demand, the higher (faster) should be the rise time setting.
      3. Pressure should not exceed the set level at the onset of inspiration.
      4. Pressure should not be concave at the onset of inspiration (Figure 21-5).
      5. A more rapid rise time results in a greater initial flow rate.
   E. Expiratory cycling criteria
      1. This control varies the end-expiratory flow that terminates the pressure support breath.

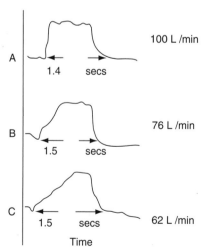

FIG. 21-4 Effect of changing rise time in a patient. **A,** The fastest rise time produces a rapid increase to set PSV level and smooth transition to the pressure plateau. As flow rate is decreased (**B** and **C**), the time to reach the pressure support ventilation (PSV) level is lengthened, and inspiratory time (T_I) increases slightly.

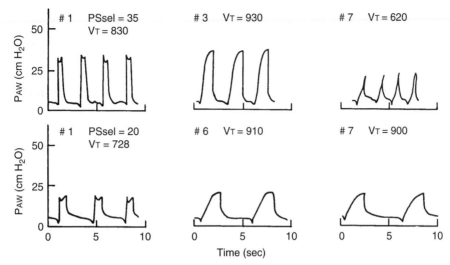

FIG. 21-5 Examples of airway pressure tracings in two patients with different rise times during pressure support. Rise times are expressed as one of seven discrete settings ranging from maximal (#1) to minimal (#7). For these two patients, a maximal, optimal, and minimal initial rise time is depicted. In the top panels, the optimal rise time for this patient was the third fastest (#3). Note that the attained pressure and tidal volume appeared highest, and the inspiratory time (T$_I$) was longest at the optimal rise time setting. In the bottom panels, the optimal rise time setting was the second slowest (#6). Again note that the attained pressure and tidal volume appeared highest, and the T$_I$ was longest at the optimal rise time setting.

    2. An increase in pressure above the set level (Figure 21-6) should not occur before exhalation in pressure support.

    3. However, this problem is common in COPD patients if their end-expiratory flow rate is higher than the flow terminating the breath.

    4. The expiratory cycling criteria should be increased (greater end-expiratory flow to cycle to exhalation) until no pressure spike is observed at end exhalation.

XII.　Weaning (see Chapter 41)

    A. COPD patients can be difficult to wean from ventilatory support.

        1. With each exacerbation COPD patients' baseline ventilatory function is more compromised.

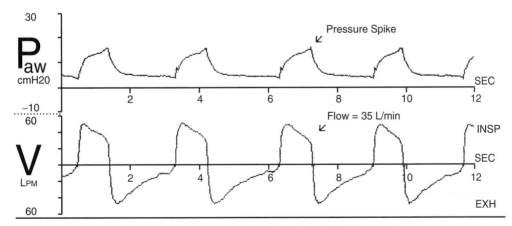

FIG. 21-6 Pressure and flow tracing in a patient with chronic obstructive pulmonary disease on pressure support ending the breath by forcing exhalation. The patient's end-inspiratory flow was 35 L/min, and the ventilator was set to cycle to expiration at an end-inspiratory flow of 5 L/min. Spike in pressure is a result of activation of accessory muscles of exhalation at the end of mechanical (pressure support) inspiration.

2. The approach to weaning that has been shown to be most successful for COPD patients is a spontaneous breathing trial.
3. Most patients can successfully be evaluated by a T-piece trial.
4. However, those with high auto-PEEP levels may need spontaneous breathing evaluation while receiving 5 cm H_2O continuous positive airway pressure.
5. Others with small endotracheal tubes or nasal intubation may need 5 cm H_2O pressure support during evaluation of spontaneous breathing.
6. A small percentage of these patients will become ventilator dependent.

B. Asthma patients do not well tolerate attempts at weaning.
1. Frequently when sedation is reversed the endotracheal tube itself can induce bronchospasm.
2. These patients once evaluated to be near baseline status can simply be extubated without a weaning trial.
3. As stated earlier patients are normally healthy and young, and once the severe asthma is reversed, they return to their baseline level.

BIBLIOGRAPHY

Albert RA, et al: *Comprehensive Respiratory Medicine.* London, Mosby, 1999.

Branson RD, Campbell RS: Patient-ventilator synchrony and ventilator algorithms. *Resp Care* 43:1045-1047, 1998.

Branson RD, Campbell RS, Davis K, et al: Altering flowrate during maximum pressure support ventilation (PSV max): Effects on cardiopulmonary function. *Respir Care* 35:1056-1064, 1990.

Chao DC, Scheinhorn DJ, Stern-Hassenpflug M: Patient-ventilator trigger asynchrony in prolonged mechanical ventilation. *Chest* 112:1592-1599, 1997.

Hess DR, Kacmarek RM: *Essentials of Mechanical Ventilation,* ed 2. New York, McGraw Hill, 2002.

Hess DR, MacIntyre NR, Mishoe SC, Galvin WF, Adams AB, Saposnick AB: *Respiratory Care Principles and Practices.* Philadelphia, WB Saunders, 2002.

Leatherman JW, Raveneraft SA: Low measured auto-positive end-expiratory pressure during mechanical ventilation of patients with severe asthma: Hidden auto-positive end expiratory pressure. *Crit Care Med* 24:541-546, 1996.

MacIntyre NR, Ho L: Effects of initial flow rate and breath termination criteria on pressure support ventilation. *Chest* 99:134-138, 1991.

Pepe PE, Marini JJ: Occult positive end-expiratory pressure in mechanically ventilated patients with airflow obstruction: The auto-PEEP effect. *Am Rev Respir Dis* 126:166-170, 1982.

Pierson DJ, Kacmarek RM: *Foundations of Respiratory Care.* New York, Churchill Livingstone, 1992.

Wilkins RL, Stoller JK, Scanlan CL: *Egan's Fundamentals of Respiratory Care,* ed 8. St. Louis, Mosby, 2003.

Chapter 22

Restrictive Lung Diseases: General and Ventilatory Management

I. **General Comments**
   A. A restrictive lung disease is any disease in which the ability to inhale is affected.
   B. Restrictive diseases of pulmonary origin are frequently associated with an increase in pulmonary fibrous tissue. The result is an overall increase in pulmonary elastance and a decrease in pulmonary compliance.
   C. Characteristic pulmonary function findings (Table 22-1)
      1. Decreased or normal tidal volume (V_T).
      2. Decreased or normal residual volume (RV).
      3. Decreased or normal expiratory reserve volume (ERV).
      4. Decreased or normal inspiratory reserve volume (IRV).
      5. Decreased total lung capacity (TLC).
      6. Decreased vital capacity (VC).
      7. Decreased inspiratory capacity (IC).
      8. Decreased or normal functional residual capacity (FRC).
      9. Flow rate studies usually are normal in pure restrictive lung diseases; however, flow rates may be decreased when an obstructive component is also present.
      10. Pulmonary and/or thoracic compliance and total compliance are usually severely decreased.
      11. There is a progressive increase in the work of breathing as the severity of the disease increases.
         a. Initially alveolar minute ventilation is normal or increased, but as the disease progresses alveolar minute ventilation progressively decreases.
         b. Arterial blood gases may follow the same pattern as that seen in obstructive lung disease. The initial presenting symptom may be chronic respiratory alkalosis with hypoxemia, but as the disease progresses chronic respiratory acidosis with hypoxemia may develop.
   D. Categories of restrictive diseases
      1. Pulmonary
      2. Thoracoskeletal
      3. Neurologic-neuromuscular
      4. Abdominal

II. **Pulmonary Restrictive Lung Diseases**
   A. Interstitial pulmonary fibrosis: A disease characterized by the excessive formation of connective tissue in the process of repairing chronic or acute tissue injury.
      1. Etiology: Any permanent injury to the lung (e.g., infection, inflammation, and allergy).

TABLE **22-1**		

Changes in Pulmonary Function Associated With Obstructive and Restrictive Lung Disease

Pulmonary Function Study	Obstructive Disease	Restrictive Disease
TLC	Normal or increased	Decreased
VC	Normal or decreased	Decreased
FRC	Increased	Normal or decreased
RV	Increased	Normal or decreased
RV/TLC ratio	Increased	Normal
$FEV_1\%$	Decreased	Normal
$MMEFR_{25\%-75\%}$	Decreased	Normal or decreased

TLC, Total lung capacity; *VC,* vital capacity; *FRC,* functional residual capacity; *RV,* residual volume; $FEV_1\%$, percentage of forced vital capacity in 1 second; $MMEFR_{25\%-75\%}$, maximum midexpiratory flow rate between 25% and 75%.

2. Type: Localized or diffuse
   a. Causes of localized fibrosis
      (1) Tuberculosis
      (2) Unresolved pneumonias
      (3) Fungal infections
      (4) Abscess formation
   b. Causes of diffuse fibrosis
      (1) Long-term exposure to various inhalants. Specific pneumoconioses are listed in Table 22-2.
      (2) Short-term exposure to toxic inhalants may also cause diffuse fibrosis (e.g., chlorine gas, ammonia, polyvinyl chloride, smoke inhalation, and radiation therapy).
      (3) Diseases of unknown etiology that often show diffuse fibrosis:
         (a) Hamman-Rich syndrome
         (b) Eosinophilic granuloma
         (c) Sarcoidosis
         (d) Familial fibrocystic dysphagia
         (e) Chronic interstitial pneumonia
         (f) Collagen diseases
3. Pathophysiology
   a. Inflammatory reaction in response to organic or inorganic foreign agents.
   b. Inflammation is followed by cellular infiltration and acute vasculitis with local hemorrhage and thrombus formation, resulting in scar tissue.
4. Clinical presentation
   a. Primary symptom: Progressive dyspnea on exertion and ultimately at rest.
   b. Nonproductive cough.

TABLE **22-2**	

Specific Pneumoconioses

Disease	Causative Agent
Silicosis	Silica dust
Farmer's lung	Moldy hay
Stannosis	Tin dust
Silo-filler's disease	Nitrogen dioxide
Coal worker's pneumoconiosis	Coal dust
Asbestosis	Asbestos
Berylliosis	Beryllium
Siderosis	Iron dust

    c. As disease continues, progressive respiratory impairment and often cor pulmonale.

    d. Physical examination findings:

       (1) Clubbing

       (2) Cyanosis

       (3) Restricted chest wall and diaphragmatic movement

       (4) Diffuse, dry, crackling rales

       (5) Increased work of breathing

       (6) Use of accessory muscles of ventilation

       (7) Tachypnea with shallow tidal volumes

    e. Chest radiography film

       (1) Small lung with large heart and elevated diaphragm

       (2) Fine reticular or nodular pattern involving entire lung but predominantly the lower lobes

    f. Arterial blood gases and pulmonary function studies as outlined in Section I, General Comments.

  5. Treatment

    a. Removal of patient from environment causing the fibrotic changes if possible

    b. Therapy for underlying disease entity

    c. Corticosteroids

    d. Immunosuppressants

       (1) Azathioprine

       (2) Cyclophosphamide

    e. Oxygen therapy: As disease progresses, increased dyspnea is reported. Many patients are relatively refractory to oxygen therapy. Continuous positive airway pressure (CPAP) is often helpful. Care must be taken when disconnecting patient from CPAP because severe acute hypoxemia may ensue.

    f. Penicillamine therapy has improved subjective assessment of patients.

    g. Cyclosporine is used in late stages.

    h. Plasmapheresis is effective in a few patients with high titers of immune complexes in later stages.

    i. Total heart-lung transplant has been successful in some patients.

    j. Mechanical ventilation: If these patients progress to mechanical ventilation, V_T delivery is limited because of decreased compliance. This results in increased inspiratory pressure that is not associated with overdistention of the lung.

       (1) V_T: 4 to 8 ml/kg

       (2) Rate: 20 to 35 breaths/min

       (3) Inspiratory time: 0.5 to 0.8 second

       (4) F_IO_2 and positive end-expiratory pressure (PEEP) settings follow normal guidelines.

       (5) See Chapters 39, 40, and 41.

B. Pleural effusion: Accumulation of fluid in pleural space.

  1. Normally the capillary network of the visceral pleural surface produces the fluid lining of the pleura, and any excess is removed by the lymphatic system.

  2. Any disturbance in production of this fluid or in its removal can lead to the development of pleural effusion.

  3. Primary causes: Inflammation and circulatory disorders.

    a. Malignancy

    b. Congestive heart failure (CHF)

    c. Infection

    d. Pulmonary infarction

    e. Trauma, including surgery

  4. The effusion compresses the lung on the affected side.

  5. The effusion is gravity dependent and may shift with positional change.

  6. Diagnosis

    a. Diagnosis is suggested by history, clinical presentation, and radiologic findings (Figure 22-1).

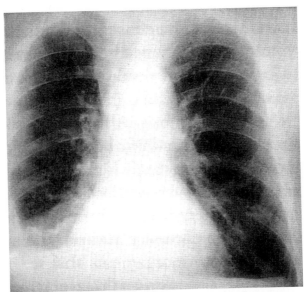

FIG. 22-1 Right-sided basal pleural effusion. Posteroanterior.

     b.   Definitive diagnosis is confirmed by thoracentesis.

  7. Types of effusions
     a.   Hydrothorax: A thin clear transudate caused by CHF, chronic nephritis, or pulmonary neoplasm.
     b.   Empyema (pyothorax): An effusion consisting entirely of pus caused by a bacterial infection.
     c.   Hemothorax: Frank blood caused by a malignancy, pulmonary infarction, or ruptured blood vessel.
     d.   Chylothorax: Accumulation of chyle resulting from the obstruction or trauma of the thoracic duct.
     e.   Fibrothorax: An accumulation of fibrous tissue normally secondary to a prolonged effusion.

  8. Treatment
     a.   Primary: Removal of fluid from pleural space.
       (1) Thoracentesis or insertion of chest tubes.
       (2) Fluid allowed to reabsorb into pulmonary lymphatic system.
     b.   Secondary: Management of underlying disease.

C. Pneumothorax: Accumulation of air within the pleural space.
  1. If air enters the pleural space, the pressure within the space changes from subatmospheric to atmospheric or supraatmospheric pressure.
     a.   The increased pressure compresses lung tissue and results in atelectasis.
     b.   Ventilation of the lung on the affected side is decreased as a result of elimination of the subatmospheric intrapleural pressure.
  2. Diagnosis
     a.   Diagnosis is suggested by history and clinical presentation.
     b.   Definitive diagnosis is confirmed by chest radiography (Figure 22-2).
  3. Types: Open and under tension.
     a.   In an open pneumothorax, there is no buildup of pressure because the gas is allowed to move freely in and out of the pleural space.
     b.   A tension pneumothorax results from the presence of a one-way valve, which allows gas only to enter the pleural space and not to leave it. This results in significant increases in pressure within the pleural space. If untreated it may quickly result in cardiac arrest.

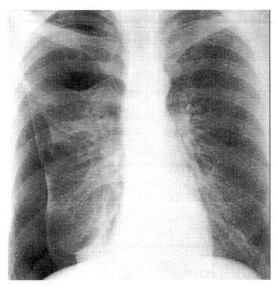

FIG. 22-2 Partial pneumothorax with adhesions.

    (1) Clinical signs
        (a) Increased difficulty in ventilation: If patient is mechanically ventilated, airway pressure increases with each breath.
        (b) Patient's vital signs begin to deteriorate as mean intrathoracic pressure increases.
        (c) Breath sounds are absent on the affected side.
        (d) The affected side is hyperresonant to percussion.
        (e) Trachea and mediastinum may be shifted toward the unaffected side as the extent of tension pneumothorax increases.
        (f) Possible pleuritic pain.
        (g) Dry, hacking cough.
        (h) These clinical signs are more predominant if the patient is using a mechanical ventilator than if he or she is ventilating spontaneously. This is because of the greater pressure gradients developed, forcing more gas into the pleural space.
    (2) Treatment: Decompression of the thorax by chest tube insertion.

D. Cardiogenic pulmonary edema: Active movement of fluid across alveolar capillary membrane into alveoli as a result of increased capillary hydrostatic pressures.
   1. Normally a fine balance exists among capillary colloid osmotic (oncotic) pressure, capillary hydrostatic pressure, interstitial hydrostatic pressure, and interstitial colloid osmotic (oncotic) pressure across the pulmonary capillary bed (see Chapter 14).
   2. Usually a small net pressure forces fluid into the interstitial space. This interstitial fluid is drained by the lymphatics.
   3. If capillary hydrostatic pressure increases significantly, the net pressure forcing fluid into the interstitial space increases, and eventually fluid moves directly into the alveoli.
   4. Primary cause: Acute left ventricular failure (CHF)
      a. The hydrostatic pressure of the pulmonary vascular bed is increased because of the inability of the left side of the heart to accept the blood presented to it.
      b. This increased pressure offsets the normal pressure dynamics at the alveolar capillary membrane.
   5. Secondary cause: Increased vascular volume causing an increase in pulmonary capillary hydrostatic pressure.

6. Acute right ventricular failure (CHF)
    a. Systemic edema develops as a result of right ventricular failure.
    b. The inability of the right side of the heart to accept the blood presented to it results in blood pooling in the periphery.
    c. Dependent edema (pedal edema), neck vein distention, and hepatomegaly are common clinical findings.
    d. It is not unlikely for patients with right-sided heart failure to eventually develop left-sided heart failure and those with left-sided heart failure to develop right-sided heart failure.
7. Treatment
    a. Primary: Pharmacologic
        (1) Furosemide (Lasix)
        (2) Morphine
        (3) Digitalis
    b. Intraaortic balloon counterpulsation
    c. Oxygen therapy: Frequently high F_IO_2 is required.
    d. CPAP, by mask, at 8 to 12 cm H_2O has been helpful in some patients and may avoid intubation if pulmonary edema can be stabilized quickly.
    e. Noninvasive positive pressure ventilation (NPPV) has also been shown to improve oxygenation. It offers the added benefit of improving ventilation in patients who begin to develop respiratory muscle fatigue.
    f. Mechanical ventilation
        (1) Mechanical ventilation with PEEP can improve or further worsen cardiac function.
        (2) The increased mean airway pressure (as with CPAP) decreases venous return in left-sided heart failure.
        (3) Marked increases in mean airway pressure can markedly reduce pulmonary perfusion and increase deadspace ventilation.
        (4) When mechanical ventilator settings are titrated, markedly increasing minute ventilation should be avoided because Pco_2 increases with hemodynamic instability.
        (5) Stabilization of cardiac function improves the deadspace volume/tidal volume (Vd/Vt) ratio and thus returns Pco_2 to normal.
        (6) If increases in minute ventilation result in no change or an increase in Pco_2, lack of pulmonary perfusion is most likely the cause of the Pco_2 increase.
        (7) Ventilator settings generally are similar to those for all patients without lung disease. Efforts should be made to improve ventilation and oxygenation without causing a secondary, ventilator-induced lung injury (see Chapters 39, 40, and 41).
        (8) These patients generally require pharmacologic control during ventilation.
        (9) Spontaneous breathing at this stage:
            (a) Diverts up to 40% of cardiac output to ventilatory muscles.
            (b) Enhances ventilation/perfusion mismatchings.
            (c) Because of marked ventilatory drive, peak airway pressure limits are frequently met or exceeded.
            (d) May contribute to cardiac instability.
E. Noncardiogenic pulmonary edema
    1. The development of interstitial or true pulmonary edema from noncardiogenic origins.
    2. Pathophysiologic etiologies
        a. Altered permeability of capillary endothelial cells, allowing an increased quantity of fluid into the interstitial space.
        b. Decreased capillary colloid osmotic pressure, which increases the pressure gradient, allowing more fluid to enter the interstitial space.
        c. Altered lymphatic function, preventing normal drainage of the pulmonary interstitium, thereby allowing fluid to accumulate.
        d. Alveolar epithelial damage, allowing fluid to enter the alveoli.

3. Clinical etiologies
   a. Neurogenic origin
      (1) Neurogenic origin is primarily a result of an acute insult to the central nervous system.
      (2) It causes an increased sympathetic discharge, leading to a sudden intravascular fluid shift into the pulmonary circulation.
      (3) The imbalance in hydrostatic and osmotic pressures created causes fluid to enter the interstitial space.
   b. Drug overdose
      (1) The exact mechanism is poorly defined.
      (2) It is presumed that drugs, especially narcotics and sedatives, have a direct effect on increasing pulmonary capillary membrane permeability.
   c. High-altitude pulmonary edema
      (1) The mechanism is poorly understood.
      (2) It is thought to be the result of severe hypoxemia and vasoconstriction of the microcirculation.
      (3) Edema develops as blood flows under high pressure through the patent portion of the microvasculature.
   d. Reexpansion edema
      (1) It develops after the sudden reexpansion of a lung that had been collapsed for several hours.
      (2) The sudden reexpansion causes a negative pressure in the interstitium, creating a large pressure gradient across the capillary membrane and an increased transudation of fluid.
      (3) The rapid removal of pleural effusion fluid (>1000 ml) may produce edema.
   e. Pulmonary edema associated with renal disease
      (1) The mechanism is poorly defined.
      (2) It may occur in patients with acute glomerulonephritis or nephrotic syndrome.
      (3) It is also seen in patients with chronic uremia and in patients requiring long-term hemodialysis.
   f. Other clinical conditions known to lead to noncardiogenic pulmonary edema:
      (1) Sepsis
      (2) Shock
      (3) Pancreatitis
      (4) Toxic gas or smoke inhalation
      (5) Aspiration
      (6) Pulmonary infections
4. Clinical presentation
   a. Responsive hypoxemia
   b. Decreased compliance
   c. Diffuse atelectasis
   d. Minimal decrease in FRC
5. Treatment
   a. Oxygen therapy
   b. Fluid therapy
   c. Diuretics
   d. Low levels of PEEP therapy
F. Acute respiratory distress syndrome (ARDS) (see Chapter 23).
G. Pneumonia: Pneumonitis caused by a microorganism.
   1. Pneumonias are a leading cause of death in the United States and account for 10% of admissions to general medical floors.
   2. Pathophysiology of pneumonia
      a. Microorganisms cause inflammation of pulmonary mucosa, resulting in edema and phagocytic infiltration.

b. Exudation and consolidation result.
c. Consolidation is typically localized, as in lobar pneumonias.
3. Bacterial pneumonia (Table 22-3)
    a. Common clinical signs and symptoms
        (1) Abrupt onset (normally)
        (2) High fevers, with chills, sometimes lasting >20 minutes
        (3) Large volumes of thick, purulent sputum
        (4) Frequently tachypnea and tachycardia, sometimes a pleuritic-type pain
        (5) Radiographic film: Consolidation
        (6) White blood cell count: Frequently >10,000/mm^3
        (7) Hypoxemia secondary to shunting
4. Nonbacterial (viral or fungal) pneumonia (see Table 22-3)
    a. Clinical signs and symptoms (occasionally mild and frequently undiagnosed)
        (1) Onset normally is gradual.
        (2) Fevers normally are low grade; chills are uncommon.
        (3) Sputum production is minimal, usually thin and mucoid.
        (4) Tachypnea and tachycardia are rare; pleuritic pain is uncommon.
        (5) Radiographic film: Consolidation is uncommon.
        (6) White blood cell count commonly is <10,000/mm^3.
5. Treatment
    a. Appropriate antibiotic therapy (bacterial and fungal)
    b. Oxygen therapy
    c. Fluid therapy
    d. Aerosol therapy, if indicated
H. Pulmonary embolism
1. Pulmonary embolism is the occlusion of the pulmonary artery or one of its branches by a substance carried in the blood, normally a blood clot.
2. A blood clot that is attached to its site of origin is referred to as a *thrombus*. Once detached it is referred to as an *embolus*.
3. The actual substance may be fat, blood, air, amniotic fluid, or a tissue fragment.
4. Etiology and pathogenesis
    a. The most common sites of thrombus formation are the deep veins of the lower extremities and pelvis and within the right side of the heart.
    b. Thrombus development is most prevalent in patients who are immobilized by pain or who are debilitated, paralyzed, or require prolonged bed rest.
    c. Factors facilitating thrombus formation
        (1) Abnormal vessel wall
        (2) Stagnation of blood
        (3) Increased coagulability
    d. Dependent lung regions are most commonly involved with pulmonary emboli.

TABLE 22-3

Comparison of Clinical and Laboratory Manifestations of Bacterial and Viral Pneumonias

Symptom	Bacterial	Viral
Onset	Abrupt	Gradual
Fever	High	Low grade
Chills	Common	Uncommon
Sputum	Purulent, thick	Mucoid, thin
Tachycardia	Frequent	Rare
Hypoxemia	Common	Uncommon
Chest radiography results	Consolidation	Consolidation rare
White blood cell count	>10,000/mm^3	<10,000/mm^3
Pleuritic pain	Occasional	Uncommon

    e.   Pulmonary infarction occurs in approximately 10% of patients with pulmonary emboli, especially if there is a history of cardiac disease.

5.   Pathophysiology
    a.   Deadspace ventilation is significantly increased.
    b.   Total ventilation markedly increases in an effort to maintain normal P_{CO_2}.
    c.   A minute volume-P_{CO_2} disparity develops (large minute ventilation with near-normal P_{CO_2}).
    d.   With large emboli pulmonary artery pressures increase, especially if there is underlying cardiac disease.

6.   Clinical presentation
    a.   Patient has dyspnea and chest pain.
    b.   Hemoptysis may develop.
    c.   Frequently cough, faintness, and anxiety accompany pulmonary embolus.
    d.   Thrombophlebitis is often noted (frequently at the site of embolus formation).
    e.   If a massive embolus is present, there may be:
        (1) Tachypnea
        (2) Tachycardia
        (3) Cyanosis
        (4) Decreased breath sounds
        (5) Wheezing and rales
        (6) Pleural friction rub
    f.   Less common findings are:
        (1) Fever
        (2) Cardiac arrhythmias
        (3) Shock

7.   Chest radiography films
    a.   In some cases decreased lung volume, atelectasis, pleural effusion, and signs of pulmonary infarction may be present.
    b.   In rare cases there is a local reduction in vascular markings and an enlarged pulmonary artery.

8.   Laboratory findings
    a.   Lung volumes and capacities are decreased.
    b.   Flow studies are usually normal.
    c.   Arterial blood gases usually reveal hypoxemia with a normal acid-base balance or a respiratory alkalosis.
    d.   Electrocardiogram may reveal arrhythmias.

9.   Radioisotope lung scanning
    a.   Ventilation/perfusion scans may help differentiate pulmonary embolism from other perfusion abnormalities.
    b.   Findings must be correlated with patient's clinical findings and history.

10.   Pulmonary angiography is considered definitive in the diagnosis of pulmonary embolism.

11.   Treatment
    a.   Anticoagulation therapy with heparin
    b.   Thrombolysis
        (1) Streptokinase
        (2) Urokinase
        (3) Recombinant tissue plasminogen activator
    c.   Oxygen therapy
    d.   Intubation and ventilation in severe cases
    e.   Occasionally embolectomy is performed; however, this procedure is controversial.

I. Pulmonary alveolar proteinosis
    1.   A disease characterized by alveoli filled with a liquid high in protein and lipid.
    2.   Alveolar walls are normal, but only scattered macrophages are noted.

3. Pathogenesis
   a. The origin is unknown, but it is theorized that type II alveolar epithelial cells produce an excess of surfactant, lipid, and protein.
   b. This substance is poorly cleared by defective macrophages.
4. Prevalence
   a. Most commonly develops in persons aged 20 to 50 years, with a 2:1 male/female ratio.
   b. Some cases have been described in infants.
5. Clinical manifestations
   a. One third of all patients are asymptomatic.
   b. Common clinical findings:
      (1) Shortness of breath on exertion
      (2) Cough
      (3) Fatigue
      (4) Weight loss
      (5) Pleuritic pain
      (6) Possible low-grade fever
      (7) Clubbing of digits
6. Chest radiographic film reveals infiltrates in perihilar regions and bases of the lung.
7. Pulmonary function studies may be normal, but diffusing capacity is decreased.
8. Diagnosis is made primarily by open lung biopsy, bronchoalveolar lavage, or the measurement of lactic dehydrogenase levels.
9. Prognosis
   a. Clinical course is variable.
   b. Disease may spontaneously resolve but reappear at a later date.
   c. One third of patients die, primarily because of predisposition to infection.
10. Treatment
    a. No specific therapy is defined.
    b. Corticosteroids are used but are controversial.
    c. Lung lavage is helpful for some patients.

III. **Thoracoskeletal Restrictive Lung Diseases**
   A. Deformities of thoracic cage that result in limited movement of the chest demonstrate pulmonary function patterns consistent with restrictive lung disease.
   B. If the deformity is severe enough, a significant increase in the work of breathing results.
   C. Increased work of breathing eventually leads to hypoxemia, hypercapnia, and possible heart failure.
   D. Most commonly encountered thoracic abnormalities leading to restrictive lung disease are:
      1. Scoliosis: Gradual curvature of vertebral column in lateral plane of body (Figure 22-3).
         a. One of the most common thoracic deformities.
         b. May occur at various levels of the vertebral column.
         c. May develop with age as a result of poor posture.
      2. Kyphosis: Posterior curvature of thoracic vertebral column, resulting in a bony hump.
         a. Frequently develops in older individuals with degenerative osteoarthritis.
         b. May develop in individuals with chronic obstructive pulmonary disease (COPD).
      3. Kyphoscoliosis: Combination of thoracic scoliosis and kyphosis.
         a. In severe cases of kyphoscoliosis, one lung becomes severely compressed and the other overdistended.
         b. Cardiopulmonary disability may be pronounced in those with severe kyphoscoliosis.
   E. Treatment
      1. No primary treatment is indicated in most cases.
      2. Scoliosis may be managed surgically.
      3. Most treatment focuses on secondary pulmonary problems (e.g., pneumonia and asthma).

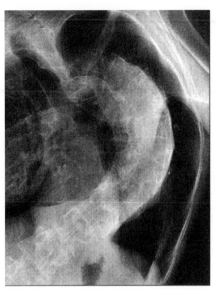

FIG. 22-3 Early-onset thoracic scoliosis.

4. Some patients with severe kyphoscoliosis develop progressive ventilatory muscle weakness and fatigue and may require nocturnal mechanical ventilatory assistance and oxygen therapy.
    a. NPPV may be helpful and is the primary mode of choice.
5. During acute pulmonary problems that require endotracheal intubation and mechanical ventilation, rates and VT settings differ from normal because of decreased lung volumes.
    a. VT: 4 to 8 ml/kg
    b. Rate: 20 to 35 breaths/min
    c. Inspiratory time: 0.5 to 0.8 second
    d. F_IO_2 and PEEP settings follow normal guidelines.
    e. See Chapters 39, 40, and 41.

IV. **Neurologic-Neuromuscular Restrictive Lung Diseases**
    A. Weakness or paralysis of the muscles of ventilation results in a pulmonary function pattern consistent with restrictive lung disease.
    B. Myasthenia gravis: A disease of the myoneural junction in which transmission of impulses across the motor endplate is inhibited.
        1. Etiology: Myasthenia gravis is most often an acquired immunologic abnormality, although some cases may be genetic. Functionally it appears that acetylcholine is improperly released, synthesized, or prematurely hydrolyzed before crossing the neuromuscular junction.
        2. The disease is most common in women aged 20 to 49 years, but it affects individuals of both sexes and all ages, with approximately 10% of patients having a tumor of the thymus gland.
        3. The disease is manifested by generalized muscle weakness and most commonly demonstrates a descending paralysis.
        4. The primary symptoms normally are ocular, progressing to facial muscle weakness or paralysis, followed by pharyngeal and laryngeal weakness and finally respiratory muscle weakness.
        5. Patients frequently have a chief complaint of easy fatigability.
        6. Diagnosis
            a. Diagnosis is based primarily on history and symptomatology.
            b. The administration of a parasympathomimetic of the cholinesterase inhibitor type confirms the diagnosis. Increased muscle strength is normally noted shortly after the administration of the drug.

7. Treatment
   a. Patients are maintained with cholinesterase inhibitor therapy.
      (1) Neostigmine (Prostigmine) is the drug of choice, but also:
      (2) Pyridostigmine (Mestinon)
      (3) Ambenonium (Mytelase)
   b. Treatment with atropine to reverse the side effects of the cholinesterase inhibitor.
   c. Thymectomy is recommended in most cases. In some patients complete remission has been reported.
   d. Corticosteroids
      (1) Adrenocorticotropic hormone; a 10-day course may be prescribed.
      (2) Prednisone
      (3) Symptoms deteriorate during administration; however, remission is frequent after a 10-day course.
   e. Immunosuppression
      (1) Azathioprine
      (2) Cyclosporine
      (3) Cyclophosphamide
   f. Plasmapheresis
   g. Intravenous immunoglobulin
   h. In severe cases, intubation and mechanical ventilation are used as supportive measures until drug therapy is titrated.
8. Myasthenic versus cholinergic crisis
   a. An acute exacerbation of the disease process producing weakness is termed a *myasthenic crisis*.
   b. An acute decrease in muscle strength as a result of the excessive use of cholinesterase inhibitors is termed a *cholinergic crisis*.
   c. The Tensilon (generic name, edrophonium chloride) test is used to differentiate between a myasthenic and cholinergic crisis. Tensilon is a short-acting (5-min) cholinesterase inhibitor.
      (1) If the patient has a myasthenic crisis, the administration of Tensilon will improve muscle strength.
      (2) If a cholinergic crisis is present, Tensilon will increase muscle weakness and exacerbate symptomatology.
      (3) Muscle strength can be evaluated using serial VC or maximum inspiratory pressure (MIP) measurements.
9. Monitoring of cardiopulmonary status
   a. Patients with acute exacerbation require close cardiopulmonary monitoring.
   b. VC and/or MIP are monitored as frequently as every hour in acute situations.
   c. Deterioration of the VC may signal the need for further medical intervention.
C. Guillain-Barré syndrome: Polyneuritis primarily affecting the peripheral motor and sensory neurons.
   1. The etiology is unclear. The disease may be viral or traumatic. An increase in the number of cases has been reported after viral infection (e.g., varicella-zoster, HIV, and cytomegalovirus) and vaccination (e.g., poliomyelitis and swine flu).
   2. The syndrome affects those of all ages but is more prevalent in adults.
   3. The signs and symptoms show a symmetric ascending pattern of sensory abnormalities that may progress to actual paralysis.
   4. The disease is normally self-limiting and is reversible with time. The amount of residual effects depends on the extent of demyelination occurring during the active disease state.
   5. Diagnosis is made by the presentation of the disease, high protein content in the cerebral spinal fluid, and the reversible nature of the disease.
   6. Treatment is purely symptomatic, the patient frequently requiring ventilatory support.
   7. As with myasthenia gravis, careful monitoring of the patient's ventilatory reserves is indicated.

   D. Other neuromuscular or neurologic diseases that may show a restrictive lung disease pattern
      1. Spinal cord diseases
         a. Paraplegia or quadriplegia
         b. Poliomyelitis
      2. Tetanus
      3. Muscular dystrophy
      4. Tick bite paralysis
      5. Congenital myotonia
   E. Ventilatory management
      1. Some of these patients require mechanical ventilation for varying time periods.
      2. Unless compounding pulmonary problems develop, the lungs of these patients are normal. As a result mechanical ventilation is relatively uncomplicated.
      3. Many of these patients want to feel the ventilator expand their lungs; thus VT should be large, <12 ml/kg.
      4. As a result the rate is frequently slow, 8 to 16 breaths/min.
      5. All other variables are titrated based on the patient's response.

V. **Abdominal Restrictive Lung Diseases**
   A. Increased size of abdominal contents results in limited movement and elevation of the diaphragm.
   B. The limited diaphragmatic movement will demonstrate pulmonary function findings consistent with those of restrictive lung disease.
   C. Conditions that may show a restrictive pattern
      1. Abdominal tumors
      2. Obesity
      3. Third-trimester pregnancy
      4. Diaphragmatic hernias
      5. Ascites
   D. Pickwickian syndrome: A complex of cardiopulmonary symptoms primarily caused by obesity.
      1. It is also referred to as obesity-hypoventilation syndrome.
      2. The syndrome is characterized by:
         a. Severe obesity
         b. Alveolar hypoventilation (more pronounced with sleep) with episodes of sleep apnea
         c. Somnolence
         d. Severe hypoxemia (more pronounced with sleep)
         e. Polycythemia
         f. Pulmonary hypertension (not related to hypoxemia)
         g. Cor pulmonale
      3. Etiology is unclear; however, the major cause appears to be extreme obesity. Genetics may also play a role.
         a. Weight loss may reverse the syndrome.
         b. A high percentage of patients experience upper airway obstruction during sleep, especially in the supine position. The obstruction is believed to be soft tissue obstruction.
      4. Frequently the hypoxemia and hypoventilation develop only during sleep (obstructive sleep apnea).

VI. **Obstructive Sleep Apnea**
   Obstructive sleep apnea causes collapse of the pharyngeal area during sleep that results in an obstruction to airflow. The patient is aroused from sleep, the obstruction clears, and the process is repeated.
   A. Usually associated with obesity.
   B. Soft tissue occludes the upper airway.

C. Respiratory efforts are present; however, airflow is blocked (Figure 22-4).
D. These apneic episodes result in hypoventilation and hypoxemia.
E. The sleep of these patients is commonly broken and restless, leading to generalized somnolence.
  1. Risk factors
    a. Increasing age
    b. Male gender
    c. Obesity
    d. Increased neck circumference
    e. Use of alcohol or other sedatives
    f. Certain craniofacial abnormalities

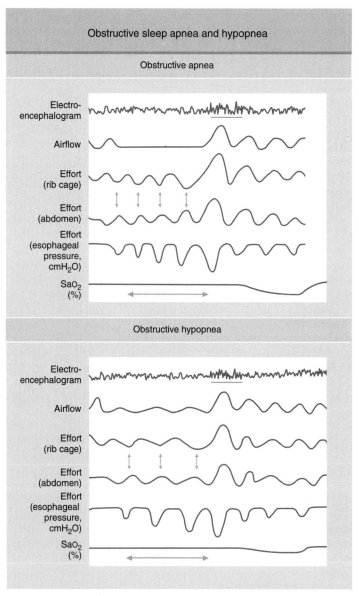

FIG. 22-4 Obstructive sleep apnea and hypopnea.

    g. Diagnosis is based on:
      (1) Patient's medical history
      (2) Physical examination
      (3) Polysomnography (Figure 22-5)
    h. Treatment
      (1) Primary treatment is weight loss.
      (2) Body positioning (i.e., sleeping on one's side or with extra pillows as adjuncts).
      (3) No alcohol or heavy meals in the evening.
      (4) Smoking cessation (to reduce airway inflammation).
      (5) Nasal CPAP helps to relieve airway obstruction and prevents arterial desaturation and hypercarbia at night.
      (6) Oral appliances
    i. Surgery
      (1) Removal of tonsils and adenoids
      (2) Uvulopalatopharyngoplasty
      (3) Tracheostomy
      (4) Laser-assisted uvuloplasty

VII. Smoke Inhalation and Carbon Monoxide Poisoning
  A. Smoke inhalation
    1. Etiology: The inhalation of by-products of a fire (i.e., smoke and other noxious gases).
      a. Aldehydes
      b. Oxides of nitrogen and sulfur
      c. Ammonia
    2. Pathophysiology
      a. Edema, congestion, sloughing of mucosal membranes of the oral and nasal pharynx, larynx, trachea, and bronchi
      b. Obliterative bronchiolitis and alveolar edema
      c. Development of pulmonary edema
      d. Atelectasis caused by airway obstruction with fibrin, edema, fluid, carbon particles, white blood cells, and epithelial debris
    3. Clinical presentation (it may take 24 to 48 hours for symptoms to develop fully)
      a. Coughing and dyspnea
      b. Hypoxemia

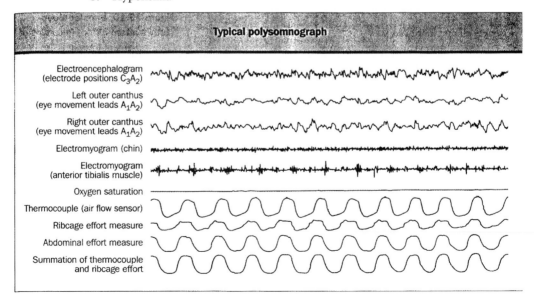

FIG. 22-5 A typical polysomnogram.

  c. Tachypnea and tachycardia

  d. Facial burns, singed nasal hairs, stridor, and grunting (all indicative of upper airway burns)

  e. Results of radiographic studies are normal for the first 24 to 48 hours; however, signs of pulmonary edema, atelectasis, and infiltrates subsequently develop.

 4. Treatment

  a. Establishment of an artificial airway. This is imperative if upper airway burns accompany the smoke inhalation. If an airway is not established early, subsequent edema may prevent cannulation of the airway.

  b. Oxygen therapy (100% if CO poisoning is also present)

  c. Fluid and electrolyte therapy

  d. Bronchodilator therapy

  e. Steroid therapy

  f. Antibiotic therapy

  g. Mechanical ventilation if pulmonary burns present

   (1) Because pulmonary burns result in severe mucosal edema, air trapping and auto-PEEP frequently develop.

   (2) As a result mechanical rates should be low, 8 to 16/min, and expiratory times should be long.

   (3) The approach generally used is similar to that for those with COPD (see Chapters 39, 40, and 41).

   (4) Some patients may develop acute lung injury and ARDS (see Chapter 23).

B. Carbon monoxide poisoning

 1. A result of inspiring by-products of the incomplete combustion of carbon or carbon-containing material

 2. Pathophysiology

  a. Carbon monoxide combines strongly with hemoglobin to form carboxyhemoglobin (hemoglobin's affinity for CO is 210 times that of O_2).

  b. The total capability of the organism to carry oxygen to the tissues is reduced (anemic hypoxia).

  c. The oxyhemoglobin dissociation curve also is shifted to the left, further limiting the amount of O_2 available at the tissue level.

  d. The likelihood of tissue hypoxia increases as COHb% saturation increases.

  e. Increased levels of carbon monoxide interfere with intracellular oxygenation, resulting in histotoxic hypoxia.

 3. Clinical manifestations (symptomatology based on carboxyhemoglobin levels):

  a. Normally asymptomatic: <20%

  b. Headache, exertional dyspnea, impaired judgment, nausea, and vomiting: 20% to 60%

  c. Loss of consciousness, convulsions, and deep coma: 60% to 80%

 4. Radiography findings: Chest radiographic film may show abnormalities consistent with pulmonary edema, usually interstitial in location.

 5. Diagnosis

  a. Analysis of arterial blood for carboxyhemoglobin levels.

   (1) A co-oximeter is required to determine actual carboxyhemoglobin and oxyhemoglobin levels.

   (2) A pulse oximeter measures the oxygen saturation of functional hemoglobin, resulting in an erroneous (high) reading.

   (3) PaO_2 is a measure of oxygen dissolved in plasma; therefore, it is not a helpful measurement.

  b. History

  c. Frequently a metabolic acidosis caused by lactic acid accumulation is noted.

 6. Treatment

  a. Oxygen therapy: One hundred percent O_2 is indicated until COHb% levels reach ≤10%. Increasing the arterial PO_2 decreases the half-life of COHb%. On inhalation of room air, the half-life of COHb is approximately 5 to 6 hours, whereas the inhalation of 100% O_2 decreases the half-life to approximately 90 minutes.

  b. Hyperbaric oxygen therapy: The inhalation of oxygen at greater than atmospheric pressure (usually 2 to 3 atmospheres). There is conflicting evidence over the use of hyperbaric oxygen therapy. It is generally indicated, where available, for patients with serious carbon monoxide poisoning. Hyperbaric oxygen therapy at 3 atmospheres can decrease the half-life of COHb to 23 minutes.

  c. With high COHb levels (>40% to 50%), intubation and mechanical ventilation may be necessary.

VIII. Drug-Induced Pulmonary Disease

  A. Many drugs used for the management of various problems have been linked to pulmonary side effects.

  B. Pulmonary response is usually one of three types:
    1. Chronic pneumonitis with fibrosis
    2. Allergic reactions
    3. Acute lung injury (e.g., ARDS)

  C. Response and magnitude of a response depend on many factors.
    1. Individual susceptibility
    2. Dose dependency
    3. Association with other therapies
      a. Oxygen
      b. Gamma irradiation

  D. The group of drugs that most commonly induce a pulmonary reaction are cytotoxic drugs used in chemotherapy for cancer. Specific agents commonly causing problems are:
    1. Antibiotics
      a. Bleomycin
      b. Mitomycin
      c. Zinostatin (neocarzinostatin)
    2. Alkylating agents
      a. Busulfan
      b. Cyclophosphamide
      c. Chlorambucil
      d. Melphalan
    3. Nitrosoureas
      a. Carmustine (BCNU)
      b. Semustine (methyl-CCNU)
      c. Lomustine (CCNU)
      d. Chlorozotocin
    4. Antimetabolites
      a. Methotrexate
      b. Azathioprine
      c. Mercaptopurine
      d. Cytarabine (cytosine arabinoside)
    5. Miscellaneous
      a. Procarbazine
      b. VM-26
      c. Vinblastine
      d. Vindesine

  E. Other agents that have been reported to produce pulmonary side effects are:
    1. Antibacterial agents
      a. Nitrofurantoin
      b. Amphotericin
      c. Sulfasalazine
    2. Acetylsalicylic acid

3. Opiates
   a. Heroin
   b. Methadone
4. Sedatives
   a. Chlordiazepoxide
5. Diuretics (hydrochlorothiazide)
6. Major tranquilizers
   a. Haloperidol
   b. Fluphenazine
7. Antiarrhythmics
   a. Amiodarone
   b. Lidocaine
   c. Tocainide
8. Miscellaneous
   a. Gold salts
   b. Penicillamine
   c. Colchicine

BIBLIOGRAPHY

Albert RK: Factors affecting transvascular fluid and protein movement in pulmonary edema and ARDS. *Semin Respir Med* 2:109-113, 1981.

Albert RA, et al: *Comprehensive Respiratory Medicine.* London, Mosby, 1999.

Bendixen HH, et al: *Respiratory Care.* St. Louis, Mosby, 1965.

Brigham KL: Primary (high permeability) pulmonary edema. *Semin Respir Med* 4:285-288, 1983.

Brigham KL: Therapy of pulmonary edema. *Semin Respir Med* 4:313-316, 1983.

Cherniack RM, Cherniack L: *Respiration in Health and Disease,* ed 3. Philadelphia, WB Saunders, 1983.

Cooper JAD, White DA, Matthay RA: Drug-induced pulmonary disease, Part 1. *Am Rev Respir Dis* 133:321-340, 1986.

Cooper JAD, White DA, Matthay RA: Drug-induced pulmonary disease, Part 2. *Am Rev Respir Dis* 13:488-505, 1986.

George RB, Light RW, Matthay RA: *Chest Medicine.* New York, Churchill Livingstone, 1983.

Griswold K, Guanci MM, Ropper AH: An approach to the care of patients with Guillain-Barré syndrome. *Heart Lung* 13:66-72, 1984.

Hudson LD: Ventilatory management of patients with adult respiratory distress syndrome. *Semin Respir Med* 2:128-139, 1981.

Hyers TM: Pathogenesis of adult respiratory distress syndrome: current concepts. *Semin Respir Med* 2:104-108, 1981.

Kacmarek RM, Stoller J (eds): *Current Respiratory Care.* Toronto, BC Decker, 1988.

Mathewson HS: Oxygen: the specific antidote to carbon monoxide. *Respir Care* 27:986-987, 1982.

Murray JF, Nadel JA: *Textbook of Respiratory Medicine,* parts 1 and 2. Philadelphia, WB Saunders, 1988.

Petty TL: Adult respiratory distress syndrome: historical perspective and definition. *Semin Respir Med* 2:99-103, 1981.

Petty TL: *Intensive and Rehabilitative Care,* ed 3. Philadelphia, Lea & Febiger, 1982.

Pore JA, Fraser RG: *Synopsis of Diseases of the Chest.* Philadelphia, WB Saunders, 1983.

Shapiro BA, Harrison RA, Kacmarek RM, et al: *Clinical Application of Respiratory Care,* ed 3. Chicago, Year Book Medical Publishers, 1985.

Snider GL: *Clinical Pulmonary Medicine.* Boston, Little Brown & Co, 1981.

Tisi GM: *Pulmonary Physiology in Clinical Medicine,* ed 2. Baltimore, Williams & Wilkins, 1983.

Urbanitle JS: Carbon monoxide poisoning. *Prog Clin Biol Res* 51:355-385, 1981.

Whitcomb ME: *The Lung: Normal and Diseased.* St. Louis, Mosby, 1982.

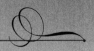
ARDS, SARS, and Sepsis

I. **Definition of Acute Respiratory Distress Syndrome (ARDS)**
    A. ARDS: A diffuse, heterogenous inflammatory response of the lungs, resulting in hypoxemia, consolidation, and decreased compliance.
    B. The American-European Consensus Conference has provided the most precise definition of this syndrome (Box 23-1):
        1. Sudden and acute onset of disease.
        2. The presence of bilateral pulmonary infiltrates in all lung regions seen on frontal chest radiograph.
        3. A pulmonary artery wedge pressure ≤18 mm Hg or a lack of clinical evidence of left atrial hypertension.
        4. Severe hypoxemia: A PaO_2/F_IO_2 ≤200 mm Hg regardless of positive end-expiratory pressure (PEEP) or F_IO_2 level.
        5. A less severe form of ARDS, referred to as acute lung injury (ALI), is defined as a PaO_2/F_IO_2 ratio ≤300 mm Hg.
    C. Although the aforementioned definition has become the most accepted definition of ALI/ARDS, it has been shown that alterations in F_IO_2 and PEEP can markedly affect the $PaO_2{:}F_IO_2$ ratio, moving patients into and out of the classification of ALI or ARDS.
    D. Others have used varying assessment mechanisms to define ARDS. The most commonly reported is the Murray lung injury score.
        1. This score is based on four areas:

	Score
a. Chest radiograph	
(1) No consolidation	0
(2) Consolidation confined to one quadrant	1
(3) Consolidation confined to two quadrants	2
(4) Consolidation confined to three quadrants	3
(5) Consolidation confined to four quadrants	4
b. Hypoxemia	
(1) $PaO_2{:}F_IO_2$ ≥300	0
(2) $PaO_2{:}F_IO_2$ 225 to 299	1
(3) $PaO_2{:}F_IO_2$ 175 to 224	2
(4) $PaO_2{:}F_IO_2$ 100 to 174	3
(5) $PaO_2{:}F_IO_2$ <100	4
c. PEEP (if mechanically ventilated)	
(1) ≤5 cm H_2O	0
(2) 6 to 8 cm H_2O	1
(3) 9 to 11 cm H_2O	2
(4) 12 to 14 cm H_2O	3
(5) ≥15 cm H_2O	4

BOX 23-1

American-European Consensus Conference Definition of ARDS/ALI

- Rapid and acute onset
- Severe hypoxemia
  - ARDS Pao_2/F_IO_2 ≤200 mm Hg
  - ALI Pao_2/F_IO_2 ≤300 mm Hg
- Chest radiograph: bilateral infiltrates on frontal chest x-ray
- Pulmonary capillary wedge pressure ≤18 mm Hg or lack of clinical evidence of left atrial hypertension

ARDS, Acute respiratory distress syndrome; *ALI,* acute lung injury.
From Bernard GR, Artigas A, Brigham KL, et al: The American-European Consensus Conference on ARDS: Definitions, mechanisms, relevant outcomes, and clinical coordination. *Am J Respir Crit Care Med* 149:650-655, 1994.

		Score
d.	Respiratory system compliance (when ventilated)	
	(1) ≥80 ml/cm H_2O	0
	(2) 60 to 79 ml/cm H_2O	1
	(3) 40 to 59 ml/cm H_2O	2
	(4) 20 to 39 ml/cm H_2O	3
	(5) ≤19 ml/cm H_2O	4

2. A score of 0 to 4 is given for each of the above available, and then scores are averaged.
3. ARDS is defined as a score >2.5; a mild to moderate injury is scored 0.1 to 2.5; and 0.0 indicates no lung injury.

E. It is important to remember that there is no test or measurement that can precisely define or identify ARDS. Diagnosis is always based on the signs and symptoms described previously.

F. Until a test is identified that can definitively diagnose ARDS there will continue to be controversy whether a patient truly has ARDS.

G. Many believe there is a genetic predisposition of ARDS and that one day an "ARDS gene" will be identified.

II. **Incidence and Mortality of ARDS**

A. Because no precise definition for ARDS exists, it is difficult to precisely identify its occurrence in the general population.

B. However, the epidemiologic data currently available indicate that approximately 3 to 19 cases of ARDS occur in every 100,000 individuals per year.

C. Similarly the reported mortality of ARDS varies widely. Early reports indicate a mortality of 80% to 90%.

D. Randomized clinical trials evaluating select populations of ALI and ARDS patients have reported mortalities as low as 25% to 30%.

E. Epidemiologic data from widely distributed intensive care units indicate that the mortality for all patients with ARDS is still approximately 50% to 60%.

III. **Long-Term Outcome of ARDS**

A. By 1 year after hospital discharge most patients have regained the majority of pulmonary function lost during the acute illness.

B. However, most have a decreased diffusing capacity, resulting in desaturation with exertion.

C. At 1 year after discharge, feelings of anxiety, depression, and posttraumatic stress also are common.

D. Quality-of-life surveys also indicate decrements in general and respiratory-associated parameters at 1 year after discharge.

IV. **Causes of ARDS**

A. Two general categories of causative factors have been defined: Direct or primary pulmonary lung injury, and indirect or secondary nonpulmonary cause of lung injury.

    B. Direct lung injury resulting in ARDS is caused by:
        1. Pneumonia: Bacterial or viral
        2. Lung trauma
        3. Smoke inhalation
        4. Near-drowning
        5. Aspiration
        6. Overly aggressive mechanical ventilation: Ventilator-induced lung injury (VILI)
    C. Indirect lung injury resulting in ARDS is caused by:
        1. Sepsis
        2. Blood transfusion
        3. Nonthoracic trauma
        4. Hypovolemic shock
        5. Hyperfusion injury
        6. Acute pancreatitis
        7. Overdose

V. Pathophysiology of ARDS
    A. ARDS is characterized by diffuse alveolar damage and microvascular injury.
    B. Three distinct phases of ARDS/ALI from a pathophysiologic perspective have been defined: Exudative phase, fibroproliferative phase, and resolution phase.
    C. ARDS does not necessarily progress to the fibroproliferative phase; many patients rapidly move from the exudative phase to the resolution phase.
    D. Exudative (acute) phase (Figure 23-1)
        1. On histologic examination of the lung the following are observed:
            a. Marked diffuse alveolar damage
            b. Increased neutrophils
            c. Vasodilatation
            d. Endothelial cell damage
            e. Pulmonary edema
            f. Presence of a hyaline membrane
        2. The adhesion and activation of neutrophils lead to the secretion of proinflammatory mediators, potentially leading to more injury (see Figure 23-1; Table 23-1).
        3. The composition of pulmonary surfactant and its quantity are altered, increasing surface tension.
        4. As the disease progresses deadspace ventilation increases.
        5. Early in this exudative phase the major gas exchange issue is oxygenation. As this phase transitions into the fibroproliferative phase, ventilation generally becomes more of a problem.
        6. The exudative phase generally lasts for approximately 3 to 7 days.
    E. Fibroproliferative phase
        1. In this stage the alveolar damage progresses, and pulmonary hypertension and pulmonary fibrosis develop.
        2. Alveolar cells, endothelial cells, and fibroblasts also proliferate.
        3. Microvascular thrombosis and vascular injury become more prominent.
        4. For those who do not improve, multiorgan system failure develops.
        5. The proinflammatory mediators released in the lung can migrate into the systemic circulation under conditions of high peak alveolar pressure and repetitive opening and closing of unstable lung units. This process is believed to be at least partially responsible for the development of multiorgan system failure.
        6. Systemic release of proinflammatory mediators in direct and indirect ARDS also occurs and can cause multiorgan system failure.
        7. Most patients with ARDS who die do so because of multiorgan system failure, not respiratory failure.
        8. The fibroproliferative phase can last for a few days or for weeks.
    F. Resolution phase (Figure 23-2)
        1. At this phase the alveolar neutrophils are replaced by macrophages.

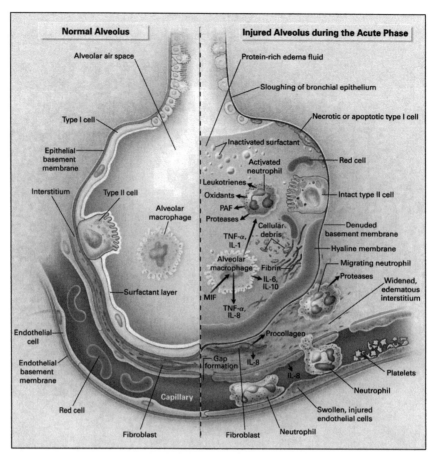

FIG. 23-1 The normal alveolus *(left side)* and the injured alveolus in the acute exudative phase of ALI and ARDS *(right side)*. In the acute phase, there is sloughing of bronchial and alveolar epithelial cells, with the formation of protein-rich hyaline membranes on the denuded basement membrane. Neutrophils are shown adhering to the injured capillary endothelium and migrating through the interstitium into the air space, which is filled with protein-rich edema fluid. In the air space, an alveolar macrophage is secreting cytokines, IL-1, -6, -8, and -10, and TNF-α, which act locally to stimulate chemotaxis and activate neutrophils. Macrophages also secrete other cytokines, including IL-1, -6, and -10. Interleukin-1 can also stimulate the production of extracellular matrix by fibroblasts. Neutrophils can release oxidants, proteases, leukotrienes, and other proinflammatory molecules, such as platelet-activating factor. A number of antiinflammatory mediators are also present in the alveolar milieu, including IL-1 receptor antagonist, soluble TNF receptor, autoantibodies against IL-8, and cytokines such as IL-1 (not shown). The influx of protein-rich edema fluid into the alveolus has led to the inactivation of surfactant. *MIF,* Macrophage inhibitory factor; *ALI,* acute lung injury; *ARDS,* acute respiratory distress syndrome; *IL,* interleukin; *TNF,* tumor necrosis factor.

TABLE 23-1

Proinflammatory Mediators Associated with the Development of ARDS/ALI

Mediator Category	Mediators
Tumor necrosis factors	TNF-α, TNF-β
Interleukins	IL-1β, IL-2, IL-6, IL-10, IL-12
Chemokines	IL-8, MIP-1, MCP-1, growth-regulated peptides
Colony-stimulating factors	G-CSF, GM-CSF
Interferon	IFN-β

From Wiedemann H: Systemic Pharmacolic Therapy of ARDS *Resp Care Clin North Am* 3:732, 1998.
ARDS, Acute respiratory distress syndrome; *ALI,* acute lung injury.

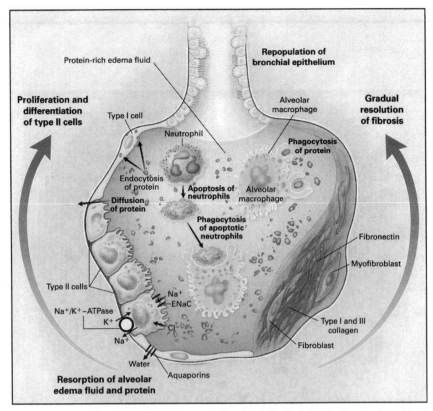

FIG. 23-2 Mechanisms important in the resolution ARDS and ALI. On the left side, the alveolar epithelium is being repopulated by the proliferation and differentiation of alveolar type II cells. Resorption of alveolar edema, sodium, and chloride occurs. Soluble protein is cleared. Macrophages remove insoluble protein and apoptotic neutrophils by phagocytosis. On the right side of the alveolus, the gradual remodeling and resolution of intraalveolar and interstitial granulation tissue and fibrosis are shown. *ALI,* Acute lung injury; *ARDS,* acute respiratory distress syndrome.

    2. In this stage the following occurs:
        a. Epithelial repopulation
        b. Reabsorption of alveolar fluid
        c. Clearing of the protein residue
        d. Resolution of fibrosis

VI. Lung Mechanics in ARDS
    A. As a result of the damage at the alveolar-capillary membrane, lung compliance decreases.
    B. Functional residual capacity also decreases.
    C. As a result respiratory time constants decrease.
    D. There is also a minor increase in airway resistance.

VII. Ventilator-Induced Lung Injury
    A. It has become increasingly clear from laboratory and clinical studies that inappropriate mechanical ventilation can cause lung injury indistinguishable from other forms of ARDS.
    B. The most common form of injury caused by the ventilator has been referred to as volutrauma, defined as end-inspiratory overdistention (Figure 23-3).
        1. The term volutrauma is used because it is believed that localized increases in end-inspiratory lung volume cause the injury.
        2. Most probably it is the localized stress and strain on the alveolar-capillary membrane associated with any tidal volume (V_T) that increases peak alveolar pressure causing the injury.

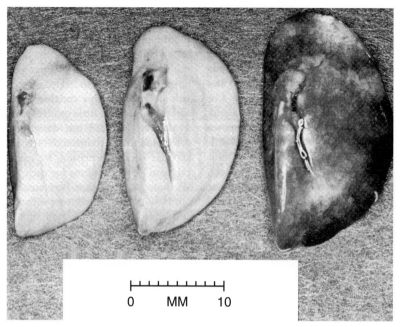

FIG. 23-3 Rat lung ventilated for 1 hour at three pressure settings: 14/0, 45/10, and 45/0 cm H_2O (first number peak alveolar pressure, second PEEP level). The lungs ventilated at 45/0 cm H_2O are markedly congested and hemorrhagic, whereas the lungs ventilated at 45/10 cm H_2O are only slightly edematous. *PEEP,* Positive end-expiratory pressure.

    3. Clearly there is debate as to the exact cause of this injury: volume or pressure.
    4. Many believe there is a safe peak alveolar pressure and that the lung is not damaged regardless of Vт if pressure is kept below this level.
    5. Available data indicate this level is approximately 25 to 30 cm H_2O.
  C. Barotrauma: Essentially the extreme of volutrauma, in which the end-inspiratory stress is so great that tears are created at the alveolar surface, allowing air to dissect through facial planes ending in various compartments (Figure 23-4).
  D. Atelectrauma: Injury that is a result of unstable lung units opening during inspiration and being allowed to close during exhalation.

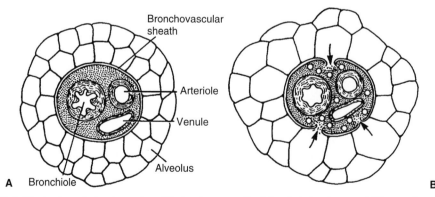

FIG. 23-4 Mechanism of alveolar rupture **(A)** showing normally distended structures and **(B)** overdistended alveoli, such as are found at peak lung inflation during mechanical ventilation. Pressures between adjacent alveoli equilibrate rapidly, even when the alveoli are unequally distended. However, pressure in the adjacent bronchovascular sheath remains somewhat lower than in the alveoli, so that when these are overdistended, a transient pressure gradient is created, and the delicate alveolar membranes may rupture.

1. The shear stress caused by this process on the walls of the unstable alveoli can exceed 140 cm H_2O when the peak alveoli pressure in adjacent open alveoli is 30 cm H_2O (Figure 23-5).
2. Many believe this injury can be as severe as volutrauma.
3. The application of PEEP should always be focused on preventing unstable lung units from collapsing once they are opened.

E. The development of volutrauma and atelectrauma causes two other mechanisms to occur that can extend the level of lung injury and cause systemic injury.
   1. Biotrauma: A term used to identify the activation of inflammatory mediators by the aforementioned injuries (i.e., in the presence of volutrauma or atelectrauma there is an increase within the lung of the release of proinflammatory mediators).
   2. Translocation of substances from the lung into systemic circulation.
      a. Injurious ventilation not only affects the alveoli epithelium but also can cause tears in the capillary endothelium.
      b. As a result organisms and inflammatory mediators can move from the lung into systemic circulation when VILI is present.
      c. Thus VILI can cause distal organ failure or sepsis.
      d. Many believe that the lung is the engine that drives the development of multiorgan system failure.

VIII. **Sepsis (Figure 23-6)**
The following are American College of Chest Physicians/Society of Critical Care Medicine (ACCP/SCCM) consensus conference (1992) definitions (used with permission).
A. Infection: A microbial phenomenon characterized by an inflammatory response to the presence of microorganisms or the invasion of normally sterile host tissue by those organisms.
B. Bacteremia: The presence of viable bacteria in the blood.
C. Systemic inflammatory response syndrome (SIRS): Systemic inflammatory response *to a variety of severe clinical insults*, defined as the presence of two or more of the following:
   1. Temperature: >38° C or <36° C
   2. Pulse: >90 beats/min at rest
   3. Tachypnea at rest: >20 breaths/min or $Paco_2$ <32 mm Hg
   4. White blood cell count: >12,000/mm^3 or <4000 mm^3 or >10% bands
D. Sepsis: Systemic response to *infection* manifested by two or more of the following:
   1. Temperature: >38° C or <36° C
   2. Pulse: >90 beats/min at rest
   3. Tachypnea at rest: >20 breaths/min or $Paco_2$ <32 mm Hg
   4. White blood cell count: >12,000/mm^3 or <4000 mm^3 or >10% bands

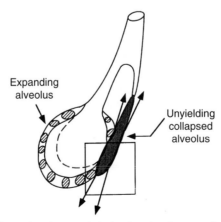

Expanding alveolus

Unyielding collapsed alveolus

FIG. 23-5 Illustration of a collapsed and expanded alveolus showing area (box) where high shear stress can develop during inflation of the expanded alveolus.

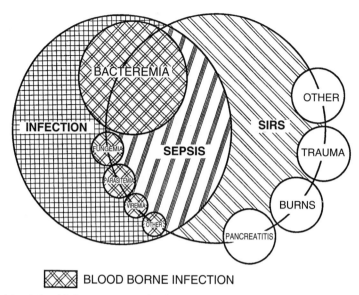

BLOOD BORNE INFECTION

FIG. 23-6 The interrelationship between systemic inflammatory response syndrome (SIRS), sepsis, and infection.

E. The definitions for SIRS and sepsis are the same except SIRS is not caused by an infection. When infection develops, SIRS becomes sepsis (see Figure 23-6).

F. Severe sepsis: Sepsis associated with organ dysfunction, hypoperfusion, or hypotension. Hypoperfusion and perfusion abnormalities may include but are not limited to lactic acidosis, oliguria, or an acute alteration in mental status.

G. Septic shock: Sepsis with hypotension, despite adequate fluid resuscitation, along with the presence of perfusion abnormalities that may include but are not limited to lactic acidosis, oliguria, or an acute alteration in mental status. Patients who are taking inotropic or vasopressor agents may not be hypotensive at the time that perfusion abnormalities are measured.

H. Hypotension: A systolic blood pressure <90 mm Hg or a reduction of >40 mm Hg from baseline.

I. Multiorgan dysfunction syndrome: Presence of altered organ function in acutely ill patients such that homeostasis cannot be maintained without intervention.

J. Approaches to managing sepsis include:
1. Appropriate antibiotic therapy addressing the underlying infection.
2. Activated protein C (Drotrecogin alfa activated) has been successful in cases of severe sepsis.
3. Antithrombin therapy, although the data supporting its use are controversial.
4. Heparin in combination with activated protein C or antithrombin therapy has demonstrated some benefit.
5. Corticosteroid therapy has also demonstrated some benefit, but again its use is controversial.
6. Many have recommended the combined use of all of these therapies in a stepwise approach. However, no definitive therapy for sepsis exists.

IX. **Severe Acute Respiratory Syndrome (SARS)**
A. SARS is an unusual atypical pneumonia that emerged in November 2002 in mainland China.
B. Approximately 20% of those diagnosed with SARS develop ARDS/ALI, and approximately 50% of these patients die.
C. Thus SARS has an overall mortality of approximately 10%.
D. The causative agent for SARS is a coronavirus (SARS-CoV) that can cause disease in animals and humans and can easily be transmitted from patient to patient and from animal to

human. This group of viruses typically was responsible for some forms of the common cold.

E. There is no rapid test that is able to identify the virus; identification may take weeks. As a result diagnosis currently is based on the patient meeting a case definition of the disease:

1. A hospitalized patient with radiographically confirmed pneumonia or ARDS without identifiable etiology.

2. One of the following risk factors within 10 days before onset of illness:

a. Travel to mainland China, Hong Kong, or Taiwan or close contact with an ill person with a history of recent travel to these areas.

b. Employment in an occupation with a high risk of SARS-CoV exposure (e.g., health care workers and individuals working with the virus).

c. Part of a cluster of cases of atypical pneumonia without an alternative diagnosis.

F. Patients with SARS should be on complete airborne and droplet precautions (see Chapter 3).

G. All health care workers treating infected patients should at least use the following:

1. N-95 respirator (mask that filters tuberculosis bacterium)

2. Gown

3. Gloves

4. Face shield

H. During high-risk procedures (e.g., intubation and bronchoscopy), an isolation hood "powered air-purifying respirator" should be worn.

I. No specific treatment is available for SARS.

X. **Pharmacologic Management of ARDS**

A. A number of different pharmacologic agents have been used to manage ARDS (Table 23-2).

B. However, none of these agents has demonstrated a decrease in mortality in ARDS.

C. Activated protein C has been shown to decrease mortality in sepsis by approximately 6% but not necessarily sepsis associated with ARDS.

D. Corticosteroids in a small trial of 24 patients with unresolved ARDS did demonstrate improved outcome (Figure 23-7) (Meduri et al, 1998).

1. This study used prolonged administration of methylprednisolone, a loading dose of 2 mg/kg, followed by 2 mg/kg/day for 1 to 14 days, followed by a tapering dose to day 32.

2. However, because the number of patients was small and a crossover design was used, these results are considered preliminary, requiring additional studies.

3. Systemic steroid therapy in patients with ARDS also has been associated with severe and prolonged paresis with muscle wasting and weakness.

E. Inhaled nitric oxide does improve Pa_{O_2} and decreases pulmonary hypertension in those with ARDS/ALI, but at least four randomized controlled trials of inhaled nitric oxide use in ARDS have been negative. Nitric oxide use in patients with ARDS/ALI is not recommended (see Chapter 34).

F. Surfactant: A number of clinical trials have evaluated surfactant therapy in adult ARDS; however, none has demonstrated benefit. Trials are ongoing, but at this time surfactant cannot be recommended for those with adult ARDS.

G. None of the other agents listed in Table 23-2 have shown improved outcome when used to manage ARDS/ALI, and none are recommended as treatment.

XI. **Ventilator Management (Table 23-3)**

A. Refer to Chapters 39, 40, and 41.

B. A lung protective strategy should always be used when ventilating patients with ALI or ARDS.

C. This strategy centers on avoiding overdistention and repetitive opening and closing of unstable lung units.

D. Overdistention is primarily avoided by maintaining plateau pressures <30 cm H_2O; the lower the plateau pressure, the greater the likelihood of avoiding VILI and increasing survival. VT also should be low, in the range of 4 to 8 ml/kg for most patients.

1. Tidal volume level is set based on the plateau pressure.

TABLE 23-2	

Proposal Pharmacologic Therapies for ARDS/ALI with "Potential" Mechanisms of Action

Drug	Mechanisms of Action
Activated protein C (rhAPC)	Inhibition of plasminogen activator inhibitor
	Inhibition of leukocyte adhesion and inflammatory cytokines
	Inhibition of neutrophil accumulation
Antiadhesion molecules	Inhibition of leukocyte adherence to endothelium
Atrial natriuretic peptide (ANP)	Activation of membrane-bound guanylate cyclase and cyclic GMP production
Corticosteroids	Inhibition of arachidonic acid metabolites
	Inhibition of complement-induced neutrophil aggregation
	Inhibition of inflammatory cytokines
	Modification of fibrogenesis
	Suppression of cytokine release from macrophages
	Suppression of platelet-activating factor and nitric oxide production
Cytokine antagonists	Inhibition of inflammatory cytokines (e.g., monoclonal antibodies and receptor antagonists)
Ketoconazole	Inhibition of thromboxane synthetase
	Inhibition of procoagulant activity by macrophages
	Blockade of 5-lipoxygenase
Lisofylline	Inhibition of TNF release
	Inhibition of neutrophil accumulation
	Inhibition of inflammatory cytokines
N-acetylcysteine, procysteine	Repletion of glufathilone stores (antioxidant activity)
Prostaglandin E$_1$	Inhibition of mediator release from granulocytes
	Pulmonary vasodilation
Nitric oxide	Increased cyclic GMP levels
	Pulmonary vasodilation
	Improved oxygenation
Surfactant	Replaces endogenous surfactant
	Improved pulmonary compliance
	Improved gas exchange

GMP, Guanosine monophosphate; *TNF,* tumor necrosis factor.
From Wiedemann HP, Arroliga AC, Komara JJ: Emerging pharmacologic approaches in acute respiratory distress syndrome. *Respir Care Clinics N Am* 9:419-435, 2003.

    2. Paco$_2$ level should be maintained by adjusting rate, not VT.

    3. Rates up to approximately 40 breaths/min may be used. Rate is only limited by the development of auto-PEEP.

    4. Once auto-PEEP develops, the benefit of increasing the rate is lost regardless of mode of ventilation.

  E. Repetitive opening and collapse of unstable lung units can be minimized by appropriate PEEP.

    1. The data to date indicate PEEP greater than the lower inflection point on the pressure-volume (P-V) curve of the respiratory system (P$_{flex}$) is the most appropriate initial level to set.

    2. This level can be determined by performing a P-V curve, or it can be estimated by a decremental PEEP trial (see Chapter 40).

    3. If neither of the above approaches is used, initial PEEP level can be set at approximately 12 to 16 cm H$_2$O.

  F. Any mode may be used, but pressure assist/control (A/C) allows for precise targeting of plateau pressure and is recommended.

  G. Inspiratory time should be set at ≤1.0 second. It should be long enough to maximize VT delivery in pressure A/C (i.e., flow should return to zero before the end of the breath).

  H. Inspiration-to-expiration (I:E) ratios should be ≤1:1; no benefit of the use of an inverse I:E ratio has been demonstrated.

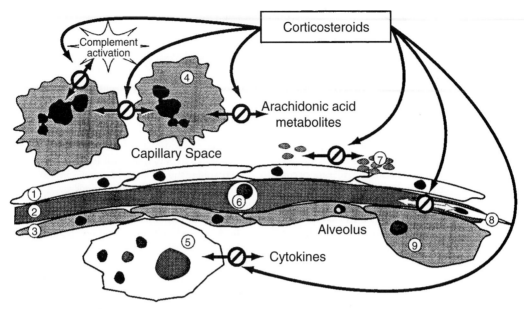

FIG. 23-7 Possible mechanism of action of corticosteroids in ARDS/ALI. Corticosteroids may decrease complement activation and associated adhesion of neutrophils (4) to the endothelium (1). They may block fibroblast proliferation and collagen deposition (8) to the interstitium (2). Corticosteroids may ameliorate release of cytokines from pulmonary alveolar macrophages (5) and lymphocytes (6). The goal of antiinflammatory therapy is to keep the type I alveolar cell layer (3) and the capillary endothelium intact. *ALI,* Acute lung injury; *ARDS,* acute respiratory distress syndrome.

TABLE **23-3**

Ventilatory Management of ARDS

Initial Setup	
Plateau pressure	<30 cm H_2O
Tidal volume	4 to 8 ml/kg PBW
Rate	≤35 breaths/min to maintain Pco_2 35 to 50 mm Hg provided auto-PEEP does not develop
Inspiratory time	≤1.0 second, in pressure A/C, allow flow to return to zero
Mode	A/C-pressure A/C recommended
I:E	≤1:1
Peak flow (volume A/C)	Sufficient to ensure inspiratory time ≤1.0 second
Flow pattern (volume A/C)	Decelerating
PEEP	≥P_{flex} or by decremental trial or at 12 to 16 cm H_2O
F_IO_2	Sufficient to maintain Pao_2 >60 mm Hg

Management of ventilation
   Hypercarbia: First increase rate, then consider permissive hypercapnia
      before adjusting VT.
   Hypocarbia: First decrease VT until plateau pressure is <28 cm H_2O,
      and then decrease rate.
Management of oxygenation
   Improving Po_2: First decrease F_IO_2 and then PEEP.
   Decreasing Po_2: First increase PEEP and then F_IO_2; consider lung
      recruitment and prone positioning.

ARDS, Acute respiratory distress syndrome; *PBW,* predicted body weight; *PEEP,* positive end-expiratory pressure; *A/C,* assist control; *I:E,* inspiration-to-expiration; *VT,* tidal volume.

  I. Set F_IO_2 high enough to ensure a PaO_2 >60 mm Hg.

  J. Management of ventilation.

    1. Ventilation is primarily managed by adjusting respiratory rate.

    2. However, if increasing rate because of hypercarbia results in auto-PEEP, permissive hypercapnia may be necessary.

    3. If patients are hemodynamically stable without head trauma, PCO_2 into the 70s and 80s is generally well tolerated if increased to this level slowly.

    4. The real concern with permissive hypercapnia is acidosis. Most patients tolerate a pH as low as 7.25.

    5. However, the older the patient, or the presence of cardiovascular or renal disease and hemodynamic instability, the less likely permissive hypercapnia will be tolerated.

    6. If patients cannot tolerate permissive hypercapnia, the V_T may be increased; however, care not to exceed a plateau pressure of 30 cm H_2O must be exercised. Allowing plateau pressures to exceed 30 cm H_2O unless the patient has decreased chest wall compliance increases the likelihood of VILI and a poor outcome (see Chapter 41).

    7. In the presence of hypocarbia V_T should be decreased first to maintain plateau pressure as low as possible; then rate can be decreased.

  K. Management of oxygenation

    1. Before setting PEEP and F_IO_2 a lung recruitment maneuver can be performed in patients who are hemodynamically stable (see Chapter 40).

    2. A recruitment maneuver ideally is performed after initial stabilization on the mechanical ventilator.

    3. PEEP and F_IO_2 are then set: PEEP $\geq P_{flex}$ or by decremental trial or at 12 to 16 cm H_2O, and then F_IO_2 is set to maintain PO_2 >60 mm Hg.

    4. If oxygenation is excessive F_IO_2 should be first reduced until the F_IO_2 is <0.50, after which PEEP may be reduced. PEEP should always be reduced once the F_IO_2 = 0.40.

    5. If oxygenation is inadequate, PEEP should be first increased, and then F_IO_2. PEEP should always be increased in small steps (2 cm H_2O), and its response assessed (both oxygenation and cardiovascular; see Chapter 40).

    6. Patients with refractory hypoxemia not responding to PEEP, F_IO_2, and recruitment maneuvers should be considered for prone positioning (see Chapter 45).

  L. Weaning from ventilatory support should be by spontaneous breathing trial (see Chapter 41).

    1. Before or between spontaneous breathing trials pressure support ventilation is frequently best tolerated.

    2. Other approaches to weaning may be tried, but a spontaneous breathing trial has been demonstrated most efficacious.

  M. Other modes of ventilation, such as high frequency oscillation, inverse ratio ventilation, and airway pressure release ventilator or bilevel ventilation, have not demonstrated benefit over the use of A/C ventilation in ARDS.

BIBLIOGRAPHY

ACCP/SCCM Consensus Conference: Definitions for sepsis and organ failure and guidelines for the use of innovative therapies in sepsis. *Chest* 101:1644-1655, 1992.

Amato MBP, Barbas CSV, Medeiros DM, et al: Effect of a protective ventilation strategy on mortality in the acute respiratory distress syndrome. *N Engl J Med* 338:347-354, 1998.

The ARDS Network: Ventilation with lower tidal volumes as compared with traditional tidal volumes for acute lung injury and the acute respiratory distress syndrome. *N Engl J Med* 342:1301-1308, 2000.

Grasso S, Mascia L, Del Turco M, et al: Effects of recruiting maneuvers in patients with acute respiratory distress syndrome ventilated with protective ventilatory strategy. *Anesthesiology* 96:795-802, 2002.

Kallet RH, Haas CF: Acute respiratory distress syndrome, part I. *Respir Care Clin N Am* 9:273-396, 2003.

Kallet RH, Haas CF: Acute respiratory distress syndrome, part II. *Respir Care Clin N Am* 9:401-509, 2003.

Lapinsky SE, Aubin M, Metha S, Boiteau P, Slutsky AS: Safety and efficacy of a sustained inflation for alveolar recruitment in adults with respiratory failure. *Intern Care Med* 25:1297-1301, 1999.

Meduri GU, Headley AS, Golden E, et al: Effect of prolonged methylprednisolone therapy in unresolved acute respiratory distress syndrome: a randomized controlled trial, *JAMA* 280:159-165, 1998.

Murray JE, Matthay MP, Luce JM, Flick MR: An expanded definition of the adult respiratory distress syndrome. *Am Rev Respir Dis* 138:720-723, 1988.

Peiris JSM, Yuen KY, Osterhaus ADM, Stöhr K: The severe acute respiratory syndrome. *N Engl J Med* 349:25, 2003.

Tugrul S, Akinci O, Ozcan PE, et al: Effects of sustained inflation and post-inflation PEEP in acute respiratory distress syndrome: focusing on pulmonary and extrapulmonary forms. *Crit Care Med* 31:738-744, 2003.

Ware LB, Matthay MA: The acute respiratory distress syndrome. *N Engl J Med* 342:1339-1349, 2000.

Chapter 24

Nutrition

I. **Metabolic Pathways**
   A. Carbohydrate (CHO) metabolism
   1. CHO usually makes up 40% to 45% of the total food intake but may reach 60%.
   2. Amylases and disaccharidases hydrolyze complex starches and sugars to monosaccharides before they are absorbed in the small intestine.
      a. One half of the ingested CHO is digested to glucose, and the rest are digested mainly to fructose and galactose.
      b. Most of the glucose circulates as blood sugar and is taken up by the body cells and metabolized for energy.
      c. Fructose, galactose, and some glucose are converted to glycogen, some in the liver and the rest in muscle.
         (1) There are approximately 500 g of glycogen stored.
            (a) Of this total, 200 g is in the liver and is available for systemic use.
         (2) The large glycogen stores in muscle are not available to provide glucose to the rest of the body.
   3. Glucose is also manufactured from amino acids and other products of intermediary metabolism by a process called gluconeogenesis, which protects the glycogen reserves.
      a. In the fasting state, liver glycogen is stimulated by catecholamine and glucagon to undergo glycogenolysis and form blood glucose.
      b. Glucose then undergoes glycolysis to pyruvate.
         (1) Pyruvate may undergo three basic metabolic processes:
            (a) It can move into the mitochondria and be converted to acetyl coenzyme A (acetyl-CoA) for oxidation in the citric acid cycle.
            (b) Diversion of pyruvate for oxidation to CO_2 and H_2O in the citric acid cycle and the respiratory chain is known as *aerobic glycolysis*.
         (2) When O_2 is not present for aerobic glycolysis, pyruvate is reduced to lactate.
            (a) This process is known as *anaerobic glycolysis*.
               i. Anaerobic glycolysis commonly occurs in periods of stress or severe exercise when demand for energy exceeds the supply of O_2.
               ii. When O_2 becomes available, lactate (which has built up in muscle and blood) can be reconverted to pyruvate for oxidation in the citric acid cycle.
         (3) Anaerobic glycolysis is a rapid method for energy production.
            (a) It does not need large quantities of O_2.
            (b) However, only limited energy production occurs via this mechanism.
            (c) Pyruvate can also be carboxylated to oxaloacetate in the mitochondria by pyruvate carboxylase.
            (d) Oxaloacetate can then form glucose in a process that is the reverse of glycolysis, known as *gluconeogenesis*.

B. Lipid (fat) metabolism
  1. Lipid is the main energy substrate in the body.
      a. Lipid provides approximately 90% of the total body caloric reserve.
          (1) In the average individual, 150,000 calories are in reserve.
          (2) In obese individuals, >150,000 calories are in reserve.
      b. Most body fat exists as fatty acids that are esterified with glycerol to form triglycerides.
          (1) Adipose tissue is approximately 90% triglycerides.
  2. Dietary lipid is hydrolyzed in the intestinal tract, absorbed, and then resynthesized to triglycerides.
      a. These are transported from the jejunal wall as lipid-protein complexes called *chylomicrons.*
          (1) Chylomicrons are a form of lipoproteins.
      b. Chylomicrons enter the blood via the intestinal lymphatics (lacteal) and thoracic duct.
      c. Short- and medium-chain free fatty acids enter directly into the portal blood without conversion into chylomicrons.
          (1) Medium-chain triglycerides are more easily hydrolyzed than long-chain triglycerides and can be easily absorbed.
  3. Lipoproteins may be modified in the liver before going to adipose tissue or may go there directly.
      a. In adipose tissue, lipoproteins are hydrolyzed, releasing fatty acids.
      b. The fatty acids are reesterified and stored as triglycerides.
  4. Triglycerides may also be formed from CHOs by lipogenesis.
      a. When CHO intake is decreased, triglycerides are mobilized to glycerol and fatty acids.
      b. The glycerol is partly converted to glucose by gluconeogenesis.
  5. The free fatty acids are oxidized to produce acetyl-CoA, which is converted to energy via the Krebs cycle.
      a. When more acetyl-CoA is produced than the Krebs cycle can oxidize, it is converted to ketone bodies.
      b. A ketone body: β-Hydroxybutyryl acetoacetate and acetone.
          (1) Ketone production and gluconeogenesis take place in the liver.
          (2) In starvation ketones are the main source of body fuel.
          (3) Ketones minimize amino acid release from muscle and aid in protein conservation.
C. Protein metabolism
  1. Protein normally comprises approximately 20% of the lean body mass or approximately 15% of the total body weight.
  2. An intake of approximately 0.8 to 1 g/kg of body weight is needed each day in a normal individual.
  3. If CHOs and lipids meet energy demands, protein is used entirely for:
      a. Protein replacement
      b. Growth and repair of tissues
      c. Maintenance of circulating proteins
      d. Manufacture of enzymes
  4. Specific enzymes in the intestinal tract hydrolyze ingested protein to peptides and ultimately to amino acids.
  5. The body cannot synthesize essential amino acids:
      a. Isoleucine
      b. Leucine
      c. Lysine
      d. Methionine
      e. Phenylalanine
      f. Threonine
      g. Tryptophan
      h. Valine

6. Amino acids not used anabolically for protein synthesis undergo catabolism (e.g., they may be transaminated or deaminated). After deamination the residue may be converted by way of either:
   a. Acetyl-CoA to lipid (ketogenesis)
   b. Or oxaloacetate to glycogen
7. The nitrogen released is excreted in the urine as urea.
   a. One gram of urinary urea nitrogen (UUN) is derived from 6.25 g of protein.
8. Branched chain amino acids (e.g., valine, leucine, and isoleucine) are used by muscle for metabolism.
   a. Valine is glycogenic.
   b. Leucine is ketogenic.
   c. Isoleucine is both.
   d. Branched chain amino acids given intravenously can be used as a source of energy for muscles and can preserve lean body mass.
9. Alanine is the major gluconeogenic amino acid.
   a. It is formed by transamination of pyruvate from branched chain amino acids.
10. CHOs have a specific protein-sparing effect.
    a. CHOs inhibit the catabolism of glycogenic amino acids.
11. Amino acids form the building blocks of proteins.
    a. One must ingest a ratio of between 100 and 150 nonprotein calories to 1 g of nitrogen to ensure protein synthesis.
    b. This ratio is much higher in those with sepsis.

D. Summary of energy metabolism
   1. Glucose is the principal energy source of anaerobic metabolism:
      a. During shock
      b. During tissue anoxia
   2. The Krebs cycle is the main source of aerobic metabolism.
      a. It requires some glucose to prime it.
      b. Total energy needs cannot be supplied by fatty acid metabolism.
   3. Glucose can be provided:
      a. From hydrolysis of CHO
      b. By glycogenolysis
      c. By hydrolysis of lipids to glycerol and gluconeogenesis
      d. By conversion of some amino acids to CHO
   4. Triglycerides can be manufactured from excess CHO, lipid, and protein intake.
   5. All fuel sources can be used for energy.

II. **Determination of Caloric and Protein Needs**
   A. Clinical energy measurement
      1. Energy is commonly measured in units of calories or joules.
         a. A calorie is the amount of energy (heat) needed to increase the temperature of 1 g of water 1° C.
         b. One kilocalorie (1 kcal) equals 1000 calories.
      2. Selected caloric requirements of various substances:
         a. Protein and CHO: 4 kcal/g
         b. Fat: 9 kcal/g
         c. Alcohol: 7 kcal/g
   B. Energy used by the body can be measured by direct or indirect calorimetry.
      1. Direct calorimetry is based on the postulate that all energy expended in the body eventually becomes heat.
         a. In a resting person, the amount of energy expended over a given time, or metabolic rate, can be determined by measuring the heat liberated.
      2. Indirect calorimetry is based on the postulate that >95% of the energy expended by a person is derived from the reaction of oxygen with food (oxidation).
         a. For the average diet, 4825 kcal is produced for every liter of oxygen consumed.

      b. Various devices have been developed for indirect calorimetry.
         (1) Metabolic cart
         (2) Gas collection hood

C. Basal metabolic rate (BMR)
  1. The BMR is defined as the rate of energy expenditure under a given set of basal conditions.
    a. Absolute rest
    b. Awake
    c. After an overnight fast
    d. Rested
    e. Reclining for 30 minutes
    f. Relaxed
  2. The BMR gives an estimate of energy expended when no extra demands are placed on a patient and would include such functions as:
    a. Ion pump
    b. Synthesis and degradation of cell constituents
    c. Substrate cycles
    d. Leakage of protons across the mitochondrial membrane
    e. Postural, respiratory, and heart muscle activity
  3. The BMR is related to body cell mass.

D. Resting energy expenditure (REE)
  1. If energy expenditure is measured after eating, energy expenditure is increased.
    a. This is known as the *specific dynamic action* (SDA) of food.
       (1) It is primarily caused by protein consumed.
       (2) It amounts to an increase of approximately 10% of the BMR.
  2. The REE is defined as the BMR plus the component of SDA of food.
  3. The Harris-Benedict equation will give an estimation of REE:

$$\text{Male REE} = 66.4230 + 13.7516W + 5.033H - 6.7750A \tag{1}$$

$$\text{Female REE} = 655.0955 + 9.6534W + 1.8946H - 4.6756A \tag{2}$$

where A = age in years, H = height in centimeters, and W = weight in kilograms.

E. Total energy expenditure
  1. The final factor that must be included to determine the total energy expenditure (TEE) is exercise or physical work performance and degree of stress.
  2. TEE = (REE × Activity factor) × Stress factor (Table 24-1)
  3. The BMR has been found to increase under certain conditions (see Table 24-1).
    a. Trauma
    b. Infection
    c. Fever
    d. Stress
    e. Burns

TABLE 24-1

Factors Indicating Increases in Basal Metabolic Rate Under Certain Physiologic Conditions

Condition	Factor
Confined to bed	1.2
Normal activity	1.3
Minor operation	1.2
Skeletal trauma	1.35
Major sepsis	1.6
Severe thermal burn	2.1

F. Protein requirement
1. The normal man engaging in an average amount of exercise requires 0.8 to 1.0 g of protein/kg body weight/day.
2. In the moderately stressed individual (e.g., infection and major surgery) protein requirement is 1.5 to 2.0 g/kg body weight/day.
3. In the severely stressed person (e.g., burns and major trauma) protein requirement is 2.0 to 4.0 g/kg body weight/day.
4. A calorie-to-nitrogen ratio of 150:1 is adequate for most catabolic patients. Higher ratios are used for those in severe stress.
5. Daily protein requirements are:

$$\text{Protein g} = 6.25 \times \frac{\text{Energy requirements}}{150} \tag{3}$$

III. **Vitamin Requirements and Deficiency States**
A. General functions of vitamins
1. Vitamins generally participate in metabolism in the interconversion and degradation of protein and amino acids.
2. They also participate in the extraction of energy from CHO and fat sources.
a. Anabolic purposes
b. Bone formation
B. Fat-soluble vitamins
1. Vitamin A (retinol)
a. Function in biochemical system
(1) Dim light vision
(2) Cell membrane stability
b. Requirement increases with increasing protein intake.
c. Deficiency symptoms
(1) Night blindness
(2) Keratomalacia
2. Vitamin D (calciferol)
a. Function in biochemical system
(1) Necessary for endochondral bone formation
(2) Intestinal Ca^{+2} absorption
b. Bile necessary for absorption
c. Deficiency symptoms
(1) Childhood rickets
(2) Adult osteomalacia
3. Vitamin E
a. Function in biochemical system
(1) Primarily an antioxidant
b. Requirement increases with increased ingestion of unsaturated oil.
c. Deficiency symptoms
(1) Muscular weakness
(2) Hemolysis
4. Vitamin K (phytonadione)
a. Function in biochemical systems
(1) Regulation of coagulation system
(2) Synthesis of prothrombin
b. Microbiologic production by intestinal flora accounts for 50% of requirement.
c. Deficiency symptom
(1) Hemorrhage
C. Water-soluble vitamins
1. Vitamin B_1 (thiamine)
a. Function in biochemical systems
(1) Ketoacid metabolism

    b. Deficiency symptoms
        (1) Beriberi
        (2) Anorexia
        (3) Ataxia
        (4) Weakness
        (5) Depression
        (6) Irritability
        (7) Lethargy
        (8) Heart failure

2. Niacin
    a. Function in biochemical systems
        (1) Cellular hydrogen transport
        (2) Component of coenzymes nicotinamide adenine dinucleotide (NAD) and nicotinamide adenine dinucleotide phosphate (NADP)
        (3) Glycolipids
        (4) Tissue respiration and synthesis
    b. Requirements vary directly with energy intake.
    c. Deficiency symptoms
        (1) Weakness
        (2) Anorexia
        (3) Dermatitis
        (4) Diarrhea
        (5) Dementia

3. Pantothenic acid
    a. Function in biochemical systems
        (1) Component of CoA
    b. Deficiency symptom
        (1) Fatigue

4. Vitamin B_2 (riboflavin)
    a. Function in biochemical systems
        (1) Oxidative enzyme systems
        (2) Combines with phosphoric acid to become part of the flavin coenzymes flavin mononucleotide (FMN) and flavin adenine dinucleotide (FAD)
    b. Deficiency symptoms
        (1) Poor growth
        (2) Alopecia

5. Pyridoxine (vitamin B_6)
    a. Function in biochemical systems
        (1) Transamination in amino acid decarboxylation
        (2) A primary coenzyme in metabolism of protein, CHO, fat, and nonoxidative degradation of amino acids
    b. Deficiency symptoms
        (1) Seborrheic dermatitis
        (2) Glossitis
        (3) Lymphopenia

6. Folic acid
    a. Function in biochemical systems
        (1) Synthesis of DNA and RNA
    b. Synthesis by intestinal flora may satisfy requirement.
    c. Deficiency symptom
        (1) Megaloblastic anemia

7. Vitamin B_{12} (cyanocobalamin)
    a. Function in biomedical systems
        (1) Synthesis of DNA
        (2) Intimate link to folate metabolism

      b. Requires gastric intrinsic factor and distal ileum for absorption
      c. Deficiency symptoms
        (1) Decreased proprioception
        (2) Megaloblastic anemia
  8. Vitamin C (ascorbic acid)
      a. Function in biochemical systems
        (1) Coenzyme or cofactor in hydroxylation of collagen
        (2) Essential to normal functioning of all cellular units, including ribosomes and mitochondria
        (3) Promotes healing of wounds
      b. Deficiency symptoms
        (1) Swollen, inflamed gums
        (2) Loosened teeth
        (3) Capillary hemorrhages
        (4) Subcutaneous and subperiosteal hemorrhages

IV. **Interrelationship Between Pulmonary Disease and Nutritional Status**
  A. Pulmonary function and nutritional status are closely interrelated.
    1. Malnutrition increases the risk of acute and chronic respiratory failure (CRF).
      a. A common complication of malnutrition is pulmonary infection.
    2. Inattention to nutritional requirements in patients with CRF results in increased morbidity and mortality.
      a. Inadequate or inappropriate nutrient intake exacerbates pulmonary dysfunction.
      b. Pulmonary distress limits nutritional intake.
  B. Providing nutrients essential for respiratory function enhances pulmonary function.
    1. Calories and protein should be provided in proportions to place the least stress on respiratory capacity.
    2. The amount of O_2 consumed and the amount of CO_2 produced are different for each major nutrient.
      a. For each calorie of CHO metabolized, 0.20 L of O_2 is consumed and 0.20 L of CO_2 is produced.
      b. For each calorie of protein metabolized, 0.24 L of O_2 is consumed and 0.19 L of CO_2 is produced.
      c. For each calorie of fat metabolized, 0.22 L of O_2 is consumed and 0.15 L of CO_2 is produced.
    3. The ratio of CO_2 produced to O_2 consumed is called the *respiratory quotient* (RQ).
    4. A diet with a decreased amount of CHO and a proportionally increased amount of fat (50%) should be provided to patients with hypercapnia.
      a. When fat replaces CHO calories, CO_2 and minute ventilation are reduced.
      b. The RQ is reduced.
  C. Protein requirements and ventilatory drive
    1. Protein intake should match requirement.
      a. Inadequate protein intake can lead to:
        (1) Protein-calorie malnutrition
        (2) Wasting of lean body mass
    2. Low protein intake and high CHO intake will:
      a. Decrease elimination of theophylline.
      b. Require adjustment in dosage to avoid theophylline toxicity.
    3. Long-term use of steroids promotes:
      a. Protein catabolism and gluconeogenesis
      b. Generalized muscle wasting
      c. A negative nitrogen balance
    4. Excessive protein intake can be detrimental to a person who is unable to increase minute ventilation.
    5. High-protein diets stimulate ventilatory drive and minute ventilation.

a. For patients without alveolar reserves, the stimulus can result in:
(1) Increased work of breathing
(2) Dyspnea
6. High-protein diets may increase the clearance of theophylline.
a. Dosage requirements will be affected.
7. Adequate protein should be provided to allow for anabolism.
a. Overfeeding of protein should be avoided.
b. A calorie-to-nitrogen ratio of 150:1 should be provided.
8. Nitrogen balance is a useful means to determine the adequacy of protein intake (see Section VII, Nutritional Assessment).

V. **Weight Loss and Pulmonary Disease**
A. Decreased body weight is a complication of chronic obstructive pulmonary disease (COPD).
1. The incidence varies between 25% and 65% of patients with COPD.
2. Body weight correlates with the percent of predicted diffusion capacity and forced expiratory volume in 1 second.
3. Sustained weight loss is associated with a poor prognosis.
a. Weight loss of ≥10% is an antecedent of heart failure in hypercapnic patients with COPD.
b. Mortality is significantly increased.
B. Factors that result in decreased calorie intake
1. Twenty percent to 25% of patients with COPD have peptic ulcers, and gastrointestinal discomfort may cause these patients to shun food.
2. Bronchodilators, both sympathomimetic and theophylline derivatives, are gastric irritants.
a. Nausea and vomiting may occur with toxic doses of theophylline.
3. Chronic sputum production may alter the desire for and taste of food.
4. A full stomach restricts descent of the diaphragm and makes breathing difficult after large meals.
5. Shortness of breath may hamper the patient's ability to prepare meals or to eat with comfort.
6. Depression is associated with decreased food intake.
C. Factors that increase caloric expenditure
1. Infections common in acute respiratory illness increase metabolic demand.
2. The respiratory disease itself is capable of increasing energy expenditure.
3. The elevated energy requirement may be related to the increased work of breathing in patients with respiratory disease.
a. With diffuse bronchial obstruction, the mechanical work necessary to overcome nonelastic resistance increases.
b. The respiratory muscles require oxygen to perform this mechanical work.
4. The caloric cost of breathing increases in patients with pulmonary disease.
a. Normal expenditure: 43 to 72 kcal/day
b. Pulmonary disease: 430 to 720 kcal/day

VI. **Muscle Mass and Strength**
A. Respiratory muscles are catabolized to meet the body's energy needs in those with malnutrition.
1. Autopsy studies provide evidence of decreased weight of the diaphragm muscle in patients with emphysema.
2. Malnutrition decreases the degree to which the diaphragm can contract.
a. Weakness of the diaphragm can contribute to respiratory failure.
B. Respiratory muscle function is decreased in those with malnutrition.
1. The loss in respiratory muscle strength occurs in inspiratory and expiratory muscles.
2. The loss in respiratory muscle strength is directly related to weight loss.
3. A major goal in the care of the patient with respiratory failure and nutritional depletion is restoration of lean body mass.

VII. **Nutritional Assessment**
   A. The systematic evaluation of a patient's current state of nutrition using physical and bio-chemical means
      1. Nutritional assessment includes three major parameters:
         a. Nutrition history
         b. Anthropometrics
         c. Laboratory analysis
   B. Nutrition history parameters
      1. Diet history and interview
         a. Dietary patterns before illness and during any past treatments
         b. Usual weight before illness
         c. Recent weight changes
         d. Changes in sense of taste or smell related to food and to past treatments
         e. Changes in appetite and food likes and dislikes related to onset of disease and to previous treatments
         f. Twenty-four-hour dietary recall
   C. Anthropometric parameters (somatic compartment) (Table 24-2)
      1. Height and weight
         a. Determine premorbid and hospital admission weights.
         b. Determine ideal body weight.
            (1) Men = 48.2 kg for 23.6 cm + 2.7 kg for each additional 2.54 cm
            (2) Women = 45.4 kg for 23.6 cm + 2.3 kg for each additional 2.54 cm
      2. Triceps skinfold (TSF; see Table 24-2)
         a. Measure of body's fat stores and nonprotein caloric reserves
         b. Measured using skinfold calipers
      3. Arm muscle circumference (AMC; see Table 24-2)
         a. Indicator of lean body mass or muscle tissue
      4. Not as reliable as originally thought; many subpopulations require additional study.
   D. Laboratory parameters (visceral compartment)
      1. Serum albumin (Table 24-3)
         a. Normal serum albumin is 3.5 to 5.0 g/dl.
            (1) Normal serum albumin level is the equilibrium point between production, distribution, and degradation.
            (2) Decreased albumin levels result from:
               (a) Inadequate synthesis
               (b) Increased catabolism
               (c) Extraordinary corporal losses of albumin
         b. Count of 2.8 g% is the cutoff point for albumin oncotic pressure; <2.8 g%, edema will usually be present.
         c. Hypoalbuminemia is more commonly a marker for systemic inflammatory response and rarely present in cases of isolated calorie malnutrition.

TABLE **24-2**

Anthropometric Standards

	Triceps Skinfold (mm)	Arm Muscle Circumference (cm)
Male	12.5	25.3
Female	16.5	23.2

% deficit in anthropometric measurements =

$$100 - \left[\frac{\text{Actual Value}}{\text{Standard Value}} \times 100 \right]$$

TABLE **24-3**

Visceral Protein Levels

	Normal	Mild Deficit	Moderate Deficit	Severe Deficit
Albumin (g/dl)	3.5-5.0	<3.5	<3.0	<2.5
Transferrin (mg%)	>200	<200	<180	<160
Total lymphocyte count (number/mm^3)	2000-4000	<1800	<1500	<900

2. Indirect calorimetry
   a. Uses gas analyzers to determine oxygen consumption ($\dot{V}O_2$) and carbon dioxide production ($\dot{V}CO_2$).
      (1) Normal $\dot{V}O_2$ is approximately 250 ml/min.
      (2) Normal $\dot{V}CO_2$ is approximately 200 ml/min.
   b. Carbon dioxide production ($\dot{V}CO_2$) divided by oxygen consumption ($\dot{V}O_2$) is RQ (e.g., RQ = $\dot{V}CO_2/\dot{V}O_2$); normal value = 0.8 to 1.0.
   c. Can be done at the bedside.
      (1) Needs a well-trained operator for consistent results.
      (2) Frequent calibration required for gas analyzers.
      (3) Incompatible with newer generation ventilators that incorporate a continuous bias flow.
   d. Indirect calorimeters require a constant inspiratory and expiratory volume for determination of $\dot{V}O_2$ and $\dot{V}CO_2$.
   e. Requires 30 to 45 minutes of an equilibrium state.
   f. Controversial whether indirect calorimetry is needed with the change in nutritional management from total parenteral nutrition (TPN) to enteral tube feeding (ETF).
      (1) TPN is characterized by "hyperalimentation" and excessive nutritional support.
         (a) Indirect calorimetry has a role in identifying individual caloric requirements and minimizing overfeeding.
         (b) Passive method of providing nutrients.
         (c) Risk of aspiration is lower with patients receiving TPN because of less content within the stomach.
      (2) ETF is a more physiologic route for providing nutritional support.
         (a) Leads to lower incidence of ileus and associated complications.
         (b) Supports stress response and prevention of complications from protein malnutrition.
         (c) Use of "trickle feeds" (rates, 10 to 30 ml/hr) insufficient to attain adequate nutritional support.
3. Bioelectrical impedance
   a. Adipose tissue has a higher water content than does lean muscle mass (LMM).
      (1) Adipose tissue comprises polymerized fatty acids.
      (2) LMM mostly comprises protein.
   b. Using electrodes spaced over the body, usually hand and ankle, a small current is passed.
      (1) Depending on the body composition, impedance to the current will change in direct proportion to the body's composition.
         (a) Assumes that there exists a uniform proportion of densities and constituents of fat-free mass (FFM).
            i. Water
            ii. Mineral
            iii. Protein
   c. Can be done at the bedside.
4. End-tidal carbon dioxide monitoring
   a. CO_2 is a by-product of metabolism.
      (1) Absorbs infrared light greater than oxygen

   b. Sensor attached to the airway uses mainstream infrared absorption of expired gases to obtain CO_2 concentration.

     (1) When paired with a pneumotachometer, it is possible to integrate airway flow and end-tidal CO_2 measurement on a breath-by-breath basis (Figure 24-1, *A*).

       (a) Allows for determination of $\dot{V}CO_2$.

          i. $\dot{V}CO_2$ is extrapolated from the graphical plot of expired gas; at the intersection point where the slope of end-tidal CO_2 is measured, and a vertical line drawn at the phase of the breath where CO_2 is beginning to be expired.

         ii. When this is matched with airway flow measurements, $\dot{V}CO_2$ is determined as the area under this curve (see Figure 24-1, *B*).

         iii. Using this technique and a partial CO_2 rebreathing method, the cardiac output can also be determined (see Figure 24-1, *C*).

   c. REE can be determined using the Harris-Benedict equation.

   d. This technique assumes either low or no intrapulmonary shunting.

     (1) Shunt can decrease the gas exchange and give false readings.

   e. Easy to use and can be performed at the bedside.

   f. Using a modified Fick equation, cardiac output can also be determined.

Example:

Fick equation:

$$CO = \frac{\dot{V}CO_2}{Cv_{CO_2} - Ca_{CO_2}} \tag{4}$$

Using CO_2 rebreathing:

$$CO_N = \frac{\dot{V}CO_{2N}}{Cv_{CO_{2N}} - Ca_{CO_{2N}}} \tag{5}$$

$$CO_R = \frac{\dot{V}CO_{2R}}{Cv_{CO_{2R}} - Ca_{CO_{2R}}} \tag{6}$$

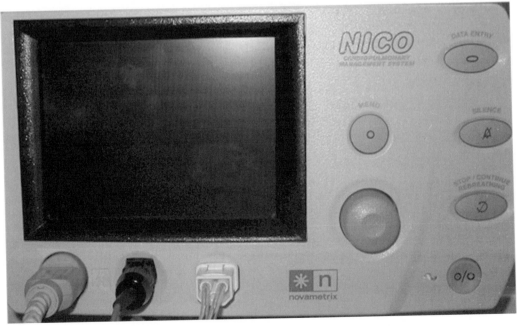

A

FIG. 24-1 A, Noninvasive cardiac output (NICO) device. It can also be used for determination of $\dot{V}CO_2$ to be used in the Harris-Benedict equations (see discussion).

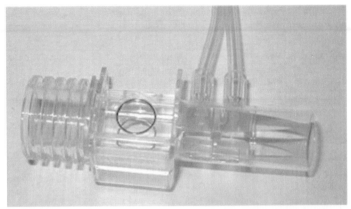

B

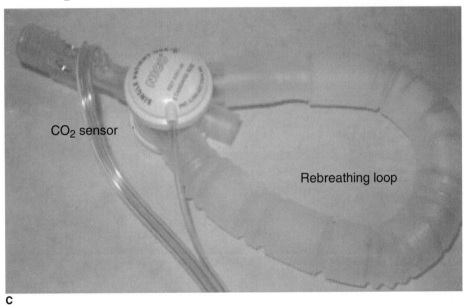

CO$_2$ sensor

Rebreathing loop

C

FIG. 24-1 cont'd B, A sample end-tidal CO$_2$ sensor incorporating a pneumotachometer for flow measurement (see discussion). **C,** A partial CO$_2$ rebreathing circuit for determination of cardiac output.

Combining the two forms:

$$CO = \frac{\left(\dot{V}CO_{2N} - \dot{V}CO_{2R} \right)}{\left(CvCO_{2N} - CaCO_{2N} \right) - \left(CvCO_{2R} - CaCO_{2R} \right)}$$

$$CO = \frac{\Delta \dot{V}CO_2}{\Delta CaCO_2} \tag{7}$$

$$CO = \frac{\Delta \dot{V}CO_2}{S \times \Delta E_T CO_2} \tag{8}$$

where:
CO = Cardiac output
R = Rebreathing
N = Normal breathing
CvCO$_2$ = Mixed venous CO$_2$ content (equivalent to E$_T$CO$_{2R}$)
CaCO$_2$ = Arterial CO$_2$ content (equivalent to E$_T$CO$_{2N}$)
$\dot{V}$CO$_2$ = CO$_2$ elimination rate

S = Slope of CO_2 dissociation curve (Figure 24-2)
E_TCO_2 = End-tidal CO_2
Assuming:
CO, $CvCO_2$, and V_D/V_T are constant during the measurement period.
A shunt correction is added to the final equation based on F_IO_2 and hemoglobin saturation.

Example:
Calculate the cardiac output using the following data:

Normal Breathing	Partial CO_2 Rebreathing
$\dot{V}co_{2N}$ = 244 ml/min	$\dot{V}co_{2R}$ = 323 ml/min
E_Tco_{2N} = 36 mm Hg	E_Tco_{2R} = 43 mm Hg
Spo_{2N} = 97%	Spo_{2R} = 97%

Using the above equation:

$$\begin{aligned} CO &= \Delta\dot{V}co_2/S \times \Delta E_Tco_2 \\ &= (323 - 244)/S \times (43 - 36) \\ &= 79/1.30 \times 7 \\ &= 8.7 \text{ L/min} \end{aligned} \tag{9}$$

Note: S is the slope of ΔE_Tco_2 by the device.
Calculate the REE for a patient with a $\dot{V}co_2$ of 279 ml/min.
Solution:
Using the following formula:

$$\begin{aligned} REE(kcal/day) &= \dot{V}co_2(L/min) \times 5.52 \times min/day \\ &= [(279/1000) \times 5.52 \times (24 \times 60)] \\ &= (0.279 \times 5.52 \times 1440) \\ &= 2217.7 \text{ kcal/day} \end{aligned} \tag{10}$$

where 5.52 is the standard number of kcal consumed to produce 1 L of CO_2.

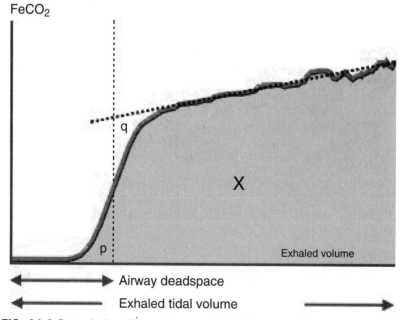

FIG. 24-2 Determination of $\dot{V}co_2$ using an end-tidal CO_2 monitor integrating airway flow.

5. Total iron-binding capacity or transferrin
   a. Values of ≤200 mg% correlate with malnutrition.
   b. Protein secreted by the liver
   c. Protein that transports iron
   d. Secretion declines in protein-depleted states.
   e. Protein is manufactured by the endoplasmic reticulum in liver cells, which depend on adequacy of amino acid, whether from diet, muscle, gut, or cutaneous tissue.
   f. First protein to increase as a result of nutritional repair.
   g. Not useful to assess malnutrition because of the metabolic half-life of transferrin.
6. Total lymphocyte count (TLC; see Table 24-3)
   a. Values of ≤1800 correlate with malnutrition.
   b. Good indication of immune response
   c. TLC = % Lymphocytes × White blood cell count/100
7. Nitrogen balance
   a. The nitrogen balance is calculated to assess whether protein is being depleted and to assess the estimated degree of hypermetabolism.
   b. Twenty-four-hour UUN is ordered.
   c. Nitrogen balance = N in − N out.
   d. In the healthy individual, nitrogen intake and nitrogen excretion are equal (approximately 11 g/day) and in balance.
   e. Positive nitrogen balance more than +2 indicates net tissue growth.
   f. Negative nitrogen balance more than −2 indicates net tissue breakdown.
      (1) Negative nitrogen balance may result from:
          (a) Trauma
          (b) Infection
          (c) Stress
          (d) Inadequate protein or CHO intake (or both):

$$\frac{\text{Protein intake}}{6.25} = (\text{UUN} + 4) \tag{11}$$

8. Creatinine height index (CHI)
   a. Creatinine is given off by muscle at a constant rate.
   b. An accurate indicator of lean body mass.
      (1) Increased creatinine in urine equals increased muscle mass.
   c. Uses 24-hour urine test for creatinine.
   d. Creatinine excreted in 24 hours is compared with normal creatinine-to-height ratios.
9. Delayed cutaneous hypersensitivity (DCH) skin testing
   a. The DCH skin test is used to evaluate the cell-mediated immunity (CMI) response.
   b. The patient is tested by injecting antigen skin tests intradermally.
   c. The CMI multitest is injected.
   d. The area of induration is read at 48 hours.
      (1) Cellular immune function is severely compromised by protein calorie malnutrition.
      (2) CMI correlates significantly with morbidity and mortality.
E. Types of malnutrition
   1. When nutrient intake is insufficient to meet requirements, malnutrition develops.
   2. Kwashiorkor (protein malnutrition)
      a. The patient who has developed kwashiorkor is one whose caloric intake was adequate or more than adequate in CHO and fat but contained little, if any, protein.
      b. The patient will have adequate somatic stores.
      c. The patient will have defects in visceral compartment.
      d. The patient may appear well nourished, even obese.
   3. Marasmus (protein calorie malnutrition)
      a. Marasmus develops in patients who cannot maintain adequate oral intake.

    b. Such patients have adequate visceral protein stores.

    c. They have depleted somatic stores.

    d. Marasmus presents with weight loss and fat and muscle wasting caused by overall calorie protein deprivation.

  4. Kwashiorkor-marasmus mix

    a. The patient has depleted somatic and visceral stores.

VIII. Dietary Intervention

  A. Basic goals of dietary intervention for patients with chronic pulmonary disease:

    1. Prevent nutritional depletion.

    2. Ensure that the mix of nutrients can be handled easily by the impaired respiratory system.

      a. Modify the level of fat and CHO.

      b. Keep RQ ≤ 1.0.

      c. Prevent overfeeding of calories, especially CHO.

      d. There is an increase in CO_2 production concurrent with the increase in RQ.

      e. The response of overfeeding CHO above energy needs is to convert the excess glucose to fat.

        (1) Conversion of CHO to fat is associated with an RQ of approximately 8.

        (2) There is a large increase in CO_2 production.

  B. General principles of tube feeding the patient with chronic respiratory disease and/or who is mechanically ventilated

    1. Provide a caloric intake to meet caloric needs of nutritional maintenance.

    2. Gradually increase the caloric intake beyond maintenance and monitor the respiratory effect when nutritional rehabilitation is the goal.

    3. Avoid overfeeding of protein.

      a. Provide enough protein so that nitrogen intake equals nitrogen output when maintenance is the goal.

      b. Provide enough protein to achieve a positive nitrogen balance if repletion is the goal.

    4. Restrict fluid and/or sodium as needed to lower pulmonary vascular pressure and decrease extravascular lung water.

      a. Use enteral formulas with high nutrient density if fluid is restricted.

    5. Monitor serum phosphate levels to avoid hypophosphatemia.

      a. Lean muscle contains approximately 100 mEq of phosphate/kg of wet tissue.

      b. Phosphate deficiency occurs when the patient's previous state of malnutrition is underestimated or if inadequate phosphate is provided.

      c. Deficiencies can develop in <48 hours.

      d. Hypophosphatemia can occur if increased requirements for phosphorus are not met.

    6. Hypercapnic and ventilator-dependent patients should have less CHO and more fat to minimize the demand on the respiratory system to eliminate CO_2.

      a. They should have $\geq 50\%$ fat calories and $\leq 30\%$ CHO calories.

      b. Sufficient CHO should be provided to prevent ketosis.

        (1) If calorie intake is adequate, 50 to 100 g of digestible CHO will prevent ketosis.

      c. The caloric distribution of the feeding can be manipulated by adding fat (corn oil) to a commercial feeding.

      d. Pulmocare, a commercial enteral product, contains >50% calories of fat.

  C. Monitoring of tube-fed patients

    1. The nutritional regimen should be continually adjusted to the patient's changing medical and nutritional condition.

      a. Hydration

        (1) Monitor fluid input and output

        (2) Monitor the specific gravity of urine

      b. Utilization of glucose

        (1) Serum and urine glucose

     c. Utilization of protein
        (1) Nitrogen balance
        (2) Blood urea nitrogen
     d. Serum electrolytes and phosphate
        (1) Sodium
        (2) Potassium
        (3) Chloride
        (4) Phosphate
     e. Respiratory function
        (1) Arterial blood gases
        (2) Minute ventilation

IX. Oral Diet Intervention
   A. Nonhypercapnic patients: dietary recommendations
     1. Make food preparation easier so fatigue does not result.
     2. Rest just before eating so respiratory demand is low.
     3. Eat in a quiet, relaxed atmosphere.
     4. Emphasize the meals early in the day if fatigue becomes worse as the day continues.
     5. Avoid foods that produce gas or bloating, which will cause distention and displacement of the diaphragm.
   B. Hypercapnic patients: dietary recommendations
     1. Eat small, frequent feedings.
       a. The demand for O_2 and the volume of CO_2 that has to be expired will be reduced.
       b. A full stomach interferes with the descent of the diaphragm and makes breathing difficult.
   C. Nutritional maintenance
     1. Provide caloric intake equal to caloric needs.
   D. Nutritional rehabilitation
     1. Gradually increase caloric intake and monitor respiratory effect.
     2. Substitute lower cholesterol fat for high CHO foods.
       a. Calories as fat: 45% to 50%
       b. Calories as CHO: 30% to 35%
       c. Monitor total calories to avoid excessive intake.
     3. Avoid overfeeding of protein.
       a. Provide enough for N balance if maintenance is the goal.
       b. Provide enough protein to achieve +N balance if repletion is the goal.
     4. Restrict intake of fluid, sodium, or both.
       a. Vascular pressure will decrease.
       b. Extravascular lung water will decrease.

BIBLIOGRAPHY

Behrends M, Kernbach M, Bräuer A, Braun U, Peters J, Weyland W: In vitro validation of a metabolic monitor for gas exchange measurements in ventilated neonates. *Intensive Care Med* 27:228-235, 2001.

Chan S, McGowen KC, Blackburn GL: Nutrition management in the ICU. *Chest* 115:145S-148S, 1999.

Chumlea WC, Guo SS, Kuczmarski RJ, et al: Body composition estimates from NHANES III bioelectrical impedance data. *J Obesity* 26:1596-1609, 2002.

Donaldson L, Dodds S, Walsh TS: Clinical evaluation of a continuous oxygen consumption monitor in mechanically ventilated patients. *Anaesthesia* 58:455-460, 2003.

Faisy C, Guerot E, Diehl J, Labrousse J, Fagon J: Assessment of resting energy expenditure in mechanically ventilated patients. *Am J Clin Nutr* 78:241-249, 2003.

Flancbaum L, Choban PS, Sambucco S, Verducci J, Burge JC: Comparison of indirect calorimetry, the Fick method, and prediction equations in estimating the energy requirements of critically ill patients. *Am J Clin Nutr* 69:461-466, 1999.

Joosten KF, Jacobs FI, van Klaarwater E, et al: Accuracy of an indirect calorimeter for mechanically ventilated infants and children: the influence of low rates of gas exchange and varying F_1O_2. *Crit Care Med* 28:3014-3018, 2000.

Kan M, Chang H, Sheu W, Cheng C, Lee B, Huang Y: Estimation of energy requirements for mechanically ventilated critically ill patients using nutritional status. *Crit Care* 7:R108-R115, 2003.

McClave SA, McClain CJ, Snider HL: Should indirect calorimetry be used as part of nutritional assessment? J Clin Gastroenterol 33:14-19, 2001.

McClave SA, Snider HL, Spain DA: Preoperative issues in clinical nutrition. *Chest* 115:64S-70S, 1999.

Persson MD, Brismar KE, Katzarski KS, Nordenstrom J, Cederholm TE: Nutritional assessment and subjective global assessment predict mortality in geriatric patients. *J Am Geriatr Soc* 50:1996-2002, 2002.

Waldau T, Larsen VH, Parbst H, Bonde J: Assessment of the respiratory exchange ratio in mechanically ventilated patients by a standard anaesthetic gas analyzer. *Acta Anaesthesiol Scand* 46:1242-1250, 2002.

Chapter **25**

Intrauterine Development and Comparative Respiratory Anatomy

I. **General Developmental Periods**
   A. Fertilization period (weeks 1 through 3)
      1. The sperm fertilizes the egg.
      2. Blood vessels first appear.
      3. Heart tubes form that will develop into the heart.
      4. Blood cells form from endothelial cells within the yolk sac.
   B. Embryonic period (weeks 4 through 7)
      1. Embryo forms a C-shaped appearance.
      2. Primitive gut is formed.
      3. Umbilical cord develops.
      4. Three primary germ layers differentiate into various organs and tissues.
      5. The brain, heart, eyes, ears, nose, and mouth are developing, giving the embryo human characteristics.
   C. Fetal period (week 8 through birth)
      1. The embryo is now called a *fetus*.
      2. Rapid body growth and organ system maturation occur.

II. **Respiratory System Development**
   A. Upper airway
      1. By the fourth week, brachial arches form and develop the maxillary (upper) and mandibular (lower) jaw.
      2. The brachial arches also form the pharynx, mouth, oropharyngeal airway, and laryngeal cartilages.
      3. The tongue develops within weeks 4 to 7.
      4. The palate starts to develop in the fifth week and is complete by the 17th week of gestation.
      5. A cleft lip may develop as a result of the lip not completely forming and extending into the nostril. A cleft palate occurs from malformation of the palate and may be unilateral or bilateral.
      6. The nasal cavity with nasal concha develops when the oronasal membrane ruptures, allowing the oral and nasal cavities to develop. This occurs during approximately the seventh week.
      7. Nasal sinuses develop during the latter part of fetal development, with further development of the ethmoid, maxillary, frontal, and sphenoidal sinuses continuing into puberty.

445

B. Lower airway
   1. An epithelial groove will give rise to the larynx, trachea, bronchi, pulmonary epithelium, and assorted glands.
   2. The tracheoesophageal septum divides into the esophagus and laryngotracheal tube.
   3. The first lung bud develops from the laryngotracheal tube by 24 to 26 days of fertilization.
   4. The laryngotracheal tube, along with the surrounding tissue, develops into the larynx, trachea, bronchi, and lungs.
   5. Visceral and parietal pleura develop from the lung buds (bronchopulmonary buds).
   6. By 5 weeks two lung buds develop.
   7. The phrenic nerve innervates the diaphragm within the fourth week, and the diaphragm is completely formed by the seventh week.
   8. By the 10th week, true and false vocal cords are formed.
   9. Further growth of the lung buds develop into secondary buds, two on the right and one on the left.
   10. This branching continues, with 24 orders of branches present at 16 weeks.
   11. By 25 weeks airways have changed from glandular to tubular and increase in length and diameter.
C. Periods of lung maturation
   1. Embryonic period (fertilization to 5 weeks)
      a. The laryngotracheal groove forms.
      b. The lung bud first appears.
      c. The lung bud divides into left and right mainstem bronchi.
      d. Branching of the airways begins.
      e. Pulmonary arteries invade lung tissue, following the airways and dividing as the airway divides.
      f. Pulmonary veins originate independently from the lung parenchyma and return to the left atrium, completing the pulmonary circuit.
   2. Pseudoglandular period (5 to 13 weeks)
      a. The conducting airways develop and are complete up to and including the terminal bronchiole.
      b. Mucous glands and goblet cells appear.
      c. Bronchi and bronchioles are lined with cuboidal epithelium.
      d. Diaphragm begins to develop.
      e. Muscle fibers, elastic tissue, and early cartilage formation can be seen along the tracheobronchial tree.
   3. Canalicular period (13 to 24 weeks)
      a. Enlargement of the conducting airways continues, with proliferation of pulmonary blood vessels.
      b. Gas exchange units develop from respiratory bronchioles.
      c. Cilia appear at 13 weeks.
      d. Meconium is present at 16 weeks.
      e. Breathing movements can be detected between 18 and 20 weeks.
      f. Elastic tissue develops beginning at 20 weeks.
      g. Airway changes from glandular to tubular and increases in length and diameter.
      h. Type I and II alveolar pneumocytes develop, with synthesis and production of surfactant starting by weeks 22 to 24.
   4. Terminal sac period (24 weeks to birth)
      a. Primitive alveoli develop from alveolar ducts.
      b. Further development of the pulmonary vasculature occurs, as does lymphatic proliferation.
      c. The fetus weighs approximately 1000 g at 26 to 28 weeks.
      d. The fetal lungs represent 2% to 3% of the total body weight. This percentage decreases as the weight of the fetus increases toward the end of gestation.
      e. The air sacs change from a cuboidal cellular configuration to a squamous epithelium, allowing greater diffusion of gases.

    f. As the lung matures, the number of alveoli increases, and the thickness of the alveoli wall decreases.

    g. At birth the number of alveoli ranges from 24 to 75 million.

    h. The number of alveoli continues to increase until there are approximately 300 to 600 million alveoli in adulthood.

    i. The size of the lung increases from approximately 1 to 2 m^2 at 32 weeks' gestation to the adult size of 70 m^2.

    j. Extrauterine life is first possible in this period.

III. **Fetal Lung Fluid**

    A. The lung begins secreting fluid by the 70th day of gestation.

    B. This fluid is composed of a combination of sodium, potassium, chloride, bicarbonate, and a small percentage of protein in water.

    C. The presence of lung fluid assists lung growth and the development of the functional residual capacity (FRC).

    D. Fetal breathing helps secrete lung fluid and mixes lung fluid with amniotic fluid.

    E. Because of this process, amniotic fluid can be analyzed to determine lung maturation (see Section V, Amniotic Fluid).

    F. Amniocentesis is the procedure in which amniotic fluid is removed from the uterus for examination.

IV. **Surfactant**

    A. Surfactant is synthesized and secreted by type II alveolar pneumocytes.

    B. Surfactant first appears between 22 and 24 weeks' gestation.

    C. Surfactant reduces surface tension, maintaining alveolar stability and preventing atelectasis.

    D. Protein makes up 10% to 20% of the surfactant, and 80% to 90% of the protein is phospholipids. A small percentage of cholesterol is also present.

    E. Two important phospholipids, lecithin and sphingomyelin, are present in surfactant.

    F. Sphingomyelin is present early in gestation and remains constant from 18 weeks to approximately 34 weeks before decreasing in concentration.

    G. Lecithin, the major phospholipid of adult surfactant, abruptly increases between 32 and 34 weeks' gestation.

    H. The increased concentration of lecithin denotes lung maturation. The increase of lecithin in surfactant reduces the incidence of respiratory distress syndrome (RDS).

    I. Without appropriate surfactant production, newborns will have reduced lung compliance, decreased FRC, increased work of breathing, and greater oxygen consumption.

    J. Inadequate surfactant levels can occur in a newborn as a result of:

        1. Prematurity

        2. Hypoxia

        3. Malnutrition

        4. Maternal diabetes

        5. Hypothermia

        6. Acidosis

V. **Amniotic Fluid**

    A. Amniotic fluid is composed of amniotic cells, maternal blood, and fetal urine.

    B. There is approximately 30 ml of amniotic fluid at 10 weeks, which increases to 1 L by term.

    C. The fetus swallows amniotic fluid, which is absorbed by the gastrointestinal tract. Every 3 hours, the placenta exchanges amniotic fluid.

    D. Amniotic fluid protects the fetus and acts as a cushion surrounding the fetus. It also allows growth and development, movement, and maintenance of a thermoneutral environment.

    E. Amniocentesis can determine sex, lung maturity, biochemical abnormalities, and chromosomal defects.

    F. Lung maturity is determined by the concentration of lecithin and sphingomyelin.

    G. The ratio of lecithin to sphingomyelin (L/S) determines the incidence of RDS.

H. An L/S ratio of ≥2.0 indicates a mature lung and low incidence of RDS.
I. An L/S ratio of 1.0 to 1.5 indicates a transitional lung with a moderate incidence of RDS.
J. An L/S ratio of <1.0 indicates a high incidence of RDS.
K. Another test to determine lung maturity is the shake test.
   1. A mixture of amniotic fluid, saline, and alcohol is placed in a test tube, shaken for 15 minutes, and then allowed to stand.
   2. A complete ring of bubbles around the tube indicates appropriate fetal production of surfactant.
   3. These results can be compared with an L/S ratio of >2.0.
   4. Absence of bubbles indicates that surfactant maturity is incomplete.

VI. **Maternal Factors**
   A. Maternal health and individual physiology, pregnancy complications, and maternal behaviors affect the health and development of the fetus.
   B. Any condition that leads to interference with placental blood flow or the transfer of oxygen to the fetus can cause adverse outcomes.
   C. Table 25-1 list maternal conditions and related neonatal outcomes.

VII. **Placenta**
   A. Major activities of the placenta include metabolism, transfer of nutrients and wastes, and endocrine secretion.
   B. Provides exchange of oxygen, carbon dioxide, and metabolic nutrients between fetal and maternal blood supplies.
   C. Blood supplies of the mother and fetus are in close proximity to one another but are not in actual contact.
   D. Fetal blood enters the placenta by way of two umbilical arteries and leaves by one umbilical vein.
   E. During birth contractions of the uterus slow blood flow to the placenta, and gas exchange may be reduced.

VIII. **Fetal Circulation (Figure 25-1)**
   A. After oxygenated blood leaves the placenta, a portion of the blood enters the portal sinus to perfuse the kidney. The remainder enters the ductus venosus, bypassing the liver and entering the inferior vena cava.
   B. The oxygen saturation of the blood (SaO_2) coming from the placenta is approximately 80%. The PaO_2 is 27 to 29 mm Hg.

TABLE 25-1

Maternal Condition and Neonatal Outcomes

Maternal Condition	Fetal or Neonatal Outcome
Previous pregnancy complication	Same outcome as previous fetus
Diabetes mellitus	LGA, congenital malformations, RDS, hypoglycemia
Pregnancy-induced hypertension	Prematurity, SGA (pre-eclampsia)
Maternal age <17 years	Low birth weight, prematurity
Maternal age >35 years	Prematurity, chromosomal defects
Placenta previa	Prematurity, bleeding, SGA
Placenta abruptio	Fetal asphyxia, bleeding
Alcohol consumption	SGA, CNS dysfunction, mental retardation, facial dysmorphology
Smoking	SGA, prematurity, mental retardation, SIDS
Drug use	Placental abruption, IUGR, prematurity, CNS abnormalities, withdrawal disorders

IUGR, Intrauterine growth retardation; *LGA,* large for gestational age; *RDS,* respiratory distress syndrome; *SGA,* small for gestational age; *SIDS,* sudden infant death syndrome; *CNS,* central nervous system.
From Wilkins RL, Stoller JK, Scanlan CL: *Egan's Fundamentals of Respiratory Care,* ed 8, St. Louis, 2003, Mosby.

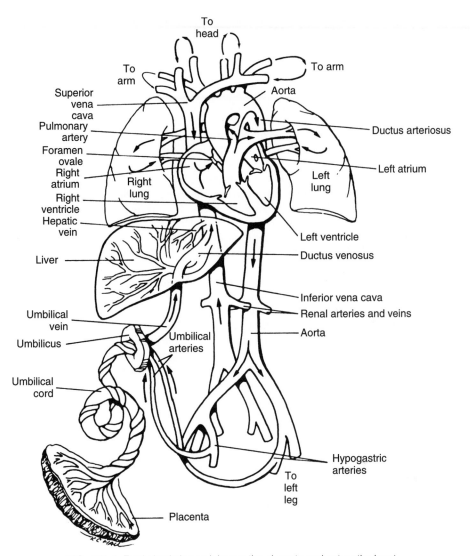

FIG. 25-1 Fetal circulation as it leaves the placenta and enters the heart.

C. Blood coming from the inferior vena cava has perfused the lower body tissues and has reduced SaO_2 and PaO_2. Thus as the oxygenated blood from the ductus venosus enters the inferior vena cava and mixes, the SaO_2 decreases to approximately 67%.
D. The blood enters the right atrium from the inferior vena cava, where it mixes with blood returning from the upper part of the body and head. This further reduces the saturation to approximately 62%.
E. The blood flow entering the right atrium is divided into two streams, with the larger stream entering the left atrium by way of the foramen ovale.
F. The foramen ovale is an opening of the interatrial septum between the right and left atria.
G. This opening remains patent because of the increase in blood pressure in the right side of the heart relative to that of the left.
H. The blood enters the left atrium and then mixes with a small amount of deoxygenated blood returning from the lungs by way of the pulmonary veins. This blood enters the left ventricle and is pumped out the aorta.
I. A portion of this blood is directed to the head and upper extremities. This flow of blood has a higher oxygen content and SaO_2 than the flow that is pumped out of the right ventricle.

J. The second stream of blood in the right atrium is pumped to the right ventricle and out the pulmonary artery. This blood has mixed with blood coming from the superior vena cava.

K. Approximately 10% of the cardiac output from the right side of the heart enters the pulmonary arteries and the lung. The lungs need little blood at this time because gas exchange occurs within the placenta.

L. The pulmonary arteries are constricted as a result of the low PaO_2 and lung fluid compressing the vessels. The pulmonary vascular resistance generally is high, and the peripheral vascular resistance generally is low.

M. A large portion of the blood volume from the right side of the heart (approximately 90% of blood entering the right heart) enters the arch of the aorta by way of the ductus arteriosus. This ductus connects the pulmonary arteries and aorta and creates a right-to-left shunt. The saturation of this blood is approximately 50%.

N. Blood flow moves out of the heart through the ductus arteriosus to the arch of the aorta, descending aorta, and thoracic aorta. Here blood is directed to the kidney, gut, and lower part of the body.

O. A major portion of the blood (approximately 50% of the cardiac output) enters the placenta and is oxygenated.

IX. **Transfer of Oxygen From Maternal to Fetal Blood (Figure 25-2)**
A. Maternal blood enters the placenta through the spiral arteries. The PaO_2 of the maternal blood is approximately 100 mm Hg.
B. Fetal blood enters the placenta through two umbilical arteries, which divide to form a vascular network. The PaO_2 of the fetal blood entering the placenta is approximately 17 mm Hg.
C. As both circulations come into proximity of one another, maternal blood releases oxygen to fetal circulation while at the same time accepts metabolic waste from the fetal circulation.

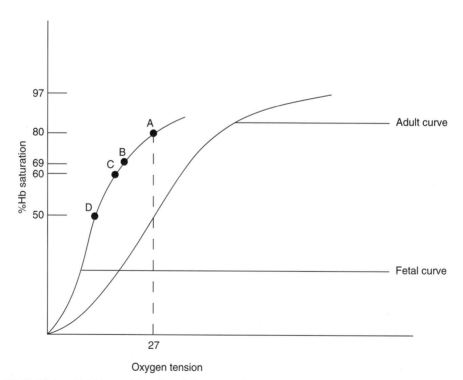

FIG. 25-2 Adult and fetal hemoglobin dissociation curve. Point A is saturation level in the umbilical artery. Point B is saturation in inferior vena cava before entering the right atrium. Point C is the SaO_2 within the right atrium, and point D is SaO_2 of the blood returning to the placenta and lower extremities.

D. The metabolic components alter the pH of maternal blood, shifting the oxyhemoglobin curve to the right, which reduces the affinity of hemoglobin for oxygen. This allows more oxygen to be released to fetal blood.

E. The fetal oxyhemoglobin dissociation curve is shifted to the left as a result of the release of metabolic waste and the presence of fetal hemoglobin (HbF).

F. Oxygen is able to combine with HbF to a greater extent than adult hemoglobin (HbA) because 2,3-diphosphoglycerate (2,3-DPG) does not affect HbF.

G. One of the primary mechanisms regulating the release of oxygen from HbA is the binding of 2,3-DPG to β chains of hemoglobin. HbF has no β chains; therefore, 2,3-DPG cannot attach to it.

H. As a result the oxyhemoglobin dissociation curve is shifted further to the left than that seen in the adult. Therefore, even with a low maternal PaO_2, HbF is able to maintain a higher SaO_2 than seen in maternal circulation. However, because the curve is shifted to the left, release of oxygen at the tissue level is impeded (see Figure 25-2).

I. Maternal blood flow leaving the placenta and returning to the mother has a PaO_2 of approximately 38 to 40 mm Hg.

J. The fetal blood flow leaving the placenta has an umbilical artery PaO_2 of approximately 29 mm Hg. The SaO_2 is 80%.

K. In contrast, an adult with a PaO_2 of 27 mm Hg would have an SaO_2 of 50%.

L. At birth approximately 77% of the total hemoglobin is HbF. Within 8 to 11 months, only 1% to 2% of the total hemoglobin will be HbF.

X. **Transition From Fetal to Newborn Circulation (Figure 25-3)**

A. By the end of the normal gestational period of 38 to 40 weeks, the fetus has completely developed and is able to assume extrauterine life.

B. After birth inflation of the lungs and transition of fetal circulation to newborn circulation occur.

C. Vaginal birth of the fetus is initiated by contraction of the uterus.

D. The fetus moves head first through the birth canal, where the chest is compressed. Intrathoracic pressures of 30 to 160 cm H_2O develop, which forces lung fluid from the airways.

E. Further presentation of the fetus allows passive recoil and the first introduction of air into the lungs. The first breath requires an opening pressure of 60 to 80 cm H_2O to overcome the surface tension at the air-liquid interphase.

F. A greater flow of blood enters the pulmonary vasculature as a result of vasodilation from the increase in PaO_2 and partial removal of lung fluid. Additional lung fluid is removed by lymphatic drainage.

G. For a short period a small left-to-right shunt exists as pulmonary artery pressure decreases and the ductus arteriosus remains patent.

H. The ductus arteriosus constricts from the increased PaO_2. This diverts more blood into the pulmonary vasculature. The ductus arteriosus remains partially open after birth but closes within 3 weeks.

I. If the newborn develops hypoxia after birth, the ductus arteriosus remains open and continues to shunt blood. This reduces the pulmonary blood flow and further reduces the PaO_2.

J. The ductus arteriosus responds by constricting to increased PaO_2 with the administration of supplemental oxygen.

K. Prostaglandin synthetase inhibitors such as indomethacin (Indocin) are used to constrict the ductus arteriosus.

L. During fetal development prostaglandin E_1 and E_2, along with the decreased PaO_2, maintain the opening of the ductus arteriosus, thus ensuring that blood with a higher saturation will be routed to the brain.

M. After complete presentation of the fetus, the umbilical cord is clamped and cut, which discontinues umbilical circulation and placental function.

N. The umbilical arteries and vein constrict.

O. The ductus venosus closes within 3 to 7 days and forms the ligamentum venosum.

P. Blood flow now follows the normal circulatory pathway through the liver.

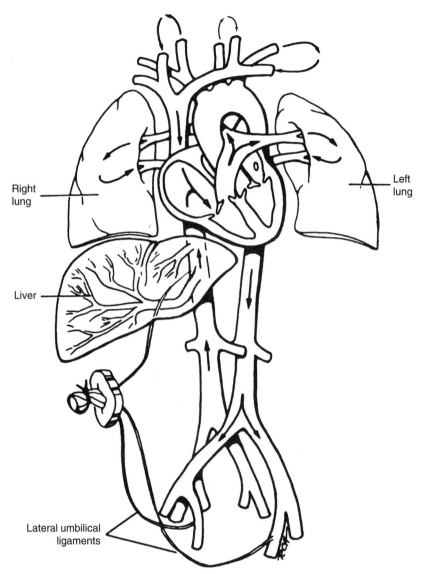

FIG. 25-3 Newborn circulation.

Q. Left atrial pressure increases as a result of greater return of blood from the pulmonary veins. This pressure change functionally closes the foramen ovale. Anatomic closure from proliferation of fibrous and endothelial tissue occurs within a few weeks of birth. Changes in pressures in the left and right sides of the heart can reopen the foramen ovale.

R. A number of factors contribute to the first and subsequent breaths of the newborn. These include:

1. Neuronal activity from the central and peripheral chemoreceptors
2. Hypoxia
3. Hypercapnia
4. Acidosis
5. Light and noise
6. Cooling of the body surface
7. Tactile stimulation

XI. **Laboratory Values of the Newborn**
  A. Normal blood gas values of a healthy term newborn are listed in Table 25-2.
  B. Blood pressure during the first 12 hours of life for various-sized newborns is listed in Table 25-3.
  C. Blood volume is 80 to 90 ml/kg of birth weight.
  D. Blood chemistry results on the first day of life are listed in Table 25-4.
  E. Glucose levels
    1. Normal newborn: 30 to 85 mg/dl
    2. Preterm: 20 to 75 mg/dl
  F. Fetal hemoglobin
    1. Newborn: 77% of total hemoglobin
    2. 6 months: 4.7% of total hemoglobin
    3. 8 to 11 months: 1% to 2% of total hemoglobin
    4. Newborn P_{50} is lower than that of the adult; however, it does approximate the adult P_{50} by 4 to 6 months.
  G. Pulmonary function values in the normal newborn
    1. Respiratory rate: 30 to 60 breaths/min, mean of 40 breaths/min
    2. Tidal volume: 5 to 7 ml/kg of birth weight
    3. Vital capacity: 45 ml/kg of birth weight
    4. FRC: 25 ml/kg of birth weight
    5. Total lung capacity: 60 ml/kg of birth weight
    6. Total lung compliance: 2.6 ml/cm H_2O
    7. Deadspace volume: 2.0 to 2.2 ml/kg of birth weight
    8. Oxygen consumption: 7 ml/kg/min
    9. Deadspace/tidal volume ratio: 0.30 to 0.35

TABLE 25-2

Normal Term Newborn Blood Gases

	Umbilical Vein	Umbilical Artery	Within 5 min after Birth	24 hr-7 days
pH	7.32	7.24	7.20-7.34	7.37
P_{CO_2} (mm Hg)	38	49	35-46	33-35
P_{O_2} (mm Hg)	27	16	49-73	72-73
HCO_3^- (mEq/L)	20	11	16-19	20
Sao_2 (%)	80	60	>80	>90

TABLE 25-3

Blood Pressure of Various-Sized Newborns During the First 72 Hours of Life

	1000-2000 g	2001-3000 g	>3000 g
Systolic	45-59	59-64	65-70
Diastolic	26-30	32-37	39-44
Mean	35-40	41-44	50-54

TABLE 25-4

Blood Chemistry Results of the Newborn

Na^+	147 mEq/L (126-159)
K^+	6.5 mEq/L (5.6-8.9)
Cl^-	104 mEq/L (98-114)
Total CO_2	20 mEq/L (18-22)

10. A-ado$_2$: 24 mm Hg
11. A-adco$_2$: 1 mm Hg

XII. **Comparative Neonatal Respiratory Anatomy (Table 25-5)**
  A. Neonatal head: Very large, approximately one fourth of total body length, in contrast to the adult head, which is approximately one eighth of body height.
  B. Neonatal tongue
    1. The neonatal tongue is large in relation to the size of the oral cavity.
    2. Tongue size is the primary factor forcing neonates to be obligate nose breathers. Normally only during crying will an infant actively ventilate through the mouth.
    3. Because of tongue size, nasal continuous positive airway pressure (CPAP) without use of endotracheal intubation can be easily accomplished.
    4. Positive end-expiratory pressure (PEEP) levels up to approximately 8 to 10 cm H$_2$O can be used; PEEP levels above this usually cause an oral leak.
  C. Neonatal neck: Short and normally is creased.
  D. Neonatal larynx
    1. The length is approximately 2 cm compared with 5 to 6 cm in the adult.
    2. The neonatal larynx is funnel shaped, whereas the diameter of the adult larynx is more or less constant.
    3. The narrowest portion of the neonate's upper airway is the cricoid cartilage; in the adult, the rima glottidis is the narrowest point. The normal anteroposterior diameter of the neonatal glottis is approximately 7 to 9 mm, and the anteroposterior diameter of the cricoid cartilage is approximately 4 to 6 mm.
      a. Endotracheal tube size must be based on the diameter of the cricoid cartilage.
      b. The larynx is much higher in relation to the oral pharynx, and the opening of the larynx is more in a straight line than in the adult.
      c. Therefore, an infant frequently extends the neck when in respiratory distress, whereas an adult will thrust the head forward.
  E. Neonatal epiglottis
    1. Stiffer, relatively longer, and U- or V-shaped compared with a flatter and much more flexible epiglottis in the adult.
    2. Located at the level of the first cervical vertebra; located in the adult at the fourth cervical vertebra.

TABLE 25-5

Comparison of Neonatal and Adult Respiratory Anatomy

Structure	Neonate	Adult
Head/body size ratio	1:4	1:8
Tongue size	Large	Proportional
Laryngeal shape	Funnel-shaped	Rectangular
Narrowest portion of upper airway	Cricoid cartilage	Rima glottidis
Shape and location of epiglottis	Long/C1	Flat, C4
Level of tracheal bifurcation	T3-4	T5
Compliance of trachea	Compliant, flexible	Noncompliant
Angle of mainstem bronchi	10 degrees right, 30 degrees left	30 degrees right, 50 degrees left
Anteroposterior transverse diameter ratio	1:1	1:2
Thoracic shape	Bullet-shaped	Conical
Resting position of diaphragm	Higher than adult	Normal
Location of heart	Center of chest, midline	Lower portion of chest, left of midline
Body surface area/body size ratio	9 times adult	Normal

  F. Neonatal trachea
1. The neonatal trachea is approximately 4 cm long compared with 10 to 13 cm in the adult.
2. The anteroposterior diameter is approximately 3.5 mm, and the lateral diameter is approximately 5 mm.
3. Normally the trachea is located to the right of the midline.
4. Bifurcation of the trachea is at the third or fourth thoracic vertebra in the neonate and at the fifth thoracic vertebra in the adult.
5. The angle of right and left mainstem bronchi widens with age. At birth the angles from the midline are 10 degrees for the right and 30 degrees for the left; in adulthood the angles are approximately 30 and 50 degrees, respectively.
6. Cartilage of the trachea may not be fully formed and often is more flexible than in the adult.
    a. As a result hyperextension of the head may cause compression of the trachea and result in airway obstruction.
    b. Thus during artificial ventilation without an endotracheal tube, the neonate's head should be maintained in a neutral position.

  G. Neonatal mainstem bronchi
1. Short and relatively wide compared with those of the adult.

  H. Neonatal thoracic cage
1. The neonatal thoracic cage has nearly equal anteroposterior and transverse diameters, and appearance generally is bullet shaped.
2. Range of movement is limited, and the ribs are basically fixed in a horizontal position.
3. The diaphragm is much higher than in the adult because of the relative size of the abdominal viscera. The diaphragm shows minimal movement during ventilation.
4. The heart is located in the center of the chest and slightly higher than in the adult. When external cardiac massage is performed, compression should be applied over the middle of the body of the sternum.

XIII. Body Surface Area
  A. The neonate's body surface area in relation to its size is about nine times that of the adult.
  B. Thus maintenance of body heat is a significant problem for the neonate and is even more so for the premature infant.
  C. The skin of the neonate plays a much greater role in water and heat balance than that of the adult. This is a result of the large body surface area-to-weight ratio, which allows significant evaporation of water. In the neonate, 80% of body weight is water; in the adult, only 55% to 60% is water.

BIBLIOGRAPHY

Aloan C: *Respiratory Care of the Newborn: A Clinical Manual.* Philadelphia, JB Lippincott, 1987.

Avery G, Fletcher MA, MacDonald MG: *Neonatalogy, Pathophysiology and Management of the Newborn,* ed 5. Philadelphia, Lippincott Williams & Wilkins, 1999.

Beard R, Nathaneilsz P: *Fetal Physiology and Medicine: The Basis of Perinatology.* Philadelphia, WB Saunders, 1976.

Eubanks D, Bone R: *Comprehensive Respiratory Care.* St. Louis, Mosby, 1985.

Gentz J, Persson B, Westin B, et al: *Perinatal Medicine. Praeger Special Studies.* New York, Praeger Publishers, 1984.

Koff P, Eitzman D, Neu J: *Neonatal and Pediatric Respiratory Care,* ed 2. St. Louis, Mosby, 1993.

Korones S: *High-Risk Newborn Infants,* ed 4. St. Louis, Mosby, 1986.

Kotecha S, Silverman M: Chronic respiratory complications of neonatal disorders. In Lansau LI, Taussing LM, eds. *Testbook of Pediatric Respiratory Medicine.* St. Louis, Mosby, 1999.

Lough M, Doershuk C, Stern R: *Pediatric Respiratory Care.* Chicago, Year Book Medical Publishers, 1985.

Murray J: *The Normal Lung,* ed 2. Philadelphia, WB Saunders, 1986.

Sinha SK, Donn SM: *Manual of Neonatal Respiratory Care.* Armonk, NY, Futura, 2000.

Thibeault D, Gregory G: *Neonatal Pulmonary Care.* New York, Appleton-Century-Crofts, 1986.

Walters DV, Strang LB, Geubelle F: *Physiology of the Fetal and Neonatal Lung.* Lancaster, UK, MTP Press, 1987.

Wilkins RL, Stoller J, Scanlon CL: *Egan's Fundamentals of Respiratory Care,* ed 8. St. Louis, Mosby, 2003.

Chapter 26

Assessment and Management of the Newborn

I.   **Clinical Evaluation of the Newborn (Table 26-1)**
   A. Respiratory rate
      1. Normal rate: 30 to 60 breaths/min
      2. Determined when newborn is not crying.
      3. Fluctuation of the respiratory rate is normal.
      4. Respirations are not necessarily regular.
      5. Preterm infants display more erratic respiratory patterns than term infants.
      6. Tachypnea: Respiratory rates >60 breaths/min
   B. Periodic breathing
      1. Defined as respiration interrupted by short periods of apnea.
      2. Apnea can last as long as 10 seconds.
      3. Not associated with other abnormalities such as cyanosis or bradycardia.
      4. Periodic breathing is common in preterm infants.
      5. Usually does not require treatment, but close monitoring is important.
      6. Little chest wall movement is observed.
      7. An accurate respiratory rate must be counted for 1 full minute.
   C. Apnea
      1. Often seen in premature newborns weighing <1500 g, with respiratory rates <30 breaths/min.
      2. May be accompanied by bradycardia, cyanosis, or both.
      3. Newborns may respond to gentle shaking or rubbing, or respirations may return spontaneously.
      4. Primary apnea may occur immediately after birth; usually associated with bradycardia.
      5. Newborns with primary apnea will resume breathing with stimulation.
      6. Newborns with secondary apnea do not resume breathing on their own.
      7. Heart rate, blood pressure, and PaO_2 level decrease during apnea.
      8. Assisted ventilation may be required.
   D. Heart rate
      1. Heart rate in the newborn is generally determined by auscultation.
      2. It can also be determined by tightly compressing the umbilicus with the index finger and thumb proximal to the abdomen.
      3. Heart rate is usually higher in preterm infants than in term infants.
      4. Normal heart rate fluctuates between 110 and 160 beats/min.
      5. Bradycardia is usually secondary to significant apnea.
      6. Palpation of the apical pulse is an important indicator of cardiac status.
      7. Palpation of the apical pulse is used to locate the position of the heart.
      8. Normally felt at the fifth intercostal space in the midclavicular line.
      9. Peripheral pulses are found by palpating the brachial, radial, and femoral arteries.

TABLE 26-1			
Normal Vital Signs of the Newborn			
	Range	Term	Preterm
Respiratory rate, breaths/min	30 to 60	Close to 30	Close to 60
Heart rate, beats/min	110 to 160	Close to 110	Close to 160
Blood pressure, mm Hg	50/35 to 65/40	65/40	50/35
Temperature, °C	36.5 to 37	36.5 to 37	36.5 to 37

    E. Blood pressure
       1. Usually measured with a Doppler apparatus and a blood pressure cuff.
       2. Blood pressure cuff must be of appropriate size for an infant to obtain an accurate pressure.
       3. A cuff ≤1-inch width is used, although larger infants may require a larger cuff.
       4. Blood pressure is usually obtained from the leg with the cuff around the thigh, although it may be obtained from the arm.
       5. Low birth weight infants' blood pressure averages 50/35 mm Hg.
       6. Infants with birth weights >2000 g have an average blood pressure of 60/35 mm Hg.
       7. Infants with birth weights >3000 g have an average blood pressure of 65/40 mm Hg.
       8. Peripheral pulses are an important and a quick indicator of blood pressure.
       9. Weak peripheral pulses commonly indicate a hypotensive state.
    F. Temperature
       1. An infant's temperature is usually taken in the axilla or obtained via a probe placed on the infant's skin.
       2. Infant temperature is a vital component in maintaining acid-base status.
       3. Maintaining thermoregulation is critical to transition after birth, more so in preterm infants than in term infants.
       4. Infant temperatures usually are maintained at 36.5° C to minimize oxygen consumption and prevent acidosis.

  II. **Signs of Respiratory Distress**
    A. Tachypnea
       1. In the newborn defined as a respiratory rate >60 breaths/min.
       2. Normal fluctuations in respiratory rate in the newborn can make initial assessment difficult.
       3. Close observation and accurate count of respiratory rate for a full minute are needed to quantify the need for further intervention.
    B. Cyanosis
       1. Cyanosis, or bluish discoloration, may be localized or generalized.
       2. Generalized cyanosis usually indicates a more serious problem.
       3. A well-lighted environment is essential for evaluation of cyanosis.
       4. Central cyanosis, involving the mucous membranes, indicates presence of excessive amounts of desaturated hemoglobin.
       5. Peripheral cyanosis (acrocyanosis) of the hands and feet is common in newborns and usually dissipates several hours after birth.
       6. Central cyanosis usually indicates an arterial oxygen tension of <40 mm Hg.
       7. Oxygen therapy usually required but may be contraindicated if a cardiac diagnosis is made.
       8. Cyanosis is more difficult to assess in nonwhite infants.
    C. Nasal flaring
       1. Involves flaring of the nostrils (alae nasi) during inspiration.
       2. Believed to be a sign of air hunger.
       3. The greater the negative intrathoracic pressure that must be generated to move air, the greater the degree of flaring.
       4. Nasal flaring may be barely discernible or obvious.

D. Expiratory grunting
   1. Is common in the infant with hyaline membrane disease.
   2. May also be seen with other disorders.
   3. Is presumed to be an attempt by the neonate to maintain positive pressure on expiration and prevent alveolar collapse.
   4. Grunting results from exhalation against a partially closed glottis.
   5. Is an obvious sound and usually heard without the aid of a stethoscope.
E. Retractions
   1. Retractions involve inward movement of the chest wall.
   2. May occur between the ribs (intercostal), above the clavicles (supraclavicular), or below the rib margins (subcostal).
   3. Retractions may also occur at the top (suprasternal) or the bottom (xiphoid) margins of the sternum.
   4. Retractions may occur in any age group but are more common in the newborn because of the high compliance of the chest wall.
   5. Retractions become more obvious and widespread as respiratory distress worsens.
   6. As the infant forcefully contracts the diaphragm in an attempt to move air, the abdomen protrudes.
   7. This increased negative pressure results in the entire anterior chest wall and sternum moving inward, producing a characteristic "seesaw" or paradoxical respiratory pattern.

III. **Apgar Score (Table 26-2)**
   A. Evaluation of the newborn begins as soon as the infant is delivered at 1- and 5-minute intervals.
   B. Standard care procedures are performed, including bulb suction of the upper airway, drying and warming of the infant, and cutting and clamping of the cord.
   C. A preliminary assessment is done during this time.
   D. The evaluation uses five factors.
      1. Heart rate
      2. Respiratory effort
      3. Muscle tone
      4. Reflex irritability
      5. Skin color
   E. The infant is given a score of 0, 1, or 2 in all categories.
   F. The 1-minute score is especially useful to identify the infant who needs immediate intervention.
      1. An Apgar score of ≤2 indicates a severely depressed infant who requires immediate resuscitation.
      2. Ventilatory assistance will be necessary.
      3. If the score is between 3 and 6 the infant may need some assistance, usually more vigorous stimulation and oxygen.
      4. Infants with scores of ≥7 are considered stable and require only routine care and close observation.

TABLE 26-2

Apgar Scoring System

Sign	Score		
	0	1	2
Heart rate (beats/min)	Absent	<100	>100
Respiratory effort	Absent	Weak, irregular	Good, crying
Muscle tone	Flaccid	Some flexion of extremities	Well flexed
Reflex irritability	No response	Grimace	Cough or sneeze
Color	Blue, pale	Body pink, extremities blue	Completely pink

5. The 5-minute score is useful to assess recovery from depression and the effectiveness of any previous interventions.
6. If the infant remains depressed at 5 minutes, with a score of ≤6, concern regarding cardiopulmonary status should be exercised, and the infant should be placed under special care.
7. These infants are at high risk for further postpartum complications:
   a. Respiratory distress
   b. Aspiration syndromes
   c. Hypoglycemia
   d. Will usually need intravenous fluids
   e. Will usually need oxygen therapy
   f. Ventilatory assistance may also be required.
8. An Apgar score at 5 minutes of ≤7 will require another Apgar assessment at 10 minutes.

IV. **Bag and Mask Resuscitation**
   A. The appropriate size mask and anesthesia (flow-inflating) bag should be used.
   B. The jaw is moved upward and away from the neck by placing a towel under the shoulders (if time allows).
   C. Ensure proper seal with mask over the infant's nose and mouth.
   D. An airtight seal between the rim of the mask and the face is essential to achieve effective positive-pressure ventilation of the lungs.
   E. An orogastric tube may be needed to aspirate air from the stomach.
   F. Effective ventilation is present when:
      1. Breath sounds are heard bilaterally.
      2. Heart rate increases to >100 beats/min.
      3. There is adequate chest rise with each manual breath.
      4. Color improves.
      5. Spontaneous movement and flexion of extremities occur.
   G. If no improvement after 30 seconds:
      1. Reposition the head, neck, and mask.
      2. Reestablish effective ventilation.
   H. If inadequate response to these maneuvers, prepare to intubate.

V. **Intubation**
   A. Intubation should be performed when:
      1. The heart rate is <100 beats/min.
      2. The Apgar score is <2.
      3. The birth weight is low.
      4. The infant is unresponsive to bag and mask ventilation.
      5. Transport of an unstable newborn is required.
   B. Estimation of endotracheal tube (ETT) sizes
      1. Weight and tube size indicated.
         a. <1000 g = 2.5-mm ETT
         b. 1000 to 2000 g = 3.0-mm ETT
         c. 2000 to 3000 g = 3.5-mm ETT
         d. 3000 to 4000 g = 4.0-mm ETT
      2. Neonatal airways do not contain cuffs.
      3. Proper placement of ETTs can be assessed by:
         a. Increases in heart rate >100 beats/min
         b. Bilateral breath sounds
         c. Adequate chest wall movement with manual breaths
         d. Confirmation with chest radiography
      4. ETTs should be securely taped after intubation.
      5. Appropriate ventilation, F_IO_2, and humidification should be provided.

VI. **Procedure for Intubation**
  A. Obtain proper equipment
    1. Resuscitation bag and mask with pressure manometer
    2. Suction catheter(s), no. 5 or 6 French
    3. Stylet
    4. Properly sized ETTs
    5. Tape
    6. Stethoscope
    7. Towel
  B. After obtaining equipment, suction the upper airway.
  C. Preoxygenate with resuscitation bag to maintain an oxygen saturation of 100%.
  D. Position infant properly with towel if necessary under the shoulders.
  E. It is important to properly align infant so that the pharynx and trachea are in the midline position.
  F. Insert appropriately sized blade, and visualize vocal cords.
  G. Insert appropriately sized ETT through vocal cords into trachea.
  H. After placement ventilate with pressures of 20 to 25 cm H_2O.
  I. Evaluate position of tube by visualizing chest wall movement and auscultating with a stethoscope.
  J. Note centimeter mark at upper lip, and secure tube with proper tape.
  K. Obtain a chest radiograph to confirm correct ETT position.
  L. If intubation is unsuccessful after 30 seconds and heart rate decreases to <100 beats/min, reestablish oxygenation with bag/mask ventilation.
  M. If no clinical improvement occurs after intubation:
    1. Check ETT for proper placement.
    2. Use of disposable end-tidal CO_2 detector to confirm tracheal or esophageal intubation.
    3. Check for possible right mainstem intubation.
    4. Withdraw ETT 1 cm, if indicated.
    5. Increase ventilatory rate.
    6. Increase ventilating pressure.
    7. Suction ETT to remove secretions.

VII. **Suctioning**
  A. Perform suctioning as needed according to breath sounds, O_2 saturation, and clinical presentation of infant.
  B. Use the appropriate size catheter.
  C. Preoxygenate infant with 100% oxygen if situation allows.
  D. Saline may be instilled into the ETT before suctioning to help thin secretions, but this should not be routine for suctioning.
  E. Suction pressure should not exceed 100 mm Hg.
  F. Remove thick secretions by repeated saline instillations.
  G. Monitor heart rate closely while suctioning, and observe for any vagal or bradycardic effects of procedure.
  H. Newer in-line suction catheters used to minimize carinal irritation and prevent vagal responses.
  I. Catheters are measured and the centimeter mark noted so that exact catheter placement is achieved each time the infant is suctioned.
  J. Apply suction only during withdrawal of catheter and for no longer than 10 seconds.

VIII. **Cardiopulmonary Resuscitation (Modified from the American Heart Association: Neonatal Resuscitation Guidelines, 2000)**
  A. Initiate chest compressions when:
    1. The heart rate remains <60 beats/min despite 30 seconds of effective positive-pressure ventilation.
    2. There is no detectable heart rate.

B. Two techniques are used for cardiac compression on any newborn.
   1. The first technique involves placing the thumbs of both hands over the lower one third of the infant's sternum while the other fingers are wrapped around the back to provide stability and support.
   2. The two-finger technique uses the index and middle fingers to compress the lower one third of the sternum while the other hand is used to support the back.
   3. The thumb technique is usually preferred.
   4. To ensure proper rate of chest compressions and ventilation, the compressor repeats "one and two and three and breathe and...."
   5. During chest compressions, the breathing rate is 30 breaths/min, and the compression rate is 90 compressions/min.
   6. This equals 120 "events" per minute; one cycle of three compressions and one breath takes 2 seconds.
C. During chest compressions ensure that:
   1. Chest movement is adequate during ventilation.
   2. 100% oxygen is being used.
   3. Compression depth is one third the diameter of the chest.
   4. Thumbs or fingers remain in contact with the chest at all times.
   5. Duration of the downward stroke of the compression is shorter than the duration of the release.
   6. Chest compressions and ventilation are well coordinated.
D. After 30 seconds of chest compressions and ventilation, check the heart rate. If the heart rate is:
   1. Greater than 60 beats/min, discontinue compressions and continue ventilation at 40 to 60 breaths/min.
   2. Greater than 100 beats/min, discontinue compressions, and gradually discontinue ventilation if the newborn is breathing spontaneously.
   3. Less than 60 beats/min, intubate the newborn, if not already done. This provides a more reliable method of continuing ventilation and a route for epinephrine administration.
E. Medications used during cardiopulmonary resuscitation (CPR) (Table 26-3)
   1. Best treatment for brief periods of bradycardia: Ventilation and 100% oxygen.
   2. Epinephrine: potent α- and β-receptor stimulation
      a. Increases perfusion pressure, coronary blood flow, and oxygen delivery to the heart.
      b. Indicated when the heart rate remains <60 beats/min, despite 30 seconds of assisted ventilation and another 30 seconds of coordinated chest compressions and ventilations.
      c. Improves cardiac contractility and increases heart rate.
      d. Given when the heart rate is 0 beats/min.
      e. Dosage is 0.1 to 0.3 ml/kg of a 1:10,000 solution in 1-ml syringe.

TABLE 26-3

Common Drugs Used During CPR

Drug	Indication	Dose	Route of Administration
Epinephrine	Low heart rate (<60 beats/min) or no heart rate	0.1 to 0.3 ml/kg of a 1:10,000 solution in 1 ml	Endotracheal tube or intravenous
Naloxone hydrochloride (Narcan)	Acute maternal narcotic depression	0.1 ml/kg of a 1.0 mg/ml solution in a 1 ml volume	Endotracheal tube or intravenous
Saline as volume expander	Evidence of blood or fluid loss	10 ml/kg given slowly over 5-10 min	Intravenous
Sodium bicarbonate (NaHCO₃)	Metabolic acidosis	2 mEq/kg of a 4.2% solution	Intravenous

CPR, Cardiopulmonary resuscitation.

        f. Given rapidly via ETT or intravenously and can be repeated every 5 minutes until an acceptable heart rate is achieved.

    3. Naloxone hydrochloride (Narcan)

        a. Indicated for infants with severe respiratory depression after positive-pressure ventilation has restored a normal heart rate and color.

        b. Mother with a history of narcotic administration within the past 4 hours.

        c. Not indicated for an infant of a mother who is suspected of being addicted to narcotics or is on methadone therapy. If given, it may result in the newborn developing acute severe seizure activity.

        d. Other drugs such as magnesium sulfate or nonnarcotic analgesics or general anesthetics will not respond to naloxone.

        e. Dosage is 0.1 ml/kg of a 1.0-mg/ml solution in a 1-ml syringe.

        f. May be administered via the ETT, but intravenous administration is preferred.

    4. Sodium bicarbonate

        a. Administered for suspected or documented metabolic acidosis.

        b. Not to be given unless the lungs are being adequately ventilated.

        c. Sodium bicarbonate is caustic and should not be given through an ETT.

        d. Recommended dosage: 2 mEq/kg (4 ml/kg of 4.2% solution)

        e. Preferred route of administration is umbilical vein, from which there is a good blood return.

    5. Volume expanders

        a. Indicated for an infant not responding to resuscitation.

        b. Evidence of blood loss (e.g., pale color, weak pulses, persistently high or low heart rate, no improvement in circulatory status despite resuscitation efforts).

        c. Normal saline volume expander of choice.

        d. Blood, albumin, or Ringer's lactate may also be used.

        e. Dosage is 10 ml/kg given slowly over 5 to 10 minutes.

    6. Drugs that can be given via an ETT are atropine, lidocaine, epinephrine, and naloxone (Narcan).

IX. Other Newborn Assessment Scales

  A. Dubowitz scoring method

    1. The Dubowitz scoring method determines gestational age when used within the first 5 days of birth.

    2. It is accurate within 2 weeks of the newborn's gestational age.

    3. Each of the following categories is assessed on a graded scale. The higher the score assigned, the greater the gestational age of the newborn (Table 26-4).

    4. Assessment is done bilaterally.

        a. External developmental signs (Table 26-5)

           (1) Edema: Finger pressure on the dorsum of the foot is done for a few seconds. Assessment compares no edema with pitting edema (score, 0 to 2).

           (2) Skin texture: Skin is assessed to determine its texture. A transparent to leathery, cracked appearance is graded (score, 0 to 4).

           (3) Skin color: Skin color is assessed during quiet time of the newborn. A pale to dark red appearance over the ears, lips, palms, and soles of the feet is used to determine scores (score, 0 to 3).

           (4) Skin opacity: Skin of the abdominal trunk is assessed. More prominent skin veins are given a lower score, and no skin veins seen are given a higher score (score, 0 to 4).

           (5) Lanugo: The amount of fine hair over the back of the newborn. Premature infants have large amounts of hair, whereas term and postterm infants have no hair. Score decreases with greater amounts of hair (score, 0 to 4).

           (6) Plantar creases: Assessment is made on the soles of the feet. No creases are given a lower score, and deep creases are given a higher score (score, 0 to 4).

           (7) Nipple formation: No nipple areola is given a low score, and areola raised and stippled is given a higher score (score, 0 to 3).

TABLE **26-4**

Dubowitz Scoring System

Score	Gestation (wk)
0-9	26
10-12	27
13-16	28
17-20	29
21-24	30
25-27	31
28-31	32
32-35	33
36-39	34
40-43	35
44-46	36
47-50	37
51-54	38
55-58	39
59-62	40
63-65	41
66-69	42

TABLE **26-5**

External Developmental Signs of the Dubowitz Scoring System

Signs	Score	Immature	Mature
Edema	0-2	None (0)	Pitting edema (2)
Skin texture	0-4	Transparent (0)	Leathery, cracked (4)
Skin color	0-4	Pale (0)	Dark red (3)
Skin opacity	0-4	Prominent skin veins (0)	No observable skin veins (4)
Lanugo	0-4	Large amounts of back hair (0)	None (4)
Plantar creases	0-4	No crease (0)	Deep crease (4)
Nipple formation	0-3	No areola (0)	Areola raised and stippled (3)
Breast size	0-3	No breast tissue (0)	>1 cm tissue (3)
Ear form	0-3	Pinna flat and shapeless (0)	Well-defined in-curving upper pinna (3)
Ear firmness	0-3	Soft, easily folded (0)	Firm with cartilage to edge (3)
Genitals male	0-2	Undescended or minimally descended testes (0)	Rugae or wrinkles in scrotal sac (3)
Genitals female	0-2	Widely separated labia majora with protruding labia minora (0)	Labia minora are covered by labia majora (2)

Number in parentheses indicates score.
From Dubowitz LMS, Dubowitz V, Goldberg C: Clinical assessment of gestational age in the newborn infant. *J Pediatr* 77:1-10, 1979.

(8)   Breast size: Assessment is done by palpating the nipple area and determining the approximate area of breast tissue. Measurements range from no breast tissue (low score) to >1 cm, which is given a higher score (score, 0 to 3).

(9)   Ear form: Increase in scoring occurs as the form of the ear develops from the pinna being flat and shapeless to a well-defined, in-curving upper pinna (score, 0 to 3).

(10)   Ear firmness: Scores increase as the ear develops from a soft, easily folded ear to a firm ear with cartilage to the edge (score, 0 to 3).

(11)   Genitals:

(a)   Boys: Scores increase as the undescended testes develop into descended testes. Rugae, or wrinkles, in the scrotal sac are seen in the mature newborn.

(b) Girls (with hips half abducted): Scores increase as the widely separated labia majora with protruded labia minora develops to where the labia minora is covered by the labia majora (score, 0 to 2).

b. Neuromuscular/neurologic signs (Figure 26-1)

(1) Posture: Increased scores are assigned when greater flexion of the newborn is observed without touching.

(2) Square window: Scores are assessed by applying enough pressure to the hand to flex it to the forearm. Scores increase as the angle between the hypothenar eminence and forearm decreases from 90 to 0 degrees.

(3) Ankle dorsiflexion: The newborn's foot is flexed against the anterior aspect of the leg. Scores increase as this angle decreases from 90 to 0 degrees.

c. Arm recoil: The newborn's arms are flexed for a few seconds and then extended fully. Recoil is then observed by releasing the hands. Scores increase as the angle of the antecubital space reduces from 180 degrees to <90 degrees.

d. Leg recoil: This assessment is done the same way as the arm recoil. The score increases as the angle between the knees and the hips decreases from 180 degrees to <90 degrees.

e. Popliteal angle: The thigh is held in the high chest position. The leg is extended with the other hand. The score increases as the angle behind the knee decreases from 180 to <90 degrees.

f. Heel to ear: The newborn's feet are drawn as close to the ears as possible. After releasing the feet, the score is then determined by assessing the popliteal angle and whether the feet can touch the ears.

g. Scarf sign: The newborn's hand is extended to the opposite shoulder. Scores increase if the elbow of the extended hand does not go past the middle of the chest.

h. Head lag: The newborn is pulled upward by both arms from a supine position. Scores increase if the newborn is able to hold the head forward. The newborn's head should be supported during this assessment.

i. Ventral suspension: The newborn, in a prone position, is suspended over one hand. The back, legs, arms, and neck are observed for extension. Scores increase as a curved back and neck with extended limp legs progress into a hyperextended back with good flexion of the arms and legs.

j. Scores indicate weeks of gestation.

B. Ballard score (Figure 26-2)

1. The Ballard score includes six neuromuscular/neurologic and six physical signs.

a. Neuromuscular signs: Posture, square window, arm recoil, popliteal angle, scarf sign, and heel to ear.

b. Physical signs: Skin, lanugo, plantar creases, breast, ears, and genitals.

c. It assesses the most useful items from the Dubowitz scoring system.

d. Gestational age is assessable from 26 to 44 weeks.

C. Silverman scoring of acute respiratory distress of the neonate (Figure 26-3)

1. Scores are based on a scale of 0 to 10.

a. Scores of 0 to 3: No respiratory distress to mild respiratory distress

b. Scores of 4 to 6: Moderate respiratory distress

c. Scores of 7 to 10: Severe respiratory distress

2. Scoring is performed in five areas and ranges from 0 to 2.

a. Upper chest movement

(1) Synchronized movement: 0

(2) Lag of upper chest on inspiration: 1

(3) Seesaw movement of upper chest: 2

b. Lower chest movement

(1) No retractions: 0

(2) Retractions just visible: 1

(3) Marked retractions: 2

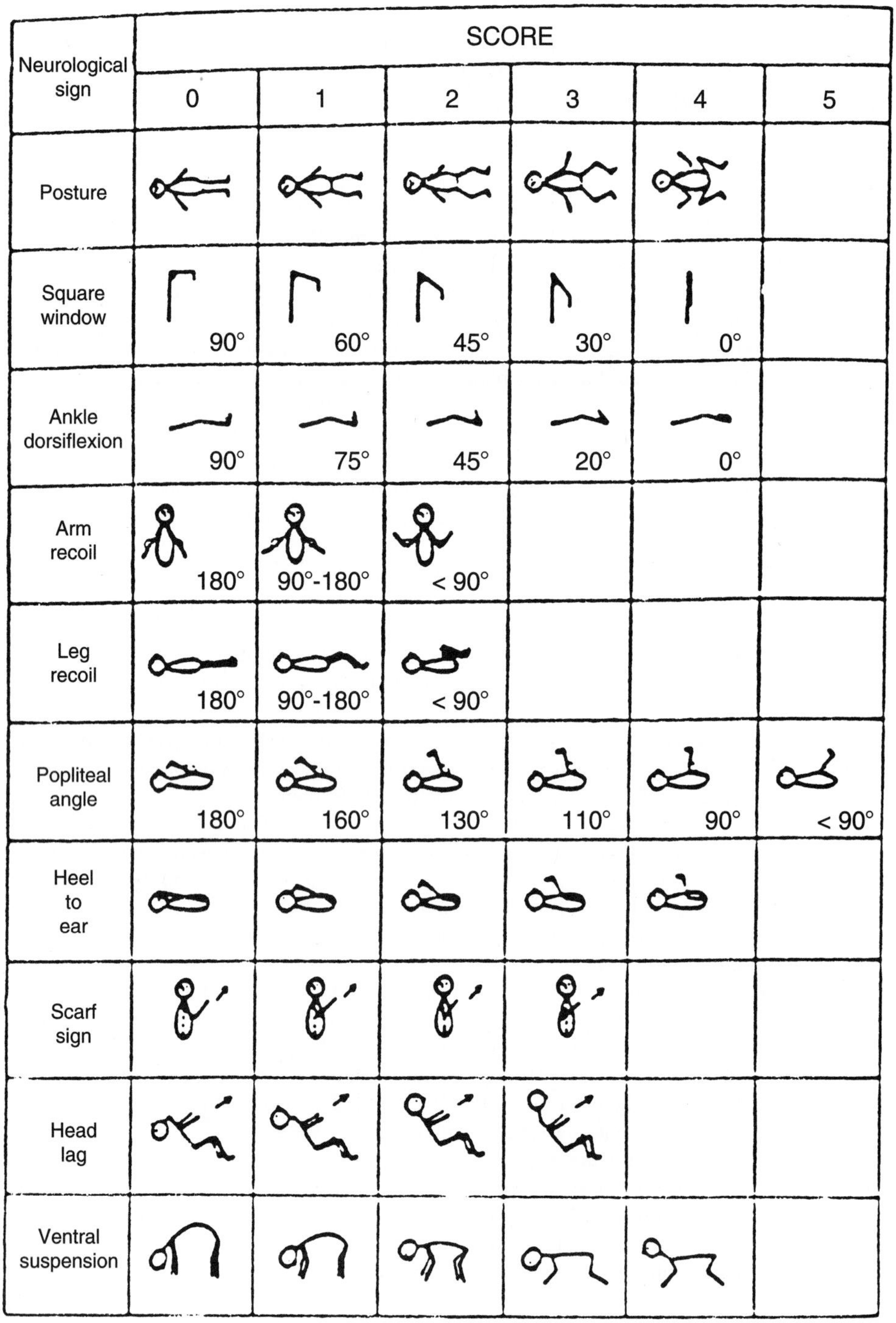

Neurological sign	SCORE					
	0	1	2	3	4	5
Posture						
Square window	90°	60°	45°	30°	0°	
Ankle dorsiflexion	90°	75°	45°	20°	0°	
Arm recoil	180°	90°-180°	< 90°			
Leg recoil	180°	90°-180°	< 90°			
Popliteal angle	180°	160°	130°	110°	90°	< 90°
Heel to ear						
Scarf sign						
Head lag						
Ventral suspension						

FIG. 26-1 Neuromuscular/neurologic signs of the Dubowitz scoring method.

Neuromuscular maturity

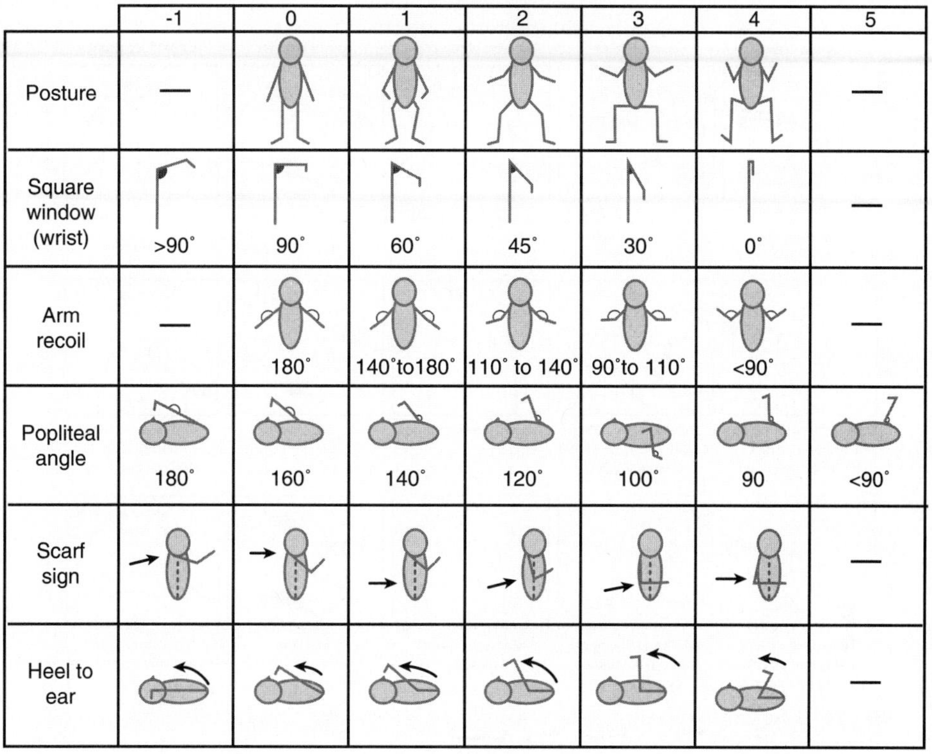

	-1	0	1	2	3	4	5
Posture	—						—
Square window (wrist)	>90°	90°	60°	45°	30°	0°	
Arm recoil	—	180°	140° to 180°	110° to 140°	90° to 110°	<90°	—
Popliteal angle	180°	160°	140°	120°	100°	90	<90°
Scarf sign							—
Heel to ear							—

Physical maturity

	-1	0	1	2	3	4	5
Skin	Sticky, friable, transparent	Gelatinous, red, translucent	Superficial peeling or rash; few visible vessels	Superficial peeling or rash; few visible vessels	Cracking; pale ares; rare visible vessels	Parchment-like; deep cracking; no visible vessels	Leathery, cracked, wrinkled
Lanugo	None	Sparse	Abundant	Thinning	Bald areas	Mostly bald	——
Plantar surface	Heel-toe 40 to 50 mm: -1; <40mm: -2	> 50 mm; no crease	Faint, red marks	Anterior transverse crease only	Creases over anterior two-thirds	Creases over entire sole	——
Breast	Imperceptible	Barely perceptible	Flat areola; no bud	Stippled areola; 1- to 2-mm bud	Raised areola; 3- to 4-mm bud	Full areola; 5- to 10-mm bud	——
Eye and ear	Lids fused, loosely: -1; tightly: -2	Lids open; pinna flat, stays folded	Slightly curved pinna; soft, slow recoil	Well curved pinna; soft but ready recoil	Formed and firm; instant recoil	Thick cartilage; ear stiff	——
Genitalia, male	Scrotum flat, smooth	Scrotum empty; faint rugae	Testes in upper canal; rare rugae	Testes descending; few rugae	Testes down; good rugae	Testes pendulous; deep rugae	——
Genitalia, female	Clitoris prominent; labia flat	Prominent clitoris; small labia minora	Prominent clitoris; enlarging minora	Major and minora equally prominent	Majora large; minora small	Majora cover clitoris and minora	——

Maturity rating

Score	−10	−5	0	5	10	15	20	25	30	35	40	45	50
Weeks	20	22	24	26	28	30	32	34	36	38	40	42	44

FIG. 26-2 The Ballard gestational age assessment system.

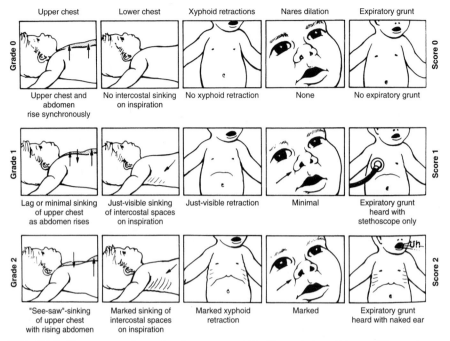

FIG. 26-3 Silverman scoring system to assess and identify respiratory distress of the newborn.

    c. Xiphoid retractions
        (1) No retractions: 0
        (2) Retractions just visible: 1
        (3) Marked retractions: 2
    d. Dilation of nares
        (1) None: 0
        (2) Minimal dilation: 1
        (3) Marked dilation: 2
    e. Expiratory grunt
        (1) None: 0
        (2) Heard only with stethoscope: 1
        (3) Heard with naked ear: 2

X. Oxygen Administration Equipment
    A. Oxyhood
      1. Most common form of short-term oxygen delivery to the newborn.
      2. Oxyhoods are clear plastic boxes or cylinders that usually surround the infant's head and have an opening for the infant's neck.
      3. For a specific F_IO_2 an oxyhood is preferred over other oxygen-delivery devices.
      4. The device is also used to provide warm humidity.
      5. It can be placed inside an isolette or on a warming table.
      6. A minimum liter flow of 8 to 10 L/min is needed to adequately prevent rebreathing of exhaled carbon dioxide.
      7. An F_IO_2 between 0.21 and 1.0 can be achieved with this device by delivering oxygen/air flow by an oxygen blender.
    B. Nasal cannula
      1. Becoming more popular for use with smaller infants.
      2. Ideal for use in infants requiring long-term oxygen therapy.
      3. Also used for infants who have been weaned and extubated from mechanical ventilation and do not tolerate nasal continuous positive airway pressure (CPAP).

   4. Should be used with flowmeters calibrated in small increments, such as quarters or tenths of a liter per minute.
   5. Flow rates used in infants and children with nasal cannulas range from 0.10 to 4.0 L/min.
   6. Easy to deliver moderate F_IO_2 with this device.
   7. Exact F_IO_2 is uncertain.
   8. Attention should be paid to oxygen saturation levels as monitored by pulse oximetry and flow titrated accordingly to achieve desired saturation.
C. Masks
   1. Simple small, tight-fitting O_2 masks can be used for short-term O_2 therapy.
   2. Difficult to apply to the infant's face.
   3. Poorly tolerated by an infant who becomes agitated with the device strapped to the head.
   4. Often used to perform hyperoxia tests.
   5. Must provide adequate flow (minimum, 6 L/min) to prevent retention of carbon dioxide.
D. Flow-inflating resuscitation bags
   1. A flow-inflating bag with mask attached is an excellent and effective way to deliver short-term, high F_IO_2 levels to an infant.
   2. Often used in the operating room and delivery room to provide a quick and consistent oxygen source for the postoperative or newborn infant.
   3. A flow of 8 to 10 L/min should be maintained for proper effect.
   4. Can also be used as a mask CPAP device if infant develops respiratory distress and does not respond to conventional O_2 therapy.
E. Mist tents
   1. These devices are used for infants and children who require a cool environment and supplemental oxygen.
   2. An F_IO_2 of 0.30 to 0.50 can be achieved.
   3. Mist is provided by a baffle system that is powered by either air or oxygen at 12 to 15 L/min.
   4. Difficult to maintain consistent F_IO_2 level because of large surface area and difficulty sealing plastic canopy around patient.
   5. The tent surrounds the bed and is tucked in under the mattress to maintain temperature and F_IO_2.
   6. Mist tents have fallen out of favor and use because of poor tolerance by patients and difficulty maintaining the unit by hospital staff.

XI. **Equipment for Thermal Control**
A. Isolette
   1. Used to maintain proper temperature of the infant's environment and to administer humidity.
   2. No longer used as a vehicle for the delivery of oxygen therapy.
   3. The temperature is monitored and maintained with a skin probe attached to the newborn (servocontrol).
   4. Isolettes are now double walled and monitor the inner surface of the isolette and the patient's skin. If either of these temperatures decreases below a preset value, the unit responds by increasing heat production.
   5. Access to the newborn is provided by hand holes on the side of the hood or the hood can be lifted for complete exposure.
   6. Humidification is provided by a system that blows air over standing water. Reduced relative humidity and infection are potential problems with this device.
B. Radiant warmers
   1. Radiant warmers use an open-bed system that provides infrared heat from an overhead source.
   2. The device allows procedures to be performed on the newborn and greater accessibility during treatment.

3. The wavelength of the infrared light does not harm the newborn's eyes.
4. A probe attached to the skin determines the amount of infrared heat. The probe has a reflective patch to prevent inappropriate temperature adjustments.
5. Heat loss can occur from evaporation and convection (personnel passing by or drafts created by vents or opening or closing of doors).
6. Side shields can be placed around the bed to prevent convection and insensible water loss; plastic wrap has also been used to shield the infant and maintain proper temperature.

XII. **Blood Gas Monitoring**
   A. Obtaining an arterial blood gas (ABG)
     1. Possible sites
       a. Radial artery
       b. Brachial, posterior tibial, and temporal arteries
       c. Capillary heal stick
       d. Femoral artery not used
     2. Radial artery site of choice
     3. Normal ABG values (1 to 7 days) after birth
       a. pH: 7.35 to 7.40
       b. Pco_2: 30 to 35 mm Hg
       c. Po_2: 60 to 80 mm Hg
       d. HCO_3^-: 16 to 20 mEq/L
       e. Percentage of oxyhemoglobin ($HbO_2\%$): >90%
     4. Arterial lines
       a. Placement of an indwelling catheter into a peripheral artery provides undisturbed access for frequent blood gas sampling.
       b. Catheter also is used for continuous real-time blood pressure monitoring.
       c. Provides clinician with unlimited access to numerous blood gas samples.
       d. Used mostly in the critically ill and unstable mechanically ventilated patient.
       e. Radial and femoral arteries are sites of choice for indwelling catheter.
       f. Umbilical artery often is used for catheter placement in the newborn.
       g. An umbilical artery line is inserted through the umbilicus into one of the two umbilical arteries.
       h. A chest radiograph must be obtained after insertion to confirm proper placement in vessel.
   B. Complications of ABGs
     1. Infection
     2. Hematoma
     3. Nerve damage
   C. Obtaining capillary blood gases (CBGs)
     1. Possible sites: heel or finger
       a. Extrinsic factors affecting results:
         (1) Improper technique
           (a) Application of pressure to puncture site
           (b) Inadequate warming of site (3 to 5 minutes for warming)
         (2) Excessive crying before puncture
       b. Intrinsic factors affecting results:
         (1) Poor peripheral perfusion
         (2) Prematurity
         (3) Hypothermia
         (4) Hyperthermia
   D. Comparison of CBG and ABG values
     1. CBG Po_2 values are approximately 10 to 15 mm Hg less than actual ABG values. The difference between CBG and ABG Po_2 values becomes greater as the Po_2 values increase.

2. The P_{CO_2} values are consistent in most circumstances but may differ up to 3 mm Hg (CBG values greater than ABG values).
3. The CBG pH values tend to be consistent with the ABG pH values but may be 0.01 to 0.02 pH unit lower.

E. Blood gas abnormalities of the newborn
   1. Respiratory acidosis
      a. Ventilatory problem
      b. Chronic respiratory acidosis is seen with bronchopulmonary dysplasia (BPD).
   2. Respiratory alkalosis
      a. Mechanical hyperventilation
      b. Persistent fetal circulation
      c. Crying during blood gas puncture
   3. Metabolic acidosis
      a. Metabolic acidosis normally is a result of hypoxemia (lactic acidosis).
      b. It is the most common acid-base problem of newborns.
      c. Other causes include:
         (1) Dietary acid
         (2) Keto acids
         (3) Diarrhea
         (4) Renal failure
      d. These acids are excreted from the kidneys, not the lungs (nonvolatile acids).
      e. Premature newborns have immature phosphate and ammonia buffer systems and cannot handle the excessive buildup of metabolic acids.
      f. Newborns may develop persistent metabolic acidosis that:
         (1) Lasts longer than 3 days
         (2) Has a base excess −7 to −15 mEq/L
         (3) Is unrelated to asphyxia
         (4) Is a dietary acid buildup
      g. Signs include:
         (1) Poor weight gain
         (2) Weight loss or adequate caloric intake
         (3) Watery stools
         (4) Lethargy in older infants
         (5) Apnea in premature infants
         (6) Gray pallor (not from anemia or hypoxia)
      h. Respiratory management includes oxygenation and ventilation if needed.
      i. Management of prolonged metabolic acidosis (not responsive to oxygenation) includes:
         (1) Giving sodium bicarbonate when the pH is <7.20 and the base deficit is >−7 mEq/L
         (2) Slowly infusing 4 ml of sodium bicarbonate/kg of a 0.5 mEq/L solution
   4. Metabolic alkalosis
      a. Metabolic alkalosis is commonly a result of:
         (1) Vomiting
         (2) Nasogastric tube
         (3) Hypokalemia
         (4) Hypochloremia
         (5) Diuretic therapy

BIBLIOGRAPHY

Aloan C: *Respiratory Care of the Newborn and Child,* ed 2. Philadelphia, JB Lippincott, 1997.
American Heart Association: *Neonatal Resuscitation.* Dallas, American Heart Association, 2000.
American Heart Association: *Pediatric Advanced Life Support.* Dallas, American Heart Association, 2000.

Ballard JL, Khoury JC, Wedig K, Wang L, Eilers-Walsman BL: New Ballard Score, expanded to include extremely premature infants. *J Pediatr* 119:417-423, 1991.

Ballard JL, Novak KK, Driver M: A simplified score for assessment of fetal maturation of newly born infants. *J Pediatr* 95:769-774, 1979.

Courtney SE: Capillary blood gases in the neonate. *Am J Dis Child* 144:168-174, 1990.

Deming DD: Respiratory assessment of neonatal and pediatric patients. In Wilkins RL, Krider SJ, Sheldon RL (eds): *Clinical Assessment in Respiratory Care,* ed 3. St. Louis, Mosby, 1995.

Dubowitz LMS, Dubowitz V, Goldberg C: Clinical assessment of gestational age in the newborn infant. *J Pediatr* 77:1-10, 1970.

Fletcher MA: Physical assessment and classification. In Avery GB, Fletcher MA, MacDonald MG (eds): *Neonatology: Pathophysiology and Management of the Newborn,* ed 4. Philadelphia, JB Lippincott, 1994.

Nugent J: *Acute Respiratory Care of the Neonate.* Durham, NC, Burroughs Wellcome, 1991.

Wilkins RL, Stoller JL, Scanlon CR. *Egan's Fundamentals of Respiratory Care,* ed 8. St. Louis, Mosby, 2003.

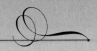
Respiratory Disorders of the Newborn

I. **Persistent Pulmonary Hypertension in the Newborn (PPHN)**
    A. Etiology
        1. Pulmonary hypertension impairs the transition from fetal to neonatal circulation.
        2. Right-to-left shunting occurs when the ductus arteriosus and foramen ovale remain open or reopen after closure.
            a. Idiopathic PPHN results from abnormal development of the pulmonary vascular system.
            b. PPHN can be the result of a pathophysiologic process, such as respiratory distress syndrome or meconium aspiration syndrome.
        3. Causative factors
            a. Hypoxia, acidosis, and asphyxia
            b. Infection (e.g., pneumonia or sepsis)
            c. Congenital heart defects
    B. Pathophysiology (Figure 27-1)
        1. Pulmonary hypertension and high pulmonary vascular resistance (PVR) impede blood flow to the lungs.
        2. The pulmonary arterioles react to the resulting hypoxemia, hypercapnia, and acidemia with vasoconstriction, further impeding pulmonary blood flow.
        3. High PVR results in right heart pressures greater than systemic blood pressure, causing right-to-left shunting through the ductus arteriosus and foramen ovale.
        4. This combination of responses leads to a cyclic pattern of decreased cardiac output, decreased pulmonary blood flow, and vasoconstriction.
    C. Clinical presentation
        1. Near-term, term, and postterm neonates
        2. Majority present within the first 72 hours after birth
        3. Refractory hypoxemia
        4. Signs and symptoms of respiratory distress to varying degrees
            a. Tachypnea
            b. Retractions
            c. Cyanosis
            d. Crying and stress are often associated with low levels of PPHN.
            e. Arterial blood gases show hypoxemia, acidosis, and hypercapnia.
    D. Diagnostic tests for PPHN
        1. Contrast or "bubble" echocardiography
            a. Demonstrates the presence of right-to-left shunt through the foramen or ductus.
            b. Used to evaluate cardiac structures and rule out cyanotic cardiac anomalies.

473

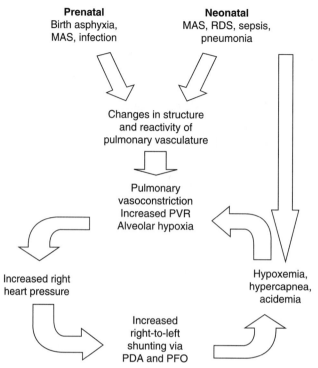

FIG. 27-1 The pathophysiology of persistent pulmonary hypertension in the newborn (PPHN) begins with the cardiopulmonary response to a prenatal or neonatal insult and results in a cyclic pattern of decreased pulmonary blood flow, right-to-left shunting, and worsening gas exchange.

2. Hyperoxia test
    a. Place infant in 100% oxygen for 5 to 10 minutes and obtain arterial blood gas.
    b. If PaO_2 does not increase, right-to-left shunting is present.
    c. Does not differentiate between PPHN and congenital heart disease.
3. Comparison of preductal and postductal arterial PaO_2
    a. Obtain simultaneous arterial blood gases from a preductal artery (right radial or brachial) and postductal artery (left radial or umbilical).
    b. A difference of >15 mm Hg in preductal and postductal PaO_2 indicates ductal shunting.
    c. A difference of <15 mm Hg indicates no ductal shunting but does not rule out PPHN or congenital heart disease.
    d. Pulse oximetry sensors can be placed at preductal and postductal sites to assess the presence of shunting and allow continuous monitoring for recurrent shunting.
4. Hypoxemia-hyperventilation test
    a. Most definitive test to detect PPHN.
    b. The patient is hyperventilated at a high rate using a manual resuscitator and 100% oxygen.
    c. Hyperventilation results in a decrease in $PaCO_2$, causing pulmonary vasodilation.
    d. PPHN is confirmed when PaO_2 is <50 mm Hg before hyperventilation and increases to >100 mm Hg during hyperventilation.
    e. For most congenital heart diseases, PaO_2 will not increase significantly during this test.
E. Management of PPHN
    1. Management goals:
        a. Stop the cyclic pattern of deterioration.
        b. Increase pulmonary blood flow by decreasing PVR or increasing systemic vascular resistance (SVR).
        c. Maintain adequate oxygenation.

2. Minimize handling and stimulation of the infant to avoid transient hypoxemia.
3. Inhaled nitric oxide (iNO)
   a. A selective pulmonary vasodilator approved for management of PPHN in neonates of gestational age >34 weeks.
   b. Initial dose is 20 parts per million (ppm).
   c. If there is no response at 20 ppm, increasing to 40 to 80 ppm will not improve oxygenation.
   d. Sustained use of 80 ppm can cause methemoglobinemia.
4. Mechanical ventilation and oxygen
   a. Conventional mechanical ventilation (CMV) and high frequency oscillatory ventilation (HFOV) have been used with success.
   b. Hyperventilation and induced alkalosis have been widely used but are controversial.
      (1) Effects of hyperventilation and alkalosis
         (a) Acute pulmonary vasodilation
         (b) Improved oxygen delivery
         (c) Cerebral vasoconstriction, which may lead to neurodevelopmental problems.
      (2) Because of the higher level of ventilator support necessary, hyperventilation carries an increased risk of lung injury.
   c. A widely practiced approach is to set the ventilator to produce mild hypocapnia and respiratory alkalosis.
      (a) $Paco_2$ = 35 to 40 mm Hg
      (b) pH = 7.40 to 7.45
   d. Success has been reported using lung protective ventilator strategies without inducing alkalinization.
      (1) Maintain $Paco_2$ <60 mm Hg
      (2) Maintain Pao_2 >50 mm Hg
      (3) Manage metabolic acidosis with sodium bicarbonate.
      (4) Use low positive end-expiratory pressure (PEEP) in the absence of parenchymal lung disease.
   e. Muscle relaxants and sedatives to prevent patient-ventilator dysynchrony and resulting fluctuations of Pao_2.
5. Administer surfactant if the infant has respiratory distress syndrome (RDS).
6. Pharmacologic treatments
   a. Increase SVR with vasopressors such as dopamine and dobutamine.
   b. Decrease PVR and hypertension with vasodilators (e.g., prostaglandin I, tolazoline, or nitroprusside).
   c. Correct hypotension using volume expanders and dopamine.
   d. PPHN is reversed when the pulmonary artery pressure is less than the arterial pressure.
7. Extracorporeal membrane oxygenation (ECMO) is used for severe cases.
   a. HFOV and iNO have reduced the number of neonates meeting criteria for ECMO.
   b. Increased survival and decreased morbidity in neonates with PPHN have been shown with ECMO compared with conventional treatments.

II. **Respiratory Distress Syndrome**
   A. Etiology
      1. RDS is a disease resulting from immature lung anatomy and physiology.
      2. The primary abnormality is surfactant deficiency.
      3. Without enough surfactant, alveoli collapse with each breath, and the lungs cannot maintain expansion.
      4. Underdeveloped alveoli and pulmonary capillary beds further compromise gas exchange.
   B. Factors that increase the risk of developing RDS
      1. Prematurity
      2. Low birth weight (<1200 g)

3. Gestational age <30 weeks
4. Male infants have twice the risk of female infants.
5. Maternal hemorrhage during delivery
6. Maternal diabetes
7. Birth asphyxia
8. Multiple births (e.g., second twin)
9. Possible association with delivery by cesarean section

C. Pathophysiology (Figure 27-2)
1. Surfactant deficiency causes atelectasis and reduced lung compliance.
2. Gas exchange is impaired, resulting in hypoxemia, hypercapnia, and acidemia.
3. Work of breathing increases, and the neonate begins to fatigue and hypoventilate.
4. Pulmonary vasoconstriction and increased PVR lead to hypoperfusion of the lung.
5. PPHN with shunting through the ductus arteriosus (right-to-left shunt).
6. Hypoxia causes damage to alveolar epithelium.
7. Pulmonary capillary permeability increases, and plasma leaks from the capillaries.
8. Fibrin present in plasma forms a hyaline membrane that lines the alveoli and bronchioles.
9. Alveolar ventilation decreases, and diffusion gradient increases.
10. High F_IO_2 and airway pressures during mechanical ventilation cause further tissue damage.

D. Clinical presentation
1. Symptoms of respiratory distress present at birth or develop 6 to 8 hours after birth.
2. Tachypnea
3. Retractions
4. Grunting
5. Nasal flaring
6. Cyanosis

E. Radiographic findings (Figure 27-3)
1. Classic appearance in the untreated newborn is reticulogranular infiltrates described as having a "ground glass" appearance.
2. Air bronchograms show collapsed alveoli surrounding air-filled bronchi.

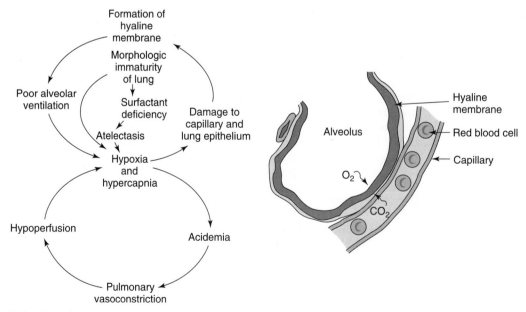

FIG. 27-2 Relationship of the factors resulting in respiratory distress syndrome (RDS). Hyaline membrane formation at the alveolar-capillary membrane in RDS.

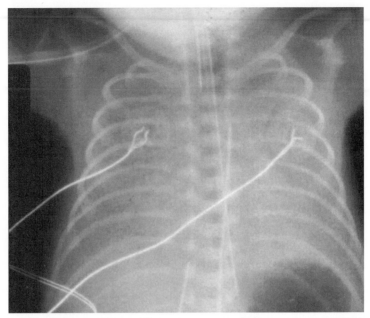

FIG. 27-3 Chest radiograph of a premature infant with respiratory distress syndrome (RDS). Note the characteristic pattern of "ground glass" infiltrates with air bronchograms.

3. Chest radiograph changes take place within 8 hours.
4. Severe RDS may progress to a "total whiteout," in which the heart border and diaphragm are indistinct because of severe atelectasis.

F. Management
  1. Monitoring of vital signs and arterial blood gases.
  2. Manage hypoxemia; maintain Pao_2 of 60 to 80 mm Hg.
  3. Continuous positive airway pressure (CPAP) may be used initially.
  4. Mechanical ventilation is usually required to manage severe acidemia, hypercapnia, and hypoxemia.
  5. High respiratory rate, F_IO_2, and airway pressures are often required.
  6. HFOV may be used either initially or in cases in which CMV is unsuccessful.
  7. Surfactant replacement therapy
    a. Synthetic and animal-derived products are available (Table 27-1).
    b. Method of administration depends on the drug used.
      (1) Can be given through a side port adaptor on the endotracheal tube (ETT).
      (2) Or through a small catheter inserted just past the tip of the ETT.
    c. Results in rapid and dramatic improvement in lung compliance and gas exchange.
    d. High levels of ventilatory support usually can be significantly reduced.
    e. Widespread use of surfactant has markedly decreased mortality from RDS.
    f. To avoid potential pneumothorax, it is important to decrease airway pressures and tidal volumes promptly when compliance improves during or immediately after surfactant administration.
    g. The most common adverse effects are transient oxygen desaturation and bradycardia.
  8. iNO
  9. Maintain normal body temperature, and minimize stimulation of infant.
  10. Provide appropriate fluid, electrolytes, glucose, and calories.
  11. Maintain blood pressure and hematocrit.
  12. Use secretion clearance techniques if necessary.
  13. ECMO is used in severe cases.

TABLE 27-1

Surfactant Replacement Therapy

Generic Name	Brand Name	Source	Characteristics	Route	Dosage
Colfosceril	Exosurf	Synthetic surfactant	No surfactant associated proteins	Side port on endotracheal tube adaptor	Initial: Two 2.5-ml/kg half-doses; avoid endotracheal suctioning for 2 hr after treatment
Beractant	Survanta	Exogenous surfactant from bovine lung extract	Contains surfactant associated proteins	Intratracheal	Initial: 4 ml/kg; if needed, 4 doses in the first 48 hr of life; ≥6 hr between each dose
Poractant alfa	Curosurf	Derived from minced porcine lung extract	Contains surfactant associated proteins	Intratracheal	Initial: 2.5-ml/kg dose divided in 2 aliquots; up to 2 more doses of 1.25 ml/kg, 12 hr apart, if needed
Calfactant	Infasurf	Derived from lavage of calf lungs	Contains surfactant associated proteins	Intratracheal	Initial: 3-ml/kg dose divided into 2 aliquots; 3 doses of 3 ml/kg, 12 hr apart, if needed

G. Prognosis
1. Most infants now recover in <14 days with minimal complications.
2. If mechanical ventilation continues >2 weeks, the incidence of bronchopulmonary dysplasia (BPD) increases.
H. Prevention of RDS
1. Education of parents about risk factors and symptoms of premature labor.
2. Pharmacologic suppression of premature labor.
3. Administration of corticosteroids to the mother to improve lung maturity of the fetus.

III. **Meconium Aspiration Syndrome (MAS)**
A. Description
1. Ten percent to 22% of newborns have meconium-stained amniotic fluid.
2. Most commonly seen in full-term and postterm newborns.
3. Rarely seen in newborns <37 weeks of gestational age.
B. Etiology
1. Meconium is a viscous fluid consisting of undigested amniotic fluid and epithelial cells.
2. Meconium is present in the colon late in gestation.
3. Meconium staining of the amniotic fluid can be a sign of fetal distress and hypoxemia.
4. Fetal responses to intrauterine hypoxemia
   a. Anal sphincter relaxes, and peristalsis increases.
   b. Meconium passes into amniotic fluid.
   c. Fetus makes gasping respiratory efforts, drawing meconium into the pharynx.
5. During the newborn's initial breaths, meconium present in the pharynx is aspirated below the vocal cords.
C. Pathophysiology
1. The effects of meconium aspiration on the lower airways:
   a. Creates an airway obstruction
      (1) Meconium acts as a ball valve in the airways, allowing inspiration but obstructing effective expiration.
      (2) The results are air trapping, hypoventilation, and atelectasis.
   b. Begins an inflammatory response in the lungs known as chemical pneumonitis
      (1) Meconium in the lower airways causes alveolar edema, production of proteinaceous exudate, and leads to alveolar collapse.
      (2) The mucosal layer is damaged and may become necrotic.
      (3) Endogenous surfactant production is inhibited.
2. During the first few hours after aspiration, hypercapnia, hypoxemia, and metabolic acidosis develop.
3. As pulmonary vascular resistance increases, the infant often develops PPHN.
4. If mechanical ventilation is required, recovery may be complicated by barotrauma and pneumothorax.
D. Radiographic findings
1. Bilateral diffuse, coarse, patchy infiltrates
2. Decreased aeration
3. Air bronchograms and consolidation in more severe cases
4. Hyperinflation with air trapping
E. Clinical presentation
1. Meconium staining of the amniotic fluid.
2. Sign and symptoms of respiratory distress
   a. Tachypnea
   b. Grunting
   c. Cyanosis
   d. Nasal flaring
3. Arterial blood gases show hypoxemia, hypercapnia, and respiratory and lactic acidosis.
4. Breath sounds are coarse with rhonchi and rales.
5. Prolonged expiratory phase
6. In severe cases the chest is hyperexpanded from air trapping.

F. Management
   1. If meconium-stained amniotic fluid is present, the mouth, nose, nasopharynx, and oropharynx are always suctioned when the newborn's head presents during birth, before the first breath is taken.
   2. If meconium is present in the oropharynx, the vocal cords are viewed under direct vision, and the airway is suctioned above the cords.
   3. If meconium is suctioned above the vocal cords, the trachea is intubated with a meconium aspirator, and the airway below the cords is suctioned.
   4. The airway must be cleared of meconium by suction before any positive pressure breaths are given.
   5. Supplemental blow-by oxygen is usually necessary.
   6. CPAP is often used to improve oxygenation.
   7. Mechanical ventilation is initiated if the infant fails to respond to oxygen with CPAP and develops worsening hypoxemia, hypercapnia, and acidemia.
   8. HFOV may be used as primary therapy or when ventilation with CMV is unsuccessful.
   9. Term infants often require sedation and sometimes muscle relaxers to maintain synchrony with the ventilator.
   10. Inhaled nitric oxide can be used if PPHN is present.
   11. Secretion clearance techniques, such as frequent endotracheal suctioning and chest physical therapy, are often useful.
   12. ECMO may be required to manage severe MAS (Table 27-2).
G. Prognosis
   1. Recovery from MAS without mechanical ventilation takes place within 3 to 7 days.
   2. When mechanical ventilation is needed, recovery increases to 7 to 10 days or may take weeks.

IV. **Pneumothorax**
   A. Etiology
      1. Stiff lungs with low compliance (e.g., RDS)
      2. Hyperinflated lungs (e.g., MAS)
      3. Hypoplastic lungs (e.g., congenital diaphragmatic hernia)
      4. Iatrogenic causes
         a. Positive pressure ventilation with high tidal volumes and peak pressures
         b. Often occurs as a complication of resuscitation
      5. Spontaneous causes
         a. Asymptomatic air leaks occur in 2% to 10% of term infants.
         b. Caused by high pressures (40 to 80 cm H_2O) that the infant generates to take its first breath.
         c. Usually minor and resolve without treatment in 24 to 48 hours.

TABLE 27-2

ECMO/ECLS Use and Survival for Neonates

Diagnosis	Number of Cases*	Percentage Survival
MAS	6263	94
CDH	4101	53
Sepsis	2307	75
PPHN	2649	79
RDS	1357	84
Others	1411	65

*Includes all cases reported to the registry.
MAS, Meconium aspiration syndrome; *CDH,* congenital diaphragmatic hernia; *PPHN,* persistent pulmonary hypertension in the newborn; *RDS,* respiratory distress syndrome.
From ELSO registry data. January 2003.

6. Surfactant replacement therapy has significantly reduced the incidence of pneumothorax.
B. Pathophysiology
1. Air trapping in obstructed airways.
2. Regional overdistention and rupture of alveoli can occur when more compliant alveoli are adjacent to atelectatic alveoli.
3. Ruptured alveoli can result in pulmonary interstitial emphysema (PIE).
a. Air from the ruptured alveoli may remain localized or may track into the interstitium surrounding the pulmonary vasculature.
b. PIE compromises ventilation and circulation and may not resolve for weeks.
C. Clinical presentation
1. Sudden cardiopulmonary deterioration
2. Tachypnea
3. Bradycardia
4. Cyanosis
5. Poor peripheral perfusion
6. Increased respiratory efforts
7. Decreased breath and heart sounds on auscultation
D. Diagnosis (Figure 27-4)
1. Chest radiography is the gold standard.
2. Transillumination is useful for critically ill infants if there is a delay in obtaining the chest radiograph.
a. Transillumination is the passage of light through body tissues for the purpose of examining a structure.
b. A fiberoptic transilluminator is placed against both sides of the infant's chest superior and inferior to the nipple.
c. If the lung is inflated the tissue will absorb most of the light.
d. A greater appearance of light through the chest suggests an abnormal amount of air in the thoracic cavity.
e. In full-term infants, pneumothorax may not be visible under transillumination.
E. Management
1. Prompt decompression by chest tube placement

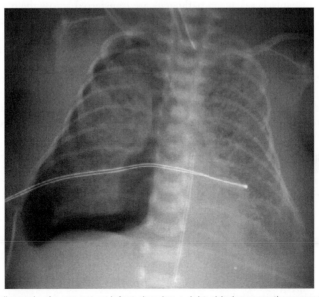

FIG. 27-4 Chest radiograph of a premature infant showing a right-sided pneumothorax and pulmonary interstitial emphysema (PIE) on the left side.

a. The tube is inserted at the second to third intercostal space lateral to the midclavicular line.

b. The tube is connected to an underwater seal drainage unit with -20 cm H_2O of suction.

2. Chest tube placement usually results in immediate improvement.

3. Needle aspiration is sometimes performed in an emergency.

    a. A small gauge scalp vein needle or angiocath is attached to a three-way stopcock and a 10- to 20-ml syringe.

    b. The needle is inserted in the chest, and air is aspirated into the syringe.

V. Pneumonia

A. Incidence of pneumonia during birth or after delivery

  1. Develops in approximately 1% of term infants.

  2. Develops in 10% of preterm neonates.

B. Etiology

  1. Bacteria usually cause the infection.

    a. Group B *Streptococcus* is the most common pathogen.

    b. Gram-negative organisms (e.g., *Escherichia coli, Klebsiella, Pseudomonas, Serratia marcescens*)

    c. Less frequently caused by *Staphylococcus aureus* or *Staphylococcus epidermis*

  2. *Candida* can cause fungal pneumonia.

  3. Viral pneumonia is less common and may be caused by

    a. Herpes

    b. Cytomegalovirus

    c. Varicella-zoster

    d. Syphilis

  4. Predisposing factors

    a. Colonization of the mother's genital and vaginal tracts with pathogens

    b. Immaturity of the immune system

    c. Prolonged rupture of the membranes

    d. Prematurity

    e. Nosocomial infections acquired in the neonatal intensive care unit

C. Pathophysiology

  1. The neonate can acquire infection via three routes.

    a. Transplacental, when pathogens are transferred across the placenta in utero.

    b. Perinatal, by aspiration of contaminated amniotic fluid during labor and delivery.

    c. Postnatal, from the mother, caregivers, or environment during the hospital stay.

  2. Rupture of placental membranes >12 hours before birth increases the chance that infectious agents will spread to the amniotic fluid and the fetus.

  3. Bacterial pneumonia causes inflamed, fluid-filled alveoli more often than viral pneumonia, and in severe cases necrosis of lung tissue develops.

  4. Sepsis can rapidly develop from gram-negative pulmonary infections.

  5. Bacterial pneumonia acquired in utero leads to stillbirth and premature delivery in many cases.

  6. Pneumonia caused by viruses and mycoplasmae involve the bronchi and interstitium, resulting in loss of ciliary function and mucus stasis.

  7. Fungal infections can produce a layer of hyphae that line the upper and lower respiratory tract, eventually leading to ulcerations in the airway.

D. Clinical presentation

  1. Signs and symptoms are similar to those of respiratory distress, transient tachypnea of the newborn, and sepsis.

    a. Low Apgar scores if the infection developed transplacentally or perinatally.

    b. Tachypnea

    c. Low SpO_2

    d. Thermal instability

    e. Periods of apnea

    2. A chest radiograph is often necessary to differentiate between diagnoses.
- **E.** Laboratory findings
  1. Chest radiographs have various patterns of infiltrates that are often characteristic of a specific causative organism (Table 27-3).
  2. Tracheal aspirates and blood cultures help identify causative organisms and diagnose sepsis.
  3. Complete blood count (i.e., neutrophil count, platelet count) may be useful to diagnose sepsis and other infections, but results from these tests are not specific enough to differentiate between causative factors.
- **F.** Management
  1. Supplemental oxygen to maintain SpO_2 at >90%.
  2. Broad-spectrum antibiotics initially (e.g., ampicillin, gentamicin).
  3. If the organism is identified, antibiotics may be changed.
  4. Manage hypotension with dopamine and fluid.
  5. Severe cases may require mechanical ventilation.
- **G.** Prognosis
  1. Mortality has been estimated at 20% for perinatally acquired pneumonia.
  2. Mortality for postnatal pneumonia is approximately 50%.
  3. The most recent reviews indicate a decrease in overall mortality to approximately 10% in perinatally acquired pneumonia attributed to perinatal use of antibiotics.

VI. Transient Tachypnea in the Newborn (TTN)
- **A.** Etiology
  1. TTN is an obstructive disease resulting from delayed reabsorption of normal fetal lung fluid.
  2. Predisposing factors
     - a. Abnormal labor or transition
       - (1) Cesarean section
       - (2) Precipitous delivery
     - b. Low Apgar scores
     - c. Pulmonary hypertension
     - d. Inadequate left ventricular function
- **B.** Pathophysiology
  1. The fetal lung is normally filled to the functional residual capacity level with fluid that is produced in the lungs (not amniotic fluid).
  2. As the neonate passes through the birth canal during a normal delivery, "thoracic squeeze" removes one third of the fluid present in the lungs at birth.
  3. The remaining fluid is removed slowly by the neonate's lymphatic system.
  4. The excessive fluid in the lungs and interstitium interferes with the ability to hold bronchioles and alveoli open.
  5. Air trapping and small airway collapse result, causing changes in pulmonary mechanics and breathing pattern of the infant.

TABLE 27-3

Chest X-ray Findings in Neonatal Pneumonia

Causative Agent	Appearance of Chest Radiograph
Group B β-hemolytic *Streptococcus* (GBS)	Diffuse opacities ("white out"), patchy infiltrates, pleural effusions
Streptococcus pneumoniae	Patchy lobar infiltrates, pleural effusion
Klebsiella	Bilateral consolidation, lung abscess, pneumatocele
Pseudomonas and *Serratia*	Parenchymal consolidation (patchy or basilar), pneumatocele
Respiratory syncytial virus	Hyperexpansion, patchy consolidation
Candida albicans	Diffuse granularity, coarse infiltrates, opacification

From Merenstein GB, Gardner SL: *Handbook of Neonatal Intensive Care*, ed 5, St. Louis, Mosby, 2002.

      a. Decreased dynamic compliance
      b. Increased deadspace
      c. Higher respiratory rate
      d. Low tidal volume
   6. TTN is usually a benign and self-limiting condition.
   7. However, TTN may be complicated by PPHN or evolve into RDS.

C. Clinical presentation
   1. Term infants with tachypnea that develops 2 to 6 hours postpartum
   2. Mild to moderate respiratory distress
      a. Grunting
      b. Nasal flaring
      c. Retractions
   3. Cyanosis may be present.
   4. Arterial blood gases show mild hypoxemia and mild acidemia.

D. Radiographic findings
   1. Fluid in fissures and effusions
   2. Streaky appearance of lung parenchyma
   3. Hyperinflation
   4. Radiographic findings may mimic cardiac problems, but in TTN these changes resolve within 72 hours.

E. Management
   1. General supportive care as fluid gradually clears via lymphatics.
   2. Usually resolves within 72 hours.
   3. Supplemental oxygen to maintain $SpO_2 \geq 90\%$.
   4. CPAP may be used if there is no response from supplemental oxygen.
   5. Mechanical ventilation is rarely necessary.
   6. Some practitioners advocate the use of diuretics.

VII. Apnea in the Neonate

A. Apnea of prematurity or primary apnea
   1. The younger the gestational age, the greater the incidence of apnea.
   2. Not caused by a specific disease entity.
   3. There are several factors that have been associated with primary apnea.
      a. Response to hypoxemia and hypercapnia
        (1) Neonatal response differs from the adult response.
        (2) Adults respond with a sustained increase in ventilation.
        (3) Infants have a brief increase in ventilation, followed by respiratory depression.
      b. Immaturity of the neurons that control respiratory rate and rhythm may contribute to primary apnea. Premature infants have fewer dendrites and synaptic connections, and this may alter transmission of impulses involved in control of breathing.
      c. Apnea in infants occurs more often during sleep, especially rapid eye movement (REM) sleep. The known neurologic effects during REM sleep include inhibition of spinal motor neurons, increased movement of the eyes, muscle twitching, and increased cerebral blood flow. There may be other effects that directly or indirectly influence drive to breathe.
      d. Respiratory muscle fatigue: The premature infant has an increased workload from the combination of a compliant chest wall and less compliant lungs.

B. Secondary apnea is caused by specific disorders that directly or indirectly lead to hypoxemia and depression of the drive to breathe.
   1. RDS
   2. Central nervous system disorders such as intraventricular hemorrhage or seizures
   3. Infection, particularly sepsis
   4. Left-to-right shunting through a patent ductus arteriosus (PDA)

C. Iatrogenic causes of apnea
1. Environmental: Sustained increases or sudden changes in temperature
2. Vagal response to endotracheal suctioning
3. Secretions or other foreign material in the oropharynx can cause apnea because of the laryngeal chemoreflex. This reflex protects against aspiration by preventing inspiration during feeding.
4. Improper neck positioning can cause obstruction of the airway.
D. Management
1. SpO_2 and heart rate should be monitored, and alarm systems should remain active.
   a. Bradycardia and desaturation often follow an apneic period.
   b. Impedance apnea monitors are not used because they do not differentiate between normal breathing and the gasping efforts seen with airway obstruction.
   c. High-risk neonates should be monitored for at least 10 to 12 days.
2. Reduce environmental stress
3. During apneic spells use the least invasive intervention that stimulates the infant to breathe.
   a. Provide gentle tactile stimulation.
   b. If stimulation is not immediately effective, use bag-mask ventilation.
      (1) Use F_IO_2 of approximately 10% above that used before the episode to manage hypoxemia.
      (2) Increasing the ambient F_IO_2 will decrease the frequency but prolong the duration of apneic periods.
   c. If necessary use nasal or nasopharyngeal CPAP.
   d. Mechanical ventilation may be needed for extremely premature or unstable neonates.
4. Manage disorders that cause secondary apnea.
5. Methylxanthines are sometimes used to manage apnea of prematurity.
   a. Caffeine citrate
   b. Theophylline

VIII. **Chronic Disorders Associated with Prematurity**
A. Bronchopulmonary dysplasia (BPD)/chronic lung disease (CLD)
1. BPD is a chronic disorder in premature infants characterized by
   a. Respiratory distress
   b. Serial radiographic changes
   c. Impaired gas exchange
2. Originally BPD described a classic progression of radiographic and functional changes in the lungs of survivors of RDS.
3. The BPD seen today is not as severe; with current treatment premature infants do not necessarily progress through all of the classic stages.
4. CLD is a term used to describe premature infants who require supplemental oxygen at 28 to 30 days of life or at 36 weeks' postmenstrual age.
5. Etiology: The causes of BPD/CLD are iatrogenic.
   a. Oxygen toxicity
      (1) Historically believed to occur because of long-term exposure to high F_IO_2.
      (2) However, BPD/CLD has been documented after short- and long-term exposure to high and low F_IO_2.
   b. Lung injury associated with positive pressure ventilation.
      (1) High peak inspiratory pressures can cause barotrauma (e.g., pneumothorax).
      (2) Large tidal volumes cause volutrauma by overdistending areas of lung.
      (3) Incidence of BPD is decreased when lower peak inspiratory pressures and tidal volumes are used.
6. Predisposing factors
   a. PDA and congestive heart failure (CHF)
   b. Poor nutrition in utero

      c.   Family history of asthma

      d.   Fluid overload in the first few days of life

  7. Pathophysiology

      a.   Developmental immaturity of the lungs makes them more susceptible to damage.

      b.   Injury to alveolar epithelium and fibrin-producing hyaline membranes occurs when the neonate develops RDS.

      c.   Repair of the lung injury requires treatment with oxygen and positive pressure ventilation, two of the factors that contribute to lung injury and development of BPD.

      d.   A cycle of constant and recurring lung injury and repair is established.

  8. The classic stages of BPD

      a.   Stage I

         (1)   Develops during the first 3 days of life.

         (2)   Chest radiography shows ground glass (reticulogranular) appearance and air bronchograms.

      b.   Stage II

         (1)   Develops during the first 3 to 10 days of life.

         (2)   Hyaline membrane formation

         (3)   Stages I and II correlate with development and resolution of RDS.

         (4)   Chest radiography shows granular opacity of the lung obscuring the cardiac borders.

      c.   Stage III

         (1)   Develops during the first 10 to 20 days of life.

         (2)   Marks the transition into chronic phase.

         (3)   Chest radiography shows opaque lungs with multiple small cysts and visible cardiac borders.

         (4)   Alveolar emphysema and interstitial fibrosis

         (5)   Right heart failure

      d.   Stage IV

         (1)   Develops after 28 days of life.

         (2)   Chest radiography shows larger, irregular cysts and areas of increased density.

         (3)   Marked respiratory distress, cyanosis, and diffuse rales.

         (4)   Hyperinflation, flattened diaphragm, and atelectasis may be evident.

         (5)   Cardiomegaly develops from cor pulmonale.

         (6)   Thickened alveolar walls and increased diffusion gradient

         (7)   Difficulty weaning from mechanical ventilation.

  9. Clinical presentation

      a.   Initially the infant presents with the signs and symptoms of RDS.

      b.   In later stages signs include

         (1)   A medical history of prematurity, moderate to severe RDS, mechanical ventilation, and difficulty weaning from the ventilator.

         (2)   Abnormal breathing pattern: Tachypnea, retractions, and nasal flaring

         (3)   Poor tolerance of feeding and handling

         (4)   Oxygen dependence

         (5)   Crackles and decreased air entry

         (6)   Pulmonary hypertension with right-sided heart failure

         (7)   Children aged <2 years with CLD are frequently readmitted to the hospital with viral respiratory infections caused by respiratory syncytial virus (RSV).

B. Management

  1. Maintain adequate oxygenation and ventilation

      a. PaO_2, 60 to 80 mm Hg, and SpO_2 90% to 95% on the lowest possible F_IO_2

      b.   Adequate PEEP to prevent atelectasis

  2. Weaning from mechanical ventilation

      a.   Infants with BPD/CLD may be able to maintain ventilation before they can maintain oxygenation.

      b.   Extubation to nasal CPAP is useful in this setting.

3. Provide adequate nutrition to facilitate healing of damaged lung tissue.
4. Drug therapy is used to improve lung mechanics.
   a. Aerosolized medications
      (1) Bronchodilators (β_2 agonists) are commonly used to manage bronchospasm in infants with BPD/CLD.
      (2) Inhaled steroids are used to decrease airway inflammation.
      (3) Histamine inhibitors (Cromolyn) are used to reduce airway reactivity and inflammatory response.
   b. Effectiveness of aerosolized medications
      (1) β_2 agonists act on bronchial smooth muscle, but this tissue is poorly developed in premature infants, thus limiting the effectiveness of these drugs.
      (2) Small ETTs baffle the aerosol, preventing 90% of the drug from reaching the lungs.
      (3) Drug delivery in intubated infants is poor from metered dose inhalers (MDI) and small volume nebulizers (SVNs).
   c. Methylxanthines are used to promote weaning from low-level ventilatory support.
   d. Diuretics can improve lung mechanics and facilitate weaning.
   e. Antenatal and postnatal steroids are widely used and have been linked to decreased mortality and faster weaning.
   f. Studies comparing the efficacy of inhaled versus systemic steroids have yielded conflicting results.
5. Unfortunately very small premature infants almost always have complications from BPD as children (Box 27-1).

IX. **Retinopathy of Prematurity (ROP)**
   A. ROP is a common complication of prematurity.
      1. Develops in approximately 85% of premature infants of <28 weeks' gestation.
      2. Develops in approximately 65% of premature infants weighing <1250 g.
      3. In 80% of the cases of ROP no intervention is necessary.

BOX 27-1
Complications of BPD

Increased mortality
Effects of long-term steroid use
Failure to gain weight, decreased head growth

Pulmonary
Acute: PIE, air leak, pulmonary hypertension, cyst formation
Chronic: Decreased pulmonary function, O_2 dependence, recurrent respiratory infections, and hospital admissions

Cardiac
Cor pulmonale, right-sided heart failure

Orthopedic problems
Fractures, rickets

Neurodevelopmental delay
Cerebral palsy, cognitive impairment, behavior problems

Sensory deficits
Hearing loss, severe ROP

BPD, Bronchopulmonary dysplasia; *PIE,* pulmonary interstitial emphysema; *ROP,* retinopathy of prematurity.

B. Etiology
   1. ROP has long been associated with lengthy exposure to high F_IO_2, but this process is not yet fully understood.
   2. Many other risk factors appear to contribute to the development of ROP.
      a. Maternal hypertension during pregnancy caused by smoking, diabetes, or other causes
      b. Prematurity, low birth weight, and multiple gestations
      c. Anemia and blood transfusions
      d. Apnea and bradycardia in the infant, along with cycles of hyperoxia and hypoxia
      e. Cytokine release caused by sepsis in the infant
      f. Intraventricular hemorrhage and/or seizures
      g. Nutritional deficiency
      h. Ethnicity: White infants are more likely to develop ROP than African-American infants.
C. Pathophysiology
   1. Most blood vessels supplying the retina are developed by 32 weeks' gestation, but those in the peripheral regions may not develop until 40 weeks.
   2. Retinal vessels constrict in response to hyperoxia.
   3. Some vessels dilate and revascularize their surrounding areas.
   4. Other vessels constrict permanently and become necrotic in a process called vasoobliteration.
   5. The remaining blood vessels begin to proliferate as they attempt to provide blood flow to the obliterated areas of the retina.
   6. If the vessels continue to proliferate, the damage can progress from hemorrhage to retinal scarring, retinal detachment, and blindness.
   7. Early changes are often seen in the temporal periphery of the retina, the region where vascularization develops in the last few weeks of gestation.
   8. ROP can no longer occur when the vascular development of the retina is complete.
D. Classification of the severity of ROP (Figure 27-5)
   1. Location on the retina
      a. The retina is divided into zones composed of two concentric circles and a crescent-shaped area lateral to the nose.
      b. Zone 1 is the interior, and zone 3 is the outermost region.
   2. Degree of vascular abnormality is classified in stages.
      a. Stage 1 describes a thin white line where the abnormal branching starts.
      b. Stage 5 describes total detachment of the retina.
   3. Area of injury or amount of the retina involved
      a. The retina is divided into quadrants corresponding to clock hours.
      b. For example, detachment occurring in the upper right quadrant would be described as "from 12 to 3 o'clock."

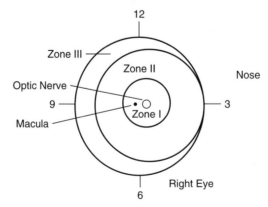

FIG. 27-5 International classification of retinopathy of prematurity (ICROP).

E. Management and prevention
   1. The most effective way to prevent ROP is to prevent prematurity.
   2. Pulse oximetry and arterial blood gases must be monitored whenever oxygen is administered.
   3. The recommended high alarm setting for preterm infants' SpO_2 is ≤96%. This decreases the risk of injury for ROP and BPD/CLD.
   4. Maintain PaO_2 of 65 to 90 mm Hg.
   5. Reduce the time of exposure to high F_IO_2 levels (>0.50).
   6. Use oxygen blenders to provide specific F_IO_2 level during procedures (i.e., suctioning, apneic spells, and endotracheal intubation).
   7. Early and frequent ophthalmic examination in premature infants, especially those weighing <1500 g.
   8. Laser surgery or cryotherapy to manage retinal detachment has yielded good results.

X. **Congenital Heart Disease (Box 27-2)**
   A. Approximately 1% of newborns are born with a heart defect.
   B. Etiology
      1. The single most important factor is family history of congenital heart defects.
      2. Approximately 8% of congenital defects are associated with specific chromosomal abnormalities (e.g., trisomy 21 or trisomy 13).
      3. Environmental factors include maternal viral infections (rubella) and maternal drug or toxic substance ingestion (e.g., seizure medications, alcohol).
   C. Newborns with severe cardiac defects generally have one or more of the following signs and symptoms.
      1. Cyanosis
      2. Respiratory distress
      3. Congestive heart failure (CHF)
   D. CHF is a syndrome characterized by decreased cardiac output and decreased tissue perfusion.
      1. Results from the inability of the myocardium to fulfill the body's metabolic needs.
      2. Causes of CHF
         a. Volume overload
         b. Pressure overload

BOX 27-2

Common Environmental Triggers and Risk Factors for Congenital Cardiovascular Disease

Drugs	**Parental Exposure to Environmental Agents**
Alcohol	Maternal exposure to solvents, hair dyes
Amphetamines	Paternal exposure to cold weather
Anticonvulsants	
Trimethadione	**Mother's Reproductive History**
Lithium	No known genetic risk but history of premature birth and induced
Valium	abortion
Corticosteroids	Genetic risk factors: family history of congenital heart disease,
Paternal exposure to cocaine	>3 previous pregnancies, an increased number of
	miscarriages
Maternal Health	
Diabetes	
Infections	
Rubella	

Modified from Merenstein GB, Gardner SL: *Handbook of Neonatal Intensive Care*, ed 5, St. Louis, Mosby, 2002.

      c. Cardiomyopathy

      d. Dysrhythmias

  3. Signs and symptoms of CHF

      a. Tachycardia as the heart attempts to increase cardiac output.

      b. Enlargement of the heart from one or both of the following

          (1) Dilation of the chambers from excess volume

          (2) Hypertrophy from increased myocardial work to overcome pressure gradients

      c. Tachypnea is the initial sign, followed by other signs of respiratory distress.

      d. Poor perfusion and mottling of extremities

      e. Decreased urine output

      f. Decreased exercise tolerance

      g. Failure to thrive and difficulty in feeding

  4. Management of CHF

      a. A positive inotrope, such as digoxin or milrinone, is administered to increase the contractility of the myocardium.

      b. Diuretics are used to decrease the amount of fluid overload.

E. PDA (Figure 27-6)

  1. Cyanosis is not present because the shunt is from left to right.

  2. The ductus arteriosus fails to close at birth.

  3. A pressure gradient exists between the aorta and the pulmonary artery; therefore, left ventricular output flows through the patent ductus into the pulmonary artery.

  4. Right ventricular work increases, resulting in CHF.

  5. PDA is common in preterm infants with RDS.

  6. Management

      a. Medical

          (1) Indomethacin, a prostaglandin inhibitor that causes constriction of the ductus arteriosus

          (2) Indomethacin is much less effective if administered after 7 days of life.

      b. Surgical ligation or clipping of the ductus arteriosus carries little risk when performed by an experienced cardiac surgical team.

F. Atrial septal defect (ASD) (Figure 27-7)

  1. Cyanosis is not present because the shunt is from left to right.

  2. When the foramen ovale fails to close or when the atrial septum does not develop normally, the result is an ASD.

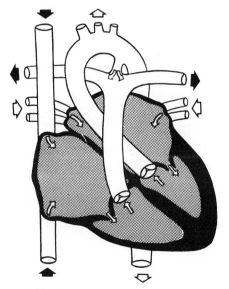

FIG. 27-6 Patent ductus arteriosus.

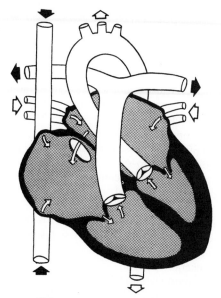

FIG. 27-7 Atrial septal defect.

3. Types of defects
   a. Ostium primum occurs low in the atrial wall and usually involves the mitral and tricuspid valves.
   b. Ostium secundum is an isolated defect occurring high in the atrial wall.
4. Because of the higher pressure in the left atrium, blood flows from the left atrium into the right atrium through the ASD.
5. Work of the right side of the heart often increases, and CHF develops.
6. Surgical closure of the defect may be necessary.

G. Ventricular septal defect (VSD) (Figure 27-8)
   1. Cyanosis is rarely present because the shunt is from left to right.

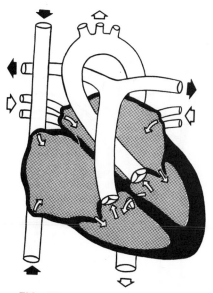

FIG. 27-8 Ventricular septal defect.

2. Defects vary considerably in size and may occur in conjunction with other cardiac defects.
3. VSD (either alone or associated with other anomalies) account for 50% of congenital heart defects.
4. Two factors influence the effect of the VSD on circulation.
    a. Size of the VSD
        (1) Small defects cause minor left-to-right shunting and may be asymptomatic.
        (2) Large defects may allow moderate left-to-right shunting, causing CHF and pulmonary edema.
    b. Degree of pulmonary hypertension
        (1) Normal pulmonary vascular resistance is approximately 20% of SVR, allowing significant left-to-right shunt.
        (2) In infants with RDS, pneumonia, and BPD, PVR is often increased, and left-to-right shunt is minimal.
5. Management
    a. Most small defects close spontaneously (50% to 75%).
    b. Large defects require surgical closure using sutures or a Dacron patch.
H. Aortic stenosis (Figure 27-9)
    1. Cyanosis is not generally present.
    2. Flow from the left ventricle into the aorta is partially obstructed.
    3. The most common obstruction is a defect in the aortic valve where the leaflets of the valve are fused.
    4. A pressure gradient of >50 mm Hg between the left ventricle and the ascending aorta indicates aortic stenosis.
    5. Left ventricular hypertrophy and CHF develop as a result of the increased resistance.
    6. Management
        a. Usually corrected surgically by performing an aortic valvulotomy.
        b. Balloon dilatation in a cardiac catheterization laboratory is an alternative treatment.
I. Pulmonary stenosis (Figure 27-10)
    1. Cyanosis is not present if this is the only cardiac lesion present.
    2. Blood flow into the pulmonary artery is obstructed, most often caused by a defect in the pulmonary valve.
    3. Right ventricular hypertrophy and CHF develop.
    4. Management
        a. Prostaglandin E_1 has been used to maintain a PDA until surgery can be performed.
        b. Surgical correction is achieved by performing a pulmonary valvulotomy.

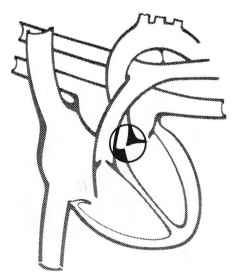

FIG. 27-9 Aortic stenosis.

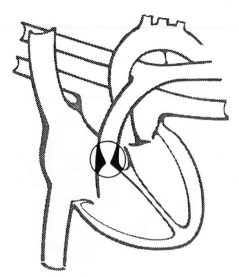

FIG. 27-10 Pulmonary stenosis.

J. Coarctation of the aorta (Figure 27-11)
   1. Cyanosis is not generally present.
   2. Characterized by a constriction in the lumen of the aorta.
   3. The most common location is near the ductus arteriosus at the junction of the transverse aortic arch and descending aorta.
   4. Therefore most of the cardiac output is to the head and upper extremities.
   5. If coarctation is present in this location, systolic blood pressure is >15 mm Hg higher in the upper extremities than in the lower extremities.
   6. Left ventricular hypertrophy and CHF often develop.
   7. Management
      a. CHF is managed with digoxin.
      b. Surgical management is resection of the area of the stricture.
K. Tetralogy of Fallot (Figure 27-12)
   1. Cyanosis is present because of right-to-left shunt.
   2. Tetralogy of Fallot is the most common cyanotic anomaly.

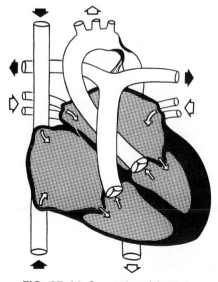

FIG. 27-11 Coarctation of the aorta.

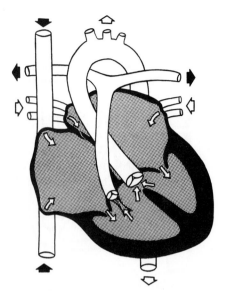

FIG. 27-12 Tetralogy of Fallot.

3. Characterized by
   a. Ventricular septal defect
   b. Pulmonary valve stenosis
   c. Positioning of the aorta directly above or overriding the VSD
   d. Right ventricular hypertrophy
4. CHF is rare.
5. Infants have occasional hypercyanotic episodes with severe cyanosis, tachypnea, irritability, flaccidity, and sometimes loss of consciousness.
6. Management
   a. Hypercyanotic episodes are managed with propranolol or sometimes morphine.
   b. Surgery in the small neonate involves building a shunt between the aorta and pulmonary artery to increase pulmonary blood flow.
   c. Total repair involves closure of the VSD and correction of the outflow obstruction at the pulmonary artery.
L. Truncus arteriosus (Figure 27-13)
   1. Cyanosis is present because of right-to-left shunt.
   2. Characterized by a common artery (truncus) originating from both ventricles and overriding a VSD.
   3. The truncus carries a mixture of oxygenated and unoxygenated blood and is the origin for the aorta, coronary arteries, and both branches of the pulmonary arteries.
   4. Pulmonary blood flow varies, depending on the location of the branching of the pulmonary arteries off the truncus and the degree of pulmonary hypertension.
   5. Pulmonary blood pressure is usually equal to systemic blood pressure.
   6. Right and left ventricular hypertrophy and CHF commonly occur.
   7. Surgical correction involves
      a. Closure of the VSD with a patch
      b. Separation of the pulmonary arteries from the truncus
      c. Reanastomosis of a graft vessel with a valve to the right ventricle and the separated pulmonary arteries
M. Complete transposition of the great vessels (Figure 27-14)
   1. Cyanosis is present because of right-to-left shunting.
   2. Characterized by reversed position of aorta and pulmonary arteries.

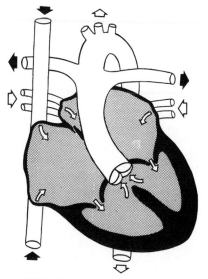

FIG. 27-13 Truncus arteriosus.

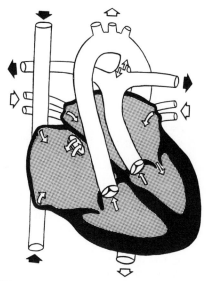

FIG. 27-14 Complete transposition of the great vessels.

    a. The aorta originates from the right ventricle and pumps unoxygenated blood to the body.

    b. The pulmonary artery originates from the left ventricle and pumps oxygenated blood back to the lungs.

    c. Thus two separate circulations occur, and mixing can only occur if there are other lesions present.

3. Venous and arterial blood may mix through an ASD, VSD, or PDA (Table 27-4).

4. Profound cyanosis may occur if the ventricular septum is intact or the ductus arteriosus begins to close.

5. In this situation oxygen therapy has a limited benefit because the only oxygenated blood reaching systemic circulation is that which is shunted through the VSD, ASD, or PDA.

6. This amount is determined by the size, position, and number of communications where shunting can occur.

7. The most common surgical repair is the arterial switch procedure.

TABLE 27-4

Congenital Heart Diseases

Cardiac Defect	Anatomic Characteristics	Direction of Shunt	Presence of CHF	Presence of Cyanosis	Treatment
Patent ductus arteriosus (PDA)	Failure of ductus arteriosus to close at birth	Left-to-right	Present	Acyanotic	Medical: Indomethacin Surgical: Ligation of PDA
Atrial septal defect (ASD)	Failure of foramen ovale to close or malformation in atrial septal wall	Left-to-right	Present	Acyanotic	Surgical closure
Ventricular septal defect (VSD)	Malformation in ventricular septal wall	Left-to-right	Present, if large VSD	Acyanotic	Large VSD requires surgical closure
Aortic stenosis	Most common type an aortic valve with fused leaflets	No shunt, if isolated lesion	Present	Acyanotic	Surgical correction is aortic valvulotomy
Pulmonary stenosis	Most common type is defect in the pulmonary valve with fused leaflets	No shunt, if isolated lesion	Present	Acyanotic	Pulmonary valvulotomy
Coarctation of the aorta	Constriction in lumen of aorta near ductus arteriosus	No shunt	Sometimes	Acyanotic	Surgical resection of the stricture
Tetralogy of Fallot	VSD with overriding aorta, outflow obstruction of RV, RV hypertrophy	Right-to-left	Rare	Cyanotic	Surgery to create shunt from aorta to PA, VSD closure, correction of outflow obstruction
Truncus arteriosus	Common artery (truncus) overriding a VSD	Right-to-left	Present	Cyanotic	VSD closure, separation of pulmonary arteries from truncus, reattachment to RV
Complete transposition of the great vessels	Aorta originates from RV; PA originates from LV, with ASD, VSD, and/or PDA	Right-to-left	Not present	Cyanotic	Most common surgical correction is arterial switch procedure
Total anomalous pulmonary venous return (TAPVR)	Pulmonary veins return oxygenated blood to the RA, ASD	Right-to-left	Not present	Cyanotic	Surgical connection of pulmonary veins to LA, ASD closure
Tricuspid atresia	Agenesis of tricuspid valve, small RV, large LV	Right-to-left	Sometimes	Cyanotic	Surgical connection of PA to RA, ASD and VSD closure

CHF, Congestive heart failure; *RA,* right atrium; *RV,* right ventricle; *LV,* left ventricle; *PA,* pulmonary artery.

N. Total anomalous pulmonary venous return (TAPVR) (Figure 27-15)
 1. Cyanosis and right-to-left shunting are present.
 2. Characterized by all pulmonary veins returning oxygenated blood to the right atrium.
 3. Several types of TAPVR are classified according to route of pulmonary venous return to the right atrium.
    a. Supracardiac TAPVR is the most common and involves return through the superior vena cava.
    b. Infracardiac TAPVR involves return through the portal venous system.
    c. Cardiac TAPVR is characterized by direct communication between the pulmonary veins and the right atrium or through the coronary sinus.
 4. To sustain life, there must be a passage between the right and left atria (ASD) so that right-to-left shunting can occur.
 5. Surgical management consists of reimplantation of anomalous pulmonary veins from the right atrium to the left atrium and closure of the ASD.
O. Tricuspid atresia (Figure 27-16)
 1. Cyanosis is present in varying degrees because of right-to-left shunt.
 2. Characterized by
    a. Failure of the tricuspid valve to form, resulting in lack of direct communication between the right atrium and right ventricle.
    b. Small right ventricle
    c. Large left ventricle
    d. Decreased pulmonary circulation
 3. Right-to-left shunting occurs through an ASD.
 4. A VSD is sometimes present.
 5. Transposition of the great arteries is also present in approximately 30% of the cases.
 6. Surgical management of the neonate consists of creating a shunt between the aorta and the pulmonary artery to increase pulmonary blood flow.
 7. Definitive repair involves connecting the pulmonary artery to the right atrium and closure of ASD and VSD if present.

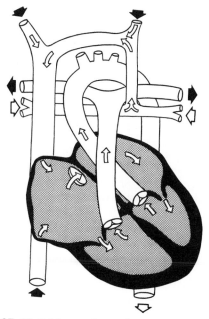

FIG. 27-15 Total anomalous pulmonary venous return.

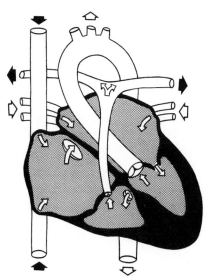

FIG. 27-16 Tricuspid atresia.

XI. **Other Congenital Anomalies with Effects on the Respiratory System**
  A. Choanal atresia
    1. Characterized by blockage, to varying degrees, of the posterior opening into the nasopharynx by a membranous tissue, usually with bony implants.
    2. Occurs in approximately 1 in 7000 live births.
    3. Can be an isolated anomaly or part of a syndrome with multiple anomalies.
    4. Clinical presentation
      a. Bilateral choanal atresia
        (1) Inability to pass suction catheter through nares
        (2) Noisy breathing
        (3) Cyanosis that worsens when the infant is at rest or during feeding but improves with crying
      b. Unilateral choanal atresia
        (1) Usually unnoticed until later in life
        (2) Nasal discharge and/or obstruction of one nostril are often the only symptoms.
    5. Computerized tomography scan usually confirms diagnosis of choanal atresia.
    6. Management
      a. Placement of an oral airway
      b. Gavage feedings
      c. Surgical repair involves transnasal puncture and placement of a stent.
  B. Esophageal atresia (EA) (Figure 27-17)
    1. Characterized by an esophagus that ends in a blind pouch before joining the stomach and usually occurs in conjunction with a tracheoesophageal fistula (TEF).
    2. There are several types; the most common involves atresia of the upper esophagus with the lower esophagus connected to the trachea or mainstem bronchi.
    3. Clinical presentation
      a. Most infants with EA have a history of maternal polyhydramnios or an abnormally high level of amniotic fluid.
      b. Excessive amounts of oral secretions, choking, and respiratory distress soon after birth
      c. Inability to swallow feedings
      d. A gastric sump tube coiled in the blind pouch of the proximal esophagus is commonly seen on radiographs.
      e. Air in the stomach and intestines seen on radiographs if TEF is present.

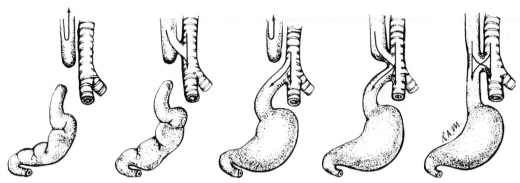

FIG. 27-17 Common forms of esophageal atresia and tracheoesophageal fistula.

    4. Management
       a. Decrease gastroesophageal reflux and decrease risk of aspiration pneumonia
         (1) Upright positioning of the infant
         (2) Suction catheter placement in the proximal pouch to drain secretions
       b. Surgical correction of EA and TEF has >97% survival in infants weighing >1500 g.
  C. Congenital diaphragmatic hernia (CDH) (Figure 27-18)
    1. Characterized by incomplete development of diaphragm, the presence of abdominal organs in the thoracic cavity, and small, underdeveloped lung(s).
    2. CDH occurs in 1 of every 4000 live births.
    3. At least 90% of occurrences of CDH involve the left side, allowing the intestines to migrate into the chest.
    4. The primary factors that influence outcome are
       a. Pulmonary hypertension
       b. Lung hypoplasia
    5. Antenatal diagnosis is confirmed by ultrasound.
    6. Early diagnosis allows the mother to plan for delivery at a high-risk perinatal center.
    7. Management

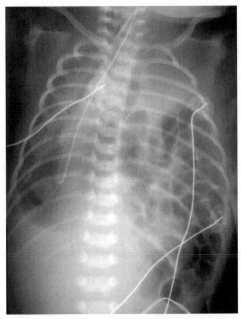

FIG. 27-18 Left-sided congenital diaphragmatic hernia. Note the loops of bowel present in the thoracic cavity.

    a. Orogastric tube placement to collapse stomach and prevent bowel distention from causing further compression of the lung.

    b. Intubation and mechanical ventilation are frequently necessary to stabilize respiratory distress.

    c. If the pulmonary dysfunction is severe, other therapies include

       (1) HFOV

       (2) iNO

       (3) ECMO

       (4) Surgical repair after 7 to 14 days

    d. Early surgical repair is sometimes performed if the CDH causes little or no pulmonary dysfunction.

  8. Prognosis

    a. Approximately 50% for those infants who require mechanical ventilation during the first day of life survive.

    b. Survival is nearly 100% for infants in whom mechanical ventilation is not needed.

XII. Nonrespiratory Disorders of Preterm Neonates

  A. Intraventricular hemorrhage (IVH)

    1. Significant cause of brain injury in premature infants, particularly those weighing <1500 g or born at <32 weeks' gestation.

    2. Incidence of IVH

      a. Occurs early in life: Nearly 90% of cases occur during the first 3 days, and 50% occur during the first 24 hours postpartum.

      b. An estimated 15% of neonates <1500 g develop IVH.

      c. Only 3% to 5% of term infants develop IVH.

    3. Etiology is multifactorial, but all risk factors relate in some way to an alteration in the infant's cerebral blood flow.

      a. Vaginal delivery, breech presentation, and birth asphyxia

      b. Severe respiratory distress, pneumothorax

      c. Seizures

      d. Blood transfusion

      e. Shock, rapid fluid resuscitation

      f. Systemic anticoagulation

    4. Pathophysiology

      a. The most common location of bleeding is in the germinal matrix, a highly vascular area of the brain that gives rise to neurons during the development of the nervous system.

      b. Preterm neonates are vulnerable to fluctuations in hemodynamics because they lack a supporting network to protect the fragile blood vessels in the germinal matrix.

      c. The network of fibers that support these capillary beds develops during the period between 24 and 32 weeks' gestation.

      d. Hemodynamic instability is common in premature neonates. Appropriate systemic blood pressure ranges are not well established.

    5. Clinical presentation of IVH varies from subtle to catastrophic.

      a. Twenty-five percent to 50% of cases are "silent" and can only be diagnosed using cranial ultrasound.

      b. Common signs may be present.

        (1) Apnea

        (2) Hypotension

        (3) Unexpected drop in hematocrit

        (4) Hypotonia

        (5) Full fontanel

        (6) Tonic posturing and seizures

      c. IVH is classified from grade 0 to grade III or grade IV depending on the system used, with higher numbers corresponding to increasing severity of bleeding.

6. Management involves supportive care to prevent extension of the IVH.
   a. Maintain cerebral perfusion
   b. Suppress seizures
   c. Correct coagulopathies
   d. Maintain gas exchange
   e. Neurosurgical interventions, such as shunt placement, are generally reserved for infants with rapid progression of increasing intracranial pressure.
   f. Other therapies remain controversial and have been used with varying success
      (1) Lumbar puncture to decrease the volume of cerebrospinal fluid.
      (2) The use of diuretics, such as furosemide and acetazolamide (Diamox), to reduce CSF formation.
      (3) The use of fibrinolytic therapy to break down clots has been studied.
7. Prognosis
   a. Outcome relates directly to the severity of the hemorrhage.
   b. Infants with mild IVH have outcomes that are similar to infants born at the same gestational age who do not develop IVH.
   c. Mortality is approximately 20% for severe IVH, and survivors generally have long-term morbidity.

B. Necrotizing enterocolitis (NEC) is an inflammatory bowel process resulting in injury to the intestinal mucosa.
   1. Etiology
      a. NEC occurs in 1 in 1000 live births and in approximately 5% of premature infants of <1500 g.
      b. Prematurity is the primary risk factor and is the only risk factor in 20% of all cases.
      c. Associated risk factors include hypoxia and gastrointestinal infection.
      d. NEC is seen in 5% of term infants and has been associated with congenital heart disease, polycythemia, and birth asphyxia.
   2. Pathophysiology
      a. The premature neonate develops inflammation and ischemia in the intestinal mucosa.
      b. Tissue damage extends to the muscular and subserosal layers of the bowel, causing areas of hemorrhage, necrosis, and accumulation of gas.
      c. The classic sign of NEC is a radiograph showing pneumatosis or air trapped in the walls of the intestine.
   3. Clinical presentation
      a. Metabolic acidosis
      b. Intolerance of feedings
      c. Abdominal distention
      d. Bloody stools
   4. Management of NEC
      a. If the infant is stable, supportive care consists of bowel rest, fluid resuscitation, and antibiotics.
      b. Up to one third of infants with NEC develop an intestinal stricture that requires surgery.
      c. Close monitoring for signs of intestinal gangrene and intestinal perforation
      d. Signs of gangrene without intestinal perforation include
         (1) Thrombocytopenia
         (2) Leukopenia
         (3) Shock
         (4) Dilated bowel loops
      e. Intestinal perforation and pneumoperitoneum require immediate surgical intervention.
   5. Prognosis
      a. Recurrent NEC is uncommon.

b. The most common complication is a requirement for long-term parenteral nutrition resulting from inadequate length of the remaining intestine after bowel resection.
c. Survival of infants >1000 g has increased from 50% to 80% in the past 20 years.

BIBLIOGRAPHY

Aloan C: *Respiratory Care of the Newborn: A Clinical Manual.* Philadelphia, JB Lippincott, 1987.

Avery G, Fletcher MA, MacDonald MG: *Neonatalogy, Pathophysiology and Management of the Newborn,* ed 5. Philadelphia, Lippincott Williams & Wilkins, 1999.

Crouse D, Phillips J: Persistent pulmonary hypertension of the newborn. *Perinatol Neonatol* 11:12-38, 1987.

Hageman J, Adams S, Gardner T: Pulmonary complications of hyperventilation therapy for persistent pulmonary hypertension. *Crit Care Med* 13:1013-1014, 1985.

International Committee for the Classification of the Late Stages of Retinopathy of Prematurity. *Pediatrics* 82:37-43, 1988.

Johnson AH, Peacock JL, Greenough A, et al. High-frequency oscillatory ventilation for the prevention of chronic lung disease of prematurity. *N Engl J Med* 347:633-642, 2002.

Koff P, Eitzman D, Neu J: *Neonatal and Pediatric Respiratory Care,* ed 2. St. Louis, Mosby, 1997.

Korones S: *High-Risk Newborn Infants,* ed 4. St. Louis, Mosby, 1986.

Kotecha S, Silverman M: Chronic respiratory complications of neonatal disorders. In Lansau LI, Taussing LM (eds): *Textbook of Pediatric Respiratory Medicine.* St Louis, Mosby, 1999.

Merenstein GB, Gardner SL: *Handbook of Neonatal Intensive Care,* ed 5. St. Louis, Mosby, 2002.

Merritt TA, Hallman M, Berry C, et al: Randomized, placebo-controlled trial of human surfactant given at birth versus rescue administration in very low birth weight infants with lung immaturity. *J Pediatr* 118:581-594, 1991.

Miller MJ, Martin RJ: Apnea of prematurity. *Clin Perinatol* 19:789-808, 1992.

Sahni R, Wung JT, James LS: Controversies in management of persistent pulmonary hypertension of the newborn. *Pediatrics* 94:307-309, 1994.

Schmidt B: Methylxanthine therapy in premature infants: Sound practice, disaster, or fruitless byway? *J Pediatr* 135:526-528, 1999.

Schwartz RM, Luby AM, Scanlon JW, Kellogg RJ: Effect of surfactant on morbidity, mortality, and resource use in newborn infants weighing 500 to 1500 g. *N Engl J Med* 330:1476-1480, 1994.

Sinha SK, Donn SM: *Manual of Neonatal Respiratory Care.* Armonk, NY, Futura, 2000.

Spear M, Spitzer A, Fox W: Hyperventilation therapy for persistent pulmonary hypertension of the newborn. *Perinatol Neonatol,* 9:27-34, 1985.

Stern L: *Diagnosis and Management of Respiratory Disorders in the Newborn.* Reading, MA, Addison-Wesley Publishing, 1983.

Vaucher YE: Bronchopulmonary dysplasia: An enduring challenge. *Pediatr Rev* 23:349-357, 2002.

Walsh-Sukys MC, Cornell DJ, Houston LN, Keszler M, Kanto WP: Treatment of persistent hypertension of the newborn without hyperventilation: an assessment of diffusion of innovation. *Pediatrics* 94:307-309, 1994.

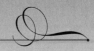

Chapter 28

Mechanical Ventilation of the Newborn

I. **Indications for Mechanical Ventilation of the Newborn Generally Fall into the Following Categories**
   A. Severe oxygenation deficit from
      1. Intrapulmonary shunting
         a. Meconium aspiration syndrome (MAS)
         b. Sepsis
         c. Neonatal pneumonia
      2. Intracardiac shunting
         a. Patent ductus arteriosus (PDA)
         b. Patent foramen ovale (PFO)
   B. Ventilatory failure with elevated PCO_2 and significant respiratory acidosis
      1. Ventilation perfusion mismatch
         a. MAS
         b. Neonatal pneumonia
      2. Apnea associated with
         a. Prematurity
         b. Sepsis
         c. Cold stress
         d. Hypoglycemia
         e. Intraventricular hemorrhage (IVH)
         f. Drugs
   C. Congenital anomalies (see Chapter 27)
      1. Lung hypoplasia
         a. Pulmonary agenesis
         b. Idiopathic bilateral pulmonary hypoplasia
      2. Congenital diaphragmatic hernia (CDH)
         a. Abdominal contents occupy thoracic cavity.
         b. May be left sided, right sided, or bilateral
      3. Tracheal anomalies
         a. Stenosis
         b. Malacia
         c. Tracheal-esophageal fistula
      4. Cardiac defects
         a. Anomalies associated with a PDA.
         b. Any anomaly preventing adequate oxygen delivery

    D. Need for surfactant administration (modified from the AARC Practice Guidelines on Surfactant Administration, 1994)
       1. Surfactant deficiency is associated with prematurity.
          a. Infants born at <35 weeks gestation may be surfactant deficient.
       2. Surfactant replacement after meconium aspiration
          a. Meconium decreases surfactant function.
          b. Replacing surfactant after meconium aspiration can be effective to improve oxygenation.

II. Goals of Mechanical Ventilation
    A. Provide adequate ventilation
       1. P_{CO_2}: 40 to 55 mm Hg, depending on underlying lung pathology
       2. pH: >7.25 to <7.45
    B. Provide adequate oxygenation
       1. P_{O_2}: 50 to 70 mm Hg
       2. SpO_2: >88% to 92% preterm infants and 90% to 95% term infants
    C. Promote patient/ventilator synchrony
       1. Appropriate ventilator mode
       2. Minimize infant's effort with appropriate inspiratory trigger
       3. Provide adequate flow rates to meet the infant's inspiratory flow demands
       4. Terminate inspiration in conjunction with the infant's desire to exhale
       5. Avoid air trapping
    D. Recruit and maintain lung volume
       1. Use positive end-expiratory pressure (PEEP)
       2. Adjust ventilating pressure to attain a tidal volume (V_T) of 5 to 7 ml/kg
       3. Assess lung volume with chest radiography
          a. Aim for lungs inflated to ninth rib bilaterally
       4. Deliver a controlled concentration of oxygen (21% to 100%)

III. Complications of Mechanical Ventilation in the Newborn
    A. Ventilator-induced lung disease
       1. Pulmonary interstitial emphysema (PIE)
       2. Chronic lung disease (CLD)
    B. Hyperoxia
       1. Retinopathy of prematurity (ROP)
       2. Oxygen toxicity
    C. Hypocarbia
       1. Periventricular leukomalacia (PVL)
          a. Softening of the white matter around the ventricles of the brain
          b. Associated with decreased P_{CO_2} in premature infants
          c. Associated with respiratory alkalosis
    D. Decreased cardiac output
       1. Increased intrathoracic pressure with decreased venous return
       2. Decreased oxygen delivery
    E. Pneumothorax
       1. Indiscriminately high ventilating pressure
       2. Nonhomogeneous lung compliance
       3. Air trapping
    F. Pneumonia
       1. Organisms may be introduced into the lungs during mechanical ventilation.
          a. Bypassed upper airway
          b. Organisms introduced during intubation
          c. Inappropriate suctioning technique
          d. Contamination of airway by caregivers

  G. Abdominal distention (gastric air)
    1. Common during bag-mask ventilation (BMV)
    2. Air should be vented through oral or nasal gastric tube.
  H. Mechanical failure
    1. Ventilator malfunction
      a. Loss of compressed gas source
      b. Electrical power loss
      c. Software malfunction
    2. Circuit disconnect
  I. Airway complications
    1. Accidental extubation
      a. Endotracheal tube (ETT) not secure
      b. Infant moving
      c. Tension from ventilator circuit
    2. Airway obstruction
      a. Secretions blocking ETT
      b. ETT against wall of trachea
      c. Kink in ETT
    3. Tracheal/laryngeal damage from ETT
      a. Stenosis
      b. Malacia
      c. Tracheal or pharyngeal tear
      d. Tracheal/esophageal fistula
    4. Bleeding
      a. Trauma during intubation
      b. Aggressive suctioning
    5. Esophageal intubation
      a. Misplaced during intubation
      b. Displaced with tube movement/repositioning

IV. Manual Ventilation

Before initiating mechanical ventilation in the newborn, manual ventilation and intubation are performed.

  A. Manual ventilation (BMV) of the neonate
    1. Equipment
      a. Non–self-inflating bag connected to an oxygen source
      b. Self-inflating bag with oxygen reservoir and PEEP device connected to an oxygen source
      c. Pressure monitoring device
      d. Appropriate size mask attached to bag
    2. Position mask on infant's face
      a. Cover nares, mouth, and tip of chin with mask
      b. Avoid contact with infant's eyes
      c. Hold mask with thumb and index or middle finger on the rim of the mask
      d. Keep infant's chin forward with fourth and fifth fingers
      e. Position head midline with neck slightly extended to optimize airway position
      f. Apply gentle downward pressure to mask to create seal
      g. Squeeze bag, and observe chest movement
      h. If no chest movement reassess the following
        (1) Mask seal on face
        (2) Head position
        (3) Secretions in oral pharynx
        (4) Mouth opening
        (5) Pressure delivered from bag
      i. Ventilate at a rate of approximately 30 to 50 breaths/min

    j.   Deliver a pressure high enough to observe chest movement

    k.   Maintain 4 to 6 cm H_2O pressure at end expiration (PEEP)

V. **Neonatal Intubation**

    A. Unlike the adult airway cuffed ETTs are generally not needed to provide mechanical ventilation to neonates.

    B. The cricoid cartilage is the narrowest point in the neonatal airway.

    C. Appropriately sized uncuffed ETTs are adequate to provide mechanical ventilation and reduce airway complications associated with cuffed tubes.

    D. Approximate ETT sizes for gestational ages and weights are listed in Table 28-1.

    E. Equipment

       1. Laryngoscope with bulbs and batteries

       2. Laryngoscope blade

          a. Miller 0, preterm infant

          b. Miller 1, term infant

       3. Size-appropriate ETTs (see Table 28-1)

       4. Neonatal stylet

       5. Resuscitation bag and size-appropriate mask

       6. Suction canister and suction regulator

       7. Appropriate-sized suction catheters (see Table 28-1)

       8. Tape

       9. Scissors

     10. Stethoscope

    F. Placing the tube

       1. Establish adequate SpO_2 with oxygen, or use BMV if apneic.

       2. Position infant on a flat surface with head midline and neck slightly extended.

       3. Turn on laryngoscope light, and hold laryngoscope in left hand.

       4. Slide the laryngoscope blade over the right side of the tongue.

       5. Advance the blade to the tip of the vallecula.

       6. Lift the tongue out of the way to expose the pharyngeal area.

       7. Observe the vocal cords.

       8. Suction if necessary to improve view of larynx.

       9. Hold the ETT in your right hand, and insert it through the vocal cords as they open.

     10. Insert tube until vocal cord guide on ETT is at the level of the vocal cords.

          a. Estimated distance to insert ETT according to gestational age and weight is outlined in Table 28-2.

     11. Stabilize the tube with one hand, and remove laryngoscope.

     12. If stylet was used withdraw it from the tube, keeping a firm hold on the ETT.

     13. Note landmark on tube associated with infant's lip or nare if nasal tube is used.

     14. With tape or ETT holder secure ETT to infant's face.

    G. Confirming ETT position

       1. Deliver positive pressure breath.

       2. Note condensate in tube.

       3. Auscultate the chest, and confirm bilateral breath sounds.

TABLE 28-1

ETT and Suction Catheter Sizes for Various Gestational Ages and Weights

Gestational Age (wk)	Weight (kg)	ETT Size (mm ID)	Suction Catheter Size (French)
<28	<1	2.5	5
28-34	1-2	3.0	6 or 8
34-38	2-3	3.5	8
>38	>3	3.5-4.0	8 or 10

ETT, Endotracheal tube; *ID*, inner diameter.

TABLE **28-2**

Approximate Distance from Infant's Lip to Tip of a Properly Inserted Oral ETT

Weight in Kilogram	Centimeter Mark at Lip
<1	6.5
1	7
2	8
3	9
4	10

ETT, Endotracheal tube.

    4. Auscultate over stomach to ensure no air entry.
    5. Obtain chest radiograph to evaluate ETT position.
    6. Position head midline in neutral position before chest radiograph.
    7. Chest radiograph should indicate ETT approximately 1 cm above the carina.
    8. Reposition ETT if tube is too high or too low.
  H. Minimize ETT length
    1. Loosen ETT adaptor.
    2. Measure 4 cm from the point where the ETT exits infant's anatomy.
    3. Cut ETT at slight angle, and reinsert ETT adaptor into tube.
    4. Reconfirm breath sounds with stethoscope.

VI. Types of Neonatal Mechanical Ventilators
  A. The condition necessitating mechanical ventilation and the goals of support should be considered when selecting the type of ventilator, ventilator mode, and settings.
  B. Neonatal ventilators are generally classified as conventional or high frequency.
  C. Approaches to conventional and high frequency ventilation are outlined below. (A detailed description of high frequency ventilation is presented in Chapter 42.)
  D. Neonatal conventional ventilation
    1. Neonates requiring mechanical ventilation are most often ventilated using pressure-limited ventilation.
    2. Pressure-limited ventilation is accomplished by setting a peak inspiratory pressure (PIP) that the ventilator targets during each mechanical breath.
    3. Pressure-limited ventilation can be accomplished using any of the following modes.
      a. Synchronized intermittent mandatory ventilation (SIMV) (Figure 28-1)
        (1) Mandatory mechanical rate is set (range generally 15 to 40 breaths/min).
        (2) Minimum PEEP is set (3 to 8 cm H_2O).
        (3) Every mechanical breath starts from the preset PEEP level to a preset inspiratory pressure (generally between 15 and 25 cm H_2O). *Total peak pressure should be less than 30 cm H_2O.*
        (4) The difference between PEEP and the inspiratory pressure target should result in a VT of 5 to 7 ml/kg.
        (5) Inspiratory time is operator controlled on all mandatory breaths (normally set between 0.3 and 0.5 second).
        (6) Continuous flow of gas is available for all nonmechanical (spontaneous) breaths (normally set between 6 and 10 L/min).
        (7) Spontaneous breaths are not supported with positive pressure >PEEP level.
        (8) Pressure support may be applied during spontaneous breaths.
        (9) Delivered oxygen concentrations vary from 21% to 100%.
      b. Assist control (AC) (Figure 28-2)
        (1) Minimum mandatory mechanical rate is set (range, 20 to 40 breaths/min).
        (2) Minimum PEEP is set (3 to 8 cm H_2O).
        (3) Every patient effort triggers a pressure-targeted breath.

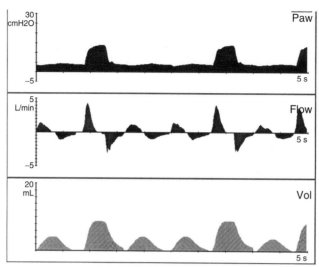

FIG. 28-1 Airway pressure (Paw), flow, and volume (vol) waveforms during synchronized intermittent mandatory ventilation (SIMV) mode using a Drager Baby Log ventilator.

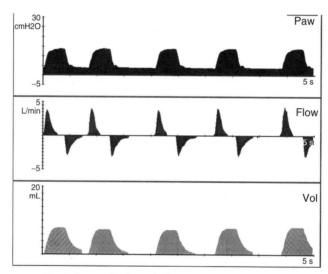

FIG. 28-2 Airway pressure (Paw), flow, and volume (vol) waveforms during pressure assist control mode ventilation using a Drager Baby Log ventilator.

 (4) The difference between PEEP and the pressure target should result in a VT of 5 to 7 ml/kg.

 (5) Inspiratory time is operator controlled for all breaths (0.3 to 0.5 second).

 (6) Delivered oxygen concentrations vary from 21% to 100%.

 (7) *The total peak pressure should be <30 cm H_2O.*

 c. Pressure support (PS) (Figure 28-3)

  (1) No set mandatory rate.

  (2) Rate controlled by patient.

  (3) Minimum PEEP is set (3 to 8 cm H_2O).

  (4) Spontaneous efforts supported with preset pressure (15 to 25 cm H_2O).

  (5) Inspiratory time determined by patient inspiratory flow rate or limited by system default to prevent prolonged inspiration (defaults are ventilator specific and are usually a set maximum time).

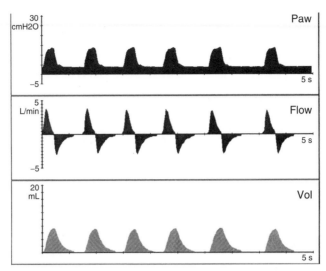

FIG. 28-3 Airway pressure (Paw), flow, and volume (vol) waveforms during pressure support mode ventilation using a Drager Baby Log ventilator.

      (6)   Delivered oxygen concentrations vary from 21% to 100%.
      (7)   *The total peak pressure should be <30 cm H_2O.*
  d. Volume guarantee (Figure 28-4)
      (1)   Specific exhaled VT is targeted on all positive pressure breaths.
      (2)   Peak pressure (PIP) varies breath to breath to maintain target VT.
      (3)   Preset maximum pressure limit *should be <30 cm H_2O.*
      (4)   Peak pressure equals the minimum pressure to deliver selected VT.
      (5)   Oxygen concentrations vary from 21% to 100%.
      (6)   May be used in conjunction with SIMV, AC, or pressure support ventilation (PSV).
      (7)   Normal VT target is 5 to 7 ml/kg.
  e. Continuous positive airway pressure (CPAP) (Figure 28-5)
      (1)   Spontaneous breathing mode
      (2)   Continuous flow through breathing circuit

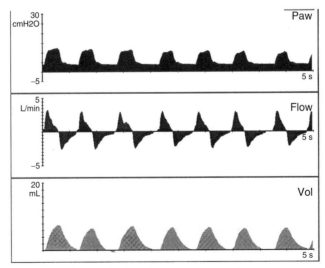

FIG. 28-4 Airway pressure (Paw), flow, and volume (vol) waveforms during pressure support with volume guarantee mode ventilation using a Drager Baby Log ventilator. Note the similarity to Figure 28-3. The only difference is when pressure level requires adjustment because VT is above or below the targeted level.

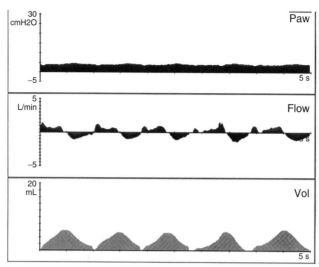

FIG. 28-5 Airway pressure (Paw), flow, and volume (vol) waveforms during continuous positive airway pressure using a Drager Baby Log ventilator.

      (3)   Level of continuous pressure preset (5 to 8 cm H_2O)

      (4)   Delivered oxygen concentration varies from 21% to 100%.

  E. Additional variables affecting neonatal conventional ventilation

    1. Inspiratory trigger is the mechanism that causes the initiation of a mechanical breath and may be a result of time, flow, or pressure.

      a. Time triggering refers to the breath being delivered as a result of a specific set time interval. A set rate of 20 breaths/min would require a time-triggered breath to occur every 3 seconds.

      b. Flow triggering indicates that a mechanical breath is delivered when patient effort is sensed by a change in inspiratory flow. Amount of flow change needed to trigger a breath is operator set and is referred to as the inspiratory sensitivity (0.2 to 0.6 liters per minute [lpm]).

      c. Pressure triggering indicates that a mechanical breath is delivered when patient effort is sensed by a decrease in pressure less than baseline (PEEP) pressure. Amount of pressure change needed to trigger a breath is operator set and is referred to as the inspiratory sensitivity (1 cm H_2O).

    2. Expiratory trigger is the mechanism responsible for cycling a mechanical breath from the inspiratory phase to the expiratory phase and may be a result of time, flow, or pressure.

      a. Time cycling refers to the change from inspiration to expiration as a result of time. If the inspiratory time is set for 0.5 second, expiration begins at the end of the 0.5-second period.

      b. Flow cycling refers to expiration occurring either as a result of a preset decrease of peak flow or an operator-selected decrease in peak flow and is referred to as the expiratory sensitivity.

      c. Pressure cycling refers to expiration being initiated as a result of the system sensing a pressure more than the desired set peak pressure. An example may be when a patient coughs during a delivered breath.

    3. Inspiratory time is from triggering of inspiration to the beginning of expiration

      a. As the inspiratory time increases mean airway pressure increases.

      b. A lengthy inspiration may interfere with expiration.

      c. Too short an inspiration may not allow sufficient time for delivery of the V_T.

    4. Mean airway pressure

      a. Average airway pressure maintained throughout the ventilator cycle.

      b. Affected by rate, inspiratory time, inspiratory flow, pressure, and PEEP.

      c.   Calculated as PEEP + (PIP − PEEP × inspiratory time) and dividing by the total cycle time during pressure-controlled ventilation.

F. High frequency ventilators are considered nonconventional ventilators and offer an alternative approach to ventilate neonates. Currently used high frequency ventilators are categorized as oscillators and flow or jet ventilators (see Chapter 42).

    1. High frequency oscillatory ventilation (HFOV)

       a.   For neonates frequency set in hertz generally ranges from 10 to 15.

       b.   1 Hz = 60 cycles/min

       c.   The higher the rate, the smaller the V_T.

       d.   Ventilation also is affected by changes in pressure amplitude (range, 10 to 45); the higher the pressure amplitude, the larger the V_T.

       e.   Lung volume is adjusted with mean airway pressure (MAP; range, 10 to 20).

       f.   Continuous gas flow allows spontaneous respirations at set MAP.

       g.   Delivered oxygen concentrations vary from 21% to 100%.

    2. High frequency jet ventilator (HFJV)

       a.   Frequency range is 150 to 600 breaths/min.

       b.   Ventilation is achieved by a rapid rate of gas pulses through an injector port.

       c.   Requires a special ETT with a jet port.

       d.   Used in conjunction with a conventional ventilator.

       e.   Delivered oxygen concentrations vary from 21% to 100%.

    3. High frequency flow interrupter ventilator (HFFIV)

       a.   Frequency from 2 to 22 Hz

       b.   Ventilation achieved by frequent short bursts of flow.

       c.   Can be used alone or in conjunction with a conventional ventilator.

       d.   Delivered oxygen concentrations vary from 21% to 100%.

VII. Initiating Ventilatory Support

A. When initiating mechanical ventilation to a neonate the pathology and gestational age of the neonate need to be considered.

B. Either conventional or high frequency ventilation (HFV) can be used as long as the ventilator is adjusted for the specific needs of the infant.

C. Avoiding damage to the lung from positive pressure ventilation is a concern for all gestational ages.

D. Careful attention to recruiting and maintaining appropriate lung volume is essential.

E. Of particular concern for the preterm neonate is retinal damage associated with hyperoxia. Oxygen should be adjusted with specific lower SpO_2 (88% to 93%) maintained to avoid retinal damage.

F. In contrast infants at risk for pulmonary hypertension (e.g., MAS, CDH, and sepsis) need higher SpO_2 (>95%) to avoid constriction of the pulmonary vasculature and pulmonary hypertension leading to an increase in shunting across the ductus arteriosus.

G. Other factors considered when initiating mechanical ventilation

    1. Gestational age

    2. Stage of lung maturity

    3. Maternal history

    4. Prenatal diagnosis

    5. Prenatal treatment

    6. Lung pathology

    7. Parenchymal disease: Unilateral or bilateral

    8. Airway concerns

    9. Current lung volumes on chest radiography

    10. Need for full or partial ventilatory support

H. Typical blood gases and saturation goals

    1. Preterm

       SpO_2: >88% and <94%

       PO_2: 50 to 60

P_{CO_2}: 45 to 60

pH: 7.25 to 7.35

2. Term or postterm

Sp_{O_2}: >95 and <100

P_{O_2}: >60 and <100

P_{CO_2}: 35 to 50

pH: 7.30 to 7.45

I. Preductal and postductal saturations

1. Term or near-term infants (>34 weeks' gestational age) at risk for pulmonary hypertension (primary disease, MAS, and sepsis) or suspected of having persistent pulmonary hypertension of the newborn (PPHN) should be monitored for differences in preductal and postductal saturations.

a. Preductal saturation monitoring is performed on the right upper extremity.

b. Postductal saturation monitoring is performed on left upper or lower extremities.

2. Postductal saturation 5% less than preductal saturation may indicate significant pulmonary hypertension. If present

a. Administer oxygen to maintain Sp_{O_2} >98%.

b. Maintain ventilator support to normalize P_{CO_2} and pH.

c. Obtain echocardiograph.

(1) Confirm pulmonary hypertension.

(2) Determine whether the PDA is essential because of congenital heart disease (see Chapter 27).

d. Establish adequate lung volume, and avoid hyperinflation.

e. Support blood pressure to maintain adequate mean arterial blood pressure.

f. Low systemic blood pressure contributes to decreased oxygen delivery.

g. Consider administering inhaled nitric oxide (iNO; see Section IX, Inhaled Nitric Oxide).

J. Initiating conventional ventilation

1. Infants with hyperinflation (e.g., CLD, PIE)

a. Pressure target to achieve a V_T of 5 to 6 ml/kg.

b. PEEP: 3 to 5 cm H_2O

c. Ventilatory rate to achieve desired P_{CO_2}: typically 25 to 40 breaths/min (monitor for adequate expiratory time)

d. F_IO_2 to achieve desired Sp_{O_2}

e. Inspiratory time: 0.25 to 0.4 second

f. Continuous flow: 5 to 10 lpm

g. Inspiratory trigger is set at minimum level without causing autocycling.

h. *Total peak pressure should be <30 cm H_2O*

2. If hyperinflation is more prominent on one side, position neonate with the more affected side dependent to direct volume to less inflated lung.

3. Reassess lung volume with chest radiography.

4. Infants with low lung volume, term or preterm infants (e.g., respiratory distress syndrome [RDS], pneumonia).

a. Pressure target to achieve V_T of 6 to 8 ml/kg.

b. PEEP: 5 to 8 cm H_2O (consider current lung volume on chest radiography).

c. Rate to achieve desired P_{CO_2}, typically 40 to 50 breaths/min.

d. F_IO_2 to achieve desired Sp_{O_2}

e. Inspiratory time: 0.3 to 0.5 second (consider total rate)

f. Continuous flow: 5 to 10 lpm

g. Inspiratory trigger is set at minimum level without causing autocycling.

h. *Total peak pressure should be <30 cm H_2O.*

K. Initiating HFOV

1. Estimate required MAP for oxygenation during manual ventilation, and increase by 2 cm H_2O when HFOV started.

2. Set pressure amplitude (ΔP) at 10 to 15 cm H_2O, and increase until visible chest wiggle is noted.

   3. Set rate at 10 to 12 Hz.

   4. Set F_IO_2 to achieve desired SpO_2.

   5. Set continuous flow at 15 to 20 lpm.

   6. Set percentage of inspiratory time at 33%.

   7. Obtain blood gas within 1 hour of initiating support.

   8. Assess lung volume on chest radiograph. Aim for nine rib expansion on chest radiograph.

L. Initiating HFJV

   1. Use in conjunction with a conventional ventilator and ETT with jet port.

   2. Set jet rate at 400 to 500 cycles/min with an inspiratory time of 0.02 second.

   3. Use relatively low conventional ventilator rates (<10 breaths/min) with an inspiratory time of 0.4 second.

   4. Set jet pressure target lower than conventional ventilator pressure target.

   5. Aim for similar MAP as on conventional ventilator.

   6. Aim for nine rib expansion on chest radiography.

M. Maintaining ventilator support in neonates requires careful attention to the following.

   1. Cardiac monitoring with alarms set for high and low heart rates

   2. Set ventilator-disconnect alarm. Brief disconnection from the ventilator may result in significant hypoxia, bradycardia, and rapid derecruitment of lung volumes or accidental delivery of higher than needed oxygen concentrations.

   3. Continuous monitoring of SpO_2 to ensure SpO_2 is in target range.

     a. Once an appropriate VT has been achieved (5 to 7 ml/kg) adjustment of F_IO_2 and PEEP should be made to achieve the targeted SpO_2.

   4. Frequent assessment of chest movement/chest wiggle with HFV

     a. Rate and VT are the primary parameters adjusted to optimize PCO_2 on conventional ventilators.

     b. Adjust rate or amplitude on HFV to affect PCO_2 level (with HFV a lower rate results in a higher VT).

     c. Assess breath sounds on conventional ventilation; less appropriate for HFV.

   5. Frequently monitor patient/ventilator synchrony.

     a. Monitor patient's ability to trigger mechanical breaths and cycle to expiration.

     b. Observe for ventilator autotriggering.

     c. Observe for adequate and appropriate inspiratory and expiratory times.

   6. Ensure adequate humidification as addressed in Section VII, N, Assessing Humidification During Mechanical Ventilation.

   7. Maintain security of ETT.

   8. Assess patient's secretions: amount, color, and consistency.

N. Assessing humidification during mechanical ventilation

   1. Evidence of condensation throughout the ventilator circuit is essential to reduce risks of humidity deficits and obstructed airways. This is necessary even with a heated wire ventilator circuit.

   2. Greater risk of ETT obstruction in neonates secondary to smaller ETT (2.5 to 4.0 mm, inner diameter [ID]) sizes than in adults.

   3. Airway temperature should be monitored and maintained at ≥36° C.

   4. Heated wire ventilator circuits reduce circuit rainout and decrease risk of inadvertently instilling condensate into the infant's airway.

     a. Adjust humidifier controls until evidence of condensate is visible throughout inspiratory and expiratory limbs of the ventilator circuit.

O. Suctioning mechanically ventilated neonates

   1. Routine/scheduled suctioning should be discouraged.

   2. Suctioning should be performed when clinically indicated, such as

     a. Decreased VT

     b. Decreased breath sounds

     c. Secretions visible in ETT

   3. Appropriately sized suction catheters should be used; French size approximately two times the ETT ID.

    4. Suction should not exceed 70 to 100 mm Hg negative pressure.

    5. Suction time should not exceed 10 seconds.

    6. Catheter should be measured and inserted to no more than 0.5 cm beyond the ETT.

    7. Complications of suctioning include

        a. Loss of lung volume

        b. Decreased SpO_2

        c. Bradycardia

        d. Increased blood pressure

        e. Increased intracranial pressure

        f. Infection

        g. Mucosal damage

        h. Tracheal bleeding

    8. Increasing F_IO_2 by approximately 0.2 before suctioning may decrease some of the risks associated with suctioning.

        a. Monitor SpO_2 and wean F_IO_2 to baseline soon after the procedure is completed.

P. Assessment for exogenous surfactant administration (Modified from AARC Practice Guidelines for Surfactant Administration)

    1. Preterm infants (<34 weeks' gestation) with evidence of RDS or infants with meconium aspiration should be considered for exogenous surfactant.

    2. The presence of two or more of the conditions outlined in Box 28-1 can be used as indications for exogenous surfactant.

    3. Potential complications of surfactant administration are outlined in Box 28-2.

    4. Guidelines for administering surfactant (specific brand may call for some modifications in these suggested guidelines)

        a. Confirm appropriate ETT position before instilling surfactant.

        b. Allow surfactant to reach room temperature before administering.

        c. Position infant on side.

        d. Divide total dose into four aliquots, and administer two aliquots to each side.

        e. Advance catheter to the tip of the ETT, and instill each aliquot directly into the ETT.

        f. Between each aliquot remove the catheter and allow the ventilator to disperse the surfactant into the lung.

        g. Monitor saturations during administration.

BOX 28-1

Relative Indications for Surfactant Administration

Oxygen concentrations of ≥30% to maintain SpO_2 >88
Low lung volumes on chest radiograph (<8 rib inflation)
Hazy diffuse ground glass appearance on chest radiograph
Compliance: <0.5 ml/cm H_2O
Meconium aspiration

BOX 28-2

Potential Complications of Surfactant Administration

Transient bradycardia
Decreased SpO_2
Tachycardia
Endotracheal tube obstruction
Hypercarbia
Acidosis
Nonuniform distribution of drug

    h. Adjust ventilator support to maintain adequate minute volume during procedure (increased rate, increased pressure) and to avoid lung derecruitment.

    i. Monitor changes in lung compliance after surfactant administration.

    j. Adjust ventilator pressure to avoid hyperinflation, hyperventilation, and hyperoxia after surfactant delivery.

    k. Endotracheal suctioning should be avoided for a minimum of 1 hour after surfactant administration unless clinically indicated.

    l. Reassess ventilator settings and oxygen requirement for potential additional doses.

    m. Consider administering second dose if ventilator and oxygen requirement remain significant (e.g., $F_IO_2 > 0.3$ and MAP > 8).

VIII. **Special Considerations for the Infant with Congenital Cardiac Disease (see Chapter 27)**
- **A.** Infants with certain cardiac lesions depend on maintaining a PDA for survival.
- **B.** Low blood oxygen levels can be essential for these infants.
  1. If sufficiently low SpO_2 cannot be maintained with room air, subatmospheric oxygen concentrations ($\geq$17% O_2) may be needed.
  2. Set continuous flow ventilator to room air.
  3. Add precise flow of nitrogen to continuous flow to reduce F_IO_2 to desired range (generally 17% to 19%).
  4. Table 28-3 outlines nitrogen and air-flow rates to obtain specific concentrations of inspired oxygen.
  5. Analyze inspired gas concentration continuously.
  6. Monitor nitrogen tank pressure.
  7. Monitor SpO_2 continuously.

IX. **Inhaled Nitric Oxide (see Chapter 34)**
- **A.** Initiate iNO at 20 ppm.
  1. Concentrations >20 ppm have not been shown to be more effective in reducing pulmonary hypertension than 20 ppm.
  2. May be administered with conventional or high frequency ventilators.
- **B.** Note preductal and postductal saturations before initiating iNO, and monitor changes after starting iNO.
  1. Effect should be evident within 5 minutes of starting drug.
- **C.** Obtain arterial blood gas after iNO initiated.
- **D.** Wean iNO when clinically indicated (sample iNO weaning protocol in Figure 28-6).

TABLE 28-3

Flow Rate of Nitrogen and Air Needed to Deliver Subatmospheric Oxygen Concentrations

Ventilator Flow	F_IO_2	Nitrogen Flow
8	0.17	1.9
9	0.17	2.1
10	0.17	2.4
11	0.17	2.6
12	0.17	2.8
8	0.18	1.3
9	0.18	1.5
10	0.18	1.7
11	0.18	1.8
12	0.18	2.0
8	0.19	0.8
9	0.19	0.9
10	0.19	1.1
11	0.19	1.2
12	0.19	1.3

iNO weaning algorithm

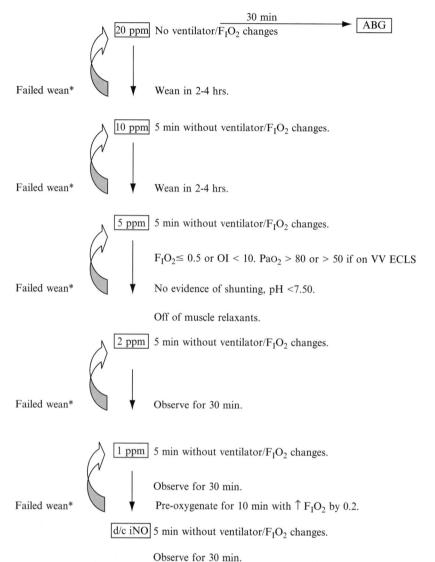

FIG. 28-6 Algorithm for the weaning of inhaled nitric oxide. *Failed wean defined as increase in preductal versus postductal oxygen saturation difference by >5% within 5 minutes of weaning with no change in vital signs/ventilator settings and isotope use. If weaning failed, return to previous inhaled nitric oxide dose and retry weaning in 8 hours. *OI,* Oxygenation index; *VV,* venovenous.

E. Avoid interrupting iNO administration once gas is initiated.
   1. Significant desaturation can occur with iNO interruptions.
F. Connect resuscitation bag to iNO system to avoid interrupting iNO administration if manual ventilation becomes necessary.
G. Monitor iNO tank pressure.
   1. Keep replacement iNO tank available.

H. Complications of iNO
1. Methemoglobinemia: Monitor methemoglobin levels every 24 to 48 hours.
2. Nitrogen dioxide: Purge system at startup, and monitor levels.
3. Rebound hypoxia can occur with discontinuation of iNO.
4. Increase F_IO_2 concentration by 0.1 to 0.2 before discontinuing iNO.

X. **Weaning Mechanical Support**
A. Assessment for weaning generally should begin as soon as the goals for instituting mechanical ventilation have been achieved, provided no new indications for maintaining support have occurred and the infant's ability to breathe is not impeded by any pharmacologic agents.
B. Goals of weaning
1. Maintain adequate oxygenation.
2. Maintain desired PCO_2.
   a. Generally desired or acceptable PCO_2 during weaning is higher than the patient's "normal" PCO_2.
3. Maintain adequate lung volume.
4. Allow infant's contribution to gas exchange to increase.
5. Minimize infant's work of breathing.
C. Weaning from SIMV pressure ventilation
1. Decrease F_IO_2 in increments of 5% to 10% as long as SpO_2 is in desired range.
2. If PEEP is >5 cm H_2O decrease by 1- to 2-cm H_2O increments to a low of 5 cm H_2O once $F_IO_2 \leq 0.3$.
3. Adjust pressure to maintain VT 5 to 7 ml/kg.
4. If PCO_2 is in desired range decrease set rate by 3 to 5 breaths/min, and assess infant's ability to maintain adequate minute ventilation.
D. Weaning from assist control pressure ventilation
1. Decrease F_IO_2 in increments of 5% to 10% as long as SpO_2 is in desired range.
2. If PEEP > 5cm H_2O decrease by 1- to 2-cm H_2O increments to a low of 5 cm H_2O once $F_IO_2 \leq 0.3$.
3. Adjust pressure to maintain VT 5 to 7 ml/kg.
4. Adjust set rate to approximately 15 breaths/min to assess for prolonged periodic breathing and the infant's ability to maintain adequate minute ventilation.
E. Weaning from HFOV
1. Wean O_2 5% to 10% as long as desired SpO_2 is maintained.
2. Decrease MAP 1 to 2 cm H_2O if O_2 concentration is <50%, and monitor for decreased SpO_2 after change.
3. Decrease ΔP in 2- to 5-cm H_2O increments as long as chest "wiggle" is maintained.
F. Weaning from PSV and pressure support volume guarantee (PSVG)
1. Wean PS in increments of 2 cm H_2O to a minimum of approximately 5 cm H_2O above PEEP ensuring VT of 5 to 7 ml/kg.
2. PSVG pressure will automatically wean. Pressure is automatically reduced as compliance improves, maintaining the set delivered VT.
3. Monitor for consistent decreases in airway pressure.
G. Extubation
1. Before extubation consider the following.
2. No significant apnea spells
   a. Methylxanthines may be beneficial for preterm infants.
   b. Sedation requirements not affecting respiratory drive.
3. Hemodynamic stability
   a. No significant bradycardia
   b. No volume or vasopressor requirement to maintain blood pressure
4. Pharmacologic support not affecting respiratory drive.
5. SpO_2 maintained in desired range with $F_IO_2 \leq 0.4$
6. PEEP: ≤6 cm H_2O with good lung volume
7. Mandatory rate: <20 breaths/min

8. MAP: ≤10 cm H_2O
9. Appropriate growth/weight pattern
10. Intact airway

H. Postextubation
1. Establish desired SpO_2, and provide appropriate support to maintain goal.
2. Continuously assess infant's respiratory rate and pattern of breathing.
3. Note signs of respiratory distress.
    a. Grunting
    b. Nasal flaring
    c. Increased respiratory rate
    d. Retractions: Sternal, substernal, and intracostal
    e. Increased oxygen requirement
4. Initiate nasal CPAP postextubation particularly in preterm infants to help maintain lung volume and decrease F_IO_2 requirements.
    a. Select CPAP prongs appropriate for infant's nares.
    b. Maintain vented oral or nasal gastric tube to avoid gastric distention.
5. Infants with more stable lung volumes may extubate to nasal cannulas.
    a. Cannula flow rate is set to maintain desired SpO_2 (typically 50 to 500 ml/min).
    b. Monitor for increased work of breathing (WOB), increased respiratory rate, and increased O_2 requirement.
    c. Wean oxygen as indicated by SpO_2.

XI. **Extracorporeal Life Support**
A. When adequate oxygenation and ventilation cannot be accomplished using the previously described methods, extracorporeal membrane oxygenation may be an option.
B. Indications for extracorporeal life support (ELSO) in neonates
1. Inadequate oxygenation/ventilation despite use of conventional ventilation or HFV and nitric oxide
    a. Oxygenation index (OI = $[MAP \times F_IO_2]/PaO_2$) > 0.4 on two or more consecutive blood gases at least 30 minutes apart
    b. PCO_2 > 65 with pH < 7.25 despite attempts to optimize ventilation
2. Evidence of barotrauma with applied support
    a. Persistent air leak through chest tubes
    b. Increasing air leaks, reaccumulating pneumothorax, and pneumomediastinum
3. Underlying condition potentially reversible
    a. MAS
    b. Neonatal sepsis
    c. Pulmonary hypertension
    d. CDH
4. Gestational age > 34 weeks
5. Weight > 2.2 kg
6. No contraindication to systemic anticoagulation

C. Methods of ECLS support
1. Extracorporeal support consists of vascular cannula(s), a circuit, pump, an oxygenator, heat exchanger, and an oxygen source (Figure 28-7).
2. Venoarterial (VA) ECLS requires cannulation of two vessels, usually the right common carotid artery and the right internal jugular vein (Figure 28-8).
3. Venovenous (VV) ECLS requires cannulation of a single vessel, the right internal jugular vein, with a double-lumen cannula (Figure 28-9).
4. With both types of support blood is drained from the right atrium to the extracorporeal circuit.
5. A pump propels the drained blood through an oxygenator.
6. The oxygenator consists of a two-sided membrane.
7. Desaturated (venous) blood flows along one side of the membrane.

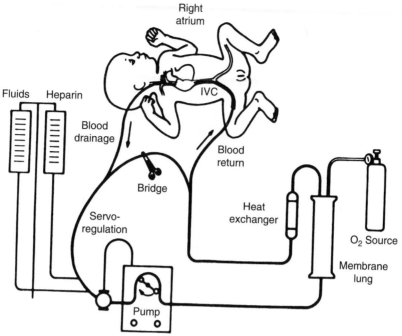

FIG. 28-7 Typical extracorporeal life support (ELSO) circuit used in neonates and pediatric patients (see text for details).

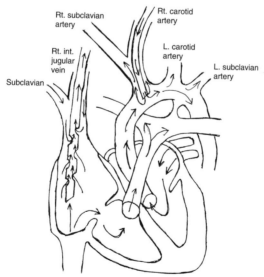

FIG. 28-8 Details of blood movement during venous-arterial (VA) extracorporeal life support (ELSO). Blood is removed from the neonate via a catheter in the right internal jugular vein extending into the right atrium. Blood returns to the neonate via a catheter in the right carotid artery.

8. Gas with a higher partial pressure of oxygen flows along the opposite side of the membrane.

9. The difference in partial pressure results in oxygen diffusing into the venous blood.

10. Similarly the venous blood has a higher partial pressure of carbon dioxide than the gas side of the membrane, resulting in carbon dioxide diffusing into the gas side of the membrane, where it is eliminated to the atmosphere.

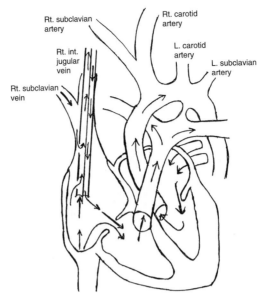

FIG. 28-9 Catheter placement during venovenous (VV) extracorporeal life support (ELSO). A double-lumen catheter is placed into the right internal jugular vein extending into the right atrium. Blood enters and leaves the neonate's circulation via this single catheter.

11. Fully saturated blood with the desired carbon dioxide level exits the membrane oxygenator.
12. The blood is warmed to the desired temperature as it flows through a blood warmer before returning to the infant.
13. During VA support the blood is returned to the infant's arterial circulation through the arterial cannula.
14. During VV support the oxygenated blood is returned through a second lumen of the venous cannula to the infant's right heart, and with adequate cardiac function the oxygenated blood is delivered to the arterial circulation.
15. Systemic anticoagulation is necessary to reduce the potential formation of clots on the artificial surfaces of the circuit, oxygenator, and cannulas.

D. Ventilator management during ECLS
1. ECLS allows significant reduction in the inspired concentration of oxygen.
   a. VA support: $F_IO_2 < 0.21$ to 0.30
   b. VV support: F_IO_2 = approximately 0.4
2. Set rate can be minimized (6 to 10 breaths/min) as CO_2 is eliminated through the oxygenator.
3. PIP is minimized to slightly more than PEEP level to allow lung rest.
4. PEEP is maintained at 8 to 15 cm H_2O to keep the lungs from total collapse.

E. ECLS course
1. Lung rest occurs while the underlying condition is reversed.
2. Changes in the native lung on chest radiographs and improvement in blood gases without increases in ECLS support are indications for weaning from ECLS.
3. Ventilator support is increased as ECLS support is decreased.
4. ECLS support is discontinued when gas exchange can be accomplished by F_IO_2 and ventilator pressures less likely to cause lung damage.
   a. PIP: <25 cm H_2O to maintain VT of 5 to 7 ml/kg
   b. Rates: 30 to 40 breaths/min
   c. PEEP: 6 to 8 cm H_2O
   d. F_IO_2: <0.4

BOX 28-3

Risks Associated with Extracorporeal Support

Bleeding
Clotting
Air embolization
Equipment failure
Infection

5. Cannulated vessels are either ligated or repaired at decannulation.
6. Systemic anticoagulation is discontinued.
7. Major risks of ECLS are outlined in Box 28-3.
8. Mechanical ventilation is weaned as the infant's condition improves.

BIBLIOGRAPHY

Branson RD, et al: *Respiratory Care Equipment,* ed 2. Philadelphia, Lippincott Williams & Wilkins, 2000.

Carlo WA, et al: Minimal ventilation to prevent bronchopulmonary dysplasia in extremely low birth weight infants. *J Pediatr* 141:370-374, 2002.

Casper CJ, et al: Cumulative metaanalysis of high-frequency versus conventional ventilation in premature neonates. *Am J Respir Crit Care* 168:1150-1155, 2003.

Cochrane National Review Group: Evaluation of the effect of surfactant administration in the treatment of term infants with meconium aspiration syndrome. Available at: *www.nichd.nih.gov.* Accessed March 1, 2004.

Courtney SE, Durand DJ, et al: High frequency oscillatory ventilation vs conventional mechanical ventilation for very-low-birth-weight infants. *N Engl J Med* 347:643-652, 2002.

Extracorporeal Life Support Organization: *ECMO Specialist Training Manual,* ed 2. Ann Arbor, MI, ELSO, 1999.

Goldsmith JP, Karotkin EH: *Assisted Ventilation of the Neonate,* ed 4. Philadelphia, WB Saunders, 2004.

Harwood R: *Exam Review and Study Guide for Perinatal/Pediatric Respiratory Care.* Philadelphia, FA Davis, 1999.

Hess D, et al: *Respiratory Care Principles and Practices.* Philadelphia, WB Saunders, 2002.

Kattwinkel J, Niermeyer S: *Neonatal Resuscitation Textbook,* ed 4. Elk Grove Village, IL, American Academy of Pediatrics/AHA, 2000.

Moriette G, et al: Prospective randomized multicenter comparison of high frequency oscillatory ventilation and conventional ventilation in pre-term infants less than thirty weeks with respiratory distress syndrome. *Pediatrics* 107:363-372, 2001.

Schreiber MD, et al: Inhaled nitric oxide in premature infants with the respiratory distress syndrome. *N Engl J Med* 349:2099-2107, 2003.

Soll RF, Morley CJ: Prophylactic versus selective use of surfactant for preventing morbidity and mortality in preterm infants. Cochrane Database Syst Rev 2:CD000510, 2000.

Surfactant Replacement Therapy. AARC Clinical Practice Guidelines. *Respir Care* 39:824-829, 1994.

Wilkins RL, Stoller JL, Scanlon CR: *Egan's Fundamentals of Respiratory Care,* ed 8. St. Louis, Mosby, 2003.

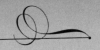

Chapter 29

Respiratory Disorders of the Pediatric Patient

I. **Pediatric Patients Are Classified by Age as Follows**
   A. Premature: <37 weeks gestational age
   B. Newborn: Up to 30 days old
   C. Infant: 30 days to 12 months
   D. Child: 1 year to 8 to 12 years
   E. Teenager: 13 to 18 years

II. **Evaluation of the Pediatric Patient for Respiratory Distress**
   A. Chief complaint
      1. Is the problem acute, recurrent, or chronic?
      2. Is the problem from ingestion, inhalation, trauma, or accident?
   B. History
      1. Current medications
      2. Medical history
   C. Physical examination
      1. Airway
      2. Breathing
      3. Cardiovascular status
      4. Activity level
      5. Conscious or unconscious
   D. Common pediatric disorders
      1. Age 1 to 24 months
         a. Cystic fibrosis
         b. Bronchiolitis
         c. Croup
         d. Epiglottitis
         e. Ingestion of poison
         f. Foreign body aspiration
      2. Age 2 to 5 years
         a. Croup
         b. Asthma (reactive airway disease)
         c. Cystic fibrosis (CF)
         d. Ingestion of poison
         e. Foreign body aspiration
   E. The majority of pediatric admissions are for respiratory-related problems.

F. Causes of respiratory problems
    1. Nasal
        a. Enlarged adenoids
        b. Deviated nasal septum
        c. Nasal polyps
    2. Oropharyngeal
        a. Enlargement of tonsils
        b. Tumors or cysts
    3. Larynx
        a. Epiglottitis
        b. Postendotracheal intubation (vocal cord problems/paralysis)
        c. Tumors or cysts
    4. Tracheal
        a. Stenosis
        b. Trauma
        c. Tumors
    5. Bronchi
        a. Excessive secretions (CF)
        b. Spasm of smooth muscle (asthma)
        c. Inflammation (bronchiolitis, asthma)
    6. Obstruction of airway
        a. Tongue
        b. Food
        c. Teeth, pins, and coins
        d. Vomitus
        e. Infection (croup, epiglottitis)

G. Clinical identification of respiratory distress
    1. Restless or irritable
    2. Nasal flaring
    3. Tracheal tug (suprasternal retractions)
    4. Retractions (intercostal)
    5. Seesaw (paradoxical) breathing
    6. Flaring of lower rib cage
    7. Decreased or absent breath sounds
    8. Tachypnea
        a. Newborn: >60 breaths/min
        b. Up to 1 year: >35 breaths/min
    9. Cyanosis
    10. Cough

H. Other signs of clinical significance
    1. Temperature
        a. Normal temperature: 36.1° C to 37° C
        b. Low-grade fever: 37.1° C to 38.4° C (normally viral infection)
        c. High-grade fever: ≥38.4° C (normally bacterial infection)
    2. Respiratory status
        a. Dyspnea
        b. Apnea
        c. Chest pain
        d. Hemoptysis
    3. Cardiovascular status
        a. Pulse: Normal
            (1) Up to age 2 years: 130 to 140 beats/min
            (2) Age 2 to 10 years: 80 beats/min
            (3) Age >10 years: 70 to 80 beats/min
        b. Pulse: Tachycardia

        (1)   Up to age 2 years: >140 beats/min
        (2)   Age 2 to 10 years: >130 beats/min
        (3)   Age >10 years: >100 beats/min
    c. Pulse: Bradycardia
        (1)   Up to age 2 years: <100 beats/min
        (2)   Age 2 to 10 years: <60 beats/min
        (3)   Age >10 years: <50 beats/min
    d. Blood pressure
        (1)   Age 1 to 24 months: 100/70 mm Hg
        (2)   >2 years of age
           (a) Upper limits for systolic pressure: $90 + (2 \times \text{years in age})$ mm Hg
           (b) Lower limits for systolic pressure: $70 + (2 \times \text{years in age})$ mm Hg

III. **Croup (Laryngotracheobronchitis or LTB)**
    A. Description
      1. Viral infection involving the larynx and subglottic area
      2. Infectious agent: Parainfluenza virus (most common) or *Mycoplasma pneumoniae* and respiratory syncytial virus (RSV)
      3. Occurs in infants and children aged 6 months to 3 years
      4. Occurs primarily in fall and winter
    B. Clinical presentation
      1. Gradual onset (1 to 3 days)
      2. Common cold–like symptoms
      3. Runny nose
      4. Hoarseness
      5. Barking cough
      6. Retractions
      7. Usage of accessory muscles
      8. Low-grade fever
      9. Stridor
    C. Radiologic presentation (Figure 29-1)
      1. Lateral neck chest radiograph shows subglottic narrowing (steeple sign).
      2. Haziness of this area indicates swelling.

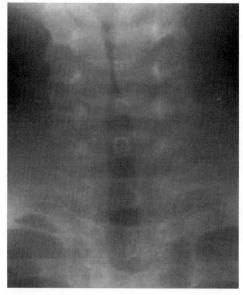

FIG. 29-1 Frontal radiograph of neck of a child with croup. Notice the narrowing of airway showing the "steeple" sign.

D. Management
1. Most children are treated at home after consult with a physician.
2. Keep child well hydrated.
3. Keep child calm, prevent agitation and crying.
4. Audible stridor and restlessness may require hospitalization.
5. Cool aerosol therapy via mask (mist/croup tents are no longer the standard).
6. Inhaled racemic epinephrine via small volume nebulizer every 1 to 2 hours.
7. Intramuscular or intravenous steroids; dexamethasone 0.6 mg/kg is the treatment of choice.
8. Severe cases may require He/O$_2$ therapy for maximum deposition of aerosolized medication.
9. Sedation is contraindicated secondary to possible respiratory depression.
10. Monitor using pulse oximetry and use of arterial or capillary blood gases once patient is stabilized.
11. Observe for signs of impending respiratory failure, including
    a. Increasing heart rate (tachycardia)
    b. Restlessness and lethargy
    c. Worsening retractions
    d. Desaturation with increased F$_I$O$_2$
    e. Decreased breath sounds
12. Intubate when
    a. Aforementioned signs of failure are present.
    b. Three percent to 6% of children with LTB require intubation.
    c. Documented acidosis/hypoxemia with a blood gas
    d. Provide good pulmonary toilet postintubation
    e. Wean ventilator parameters to baseline
    f. Extubate usually within 2 to 5 days.

IV. **Epiglottitis**
A. Description
1. Bacterial infection affecting the supraglottic structures
2. Causative agent in >80% of cases is *Haemophilus influenzae* type B bacteria.
3. Produces an enlarged cherry red epiglottis, which can either partially or completely obstruct the airway
4. Decreased incidence of complete obstruction secondary to conjugate *H. influenzae* vaccinations
5. Usually manifested in children aged 3 to 7 years
B. Clinical presentation
1. Abrupt onset: 4 to 8 hours
2. Noticeable signs of upper airway obstruction
3. Fever
4. Hoarseness
5. Cough
6. Lethargic or irritated
7. Sore throat
8. Drooling (inability to swallow)
9. Hyperextension of the neck and chest thrust forward (characteristic sitting or tripod position)
10. Stridor
11. Suprasternal retractions and nasal flaring
C. Radiologic findings (Figure 29-2)
1. For typical clinical presentations, radiographs may not be needed.
2. A lateral neck film may differentiate croup from epiglottitis.
3. Lateral neck radiograph revealing classic "thumb sign" of a swollen epiglottis and enlarged aryepiglottic folds.
4. Vallecula is obliterated on lateral neck radiograph.

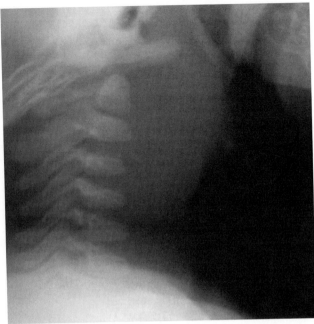

FIG. 29-2 Lateral radiograph of the neck of a child with epiglottitis. Notice the enlarged epiglottis showing the "thumb" sign.

D. Management
1. Keep child as calm as possible.
2. Deliver cool mist aerosol to patient as tolerated.
3. Have parent or guardian hold child if possible to keep calm.
4. Have intubation and resuscitation equipment ready at the bedside.
5. Child's mouth, tonsils, or oropharynx should not be examined unless under controlled situation.
6. If intubation required, patient should be taken to an operating room.
7. Only skilled anesthesiologists should intubate.
8. Standby tracheotomy/cricothyroidotomy equipment should also be available.
9. Use of an oral or nasal endotracheal tube (ETT) should be 0.5 mm smaller than predicted to prevent possible trauma.
10. After the airway is secured, provide patient with good pulmonary toilet.
11. Sedate patient as necessary.
12. Obtain sputum and blood cultures.
13. Hydrate patient intravenously.
14. Initiate antibiotic therapy.
15. Maintain patient intubated for 24 to 48 hours.
16. Assess for extubation.
17. Extubate only when an audible leak is heard around the ETT.
18. Aerosolized racemic epinephrine may be required after extubation.
19. Also provide patient with cool mist aerosol, and look for signs of possible tracheal/glottic swelling postextubation.
20. Table 29-1 compares and contrasts the signs and etiology of croup and epiglottitis.

V. **Bronchiolitis (Box 29-1)**
A. Description
1. An inflammatory disease of the bronchioles
2. The most common cause of lower respiratory tract obstruction in the young child
3. Most common in children aged <2 years

TABLE **29-1**		

Comparison of Croup and Epiglottitis

Factor	Croup	Epiglottitis
Etiology	Virus: Parainfluenza	Bacteria: *Haemophilus influenzae*
White blood cell count	Normal	Elevated
Onset	Gradual	Sudden
Cough	Dry, barking	Muffled
Lateral neck radiographic film	Subglottic inflammation	Supraglottic inflammation
Treatment	Symptomatic	Symptomatic, artificial airway frequently required

BOX 29-1

Presentation, Clinical Features, and Treatment of Bronchiolitis

- Most common in children aged <2 years
- Most common infectious agents:
  - Respiratory syncytial virus (RSV)
  - Parainfluenza virus
- Affects the lower respiratory tract
- Diagnosis: Nasopharyngeal cultures
- Management of mild cases:
  - Albuterol
  - Racemic epinephrine
  - Atrovent
  - RSV-specific immunoglobulin therapy
- Management of severe cases:
  - All of the above
  - Ribavirin (virazole): Controversial, currently infrequently used
  - Intubation and mechanical ventilation
- Symptoms resolve in 3 to 5 days

   4. Most common infectious agents are RSV and parainfluenza viruses.
   5. Other infectious agents include parainfluenza types 1 and 3, adenovirus, and *M. pneumoniae*.
   6. Chemical factors may also precipitate condition (e.g., cigar, cigarette smoke).
   7. Occurs most frequently in the fall and winter
   8. Viruses are transmitted via contact with infected secretions.
   B. Clinical presentation
      1. A lower respiratory tract infection after 2 to 3 days of
         a. Cough
         b. Tachypnea, respiratory rate >50 breaths/min
         c. Low-grade temperature
         d. Intercostal retractions
         e. Wheezing
         f. Fine rales
         g. Poor appetite
         h. Cyanosis
      2. It may be difficult to differentiate bronchiolitis from asthma in the younger patient.
   C. Radiologic findings
      1. Hyperinflation
      2. Consolidation in lower lobes
      3. Peribronchiolar thickening
   D. Diagnosis
      1. Usually made by analysis of nasopharyngeal cultures
      2. Medical history

   3. Clinical signs and symptoms
   4. Use immunofluorescent staining techniques for presence of RSV antigen.
   5. Rule out CF, and perform sweat test.
E. Management of mild symptoms
   1. Symptoms
      a. Respiratory rate: 30 to 45 breaths/min
      b. Wheezing
      c. Blood gases (capillary or arterial)
      d. Mild retractions
   2. Isolation
   3. Frequent suctioning
   4. Cool mist aerosol therapy
   5. Bronchodilators
      a. Albuterol
      b. Racemic epinephrine
      c. Atrovent
   6. RSV-specific immunoglobulin therapy
F. Management of severe symptoms
   1. Symptoms
      a. Respiratory rate: >45 breaths/min
      b. Distant or inaudible breath sounds
      c. Cyanosis
      d. Worsening arterial or capillary blood gas
      e. Severe retractions
   2. Ribavirin (Virazole)
      a. Its use in the clinical arena is highly controversial and has fallen out of favor in most institutions.
      b. Ribavirin is delivered via small particle aerosol generator (SPAG) unit.
      c. Patient must have underlying cardiac disease.
      d. Underlying chronic lung disease (e.g., bronchopulmonary dysplasia [BPD])
      e. Immunosuppressed children (e.g., HIV, organ transplant)
      f. Can be used in conjunction with mechanical ventilator
      g. Not recommended
   3. Monitor the PaO_2 and $PaCO_2$ for impending respiratory failure.
   4. Monitor patient's fluid status.
   5. Follow weight loss and gain closely.
   6. Intubate when
      a. Breath sounds are absent.
      b. The patient is lethargic and difficult to arouse.
      c. The patient appears exhausted.
      d. Desaturation continues despite increased F_IO_2 requirement.
      e. Periods of apnea are observed.
   7. Once intubated
      a. Provide patient with adequate sedation.
      b. Vigorous chest physiotherapy (CPT) should be performed.
      c. Continue bronchodilator treatment through mechanical ventilator.
      d. Maintain appropriate fluid status.
      e. Monitor input and output closely.
      f. Look for resolution of symptoms 3 to 5 days postintubation.
      g. May take longer if patient has underlying disease process.

VI. **Cystic Fibrosis (Box 29-2)**
   A. Description
      1. Inherited as a recessive disorder that involves the exocrine glands
      2. Disorder prompted by mutations of a single gene pinpointed on the seventh chromosome

BOX 29-2

Presentation, Clinical Features, and Management of Cystic Fibrosis

- Inherited: Recessive exocrine gland disorder
- Excessive viscid secretion from exocrine glands
- Diagnosis: High sweat electrolyte concentration
- 60% diagnosed by 1 year, 90% by 5 years
- Survival: >30 years
- Pulmonary problems:
  - Chronic infection: Common pathogens, *Pseudomonas aeruginosa*, and *Staphylococcus aureus*
  - Excessive thick, tenacious mucus
- Other early clinical features
  - Inability to pass meconium within 12 hours of birth
  - Digital clubbing
  - Airway obstruction
  - Chronic pancreatic insufficiency
  - Fatigue, anorexia, and weight loss
  - Growth retardation
- Treatment
  - Airway clearance
  - Aerosolized Pulmozyme
  - Bronchodilators
  - Antiinflammatory agents
  - Lung transplantation
- Death almost always from acute or chronic respiratory failure

3. *Autosomal recessive* means that the CF gene can occur in either male or female children.
4. Disease affects nearly every organ system in the body that contains epithelial surfaces.
5. CF causes exocrine glands to produce abnormally viscid secretions, as well as pancreatic deficiency and a high sweat electrolyte concentration.
6. Sixty percent of patients are diagnosed during the first year of life, and 90% are diagnosed by age 5 years.
7. Median survival age greatly increased because of newer treatment modalities, now >30 years of age.

B. Clinical manifestations result from abnormal secretions from the sweat glands, bronchial glands, mucosal glands, small intestine, pancreas, and bile ducts of the liver.
1. Sweat glands: There is abnormal absorption of sodium and chloride (two to five times normal), but water reabsorption is normal.
2. Pancreas: Eighty percent of patients with CF have pancreatic deficiency. A low-volume, highly viscid fluid that has few enzymes to break down ingested fat is secreted. Insulin secretion is impaired as a result of fibrosis. Diabetes is often present in older children.
3. Intestine: Mucous glands of the intestine are involved, causing tarry, viscous feces in the newborn. A distended abdomen results from failure to pass feces.
4. Liver: Lesions found in the liver are similar to those of the pancreas. Blockage of bile ducts and fibrosis results.
5. Bronchial glands: Excessive thick, tenacious mucus is produced, which obstructs small airways and produces respiratory insufficiency and pulmonary hypertension.

C. Pulmonary pathophysiology
1. At birth the size of the bronchial glands is normal, but hypertrophy and hypersecretion quickly develop.
2. Obstruction of small bronchi and bronchioles from thick, tenacious secretions occurs.
3. Overdistention of the lung and dilation of airways follow.
4. Infection from stagnant mucus, *Pseudomonas aeruginosa*, and *Staphylococcus aureus* is common.
5. Progression of the disease results in
   a. Consolidation and atelectasis

      b. Destruction of respiratory epithelium and simple squamous epithelium

      c. Pneumonitis

      d. Fibrosis

      e. Abscesses

  6. Progressive respiratory failure occurs with marked hypercapnia, hypoxemia, and pulmonary hypertension.

  7. Congestive heart failure follows.

  8. Ninety-eight percent of patients die from cardiorespiratory failure.

D. Diagnosis

  1. Diagnosis is based on clinical symptoms and family history.

  2. In the newborn failure to pass meconium (first feces) within 12 hours of birth is common.

  3. *CFTR* is the gene responsible for CF.

  4. Diagnosis is based on the combination of one or more typical phenotypic features and evidence of *CFTR* malfunction.

      a. Chronic sinopulmonary disease

      b. Persistent infection with typical CF pathogen (e.g., *S. aureus*, *P. aeruginosa*)

      c. Chronic cough, sputum

      d. Persistent chest radiographic abnormality (e.g., bronchiectasis, hyperinflation, and atelectasis)

      e. Airway obstruction (e.g., wheezing, decreased expiratory flows)

      f. Nasal polyps or radiographic sinus involvement

      g. Digital clubbing

  5. Gastrointestinal, nutritional abnormality

      a. Intestinal: Meconium ileus, rectal prolapse, and distal intestinal obstruction syndrome

      b. Pancreatic: Pancreatic insufficiency, recurrent pancreatitis

      c. Hepatic: Focal biliary cirrhosis

      d. Nutritional: Malnutrition, hypoproteinemia, and fat-soluble vitamin deficiency

  6. Salt loss syndrome

      a. Acute salt depletion

      b. Chronic metabolic alkalosis

  7. Male urogenital abnormality

      a. Obstructive azoospermia resulting from congenital bilateral absence of the vas deferens (CBAVD)

  8. Presence of the *CFTR* gene abnormality

      a. Determined by a sweat chloride test

      b. A result >60 mmol/L on two occasions (minimum 75 mg of sweat collected during 30 minutes) indicates a positive presence.

      c. *CFTR* mutational analysis

      d. Two mutant *CTFR* alleles required

      e. Nasal potential difference (PD) testing

      f. Higher basal PD

      g. Greater amiloride-sensitive PD

      h. Absent or minimal change in PD after isoproterenol in chloride-free perfusion solution

E. Physical presentation

  1. Earliest pulmonary symptoms

      a. Dry, hacking cough

      b. Progression of cough to more frequent coughing spells with production of large quantities of secretions

      c. Cough is paroxysmal

      d. Fatigue, anorexia, and weight loss

      e. Chest radiograph shows hyperinflation (with flattened diaphragms in the older child).

      f. Recurrent wheezing

      g. Dyspnea on exertion

      h. Airways become persistently infected with gram-negative pathogens, such as *P. aeruginosa*.

      i. Symptoms recur more often than usual and become less responsive to intensive and aggressive therapy.

  2. The older child has muscular weakness and growth retardation, short stature, reproductive tract underdevelopment, and clubbing of the digits.

  3. Development of subpleural air cysts is likely responsible for increased incidence of spontaneous pneumothorax; 5% to 8% in children and 16% to 20% in adults.

  4. Hemoptysis (>240 ml in 24 hours) can occur, although it is now less common, occurring in approximately 5% of patients.

  5. Respiratory failure caused by progressive airway obstruction and destruction is the universal cause of death in 98% of CF patients.

F. Pulmonary function studies

  1. Pulmonary function testing is a sensitive and reliable way to evaluate the severity of CF lung disease.

  2. It is an objective means to determine when a patient's clinical status has deteriorated and requires more intensive therapy.

  3. Primary alteration is a decrease in compliance and an increase in respiratory rate.

  4. The $PaCO_2$ level is reduced or near normal in the early stages of the disease, progressing to hypercapnia.

  5. The first abnormality detected is obstruction of small airways.

  6. Indicated by reduced flow rates at low lung volumes (FEF 25% to 75%).

  7. Elevation of residual volume-to-total lung capacity ratio also seen (RV/TLC).

  8. FEV_1 is the best indicator of exercise capacity and disability and somewhat predictive of length of survival.

  9. Hypoxemia develops as airway obstruction worsens as a result of ventilation/perfusion mismatching.

  10. Spirometric parameters are poor predictors for the need of oxygen therapy.

  11. Supplemental oxygen is most always required in later stages of disease.

  12. Oxygen therapy generally is effective for the prevention of pulmonary hypertension and cor pulmonale.

  13. Severe airway disease causes retention of carbon dioxide because of an increased dead space-to-tidal volume ratio (VD/VT), which in turn may worsen hypoxemia.

  14. Carbon dioxide retention and severe airway obstruction along with resting hypoxemia are negative predictors of survival.

  15. Lung transplantation is another option for those with deteriorating pulmonary function tests (PFTs).

  16. FEV_1 of approximately 30% of predicted maximum FEV_1 considered an indication for lung transplantation, although other factors should be considered.

G. Radiologic findings

  1. Often normal in the early course of the disease

  2. Hyperinflation may be the first radiologic finding in children.

  3. Increased interstitial markings are common.

  4. These progress to typical findings of cystic bronchiectasis.

  5. Atelectasis in the right upper lobe frequently is seen.

  6. Progression of the disease leads to hyperinflation and flattening of the diaphragms and increased anteroposterior diameter.

  7. The heart shadow is narrowed.

  8. Chest computerized tomography (CT) scans may be useful to detect earlier physiologic changes not visible on routine chest radiographs.

  9. Chest CT indicated for the CF patient suspected of having nontuberculous mycobacterium (NTM). NTM infection demonstrates multiple small parenchymal nodules primarily in the middle and lower lobes and patchy airspace disease.

H. Management

  1. Airway clearance techniques (see Chapter 36)

a. Physical maneuvers to promote the movement of airway secretions from small toward central airways where they may be removed by cough.
b. Chest percussion and postural drainage are most effective.
c. Postural drainage uses multiple body positions to facilitate drainage of individual lung segments via gravity.
d. Performed in conjunction with chest percussion and vibration
e. Has been shown to improve mucus clearance and pulmonary function in otherwise stable patients
f. Time consuming and often difficult for patient to tolerate
g. Mechanical percussors are sometimes used.
h. Forced expiratory maneuvers, positive expiratory pressure (PEP) devices, the flutter valve, and exercise all assist in airway clearance.
i. The high frequency chest compression vest (ThAIRapy vest), autogenic drainage, and the active cycle of breathing technique are also used.
j. Exercise has been shown to assist secretion removal, but the need for oxygen therapy during exercise should be assessed periodically.

2. Aerosolized recombinant human DNase (rhDNase; Pulmozyme) (see Chapter 17)
   a. Used to modify the transportability of secretions
   b. DNA is a major component of CF secretions, which are extremely viscous and poorly transportable within the airway.
   c. rhDNase was developed and approved for use in patients with CF in 1994.
   d. A single daily use has been shown to improve FEV_1 by 6% and to decrease exacerbations by 28%, but response can be variable.
   e. Most patients show a response within 1 to 3 months after initiation of drug use.
   f. Efficacy of rhDNase over longer periods and its impact on mortality remain unknown.

3. Other mucus-modifying agents
   a. N-acetyl-L-cysteine (Mucomyst) is most commonly used.
   b. Agent reduces disulfide bonds in mucins, thus making them less viscous.
   c. This agent is known to increase epithelial injury or inflammation.
   d. Despite its common use it is not approved for inhalation, and no data demonstrate it improves secretion removal when aerosolized.
   e. Most effective when instilled during bronchoscopy
   f. Not recommended for aerosol use

4. Hypertonic saline solutions are used to promote hydration of inspissated mucous secretions.
   a. Three percent NaCl is used after albuterol pretreatment.
   b. Can induce bronchospasm in those with reactive airways
   c. Normally not recommended

5. Antibiotics
   a. Oral and inhaled antibiotics are an important part of a standard CF regimen.
   b. Oral antibiotics are used episodically when new respiratory symptoms develop.
   c. Ciprofloxacin is the primary oral agent to manage *P. aeruginosa*, but rapid development of resistance should be considered.
   d. There are a limited number of oral agents available for management of *P. aeruginosa*.
   e. Inhaled aminoglycosides and other parenteral antibiotics are now used.
   f. Inhaled route of administration has the benefit of achieving high drug levels in airway secretions.
   g. Minimal systemic levels are developed during inhalation, avoiding toxicity.
   h. High drug concentrations in secretions, beneficial for the management of organisms resistant to antibiotic concentrations, are achieved intravenously.
   i. The most effective inhaled antibiotic is high-dose tobramycin (300 mg, twice daily).
   j. An alternative to inhaled tobramycin is inhaled colistin (75 to 150 mg, twice daily), good in vitro activity against *P. aeruginosa*.

      k. Colistin is less well studied in clinical trials, and bronchospasm is a more common side effect with its continued use.

  6. Bronchodilators

      a. Inhaled bronchodilators are commonly prescribed for management of CF.

      b. Twenty-five percent of CF patients have bronchial reactivity and do respond to bronchodilator therapy.

      c. Bronchodilators may improve respiratory symptoms and airway secretion clearance.

      d. Inhaled anticholinergic agents, especially ipratropium bromide, may also have a role in CF.

  7. Antiinflammatory agents

      a. Used to lessen neutrophilic inflammation and harmful effects of neutrophil products

      b. Use of high-dose corticosteroids has yielded mixed results.

      c. Patients receiving 1 to 2 mg/kg of prednisolone on alternate days have shown a slowed decrease in lung function.

      d. Inhaled steroids have been studied in patients with CF, and their efficacy is yet to be determined.

      e. High-dose ibuprofen is used to lessen neutrophilic inflammation, although further studies are needed to determine benefit of such therapy.

  8. Lung transplantation

      a. Has become an accepted therapy for end-stage CF lung disease

      b. Waiting times >2 years at some centers

      c. Indications for transplantation

          (1) Accelerated clinical decline

          (2) Exacerbations not responding to aggressive therapy

          (3) Recurrent pneumothoraces, recurrent hemoptysis, and presence of pan-resistant organisms should prompt consideration for early referral.

      d. Optimal candidates should not have significant other organ dysfunction (e.g., kidney, liver).

      e. Candidate should be motivated and compliant with therapy.

      f. Candidate should have adequate psychosocial support.

      g. Five-year survival rate is approximately 48%. Survival is limited by opportunistic infections and chronic graft rejection, manifesting as bronchiolitis obliterans.

VII. Foreign Body Aspiration (FBA)

  A. Description and etiology

    1. Children aged 7 months to 4 years are at risk for aspirating a foreign body.

    2. Foreign bodies usually obstruct the larynx, trachea, or bronchi.

    3. Majority of materials aspirated are radiolucent and cannot be seen on typical chest radiographs.

    4. The major cause of death in children aged <6 years

    5. Common aspirated objects include small toys, balloons, hot dogs, beans, peanuts, coins, nuts, raisins, and buttons.

  B. Manifestations

    1. Aspirated material obstructing the trachea is a medical emergency. Symptoms include

      a. Choking

      b. Retractions

      c. Struggling and fighting for air

      d. Gagging

      e. Breath sounds that may vary from absent to rhonchi

    2. Aspirated material lodged in the trachea or bronchus usually stimulates a violent cough, sneezing, and possibly bloody sputum if the material is sharp.

      a. Foreign bodies may create a partial or complete obstruction.

      b. Foreign bodies lodged in the trachea or larynx that completely occlude the airway are most life threatening.

  c. Can lead quickly to respiratory arrest and death if object cannot be removed quickly.

  d. Heimlich maneuver is most effective or by other means available to trained health care personnel.

  e. For more definitive management of upper airway obstruction in children refer to the American Heart Association Basic Life Support Guide.

 C. Management and complications

  1. Children who aspirate foreign bodies seldom cough up the object spontaneously.

  2. Objects deposited in the laryngeal area may be removed via direct laryngoscopy by a skilled physician.

  3. The presence of a foreign body in the trachea or bronchi can be confirmed with the use of a flexible fiberoptic bronchoscope.

  4. Definitive management and removal of a foreign body located distal to the larynx should be done with a *rigid* bronchoscope while the child is under general anesthesia.

  5. Potential complications of FBA include pulmonary air leak if object is lodged distal to the trachea.

  6. Cardiopulmonary arrest and death may occur if foreign body is dislodged from the lower airway and then occludes the opposite mainstem bronchus or trachea.

  7. Bronchiectasis can develop if the object is left in the airway for an extended period.

  8. Pneumonia can develop if certain materials are aspirated or if incomplete removal occurs during bronchoscopy.

  9. Repeat bronchoscopy, antibiotic therapy, and postural drainage/CPT may also be necessary as adequate treatment modalities.

VIII. **Asthma**

 A. Etiology (Modified from National Asthma Education and Prevention Program of the National Institutes of Health, 1997)

  1. Asthma is a condition caused by hyperactive airways.

  2. The patient can have an exacerbation triggered by various allergic and nonallergic stimuli.

  3. The most common mechanism for asthma is allergy.

  4. Other mechanisms include cold exposure, stress, exercise, infection, and other nonspecific inhaled irritants, cigarette smoke, pollen, animal dander, viruses, and exhaust fumes.

  5. Pediatric asthma affects 5% to 10% of all children in the United States.

  6. Common cause of absenteeism in school-aged children

  7. Hospitalization and mortality rates in pediatric asthma have increased dramatically in the past decade.

  8. Exacerbations are often reversible either spontaneously or with treatment.

 B. Pathophysiology

  1. Hyperresponsive lower airways to various allergic and nonallergic stimuli

  2. Classic presentation is an "attack" or spasm of bronchial smooth muscle.

  3. Bronchospasm occurs within the first hour after exposure to airway stimuli.

  4. Histamine and other mast cell mediators are released to prolong reaction.

  5. Airways release a host of inflammatory mediators leading to hypersecretion of mucus.

  6. Airway response includes goblet cell hyperplasia, smooth muscle hypertrophy, and other inflammatory reactions.

  7. Increased volume of mucus mixes with inflammatory cells to form thick, tenacious plugs that occlude small airways.

  8. Combination of bronchospasm and inflammation causes a significant degree of airway obstruction.

  9. Resultant obstruction leads to air trapping and a potential auto-positive end-expiratory pressure effect.

  10. This produces ventilation/perfusion abnormalities with hypoxic vasoconstriction.

  11. Air trapping and hyperinflation can occur.

  12. Changes in pulmonary mechanics include reduced compliance, increased airway resistance, and increased functional residual capacity.

C. Clinical manifestations
   1. A child with an asthma exacerbation may first present with a cough and dyspnea.
   2. Wheezing with decreased air entry is heard on auscultation.
   3. Audible wheezing without use of a stethoscope indicates possible moderate or severe attack.
   4. Child may be diaphoretic or cyanotic.
   5. Absence of wheezing does not rule out attack because poor airflow may be severe enough as to not elicit audible wheeze.
   6. Cyanosis is a late grave sign of respiratory insufficiency that must be managed immediately.
   7. Tachypnea and tachycardia are almost always present.
   8. Use of accessory muscles is common.
   9. Pulsus paradoxus is present in moderate and severe attacks.
  10. Blood gases
     a. Hypoxemia and hypocarbia (mild asthma)
     b. Hypoxemia and hypercarbia (severe asthma)
  11. Hypercarbia, PCO_2 >50, should alert clinician of a deteriorating condition, usually in need for intubation.
  12. Inability to speak in complete sentences in older children is another sign of pulmonary insufficiency.

D. Pulmonary function
   1. Increased TLC
   2. Greatly increased RV
   3. Reduced ventilatory capacity
   4. Reduced FEV_1 and forced vital capacity
   5. Greatly reduced peak flow rate
     a. None of the above should be measured if patient is grossly symptomatic because maneuver(s) can/will exacerbate patient condition.

E. Radiologic findings
   1. Initial chest film reveals hyperinflated lungs with flattened diaphragms.
   2. Lungs fields may otherwise appear relatively clear.
   3. Follow-up films may show increased opacity with consolidated lung.
   4. If inflammatory process is allowed to continue, infiltrates can develop.
   5. Often seen in children aged <6 years

F. Risk factors
   1. Atopy (familial or genetic)
     a. Strongest identifiable predisposing factor for development of asthma
     b. Familial or genetic predisposition to develop an immunoglobulin E (IgE)-mediated response to allergens in the environment
     c. More prevalent in pediatric or allergic asthma
     d. Easiest diagnosis is through skin-prick testing.
     e. Most common method is the radioallergosorbent (RAST) test, which measures antigen-specific IgE.
     f. Highest risk factors of atopic asthma are for inner-city children, where cockroach antigen, animal dander, and dust mites are common.
     g. Other factors that may contribute to development of asthma include environmental pollution, low birth weight, tobacco smoke, diet, or viral infections.
   2. Allergens
     a. Attacks are exacerbated by inhalation of an allergen.
     b. Indoor allergens include mold, animal dander, cleaning chemicals, cockroach antigen, and dust mites.
     c. Outdoor allergens include cold air, noxious fumes, grass, and tree pollens.
   3. Pollution
     a. Role of indoor and outdoor air pollution in development of asthma remains unproved and controversial.
     b. Research has failed to develop a direct link between air pollution and asthma.

    c. Mainly associated with industrialized nations with large amounts of industrial or photochemical smog

    d. Indoor air pollutants have a higher association with development of respiratory symptoms.

    e. Smoking has not been indicated as a general risk factor for development of asthma.

    f. Smoking does seem to play a role in eliciting exacerbations in patients with asthma who are exposed.

    g. Other potential sources of indoor air pollution include nitric oxide, carbon dioxide, carbon monoxides, sulfur dioxides, formaldehydes, and biologic endotoxins.

4. Food and drug additives

    a. Patients with food allergies increase their potential to develop exacerbations.

    b. Foods containing salicylates, certain food-coloring agents, food preservatives, and monosodium glutamate are substances known to trigger responses.

    c. Many drugs are associated with an increased likelihood of a response.

    d. Primary risk is with nonsteroidal antiinflammatory agents and aspirin.

    e. Patients with sensitivity to aspirin have increased risk of developing asthma later in life.

    f. Asthmatic patients also are sensitive to β-blockers.

5. Viral agents

    a. Viral illness seasons (October through December and February through April) are the most prevalent periods for hospitalizations for asthma in children and adults.

    b. Evidence of respiratory tract infection is indicative of a viral response.

    c. Often called intrinsic asthma

    d. Inflammatory responses to viral infections may start a cascade of symptomatic wheezing and excessive mucous production in the airways.

    e. Induced sputum analysis can be a useful marker of the effects of natural colds and influenza on the airways of the lungs.

    f. A relationship exists between respiratory viral infections in early childhood and the development of asthma.

    g. Most prominent viral infection is RSV.

    h. Respiratory tract infections are a significant risk factor for the initiation of an asthma exacerbation.

    i. Families of children with asthma have benefited from written treatment plans that initiate more aggressive outpatient treatment with the onset of coldlike symptoms.

G. Diagnosis

1. Asthma in the child is primarily based on a history of recurrent episodes of reversible airway obstruction triggered by certain allergic or nonallergic stimuli.

2. A family history of atopy predisposes a child to the development of asthma.

3. Children with history of repeated episodes of viral bronchiolitis, pneumonia, and gastroesophageal reflux are at increased risk to develop reactive airways.

4. Children with a history of BPD are also at higher risk to develop reactive airways.

5. A definitive diagnosis is difficult to obtain in the young child.

6. PFTs may prove useful to detect small airway obstruction in the older child.

7. Reversibility of a child's airway obstruction can be assessed with pre- and post-bronchodilator spirometry.

8. Degree of airway responsiveness may also be assessed through the use of a metacholine challenge.

    a. Child inhales a small amount of aerosolized metacholine.

    b. After inhaling the irritant the child performs a forced vital capacity maneuver.

    c. The more responsive the child's airways, the smaller the amount of metacholine required to produce a significant decrease in pulmonary function.

    d. Test is limited to children aged ≥5 years.

9. Another measurement is a test for the presence of specific IgE antibodies; many children with asthma and atopy have elevated levels of IgE present in their serum.

H. Management (Refer to Chapter 20 for exact details of the NHLBI Global Strategy for asthma management and prevention guidelines.)
1. Treatment of a child with an asthma attack is based on relief of airway obstruction.
2. The second objective is to prevent "late phase" inflammatory reactions through the use of certain antiinflammatory agents.
3. Primary medications used for the management of asthma in children are inhaled β-adrenergic bronchodilators and corticosteroids.
4. Oxygen therapy also is used to keep PaO_2 at 60 to 70 mm Hg and SaO_2 at >90%.
5. "Quick relief" medications are primarily short acting β-agonists used to combat acute exacerbations of bronchoconstriction.
6. "Controller medications" are taken daily in an attempt to control mediator release in the airways.
7. Management of severe asthma (status asthmaticus) (Tables 29-2 and 29-3)

TABLE 29-2

Stepwise Approach for Treating Infants and Young Children (≤5 Years of Age) With Acute or Chronic Asthma Symptoms

Severity Level	Symptoms/Day Symptoms/Night	Daily Medications*
Step 4 Severe Persistent	Continual Frequent	• Preferred treatment: • High-dose inhaled corticosteroids AND • Long-acting inhaled $β_2$-agonists AND, if needed, • Corticosteroid tablets or syrup long term (2 mg/kg/day, generally do not exceed 60 mg/day). (Make repeated attempts to reduce systemic corticosteroids and maintain control with high-dose inhaled corticosteroids.)
Step 3 Moderate Persistent	Daily >1 night/week	• Preferred treatment: • Low-dose inhaled corticosteroids and long-acting inhaled $β_2$-agonists OR • Medium-dose inhaled corticosteroids. • Alternative treatment: • Low-dose inhaled corticosteroids and either leukotriene receptor antagonist or theophylline (If needed [particularly in patients with recurring severe exacerbations]: • Preferred treatment: • Medium-dose inhaled corticosteroids and long-acting $β_2$-agonists • Alternative treatment: • Medium-dose inhaled corticosteroids and either leukotriene receptor antagonist or theophylline)
Step 2 Mild Persistent	>2/week but <1×/day >2 nights/month	• Preferred treatment: • Low-dose inhaled corticosteroids (with nebulizer or MDI with holding chamber with or without face mask or DPI) • Alternative treatment (listed alphabetically): • Cromolyn (nebulizer is preferred or MDI with holding chamber) OR leukotriene receptor antagonist
Step 1 Mild Intermittent	≤2 days/week ≤2 nights/month	• No daily medication needed

*Medications required to maintain long-term control.
MDI, Metered dose inhaler; *DPI*, dry powder inhaler.
From *Making a Difference in the Management of Asthma: A Guide for Respiratory Therapists.* Washington DC, U.S. Department of Health and Human Resources, 2003, NIH publication no. 02-1964.

TABLE **29-3**

Dosages of Drugs for Asthma Exacerbations in Emergency Medical Care or Hospital

	Child Dose*	Comments
Albuterol		
Nebulizer solution (5.0 mg/ml, 2.5 mg/3 ml, 1.25 mg/3 ml, 0.63 mg/3 ml)	0.15 mg/kg (minimum dose, 2.5 mg) every 20 min for 3 doses, then 0.15-0.3 mg/kg up to 10 mg every 1-4 hr as needed, or 0.5 mg/kg/hr by continuous nebulization	Only selective β_2-agonists are recommended. For optimal delivery, dilute aerosols to minimum of 3 ml at gas flow of 6-8 L/min
MDI (90 µg/puff)	4-8 puffs every 20 min for 3 doses, then every 1-4 hr. Use spacer/holding chamber.	As effective as nebulized therapy if patient is able to coordinate
Bitolterol		
Nebulizer solution (2 mg/ml)	See albuterol dose; thought to be half as potent as albuterol on a milligram basis	Has not been studied in severe asthma exacerbations; do not mix with other drugs
MDI (370 µg/puff)	See albuterol dose	Has not been studied in severe asthma exacerbations
Levalbuterol (R-albuterol)		
Nebulizer solution (0.63 mg/3 ml, 1.25 mg/3 ml)	0.075 mg/kg (minimum dose, 1.25 mg) every 20 min for 3 doses, then 0.075-0.15 mg/kg up to 5 mg every 1-4 hr as needed, or 0.25 mg/kg/hr by continuous nebulization.	0.63 mg of levalbuterol is equivalent to 1.25 mg of racemic albuterol for efficacy and side effects
Pirbuterol		
MDI (200 µg/puff)	See albuterol dose; thought to be half as potent as albuterol on a milligram basis	Has not been studied in severe asthma exacerbations
Systemic (Injected) β_2-Agonists		
Epinephrine 1:1000 (1 mg/ml)	0.01 mg/kg up to 0.3-0.5 mg every 20 min for 3 doses subcutaneous	No proven advantage of systemic therapy over aerosol
Terbutaline (1 mg/ml)	0.01 mg/kg every 20 min for 3 doses, then every 2-6 hr as needed subcutaneous	No proven advantage of systemic therapy over aerosol
Anticholinergics		
Ipratropium bromide		
Nebulizer solution (0.25 mg/ml)	0.25 mg every 20 min for 3 doses, then every 2-4 hr	May mix in same nebulizers with albuterol. Should not be used as first-line therapy; should be added to β_2-agonist therapy
MDI (18 µg/puff)	4-8 puffs as needed	Dose delivered from MDI is low and has not been studied in asthma exacerbations
Ipratropium with Albuterol		
Nebulizer solution (Each 3-ml vial contains 0.5 mg ipratropium bromide and 2.5 mg albuterol)	1.5 ml every 20 min for 3 doses, then every 2-4 hr	Contains EDTA to prevent discoloration; this additive does not induce bronchospasm

TABLE **29-3**		
Dosages of Drugs for Asthma Exacerbations in Emergency Medical Care or Hospital —cont'd		
	Child Dose*	**Comments**
Ipratropium with Albuterol—cont'd		
MDI (Each puff contains 18 µg ipratropium bromide and 90 µg of albuterol)	4-8 puffs as needed	Combivent MDI
Systemic Corticosteroids		
Prednisone, methylprednisolone, prednisolone[†]	1 mg/kg every 6 hr for 48 hr, then 1-2 mg/kg/day (maximum = 60 mg/day) in 2 divided doses until PEF 70% of predicted or personal best	For outpatient "burst" use 40-60 mg in single or 2 divided doses for adults (children, 1-2 mg/kg/day; maximum, 60 mg/day) for 3-10 days

*<12 years of age.
[†]Dosages and comments apply to all three corticosteroids.
MDI, Metered dose inhaler; *EDTA,* ethylenediaminetetraacetic acid; *PEF,* peak expiratory flow.
From *Making a Difference in the Management of Asthma: A Guide for Respiratory Therapists.* Washington, DC, U.S. Department of Health and Human Resources, 2003, NIH publications no. 02-1964.

a. Inhaled β_2-specific bronchodilators first-line therapy for management of an attack
b. Inhaled albuterol, as well as intravenous terbutaline, has proved safe and effective for the management of childhood asthma.
c. Recommended frequency of albuterol is every 4 to 6 hours with a maximum dosage of 5 mg.
d. However, albuterol aerosols may be given every 20 minutes to the unstable patient in the emergency department under constant monitoring.
e. Newer guidelines suggest the use of continuous bronchodilator therapy for the severely exacerbated patient not responding to conventional care.
f. Pediatric patients are more tolerant of specific side effects associated with aggressive treatment: tachycardia, tachypnea, and increased work of breathing.
g. A small volume nebulizer (SVN) is the most effective way to deliver aerosolized medication to the child.
h. Depending on the patient's age the parent may have to hold the nebulizer to the child's face.
i. Additional intravenous medications are also used to manage exacerbations.
   (1) Intravenous corticosteroids are effective; initially high doses are given, but they may take several hours to demonstrate effects.
   (2) Intravenous magnesium sulfate is also used.
   (3) Magnesium is a calcium channel blocker in the airway smooth muscle and an inhibitor of acetylcholine and histamine release.
   (4) Onset of action can occur within minutes, but effectiveness is difficult to quantify.
   (5) Use of magnesium sulfate for the management of status asthmaticus remains controversial.
j. Usual signs of improvement after treatment(s) include decreased wheezing, improved work of breathing, improved O_2 saturations, improved peak flow, and overall improvement in patient's mental and anxiety status.
k. Signs of failure or nonresponse to therapy include $Paco_2$ >40 mm Hg, refractory hypoxemia (Pao_2, <60 mm Hg and F_Io_2, >50%), mental status deterioration, decreased or absent breath sounds, and apneic episodes.
l. Heliox therapy (≥50% He)

I. Controller medications
1. Corticosteroids are considered the most potent antiinflammatory agents available.
    a. Daily antiinflammatory therapy has shown to actively control severe cases of asthma.
    b. Corticosteroids have been shown to suppress the release of certain inflammatory mediators.
    c. Shown to decrease airway hyperresponsiveness
    d. Can be inhaled, taken orally, or administered intravenously
    e. Dosage and frequency can vary depending on patient condition and present physiology.
    f. Some studies have demonstrated that once-daily dosing can be effective therapy for patients with mild, persistent asthma.
    g. The effect of corticosteroids on the growth of preadolescents who are taking this type of medication is controversial.
2. Nonsteroidal antiinflammatory medications
    a. Most common type of long-term controller medications used in adolescents and children
    b. The two most popular are cromolyn sodium (Intal) and nedocromil (Tilade).
    c. Similar method of action; chloride channel blocker acting to disrupt mast cell mediator release and promote eosinophil release
    d. These medications can reduce the need for quick relievers and reduce bronchial hyperresponsiveness.
    e. They can also improve morning peak flows and decrease symptoms of nocturnal asthma.
3. Long-acting β_2-agonist
    a. Considered a long-term controller medication
    b. Not intended for acute bronchospasm relief
    c. Medication acts as a stimulant to increase cyclic adenosine monophosphate and produce antagonistic reactions to bronchoconstriction.
    d. Long-acting β_2-agonists appear to target asthma symptoms that seem to worsen at night.
    e. Duration of effect: approximately 12 hours
    f. Salmeterol (Serevent) is the drug of choice for this group of patients.
4. Methylxanthines
    a. Long-term controller used predominantly to provide mild to moderate bronchodilation.
    b. Principal medication in this class is theophylline.
    c. Slow-release theophylline is used as an adjunctive therapy for nocturnal asthma.
    d. Acts as a nonselective phosphodiesterase inhibitor
    e. The drug is relatively safe but requires frequent monitoring of serum drug levels to keep patient within therapeutic range for maximum effect.
    f. Increased serum drug levels are associated with tachycardia, nausea and vomiting, headache, seizures, hyperglycemia, and hypokalemia.
    g. Therapeutic serum range has recently been decreased to 5 to 15 mcg/L.
5. Leukotriene modifiers
    a. Newest class of medications introduced to clinicians in >20 years
    b. Considered controller medications
    c. Leukotrienes are considered inflammatory mediators.
    d. They are mediators responsible for release of chemicals from inflammatory cells, mast cells, eosinophils, and basophils.
    e. These reactions lead to bronchoconstriction, increased vascular permeability, and secretion production.
    f. Leukotriene modifiers appear to work via two routes: leukotriene modifiers (zafirlukast/montelukast) and a leukotriene receptor antagonist.
    g. Other agents (zileuton) act as inhibitors of leukotriene release.

    h. They both act to block leukotriene receptor sites.

    i. Can be an oral alternative therapy to inhaled corticosteroids.

    j. Zileuton is more controversial because of its potential to induce liver toxicity.

J. Asthma education

    1. Begins at diagnosis and is reinforced with each visit

    2. Teach patient or parent of a child the basic facts about asthma.

    3. Teach necessary medication skills, techniques, delivery devices, and dosing regimens.

    4. Teach self-monitoring skills and symptom-based, peak flow monitoring.

    5. Teach relevant environmental control and avoidance strategies.

    6. Provide a written asthma exacerbation treatment plan.

    7. Children as young as 2 years of age can begin learning about asthma and its management.

    8. The asthma educator must be prepared to intervene and solve problem areas that may appear to be neglected by the patient.

    9. Educator should be well versed in knowledge of medications, level of treatment, trigger avoidance, compliance, and self-management skills.

BIBLIOGRAPHY

Aloan CA, Hill TV: *Respiratory Care of the Newborn and Child,* ed 2. Philadelphia, Lippincott Williams & Wilkins, 1997.

Expert Panel Report 2: *Guidelines for the Diagnosis and Management of Asthma.* Bethesda, MD, National Asthma Education Program, National Heart, Lung and Blood Institute, National Institutes of Health, 1997, publication no. 97-4051.

Global Initiative for Asthma: *Global Strategy for Asthma Management or Prevention. NHLBI/WHO Workshop Report.* Bethesda, MD, National Institutes of Health, 1995, publication no. 95-3659.

Hess DR: Aerosol therapy. *Respir Care Clin N Am* 1:239, 1995.

Hess DR, MacIntyre NR: *Respiratory Care Principles and Practice.* Philadelphia, WB Saunders, 2002, p. 896-913.

Katz RW, Kelly HW, Crowley MR, et al: Safety of continuous nebulized albuterol for bronchospasm in infants and children. *Pediatrics* 92:666-669, 1993.

Making a Difference in the Management of Asthma: A Guide for Respiratory Therapists. Washington, DC, U.S. Department of Health and Human Services, 2003, NIH publication no. 02-1964.

Skobeloff EM, Spivey WH, McNamara RM, et al: Intravenous magnesium sulfate for the treatment of acute asthma in the emergency department. *JAMA* 262:1210-1213, 1989.

Whitaker K: Pediatric diseases requiring respiratory care. In *Comprehensive Perinatal & Pediatric Respiratory Care,* ed 2. Albany, NY: Delmar Publishers, 1997, p. 425-431.

Wilkins RL, Stoller JT, Sanlon CL: *Egan's Fundamentals of Respiratory Care,* ed 8. St. Louis, Mosby, 2003.

Chapter 30

Assisted Ventilation for Pediatric Patients

I. **General Concepts of Ventilation (Box 30-1)**
   A. Alveolar ventilation: The measure of the adequacy of ventilation; CO_2 removal is directly related to alveolar ventilation.
   B. Compliance: The measure of distensibility of the lungs and thorax expressed as the volume change in the lung per unit of pressure change. The higher the compliance, the greater the volume change in the lungs for a given change in pressure. With a reduction in compliance, a greater pressure gradient is required to move a given volume of gas into the lungs.
   C. Resistance: The measure of the tendency for the airways and lung tissue to resist the flow of gas expressed as the change in pressure per unit of gas flow: the greater the resistance to gas flow, the greater the pressure gradient necessary to deliver a volume of gas in a given time interval.
   D. Time constant: The relationship between compliance and resistance and pressure equilibration between patient and ventilator circuit, or filling and emptying of the lungs during inspiration and expiration. One time constant is the measure of the time necessary for alveolar pressure to equilibrate to 63% of a change in airway pressure; 99% pressure equilibration occurs in lungs with normal compliance and resistance in approximately five time constants.

II. **Continuous Positive Airway Pressure (CPAP)**
   A. General description
      1. Continuous distending pressure maintained throughout respiratory cycle.
      2. Prevents alveolar collapse during expiration, and reduces the pressure required to open alveoli during inspiration.
      3. Improves and maintains functional residual capacity (FRC) and ventilation-perfusion relationship.
      4. Typically provided noninvasively by facial apparatus.
   B. Clinical applications
      1. Overcomes resistive forces of dilator muscles of the pharynx and upper airway in patients with obstructive sleep apnea.
      2. Helps preserve lung volume (FRC) in patients with chronic pulmonary or neuromuscular disease.
      3. Noninvasive facial or nasal appliances interface CPAP generator to patient.
   C. CPAP generators
      1. Fluidic systems
      2. Simplified stand-alone units used for long-term care
      3. Bilevel or BiPAP unit set in CPAP mode
      4. Mechanical ventilator set in CPAP mode

BOX 30-1

Equations for General Concepts of Ventilation

Alveolar ventilation (L/min) = f × (V_T – anatomic deadspace)
Compliance (L/cm H_2O) = Δ volume (L)/Δ pressure (cm H_2O)
Resistance (cm H_2O/L/sec) = Δ pressure (cm H_2O)/flow (L/sec)
Time constant (sec) = compliance (L/cm H_2O) × resistance (cm H_2O/L/sec)

III. Types of Ventilation
   A. Control variables
      1. The variable that a ventilator controls to effect inspiration
      2. Pressure, flow, or volume
      3. Mandatory and spontaneous ventilator-supported breaths are classified as pressure controlled or volume controlled.
   B. Pressure-control ventilation (PCV)
      1. Pressure is the variable that the ventilator controls to effect inspiration.
      2. The shape of the inspiratory pressure waveform remains consistent breath to breath as compliance and resistance change.
      3. Flow pattern and delivered tidal volume (V_T) vary depending on changes in compliance and resistance.
      4. Volume delivery primarily depends on the change in pressure from baseline to peak pressure, referred to as delta-P (ΔP).
      5. As the lungs fill and lung pressure approaches the set pressure target or limit (circuit pressure), the inspiratory gas flow rate to the patient decreases or decelerates.
      6. Time-cycled, pressure-limited (TCPL)
         a. Most common type of ventilation used to support infants weighing <10 kg
         b. Pressure-controlled, incorporating a continuous flow of gas through the breathing circuit, a pneumatic exhalation valve, and a timing mechanism
         c. The breath rate setting determines a fixed time interval to trigger mandatory breaths.
         d. During inspiration the exhalation valve closes; flow is diverted to the inspiratory limb; pressure builds to a preset limit; and the breath is cycled after a preset inspiratory interval.
   C. Pressure support ventilation (PSV)
      1. PSV is used to support spontaneous breaths.
      2. Triggered by patient inspiratory effort, the ventilator provides the inspiratory flow necessary to reach and maintain a set pressure support level (pressure limit) for the duration of inspiratory time.
      3. Breaths are terminated (cycled) when inspiratory flow decreases to a predetermined level, usually a percentage of peak inspiratory flow rate.
      4. The change in inspiratory flow rate depends on patient demand and lung mechanics.
      5. Inspiratory time and V_T may vary from breath to breath.
   D. Volume-control ventilation (VCV)
      1. Volume and flow, which are functions of each other, are the control variable.
      2. A set V_T is delivered in an inspiratory time that is either directly set or set indirectly as the result of setting a peak inspiratory flow rate.
      3. Volume is constant from breath to breath, and the pressure gradient required to deliver a given volume varies with changes in compliance and resistance.
   E. Dual control
      1. Two variables are controlled.
      2. Volume-targeted breaths
         a. PCV and PSV breaths can be delivered with a guaranteed or targeted V_T.
         b. May be beneficial to patients with dynamic pulmonary compliance and airway resistance in which minute volume is highly variable.

IV. **Modes of Ventilation**
  A. Assist control (AC)
    1. All breaths are mandatory and are time triggered by the ventilator at an interval determined by the breath rate setting or patient triggered if the patient's inspiratory effort meets the set-triggering criteria.
    2. All delivered breaths can be either volume controlled (e.g., AC-VCV) or pressure controlled (e.g., AC-PCV).
  B. Synchronized intermittent mandatory ventilation (SIMV)
    1. A preset number of mandatory breaths per minute are provided as volume-controlled (e.g., VCV-SIMV) or pressure-controlled (e.g., PCV-SIMV) breaths.
    2. Spontaneous breathing is allowed between mandatory breaths.
    3. Mandatory breaths are synchronized with the patient's spontaneous breathing.
  C. Spontaneous modes
    1. CPAP
    2. PSV
  D. Combined modes
    1. PCV/SIMV + pressure support (PS)
    2. VCV/SIMV + PS

V. **Indications for Mechanical Ventilation (Box 30-2)**
  A. Overall goals of mechanical ventilation
    1. Support muscles of ventilation
    2. Ventilation, CO_2 elimination
    3. Oxygenation, improve Po_2
    4. Recruitment and preservation of lung volume
  B. General indications
    1. Respiratory failure as indicated by a respiratory acidosis (pH, <7.20 to 7.25)
    2. Hypoxemia (Pao_2, <50 mm Hg)
    3. Clinical signs of respiratory failure, including
      a. Tachypnea
      b. Substernal and intercostal muscle retractions
      c. Expiratory grunting
      d. Nasal flaring
      e. Cyanosis

VI. **Pediatric Ventilator Settings**
  A. Initial assessment
    1. The disease process and the size of the child are considered when selecting ventilator settings.

BOX 30-2

Common Diagnoses Requiring Assisted Ventilation

Respiratory disorders	**Neurogenic**
Pneumonia (infectious, aspiration)	Seizure disorders
Bronchopulmonary dysplasia	Central apnea
Cystic fibrosis	Head injury
Asthma	
Acute respiratory distress syndrome	**Cardiac**
Bronchiolitis	Congenital heart disease
Near drowning	Primary pulmonary hypertension
Neuromuscular disease	**Postanesthesia**
Spinal muscle atrophy	
Muscular dystrophy	**Trauma/shock**

2. Manual ventilation is useful to assess the compliance of the lungs while observing the chest excursion and evaluating breath sounds.
3. Peak inspiratory pressure (PIP) and positive end-expiratory pressure (PEEP) observed on an airway manometer during manual ventilation are noted and used as a guide to select the initial ventilator settings.

B. Mode
1. SIMV volume or pressure controlled
   a. Allows the patient to perform some of the ventilator work with the guarantee that an adequate minute volume (VE) may enhance patient-ventilator synchrony.
   b. VCV-SIMV is typically used as the initial mode to ventilate older pediatric patients.
   c. One disadvantage of VCV is the potential for excessive airway pressures that can lead to barotrauma/volutrauma, hemodynamic compromise, and patient-ventilator dysynchrony.
   d. PCV-SIMV is used when high inflation pressures are observed, such as in patients with decreased lung compliance and/or increased airflow obstruction in which PIP >35 cm H_2O is required during VCV.
2. PSV
   a. May be added (i.e., SIMV-VC + PSV) to augment spontaneous respiratory efforts and decrease the work of breathing imposed by the ventilator and circuit
   b. Used to assess the need for weaning and tolerance of extubation

C. VT
1. Adjusted in VCV and measured in PCV
2. Consider patient size and underlying condition
3. Effective VT of 7 to 10 ml/kg is considered a good starting point.
4. VT >10 ml/kg may be potentially deleterious.
5. Larger VT may require the use of higher PIP, which may increase compressible volume loss and lower effective VT delivery; the set VT may not reflect the true or effective VT.
6. PCV VT
   a. Determined by the set PIP
   b. PIP is generally comparable with the plateau pressure (P_{plat}) measured during VCV and used as a starting point.
   c. If P_{plat} is not available, the initial PIP should be set 2 to 5 cm H_2O lower than the PIP that was measured during VCV.
   d. Because PIP is constant, the risks of barotrauma are somewhat minimized; however, if delivered VT or PIP is excessive, volutrauma may occur.

D. Frequency
1. Generally set at 10 to 25 breaths/min
2. Frequencies >30 breaths/min are rarely used in children because of the potential for gas trapping.
3. Patients with obstructive lung disease (e.g., asthma) will benefit from slower ventilator rates that allow more time for expiration.
4. Patients with elevated intracranial pressures are treated with hyperventilation and ventilated with faster rates.

E. Inspiratory time (TI)
1. TI is adjusted to establish the inspiration/expiration (I:E) ratio.
2. TI affects patient comfort and patient/ventilator synchrony. When selecting a TI, patient age, breathing pattern, and disease process are considered.
3. General range is approximately 0.5 second for small children to approximately 1.0 second for large children.
4. Set directly or indirectly by adjusting inspiratory flow rate.
5. As TI is lengthened in VCV, flow is decreased, and a more laminar flow pattern is created, decreasing PIP.
6. An I:E ratio of 1:2 or 1:3 is commonly set.
7. Prolonged TI can be used to increase mean airway pressure (P_{aw}) and improve oxygenation in those with acute respiratory failure, provided that the time for expiration is sufficient to avoid stacking of breaths and associated complications.

8. In the lung recovery phase and in the patient who is spontaneously breathing, a long T_I may result in patient/ventilator dysynchrony because the patient may begin to exhale before the mandatory breath cycles to exhalation.
9. Shortened T_I should be used when severe airflow obstruction is present, thus providing a longer expiratory phase.

F. Inspiratory flow rate
1. VCV inspiratory flow rate is either set directly or indirectly as a result of setting inspiratory time.
2. Adequate inspiratory flow meets patient demand, whereas insufficient inspiratory flow may lead to increased work of breathing if spontaneous inspiratory flow demand is greater than the inspiratory flow rate provided.
3. PCV inspiratory flow is variable depending on PIP, lung mechanics, and patient demand.

G. PEEP
1. Provides alveolar recruitment and varies depending on the severity of lung disease
2. Generally started at 3 to 5 cm H_2O
3. Increases are made in increments of 2 cm H_2O in patients with conditions with low lung compliance (e.g., acute respiratory distress syndrome) to improve lung recruitment and oxygenation.
4. Optimal PEEP is considered the level that achieves the best lung compliance and oxygenation with the fewest cardiovascular side effects.
5. PEEP >15 cm H_2O should be avoided because of the risk of cardiovascular compromise.
6. Lung hyperinflation leading to decreased compliance, increased pulmonary vascular resistance, increased deadspace, and decreased oxygen delivery may result from excessive PEEP.
7. PEEP is applied judiciously in patients with airflow obstruction (e.g., asthma) because lung hyperinflation may be exacerbated.

H. Oxygen concentration (F_IO_2)
1. F_IO_2 is set to the lowest concentration that provides acceptable arterial oxygenation.
2. By increasing PEEP or other ventilator manipulations to reduce the F_IO_2 to <0.60 in those with severe lung disease, P_{aw} is typically increased.
3. Additional strategies to minimize adverse effects of high F_IO_2 include accepting PaO_2 of 50 to 70 mm Hg or SpO_2 >85%, provided that hemoglobin levels are adequate, cardiovascular status is stable, and metabolic acidosis does not develop secondary to tissue hypoxia.

I. Lung protective ventilation
1. Permissive hypercapnia (allowing PCO_2 to increase >45 cm H_2O) is achieved by limitation of ventilator support (P_{aw} and V_T) to avoid lung overdistention.
2. Used to prevent or reduce the severity of ventilator-induced lung injury
3. Peak alveolar pressures (end-inspiratory P_{plat}) should be maintained <30 cm H_2O.
4. PEEP is applied as needed to maintain adequate lung volume.
5. V_T: range 5 to 7 ml/kg
6. If necessary $PaCO_2$ is allowed to gradually increase above the normal clinical range to ≥50-100 mm Hg, provided that pH is maintained >7.25 with metabolic compensation.

VII. **Monitoring Mechanical Ventilation in the Pediatric Patient**
A. Arterial blood gases
1. Clinically acceptable blood gas parameters are established depending on the disease state and level of acuity.
2. Used as a guide to select and modify ventilator settings.
3. Permissive hypercapnia ($PaCO_2$, 50 to 100 mm Hg; pH, ≥7.25) is considered when the risk of ventilator-induced lung injury is high.
4. Arterial oxygen tensions of 50 to 70 mm Hg are frequently tolerated and permit the use of lower, less toxic, oxygen concentrations, provided that metabolic acidosis from tissue hypoxia does not occur.

B. Noninvasive measures of gas exchange
1. Continuous SpO_2 monitoring
2. Periodic or continuous $ETCO_2$ monitoring provides a guide for changes in ventilation.
C. Physical examination
1. Changes in vital signs alert clinicians of physiologic responses to changes in ventilator settings.
2. Respiratory effort and evaluation of work of breathing
3. Breath sounds
D. Patient-ventilator interaction
1. Airway pressure measurements, including PIP, P_{aw}, and P_{plat}
a. Increased PIP in VCV is commonly attributed to decreased lung compliance, increased airway resistance, patient-ventilator dysynchrony, or airway secretions.
b. $P_{aw} > 15$ indicates worsening lung disease and is associated with barotrauma.
c. Because increasing P_{aw} is required to maintain adequate oxygenation, alternative ventilator management strategies, such as permissive hypercapnia or high frequency ventilation, should be considered.
d. P_{plat} (an indication of peak alveolar pressure) is used to calculate static compliance, which can be trended when adjusting ventilator settings.
e. Auto-PEEP should be monitored if there is a suspicion of air trapping.
E. Effective VT
1. The VT delivered to the patient minus the amount compressed in the ventilator circuitry
2. (PIP − PEEP)(ventilator-specific compression factor) = volume lost to compression (Box 30-3)

VIII. **Weaning the Pediatric Patient from Mechanical Ventilation**
A. Readiness to wean
1. Stable cardiovascular system with minimal or no vasopressor support
2. Acceptable respiratory mechanics
3. Stable respiratory rate
4. Adequate spontaneous VT (e.g., 3 to 5 ml/kg)
5. Minimal work of breathing
6. Maximum inspiratory pressure can be obtained in older children as a gauge of muscle effort and should be at least −20 cm H_2O.
7. Forced vital capacity (FVC) may also be obtained and should be 10 ml/kg.
8. Improved chest radiographic findings
9. Reduced sedation requirement
10. Acceptable ventilator parameters
a. F_1O_2, <0.50; PEEP, <8 cm H_2O; P_{aw}, <12 cm H_2O; PIP, <25 cm H_2O; and a ventilator frequency, <15 breaths/min

---

BOX 30-3
Calculating Effective VT

Effective VT = set VT − volume lost to compression

Example:
Patient weight: 30 kg
VT set: 200 ml
PIP/PEEP: 28/8 cm H_2O
Compressible volume: 1 ml/cm H_2O
(28 − 8 cm H_2O)(1 ml/cm H_2O) = 20 ml
200 ml − 20 ml = 180 ml/30 kg
Effective VT = 6 ml/kg

VT, Tidal volume; *PIP,* peak inspiratory pressure; *PEEP,* positive end-expiratory pressure.

B. Weaning process
   1. Reduce mandatory frequency incrementally by 2 to 5 breaths/min over time.
   2. Observe for signs of distress.
      a. Tachypnea, retractions, nasal flaring, agitation, increased heart rate, and blood pressure
C. Weaning with PSV
   1. PSV assists spontaneous respiratory efforts.
   2. Decreases the work of breathing imposed by artificial airways, ventilator circuits, and demand systems
   3. Improves patient/ventilator synchrony
   4. May prevent respiratory muscle fatigue
   5. Titrated to maintain a VT of 5 to 7 ml/kg
   6. Decreased in increments of 1 to 2 cm H_2O while observing delivered VT
   7. Slowly returns work of breathing to patient
   8. Used in conjunction with extubation readiness evaluation (Box 30-4)
      a. Patient is changed to PSV and observed over time.
      b. Minimal level of PSV is used to overcome endotracheal tube (ETT) resistance without increasing VT.
      c. Successful evaluation permits earlier extubation without the need for prolonged weaning.

IX. **Complications**
   A. Barotrauma
      1. Alveolar rupture and the dissection of air into various thoracic compartments
      2. Causes
         a. Overdistention of the lungs and lung injury
         b. High airway pressures
         c. Large VT
         d. Excessive PEEP
         e. Patient-ventilator dysynchrony
      3. Air leak syndromes
         a. Pneumothorax
         b. Pneumomediastinum

BOX 30-4

Extubation Readiness Test (Children's Hospital, Boston)

Criteria: Confirm spontaneous breathing
Level of consciousness acceptable
F_1O_2, ≤0.50; PEEP, ≤5 cm H_2O

ETT size	PSV level
3.0-3.5 mm	10 cm H_2O
4.0-4.5 mm	8 cm H_2O
≥5.0 mm	6 cm H_2O

Consider extubation if:
SpO_2, >95%
Effective VT, >5 ml/kg
RR goal achieved
   <6 mo: 20-60 breaths/min
   6 mo to 2 yr: 15-45 breaths/min
   2-5 yr: 15-40 breaths/min
   >5 yr: 10-35 breaths/min

From *Respiratory Care Procedure Manual,* Children's Hospital, Boston, MA, 2004.
PEEP, Positive end-expiratory pressure; *ETT,* endotracheal tube; *PSV,* pressure support ventilation; *VT,* tidal volume; *RR,* respiratory rate.

        c. Pneumopericardium
        d. Pneumoperitoneum
   B. Pulmonary complications
      1. Ventilator-induced lung injury
      2. Ventilator-associated pneumonia
   C. Airway complications associated with ETT
      1. Malpositioned ETT
      2. Unplanned extubation
      3. Kinking of ETT
      4. Occluded ETT
      5. Infection
      6. Tracheal damage
   D. Cardiovascular effects
      1. Decreased venous return
      2. Decreased cardiac output
      3. Increased pulmonary vascular resistance

X. High Frequency Oscillatory Ventilation
   A. Goals
      1. Recruit and maintain lung volume above alveolar closing volume
      2. Improve gas exchange without allowing lungs to open and close with each breath (Box 30-5).
   B. Indications
      1. Diffuse alveolar disease
         a. Acute respiratory distress syndrome
         b. Pneumonia
      2. Pulmonary air leak syndrome

BOX 30-5

High Frequency Oscillatory Ventilation Pediatric Guidelines (Children's Hospital, Boston, MA)

Pre-HFOV
ETT in proper position
BP/cardiac output adequate
Sedation and/or paralysis

Initial HFOV Settings

P_{aw}:	5-8 cm H_2O > conventional ventilator
Frequency:	<10 kg: 10-12 Hz
	10-20 kg: 8-10 Hz
	20-40 kg: 6-8 Hz
F_IO_2:	1.0

Clinical management

Diffuse alveolar disease:	Increase P_{aw} 1-2 cm H_2O until F_IO_2 <0.60
Air leak syndrome:	Minimize P_{aw}, tolerate F_IO_2 0.8-1.0
Amplitude:	Adjusted in 3-5 cm H_2O to change $P{CO_2}$
CXR:	2 hr after initiation, then daily
	Ideal expansion 8-9 ribs
Suctioning:	Every 12 hr daily, minimize disconnections

Weaning
Consider trial of conventional ventilation when CXR and lung compliance improve, and P_{aw} is weaned to 15-18 cm H_2O

From *Respiratory Care Procedure Manual,* Children's Hospital, Boston, MA, 2004.
HFOV, High frequency oscillatory ventilation; *ETT,* endotracheal tube; *BP,* blood pressure; *P_{aw},* mean airway pressure; *CXR,* chest radiograph.

BOX 30-6
Common Diagnoses Requiring Extracorporeal Membrane Oxygenation

Congenital diaphragmatic hernia
Persistent pulmonary hypertension of the newborn
Acute respiratory distress syndrome
Air leak syndromes
Septic shock
Congenital heart disease
Cardiomyopathy

---

  3. Failure of conventional ventilator strategies
     a. P_{aw}: >15 cm H_2O
  C. Failure of lung protective ventilator strategies
     1. VT requirements: >7 ml/kg
     2. P_{plat}: >30 cm H_2O
     3. Permissive hypercapnia

XI. **Extracorporeal Membrane Oxygenation**
  A. Goals
     1. Provide complete lung rest and recovery
     2. Support gas exchange
     3. Provide adequate tissue perfusion
     4. Support cardiac function
  B. Indications (Box 30-6)
     1. Failure of advanced ventilator strategies
        a. High frequency oscillatory ventilation
        b. Lung protective ventilation
     2. Respiratory failure
        a. Acute respiratory failure
        b. Pneumonia
     3. Cardiac failure
        a. After palliative or corrective surgery for congenital heart disease
        b. Resuscitation when conventional resuscitative measures fail
        c. Support while awaiting cardiac transplantation

BIBLIOGRAPHY

Carlo WA, Martin RJ: Principles of neonatal assisted ventilation. *Pediatr Clin North Am* 33:221, 1986.

Chatburn RL: Similarities and differences in the management of acute lung injury in neonates (IRDS) and in adults (ARDS). *Respir Care* 33:539, 1988.

Chatburn RL: A new system for understanding mechanical ventilators. *Respir Care* 36:1123, 1991.

Chatburn RL: Principles and practice of neonatal and pediatric mechanical ventilation. *Respir Care* 36:569, 1991.

Cheifetz IM: Invasive and noninvasive pediatric mechanical ventilation. *Respir Care* 48:442, 2003.

Donn SM, Sinha SK: Invasive and noninvasive neonatal mechanical ventilation. *Respir Care* 48:426, 2003.

Hansell DR: Extracorporeal membrane oxygenation for perinatal and pediatric patients. *Respir Care* 48:321, 2003.

Priebe GP, Arnold JH: High-frequency oscillatory ventilation in pediatric patients. *Respir Care Clin N Am* 7:633, 2001.

Chapter 31

Pulmonary Rehabilitation

I. The following definition of pulmonary rehabilitation was drafted and adopted in 1999 by the American Thoracic Society:

"Pulmonary rehabilitation is a multi-disciplinary program of care for patients with chronic respiratory impairment that is individually tailored and designed to optimize physical and social performance and autonomy."

II. Pulmonary Rehabilitation Program

A pulmonary rehabilitation program is structured according to the individual needs of the patient population being serviced in conjunction with the resources available to the program.

A. Community assessment and planning before a program is started are crucial.
1. Assess the demographic profile of patients in the target community.
2. Evaluate medical (physician) interest and awareness.
3. Identify potential competition.
4. Develop a marketing plan.
5. Investigate transportation options for outpatients.

B. Assessment of program resources
1. Determine available versus needed space and equipment.
2. Identify clinical personnel desired versus personnel available.
3. Discuss financial expectations of the program.

C. Alternatives in program structure
1. Inpatient pulmonary rehabilitation, which may include hospital, skilled nursing facility, or rehabilitation hospital
a. Individual or group education and breathing retraining are scheduled for the patient in a general acute care unit 5 to 7 days/week.
b. Individual low-level bedside or ambulatory exercise is instituted.
c. Patients may be prepared for follow-up evaluation in an outpatient rehabilitation setting.
d. Few are structured as comprehensive multidisciplinary 1- to 2-week inpatient programs because of reimbursement limitations, time constraints, and patient acuity.
e. Most commonly created to serve rehabilitation needs of patients with greatest acuity and complex long-term needs.
2. Outpatient pulmonary rehabilitation, conducted in outpatient hospital-based clinic, comprehensive outpatient rehabilitation facility (CORF), or extended care facility
a. These are the most common formats used for pulmonary rehabilitation.

    b. Usually these programs involve two or five visits per week, but program lengths vary from 4 to 12 weeks, with 6 to 8 weeks the norm.

    c. Individual or small group (two to five patients) exercise and educational sessions are instituted.

    d. These programs are usually multidisciplinary.

3. Outpatient office-based pulmonary rehabilitation

    a. These programs may include some components of outpatient programs, such as education, breathing retraining, and exercise testing and prescription.

    b. A pulmonary physician, pulmonary nurse specialist, and/or respiratory care practitioner usually implements the program.

4. Home-based pulmonary rehabilitation

    a. These programs may include education, breathing retraining, and a simple exercise routine.

    b. They may be included in the home care services of visiting nursing agencies or occasionally by the respiratory equipment providers.

    c. They are generally less comprehensive in scope than hospital- or clinic-based programs, with visits often fewer than once per week.

    d. They may be the only alternative for the homebound patient or when nearby hospitals do not have a pulmonary rehabilitation program.

    e. Such programs may serve as a final rehabilitative transition from other more comprehensive and intensive program formats.

D. Advantages and disadvantages of various pulmonary rehabilitation settings

  1. Inpatient rehabilitation advantages

    a. Reserved for the most acute patients with the greatest functional deficits, monitoring by professional staff is available 24 hr/day.

    b. Allows staff to teach and observe family/patient interaction during therapies.

    c. Best for patients requiring assistive devices, suctioning, tracheostomy care, or long-term ventilation.

  2. Inpatient rehabilitation disadvantages

    a. Most labor intensive and costly format

    b. Transportation/availability of family members may be problematic.

    c. Staff is precluded from observation of home activities.

  3. Outpatient rehabilitation advantages

    a. Most efficient use of professional staff

    b. Typically greatest scope of professional staff is available.

    c. Largest exposure (availability and accessibility) to target patient population

    d. Most well accepted for reimbursement

  4. Outpatient rehabilitation disadvantages

    a. Requires a certain base level of functional ability to access program

    b. Transportation and availability of patient and/or family members may be issues.

    c. External variables such as weather and pollution alerts may present barriers.

    d. Staff is precluded from observation of home activities.

  5. Home-based pulmonary rehabilitation advantages

    a. Most convenient for patient and family

    b. Transportation and availability of patient/family generally are nonissues.

    c. Adaptation of exercises to a familiar environment may lead to greater compliance and offer identification by staff of home limits/barriers.

  6. Home-based pulmonary rehabilitation disadvantages

    a. Limited availability of sophisticated monitoring, testing, and exercise equipment

    b. Most labor intensive, being one on one, and requires professional staff travel

    c. The smallest scope of professional staff generally is available.

    d. Usually the most questionably reimbursed rehabilitation format

E. Multidisciplinary team approach

  1. Clinicians from a variety of health care disciplines are necessary participants in a pulmonary rehabilitation program.

2. The number of contributing disciplines varies with the size, scope, availability, and setting of the pulmonary rehabilitation program.
3. If some or all of these disciplines are not available, a simple team composed of the physician and respiratory care practitioner, nurse, or physical therapist can provide thorough pulmonary rehabilitation in any of the previously mentioned settings.
4. Team members should have special interest or training in meeting the needs of patients with pulmonary disease.
5. Each team member should be qualified in their area of expertise to assess the patient's needs, provide appropriate intervention, and monitor patient outcomes.
6. Each team member must be fully versed in their role and educational content, as well as completely aware of the role and content of each of the other disciplines represented.
7. All team members should be minimally trained in basic cardiac life support and ideally trained in advanced cardiac life support.
8. Team conferences:
   a. Are attended by all team members at regular intervals (e.g., weekly or monthly)
   b. Provide a forum for initial goal setting, plan formation, and ongoing discussion of patients' progress and discharge goals
   c. Facilitate dissemination of general program information to team members (e.g., quality assurance findings, policy and procedure changes)

F. Team members and their roles
1. Medical director
   a. A licensed physician with an interest in and knowledge of pulmonary rehabilitation, pulmonary function, and exercise evaluation
   b. A pulmonary physician commonly fills this role.
   c. Reviews and oversees all policies and procedures of the program
   d. Reviews and oversees all billing and reimbursement practices
   e. Participates in the initial screening of patients
      (1) Reviews the medical history, medications, and diagnostic test results
      (2) Supervises and interprets all exercise testing
      (3) Performs or reviews the physical examination
   f. Performs an educational and administrative role in advanced medical care planning/advanced directives
   g. Represents the program to hospital administration, medical staff colleagues, and the community
   h. May initiate, review, participate in, and evaluate pulmonary rehabilitation research
2. The program coordinator should be trained in a health-related profession and have demonstrated clinical experience and expertise in the care of patients with chronic pulmonary disease.
   a. A respiratory care practitioner, registered nurse, or registered physical therapist commonly fills this role.
   b. May serve a combined role as program coordinator and primary patient care provider/educator with responsibilities to
      (1) Develop and revise program policies and procedures
      (2) Implement and oversee daily program activities
         (a) Assess weight, heart and breath sounds, respiratory and other symptoms, sleep, appetite, and adherence to home medication and exercise regimen at each patient visit
         (b) Carry out monitored exercise sessions
      (3) Maintain written and verbal communication with each patient's referring physician
      (4) Participate in the development and implementation of program marketing plan
      (5) Collect and report program quality assurance data
      (6) Collect and report billing and reimbursement data
      (7) Review current pulmonary rehabilitation literature and update protocols and equipment as indicated

(8) Represent the program to other hospital departments and to the community

 c. Provides patient education on select topics

  (1) Medications, with emphasis on indications, actions, side effects, drug interactions, and prescription compliance

  (2) Respiratory anatomy and pathophysiology of chronic pulmonary disease

  (3) Sequelae of chronic pulmonary disease

  (4) Sleep disorders common to chronic pulmonary disease

  (5) Description of medical procedures and test results used in pulmonary medicine

  (6) Exercise testing, techniques, and conditioning

  (7) Activities of daily living (ADLs)

  (8) Breathing retraining, relaxation, and stress management techniques

  (9) Oxygen therapy and bronchial hygiene techniques

  (10) Functional self-management (e.g., self-assessment and management of symptoms, early intervention, and seeking medical attention)

  (11) Smoking cessation

  (12) Sexuality

  (13) Travel

 d. Commonly participates in exercise testing

 e. Performs assistance as needed with ADLs

 f. Assesses the need for home care equipment/supplies and personnel

3. Dietitian

 a. Evaluates nutritional status of patients

  (1) Weight

  (2) Interview (diet history)

  (3) Review of food record or calorie count

  (4) Laboratory indices (e.g., total protein, albumin, cholesterol, phosphate, magnesium, transferrin, and calcium values)

  (5) Anthropometric measurements (e.g., skinfold thickness, arm muscle circumference)

 b. Recommends individual dietary modifications, including calories, components, supplements, and meal scheduling as indicated

 c. Instructs patient and family on diet

 d. Develops individualized sample menus

4. Social worker

 a. Screens patients and families for evidence of psychosocial problems warranting referral or further treatment

 b. Assesses and discusses with patients and families the impact of pulmonary disease on self-esteem, lifestyle, and relationships

 c. Provides information on community resources to meet social, vocational, financial, transportation, and counseling needs

 d. Assists physician and clergy in performing an educational and administrative role in advanced medical care planning/advanced directives

5. Psychologist or psychiatrist

 a. Most often serves the pulmonary rehabilitation program on a consultant basis for select patients and families

 b. Administers and interprets psychological tests

 c. Conducts ongoing group or individual therapy

 d. Recommends or prescribes psychotropic medications (e.g., anxiolytics, antidepressants, and sedative hypnotics)

6. Occupational therapist

 a. Evaluates the impact of chronic pulmonary disease on the patient's ability to perform ADLs and home maintenance, social, and vocational activities

 b. Provides instruction and opportunities for practice in energy conservation and work simplification techniques

    c. Recreational and leisure activity assessment and education
    d. Includes instruction on coordinated breathing strategies
    e. Recommends vocational alternatives or modifications for continued employment in the same setting

7. Physical therapist
    a. Serves as program coordinator and primary patient caregiver in some institutions
    b. Teaches relaxation and biofeedback techniques
    c. Provides consultation, treatment, and modified exercise recommendations for pulmonary rehabilitation patients with specific neuromusculoskeletal conditions
    d. May design warm-up, strengthening, and toning exercise routines

8. Pharmacist
    a. Provides consultation to program staff on medication selections, actions, and interactions
    b. May provide group education to patients and families on medications

9. Exercise physiologist
    a. Participates in exercise testing and prescription
    b. May assist in conducting or monitoring group exercise sessions

10. Clergyman
    a. May receive referrals as a consultant for patients and families with identified spiritual concerns
    b. Provides spiritual counseling on issues such as death, dying, and quality of life, assisting physician and social worker in performing an educational and administrative role in advanced medical care planning/advanced directives

III. **Evaluation of the Pulmonary Rehabilitation Candidate**
    A. Thorough screening of each patient is essential to the optimal planning and success of the individual treatment program.
    B. Pulmonary rehabilitation is indicated for patients with chronic respiratory impairment who, despite optimal medical management, remain dyspneic, have reduced exercise tolerance, or a restriction in activities. It is therefore not exclusionary on a disease-specific basis.
    C. The ideal candidate meets the following criteria.
      1. Correctly diagnosed with symptomatic chronic pulmonary disease (most commonly chronic obstructive pulmonary disease [COPD]); however, with recent expansion to also include
        a. Asthma
        b. Bronchiectasis
        c. Chest wall diseases
        d. Cystic fibrosis
        e. Interstitial lung disease
          (1) Post–acute respiratory distress syndrome
          (2) Pulmonary fibrosis
        f. Lung cancer
        g. Selected neuromuscular disease
        h. Thoracic/abdominal surgical perioperative state
        i. Post-polio syndrome
        j. Pre- and post-lung transplant and/or reduction
        k. Chronic ventilator dependence
      2. Willing and motivated to participate in the program
      3. Free from concurrent medical problems precluding safe, successful program participation, such as
        a. Recent myocardial infarction or ischemic heart disease
        b. Uncontrolled dysrhythmias
        c. Acute cor pulmonale
        d. Severe pulmonary hypertension
        e. Febrile or symptomatic infectious illness

    f.   Significant hepatic dysfunction

    g.   Renal failure

    h.   Recent gastrointestinal (GI) bleeding

    i.   Severe disabling neuromusculoskeletal condition

    j.   Metastatic cancer

    k.   Psychiatric disorder or substance abuse, with significant impairment in concentration, motivation, judgment, or mood

    l.   Physical limitations secondary to poor eyesight, hearing, or orthopedic impairment may require modified techniques but should not represent a barrier to participation in pulmonary rehabilitative programs.

D. The program medical director and primary patient caregiver (usually the program coordinator) should participate in the initial evaluation visit.

    1. The patient should undergo a physical examination (see Chapter 18).

    2. A patient and family medical history interview is conducted with assessment of the following

        a.   Respiratory symptoms: Onset, duration, severity, and ameliorating or aggravating factors

        b.   Family history of respiratory problems

        c.   Childhood respiratory health and illness

        d.   Environmental history

           (1) Travel

           (2) Occupations

           (3) Smoking

           (4) Allergies

        e.   General medical and surgical history

        f.   Effects of pulmonary disease on quality of life

        g.   Exercise/activity abilities

        h.   Dependence versus independence in ADLs

        i.   Impairment in occupational performance

        j.   Current medications and schedule

        k.   History of psychosocial issues, such as depression and/or anxiety

        l.   Patient social support network

        m. Use of assistive devices, such as cane, walker, or wheelchair

        n.   Requisite availability of transportation

        o.   Financial resources/reimbursement

    3. The goals and expectations of the patient and family are determined.

        a.   Symptom control

        b.   Psychosocial improvement

        c.   Functional improvement

    4. The program's overall goals, activities, and expected benefits (Box 31-1), as well as limitations and risks, should be explained verbally and detailed on an informed written consent or program contract form.

        a.   Program risks/hazards are typically precipitated by exercise and are usually either

           (1) An acute cardiac or respiratory event

           (2) Skeletal muscular/ligamental injury

E. Preentry diagnostic tests should include

    1. Complete pulmonary function test

        a.   To establish correct diagnosis and severity of lung disease

        b.   To assess response to bronchodilators

        c.   To establish occupational disability

    2. Chest radiography

        a.   To rule out acute cardiopulmonary congestion related to infection, heart failure, or interstitial lung disease

        b.   To assist in the diagnosis of cor pulmonale

        c.   To assist in assessment of the severity of hyperinflation and diaphragmatic flattening

BOX 31-1

Benefits of Comprehensive Pulmonary Rehabilitation

Increased physical energy and endurance
Increased exercise capacity
Improved ability to perform daily activities

Decreased anxiety and depression
Improved understanding of the condition and its management
Enhanced self-care and family support
Acquisition of new coping skills

Improved quality of life
Decreased respiratory symptoms
Decreased hospital days
Decreased mortality

   3. Laboratory data
      a. Arterial blood gas analysis with baseline oximetry (SaO_2)
      b. Laboratory and blood chemistry indices
         (1) Complete blood cell count
         (2) Electrolyte values
         (3) Nutritional-metabolic indices
   F. Quantification of dyspnea is an essential component of evaluating the effectiveness of pulmonary rehabilitative efforts in patients. A number of reliable and valid tools exist to assess dyspnea in a given patient.
      1. The Borg Scale for Breathlessness (BORG) uses a 10-point scale with a nonlinear scaling scheme with descriptive terms to pinpoint patient responses.
      2. The visual analog scale (VAS) is a vertical or horizontal line with anchors to represent extremes of sensation. Patients physically mark the scale (commonly 100 cm long) during exercise to quantify their dyspnea.
      3. The Baseline Dyspnea Index (BDI) is completed by an interviewer and measures three elements affected by dyspnea: functional impairment, magnitude of effort, and magnitude of task that provokes dyspnea.
      4. The Transitional Dyspnea Index (TDI) is also completed by an interviewer comparing changes in dyspnea reported by the patient with BDI data.
      5. The Chronic Respiratory Disease Questionnaire (CRQ) administered by an interviewer assesses dyspnea, fatigue, emotional function, and mastery of breathing.
      6. The Pulmonary Functional Status and Dyspnea Questionnaire (PFSDQ) rates six categories: self-care, mobility, eating, home management, social, and recreational activities independently and in association with level of dyspnea.
      7. The University of California, San Diego Shortness of Breath Questionnaire (SOBQ) assesses dyspnea on a six-point scale for each of 21 ADLs associated with varying exertional demands.
   G. A variety of reliable and valid tools can be used to assess psychological status, motivation, and several aspects of quality of life in patients with chronic pulmonary disease.
      1. The St. George's Respiratory Questionnaire (SGRQ) is a patient-completed quality of life questionnaire that assesses the three areas of illness, namely symptoms, activity, and impact on daily life.
      2. The Medical Outcomes Study Short Form 36 (SF-36) consists of a 36-question questionnaire that assesses physical functioning, role functioning, bodily pain, general health, vitality, social functioning, and mental health.
      3. The Minnesota Multiphasic Personality Inventory (MMPI) assesses 10 major dimensions of emotional distress and personality disturbance.

4. The Profile of Mood States (POMS) is a list of adjectives rated on a Likert-type scale to indicate recent mood.
5. The Katz Adjustment Scale (KAS) is composed of five subscales that focus on social adjustment, recreational activities, and general psychological disturbance.
6. The Sickness Impact Profile (SIP) measures the effect of illness on behavioral function in 12 areas of daily living, such as ambulation, home maintenance, social interaction, communication, alertness, and recreational pastime.
7. The Quality of Well-Being Scale (QWBS) is a subcomponent of the General Health Status index. The scaled score is derived based on symptom complexes and weighted functional level and indicates health-related life quality at one point in time.
8. The Eysenck Personality Inventory (EPI) is a simple instrument used to assess basic pertinent personality traits, such as extroversion and neuroticism.
9. The Additive Daily Activities Profile Test (ADAPT) is a self-administered test on which patients identify which of 105 activities (listed in order of descending estimated volume of oxygen utilization [$\dot{V}o_2$] requirement) they currently perform and which they have stopped because of respiratory limitations.
10. Rotter's Locus of Control Scale evaluates the extent to which an individual perceives internal or external factors as responsible for outcomes and events in his or her life.

H. Exercise testing in pulmonary rehabilitation should include
1. Indications and purposes
   a. To diagnose the etiology of exercise limitation
      (1) Rule out primary or concomitant cardiac disease (e.g., exercise-induced ischemia or dysrhythmias)
      (2) Assess ventilatory response to exercise
      (3) Identify exertional hypoxemia (oxygen desaturation)
      (4) Rule out exercise-induced asthma
   b. To determine the functional capacity and severity of exercise impairment
      (1) Document baseline exercise capacity
      (2) Obtain data for exercise prescription
      (3) Establish occupational disability
   c. To assess the effects of therapy
      (1) Document postprogram exercise capacity (i.e., measure results of training effect)
      (2) Assess symptomatic or objective response to specific therapy (e.g., medication, oxygen therapy, and changes in exercise-induced bronchospasm)
2. Contraindications
   a. Absolute
      (1) Heart failure
      (2) Unstable angina
      (3) Acute myocarditis
      (4) Uncontrolled hypertension (resting systolic pressure >190 mm Hg, diastolic pressure >120 mm Hg)
      (5) Myocardial ischemic changes on electrocardiography (ECG) not attributable to medications
      (6) Acute exacerbation of COPD
      (7) Other acute medical illnesses (e.g., febrile condition, recent pulmonary embolism or thrombophlebitis, GI bleeding)
   b. Relative
      (1) Aortic valve disease
      (2) Recent myocardial infarction (<6 weeks earlier)
      (3) Medication effects (e.g., tachycardia >120 beats/min, ST segment abnormalities)
      (4) Seizure disorder
      (5) Respiratory failure or insufficiency
      (6) Cerebrovascular disease

3. Patient safety and monitoring during exercise testing
   a. Two experienced clinicians, including a physician and respiratory care practitioner, exercise physiologist, or cardiopulmonary diagnostic technician, conduct most exercise tests.
   b. All persons should be certified in basic cardiac life support and ideally in advanced cardiac life support measures.
   c. Emergency resuscitation equipment should be available.
   d. Minimum requirements for noninvasive monitoring during exercise testing of the patient with chronic pulmonary disease include
      (1) Patient's physical appearance
      (2) Perceived levels of dyspnea using a dyspneic rating tool (e.g., BORG)
      (3) Blood pressure values, heart rate, and respiratory rate: Baseline, every 2 to 3 minutes, at the end of exercise, and 3 to 5 minutes after exercise
      (4) Continuous ECG monitoring
      (5) Oxygen saturation: Baseline, continuous during exercise, and for 3 to 5 minutes after exercise
   e. Derived additional exercise diagnostic measurements and information (Table 31-1); such data may not be available because of equipment, setting, and financial limitations of the program.
      (1) Expiratory flow measurements, such as peak expiratory flow rate (PEFR), minute volume (V_E), and tidal volume (V_T), provide information regarding airflow limitation to exercise and the anaerobic threshold.
      (2) Measurements of exhaled gases (breath by breath, end-tidal carbon dioxide and oxygen) allow calculation of the maximal oxygen consumption ($\dot{V}_{O_2}$ max), respiratory quotient (RQ), and ventilatory equivalents for oxygen and carbon dioxide. These values indicate work efficiency and anaerobic threshold, as well as the physiologic efficiency for oxygen transport and the adequacy of ventilation during exercise.
4. General exercise testing schemes
   a. *Constant time tests* require exercise at the highest possible work rate for a given period.
   b. *Single-stage tests* require exercise at a constant work rate for as long as possible; careful selection of the steady-state, submaximum exercise level is important to allow test completion in approximately 8 to 12 minutes.
   c. In *discontinuous tests*, patients exercise at increasing work rates for constant periods with rests of 15 minutes to 24 hours between exercise periods.
   d. *Continuous incremental tests* are used most commonly and use stages that are 1 to 3 minutes long. The increase in workload between each stage may vary, and a 3-minute stage is required for steady-state measurements.
5. Specific protocols
   a. The standard Bruce protocol consists of five 3-minute stages beginning at 1.7 miles/hr (mph) and 10% grade but has been modified for use in pulmonary patients by decreasing the starting grade and maximum speed. This protocol is used commonly in stress testing for cardiac disease.
   b. The lower-level Naughton protocol begins at 0% grade and 1 or 2 mph and after seven 2-minute stages reaches the maximal level, 2.0 mph, 17.5% grade, or approximately a level of seven metabolic equivalents of the task, or 7 METs. The metabolic energy equivalent unit represents approximately 3.5 ml/kg of oxygen consumption at rest. Multiples of the MET unit are used to roughly indicate energy (oxygen consumption) required to perform various activities.
   c. A variety of continuous cycle ergometer protocols are each designed with workload increments of equal size (usually 8 to 25 W) imposed every 30 seconds to 4 minutes (1 W equals 1 joule).
   d. The 12-minute walking test requires that the patient cover as much distance as possible in a measured level corridor, resting only if necessary. At least two baseline

TABLE **31-1**

Selected Exercise Test Information: Results in Health and in COPD

Term	Explanation	Normal Values	Lung Disease
Maximal heart rate achieved	During exercise, heart rate normally increases linearly with increasing work rate up to an age-related maximum.	≥85% of maximum	Decreased
$\dot{V}O_2$ maximum (L/min or ml/kg/min)	Maximal O_2 consumption indicates a subject's maximal exercise capacity or energy expenditure; it is expressed in volume per unit time and may be roughly predicted based on exercise test work levels or directly calculated from exhaled gas measurements. $\dot{V}O_2$ maximum occurs when $\dot{V}O_2$ reaches a plateau despite continued increase in work rate.	Average adult, ≥24 ml/kg/min	Significantly below normal because ventilatory limitations end exercise at low levels of work; $\dot{V}O_2$ max recorded as symptom-limited $\dot{V}O_2$.
Anaerobic threshold	It is the level of work (exercise $\dot{V}O_2$) above which blood lactate levels show a sustained increase and may occur at the exercise level (work rate) at which respiratory minute volume ($\dot{V}E$) and CO_2 output ($\dot{V}CO_2$) markedly increase but $\dot{V}O_2$ does not	50-60% of $\dot{V}O_2$ maximum	Threshold normal in COPD or may not be reached because of low maximal work capacity.
VD/VT	This is the deadspace/tidal volume ratio; it normally decreases during exercise because of increased tidal volume and pulmonary blood flow flow and distribution.	Resting, 0.30-0.40 Exercise, 0.15-0.20	Above normal at rest and fails to decrease with exercise as VT fails to increase significantly.
$\dot{V}E$ max/MVV	This is the ratio of maximum exercise minute ventilation to maximum voluntary ventilation.	Approximately 60%	Increased: may reach or exceed 100% of calculated MVV.
MVV-$\dot{V}E$ max	The difference between maximum voluntary ventilation and minute ventilation at maximum exercise reflects breathing reserve.	20-40% MW	Significantly below normal (i.e., may be close to zero, indicating little or no ventilatory reserve).
$\dot{V}E/\dot{V}O_2$	This is the ventilatory equivalent for oxygen (liters of ventilation for each liter of oxygen used) and reflects physiologic efficiency for ventilation.	30 L$\dot{V}E$/L$\dot{V}O_2$	Increased up to 60 because of ventilation/perfusion mismatch

COPD, Chronic obstructive pulmonary disease.

measurements are recommended to account for a learning effect; through practice and pacing improvements subjects may show a significant increase in distance even before true training begins.

e. The 2- or 6-minute variation of the 12-minute walking test is useful for patients unable to complete the latter.

f. Many pulmonary rehabilitation teams design their own treadmill or cycle protocols; however, common to most are a work rate increment and intensity that achieve the symptom-limiting end point in 10 to 15 minutes.

g. Advantages and disadvantages of common exercise testing equipment are highlighted in Table 31-2.

TABLE **31-2**

Exercise Testing Equipment: Advantages Versus Disadvantages

Type of Exercise Equipment	Advantages	Disadvantages
Level course, variable distance	Practical (uses walking, a familiar skill); inexpensive; no calibration after course measured; useful in repeated measurements in pulmonary rehabilitation programs; able to test more than one patient at a time	Difficult to perform certain physiologic assessments during testing (blood pressure, ECG, ventilation); difficult to quantify workload
Steps	Simple, practical, applicable to daily living; inexpensive, relatively, safe, and transportable	Unable to vary workload; difficult to control patient's center of gravity to ensure full stepping excursion; some measurements difficult (e.g., blood pressure, ventilation)
Treadmill	Uses familiar exercise; easily calibrated; allows measurement of all important physiologic variables; use of incline allows stress to $\dot{V}o_2$ max in a relatively short period	Work rate depends on body size; most expensive; noisy; motion may cause measurement artifact
Cycle ergometer	Safest; work rate independent of body size; less costly than treadmill; less artifact than treadmill; allows measurement of all important physiologic variables	Inability to pedal smoothly may affect determination of work rate; weak quadriceps muscles may stop test prematurely

ECG, Electrocardiography.

IV. **Exercise Training**
  A. Components of an exercise prescription: Type of exercise, frequency, intensity, and duration
    1. The type of exercise prescribed should parallel the desired outcome (the goals of training) as closely as possible and should be further determined by the patient's abilities, preferences, and availability of equipment.
      a. Aerobic exercise aims to improve cardiopulmonary fitness through sustained activity of large muscle groups at an intensity increasing the heart rate to a safe target range.
      b. Strengthening exercises aim to improve the tone and function of select muscle groups. Isolated muscle movements are repeated 10 to 30 times often against resistance.
      c. Most pulmonary rehabilitation programs emphasize lower extremity muscle training. However, many of the ADLs involve use of the arms; therefore, upper extremity muscle training should additionally be incorporated into the program.
    2. Equipment and exercises commonly used in pulmonary rehabilitation include
      a. Treadmill
      b. Cycle ergometer
      c. Level walking
      d. Stair climbing
      e. Rowing
      f. Arm ergometer
      g. Light weights
      h. Pulleys
      i. Elastic bands
    3. The intensity of exercise is traditionally prescribed based on the heart rate or workload achieved on the baseline exercise test.
      a. The initial target heart rate (THR) is 60% to 70% of the maximum age-predicted heart rate (males, 205 – one half their age; females, 220 – their age) unless it exceeds the maximum heart rate achieved during exercise testing.
      b. The Karvonen method is an alternative means to calculate exercise THR.

(1) Maximum heart rate achieved on the exercise test (MHR) minus the resting heart rate (RHR) equals the heart rate range (HRR):

$$MHR - RHR = HRR \tag{1}$$

$$HRR \times 0.70 = Product \tag{2}$$

(2) In this equation 0.60 or 0.80 may be substituted to set the THR at lower or higher levels.

(3) Adding the *product* from equation 2 to the RHR will determine the THR:

$$Product + RHR = THR \tag{3}$$

4. Intensity of exercise may also be selected based on the exercise test workload (treadmill speed and grade or cycle load) corresponding to the following measurements.
   a. 50% $\dot{V}o_2$ max
   b. 50% $\dot{V}_E$ max
5. Home or supervised exercise performed at any of these levels for 30 minutes three to four times per week generally will produce training effects in 4 to 6 weeks.
6. Some patients with chronic pulmonary disease may be unable to tolerate this traditional exercise-conditioning scheme; some may fail to achieve target heart rates, whereas others achieve high heart rates at relatively low levels of exercise.
   a. Exercise schemes should be modified to each patient's tolerance.
   b. If necessary, begin with short exercise periods at a low intensity (e.g., 3 to 5 minutes walking or unloaded cycling) and aim to increase endurance before increasing the intensity of exercise.
7. Box 31-2 lists potential benefits from exercise reconditioning.
B. Implementation of pulmonary rehabilitation exercise sessions
   1. Patients are taught 10- or 15-second pulse taking.
   2. Each session begins and ends with stretching and warm-up or cool-down exercises.
      a. Rhythmic controlled breathing with head, neck, and shoulder exercises
      b. Arm lifts (small 1- to 5-lb weights optional)
      c. Side stretches for rib cage mobility
      d. Calf stretches
      e. Leg lifts (to forward, back, and sides)
   3. The following parameters are monitored.
      a. Heart rate, blood pressure, and respiratory rate at rest, at the end of exercise, and 3 minutes after exercise
      b. Oxygen saturation (Sao_2) as needed
      c. ECG rhythm as needed in patients with known (or at high risk for) cardiac arrhythmias using conventional lead or telemetry
   4. The main exercise should be continuous and should involve large muscle groups of the upper and lower extremities.
      a. Level walking

BOX 31-2

Benefits from Exercise Reconditioning

- Increased endurance and strength
- Increased maximum O_2 consumption
- Increased skill in performance, with decreased ventilation, O_2 consumption, heart rate, and increased anaerobic threshold
- Improved function capabilities for ambulation
- Delayed onset and/or decreased dyspnea
- Increased perception of quality of life/sense of well-being

  b. Treadmill with or without incline

  c. Cycle ergometer

  d. Stair climbing

 5. Supplemental oxygen is given during exercise.

  a. The use of supplemental oxygen during exercise is mandatory for patients who receive oxygen at rest.

  b. Flow rate or F_IO_2 is titrated to achieve SaO_2 of at least 90% with exercise.

  c. It is indicated for patients not otherwise receiving oxygen if the SaO_2 level decreases to <90% with exercise.

  d. Traditionally it is provided via nasal cannula.

  e. Portable oxygen should be used when warranted by the mobility demands of the exercise.

  f. Oxygen-conserving systems (see Chapter 34) should always be used when the patient is using such a device at home for portability. Some of the devices may not provide adequate F_IO_2 with the increased minute ventilation resulting from exercise. Doing so provides documentation that oxygen requirements during exercise are or are not being met by the system, and changes should be made accordingly.

V. Ventilatory Muscle Training

A. Clinical assessment of ventilatory muscles

 1. Maximal inspiratory pressure (MIP) and maximal expiratory pressure (MEP)

  a. Measured during maximal static inspiratory or expiratory efforts into a mouthpiece connected to a pressure gauge

  b. Indicate ventilatory muscle strength

  c. Measured from near residual volume and total lung capacity, respectively

  d. Normal values for MIP in those aged 20 to 54 years

   (1) Men: Approximately 100 to 150 cm H_2O

   (2) Women: Approximately 75 to 125 cm H_2O

  e. Normal values for MEP in those aged 20 to 54 years

   (1) Men: Approximately 200 to 250 cm H_2O

   (2) Women: Approximately 150 to 200 cm H_2O

  f. MIP and MEP measurements decrease with age, chronic pulmonary disease, neuromuscular conditions, and nutritional depletion.

 2. Diaphragmatic excursion

  a. Measured as the distance between percussed levels of dullness on full inspiration and full expiration

  b. Normally approximately 3 to 5 cm

  c. May be reduced in those with chronic pulmonary disease because of diaphragmatic weakness, severe hyperinflation, or both

 3. Sustainable inspiratory pressure (SIP)

  a. Defined as the highest inspiratory pressure (or %MIP) a patient can generate repeatedly over time (e.g., every breath for 10 minutes)

  b. Indicates inspiratory muscle endurance

 4. Maximal sustained ventilatory capacity (MSVC)

  a. Defined as the highest level of ventilation (L/min or % maximum voluntary ventilation) a patient can sustain over time (usually 10 to 15 minutes)

  b. Indicates ventilatory muscle endurance

B. Types of training

 1. Isocapneic hyperpnea: Rapid deep breathing into a circuit maintaining end-tidal carbon dioxide level within normal limits

  a. Ventilatory muscle endurance training: Subject performs near-maximal breathing (rate and depth) for 15 to 30 minutes 3 to 5 days/week.

  b. Sophisticated equipment and supervision are required to regulate F_IO_2 and prevent hyperventilation and respiratory alkalosis; *thus it should not be performed at home or in any other unmonitored setting.*

    2. Inspiratory resistive breathing (IRB)

        a. The variable-orifice, flow-dependent device has multiple openings ranging from 1.8 to 5.3 mm in diameter.

        b. With the spring-load, flow-independent device, the patient must generate a pre-scribed threshold pressure to open a vent and allow inspiration.

        c. Optimal candidates and protocols for IRB are not firmly established.

            (1) One should begin with inspiratory resistive load corresponding to 30% of the MIP, or the smallest orifice tolerated, and monitor the SaO_2 and respiratory rate.

            (2) Frequency and duration are 10 to 15 minutes once or twice daily for 4 to 8 weeks, and then the resistance or threshold pressure is increased gradually to 60% to 70% of the MIP.

C. Reported benefits of ventilatory muscle training

    1. Increased inspiratory muscle strength (MIP)

    2. Increased inspiratory muscle endurance (SIP, MSVC)

    3. Improvement in dyspnea

    4. Increased exercise performance

    5. Improved ability to perform ADLs

    6. There is conflicting scientific evidence supporting the routine use of ventilatory muscle training as an essential component of pulmonary rehabilitation. However, it is reserved for individual consideration in select patients with COPD who have decreased ventilatory muscle strength and dyspnea.

VI. Patient and Family Education

A. Major objectives of patient education in pulmonary rehabilitation

    1. Identifying and explaining the physical and psychosocial changes related to chronic pulmonary disease to set realistic individual goals

    2. Identifying and developing skills in self-care techniques for optimal symptom management and overall health maintenance

B. Factors that influence learning

    1. Acceptance of diagnosis

    2. Motivation and perceived need to learn

    3. Physical energy level

    4. Patient-professional relationship (learner-educator relationship)

    5. Cognitive functional level

    6. Psychomotor abilities

    7. Health beliefs and values (e.g., locus of control)

    8. Level of emotional stability

C. Teaching techniques used in pulmonary rehabilitation programs

    1. Lecture or panel presentation to group

    2. Individualized patient and/or family education sessions

    3. Demonstration of skills, practice, and return demonstration

    4. Group/family discussion

    5. Reading or written assignments

    6. Workbooks

    7. Normal anatomy and pathology posters

    8. Three-dimensional lung and skeletal models

    9. Audio and/or videotaped materials

D. Content of pulmonary rehabilitation education as modified from the AARC Clinical Practice Guidelines on Pulmonary Rehabilitation

    1. Respiratory anatomy and physiology and pathophysiology of the specific chronic pulmonary disease

        a. Upper and lower airway structures

        b. Respiratory muscles and the act of breathing

        c. Anatomic and functional changes in chronic pulmonary disease

        d. Diagnostic tests and expected findings

e. Origin of symptoms
f. Common complications of chronic pulmonary disease (e.g., infection, cor pulmonale)
2. Breathing retraining
   a. Techniques
      (1) Diaphragmatic breathing is generally not recommended; however, it may have application in a non-COPD patient population.
      (2) Pursed lip breathing with prolonged controlled exhalation
      (3) Relaxation of accessory muscles
   b. Use of breathing retraining techniques at rest, during exercise, and with daily activities
   c. Benefits
      (1) Decreased respiratory rate
      (2) Increased V_T
      (3) Decreased work of breathing
      (4) Improved subjective sense of control over breathing, especially during episodes of dyspnea or exertion
      (5) Decreased air trapping
      (6) Decreased airway closure
      (7) Improved exercise/exertional Sao_2
3. Stress and relaxation
   a. Causes and effects of stress
   b. Techniques for stress reduction and relaxation
      (1) Jacobsen's progressive relaxation technique: Selected muscle groups are consciously relaxed in a systematic manner. The patient tenses and then relaxes muscles from head to toe, including face, neck, shoulders, arms, back, abdomen, legs, and feet.
      (2) Guided imagery: The coach (nurse, therapist, or family member) uses descriptive statements to aid the patient in visualizing relaxing scenes.
      (3) Biofeedback: Instrumentation is used to provide patients with signals regarding their control of select physiologic functions, such as respiratory rate and muscle tension.
      (4) Physical exercise
      (5) Simple body positioning and controlled breathing
      (6) Self-relaxation using tapes, music, or self-talk
      (7) Yoga
4. Medications
   a. Drug types
   b. Indications and actions
   c. Adverse effects
   d. Drug interactions
   e. Prescription compliance
   f. Over-the-counter medications
5. Energy conservation in ADLs
   a. Simplifying work tasks
   b. Planning daily schedules
   c. Using correct body mechanics
   d. Balancing work and recreation
   e. Getting adequate sleep and rest
6. Bronchial hygiene measures
7. Smoking cessation: Importance and methods available
   a. Behavior modification techniques (e.g., desensitization, gradual reduction, and stimulus control)
   b. Individual counseling or psychotherapy
   c. Group smoking-cessation clinics
   d. Hypnosis
   e. Cognitive approach (e.g., medical information, physician order)

      f. Acupuncture
      g. Relaxation
      h. Exercise
      i. Pharmacologic aids
  8. Oxygen therapy (see Chapters 33 and 34)
      a. Indications and expected benefit
      b. Use/prescription (dose, hours, adjustment with sleep and exercise)
      c. Prescription compliance
      d. Care of equipment
      e. Safety information
  9. Nutrition (see Chapter 24)
 10. Fluid management
 11. Sexuality and lung disease
      a. Sexuality and self-esteem
      b. Expected sexual changes with aging
      c. Effects of medications
      d. Techniques for sexual expression and energy conservation
 12. Sleep abnormalities commonly associated with chronic pulmonary disease
      a. Obstructive sleep apnea
      b. Central sleep apnea
      c. Mixed components of obstructive and central sleep apnea
 13. Advanced medical care planning/advanced directives
 14. Infection control
      a. Influenza immunization
      b. Avoidance of settings with high density of respiratory infections
      d. Cleaning and disinfecting home respiratory equipment
      e. Prompt access of medical attention with symptom occurrence
 15. Miscellaneous
      a. Environmental influences on breathing (e.g., temperature, humidity, indoor and outdoor pollutants, allergens, and second-hand smoke)
      b. Handling medical emergencies (e.g., knowing when to call the physician or emergency medical services)
      c. Community resources
      d. Travel tips
      e. Better Breathers Clubs

VII. Psychosocial Support
Psychosocial support in pulmonary rehabilitation aims to assist patients and families toward optimal understanding of and coping with chronic pulmonary disease.
A. Specific goals
    1. Help patients accept their condition and realistically assess strengths and limitations.
    2. Identify specific strategies to enlist for coping with stress, anxiety, and depression.
B. Intervention methods
    1. Individual counseling
    2. Couple counseling
    3. Role playing
    4. Group discussion or therapy
    5. Better Breathers Clubs
    6. Spouse support group
C. Activities and benefits of group support sessions
    1. Explore changes in individual image, family structure, and role functioning
    2. Share problems and coping methods
    3. Mobilize passive patients to participate
    4. Enhance social interaction opportunity and skills

VIII. Program Evaluation and Quality Assurance
  A. Program activities and goals should be monitored regularly in quality assurance audits (e.g., monthly or quarterly).
  B. Sample criteria include assessment of subjective and objective elements of pulmonary rehabilitation.
    1. Patient satisfaction assessments (postprogram interviews or questionnaires)
    2. Survey of patient's perceived achievement of goals
    3. Preprogram and postprogram comparison of
      a. Ability to perform ADLs
      b. Exercise (tolerance) testing data
      c. Indicators of quality of life, including reduction in dyspnea
      d. Frequency of respiratory symptoms (e.g., cough, sputum production, wheezing)
      e. Tests of educational content presented
      f. Patient reemployment rate
    4. Program attrition rates and reasons
    5. Preprogram and postprogram hospitalization days and need to access other medical services

IX. Postprogram Patient Follow-up Evaluation
  A. A summary letter is sent from the program coordinator to the primary or referring physician detailing the patient's goals, progress, and achievements.
  B. The patient is encouraged to continue ongoing physician office visits for periodic medical assessment and regulation of medications.
  C. Many outpatient pulmonary rehabilitation programs offer reevaluation visits at 3-, 6-, and 12-month intervals to assess and reinforce compliance with home exercise and activity plans and to provide remediation as warranted.
  D. Ongoing education, support, and contact among patients are available through groups such as Better Breathers Clubs or other local lung association groups.
  E. Home respiratory equipment providers commonly participate in patient follow-up evaluation through written or verbal reports to program coordinators and physicians.
  F. Long-range follow-up evaluation is warranted to evaluate adherence, progression of underlying disease and comorbidity, hospitalization, and survival rates.

BIBLIOGRAPHY

AARC: AARC Clinical Practice Guideline Pulmonary Rehabilitation. *Respir Care* 47:617-625, 2002.

ACCP/AACVPR Pulmonary Rehabilitation Guidelines Panel, American College of Chest Physicians, American Association of Cardiovascular and Pulmonary Rehabilitation: Pulmonary rehabilitation: joint ACCP/AACVPR evidence-based guidelines. *Chest* 112:1363-1396, 1997.

American Thoracic Society: Pulmonary rehabilitation, 1999. *Am J Respir Crit Care Med* 159:1666-1682, 1999.

Antonucci R, Berton E, Huertas A, Laveneziana P, Palange P: Exercise physiology in COPD. *Monaldi Arch Chest Dis* 59:134-139, 2003.

Boueri FM, Bucher-Bartelson BL, Glenn KA, et al: Quality of life measured with a generic instrument (Short Form-36) improves following pulmonary rehabilitation in patients with COPD. *Chest* 119:77-84, 2001.

British Thoracic Society: Pulmonary rehabilitation. *Thorax* 56:827-834, 2001.

Brusasco V, Pellegrino R: Oxygen in the rehabilitation of patients with chronic obstructive pulmonary disease: an old tool revisited. *Am J Respir Crit Care Med* 168:1034-1042, 2003.

Carter R, Holiday DB, Stocks J, Tiep B: Peak physiologic responses to arm and leg ergometry in male and female patients with airflow obstruction. *Chest* 124:511-518, 2003.

Elpern EH, Stevens D, Kesten S: Variability in performance of timed walk tests in pulmonary rehabilitation programs. *Chest* 118:98-105, 2000.

Gimenez M, Servera E, Vergara P, et al: Endurance training in patients with chronic obstructive pulmonary disease: a comparison of high versus moderate intensity. *Arch Phys Med Rehabil* 81:102-109, 2000.

Hernandez MT, Rubio TM, Ruiz FO, et al: Results of a home-based training program for patients with COPD. *Chest* 118:106-114, 2000.

Mannino DM, Ford ES, Redd SC: Obstructive and restrictive lung disease and functional limitation:

data from the Third National Health and Nutrition Examination. *J Intern Med* 254:540-547, 2003.

Martin UJ: Whole-body rehabilitation in long-term ventilation. *Respir Care Clin N Am* 8:593-609, 2002.

Nandi K, Smith AA, Crawford A, MacRae KD, Garrod R, Seed WA, Roberts CM: Oxygen supplementation before or after submaximal exercise in patients with chronic obstructive pulmonary disease. *Thorax* 58:670-673, 2003.

Nazarian J: Cardiopulmonary rehabilitation after treatment for lung cancer. *Curr Treat Options Oncol* 5:75-82, 2004.

Ramirez-Sarmiento A, Orozco-Levi M, Guell R, Barreiro E, Hernandez N, Mota S, Sangenis M, Broquetas JM, Casan P, Gea J: Inspiratory muscle training in patients with chronic obstructive pulmonary disease: structural adaptation and physiologic outcomes. *Am J Respir Crit Care Med* 166:1418-1419, 2002.

Revill SM, Singh SJ, Morgan MD: Randomized controlled trial of ambulatory oxygen and an ambulatory ventilator on endurance exercise in COPD. *Respir Med* 94:778-783, 2000.

Ries AL: Perspectives on pulmonary rehabilitation: no longer out in right field. *J Cardiopulm Rehabil* 23:78-83, 2003.

Chapter 32

Home Respiratory Care and Mechanical Ventilation

I. **Overall Goals of Home Respiratory Care**
   A. Reduce mortality
   B. Enhance the quality of life
   C. Reduce morbidity associated with disease
   D. Arrest the progress of chronic diseases
   E. Improve overall physiologic and psychological function
   F. Provide an environment to enhance individual potential
   G. Provide independence/autonomy
   H. Patient self-care
   I. Provide cost-effective medical care

II. **Home Care Coverage: Financial Considerations**
   A. Federal programs such as Medicare Part B DME provision, Veterans Administration, Social Service Block Grants, or Medicare Hospice
   B. State programs such as Medicaid
   C. Local community organizations and chapter affiliates of large organizations such as American Cancer Society, National Easter Seal Society, Amyotrophic Lateral Sclerosis Association
   D. Private third-party payers, which include commercial health insurance companies, health maintenance organizations (HMOs), managed care organizations (MCOs), participating provider organizations (PPOs), and worker's compensation
   E. Payment directly by patient and/or family, which may satisfy deductible, copayment, or total payment for uninsured or uncovered services

III. **Primary Forms of Home Respiratory Care**
   A. Oxygen therapy
   B. Aerosol therapy
   C. Bronchial hygiene
   D. Nasal continuous positive airway pressure (CPAP)/bilevel positive airway pressure (BiPAP)
   E. Mechanical ventilation
      1. Positive pressure
      2. Negative pressure
      3. High frequency oscillation

IV. **Oxygen Therapy**
   A. Indication: Any cardiopulmonary disease resulting in significant, chronic hypoxemia in the patient's chronic stable state.

B. Chronic hypoxemia in the home care setting is defined by Health Care Financing Administration (HCFA) reimbursement criteria and is scientifically supported by the Nocturnal Oxygen Therapy Trial (NOTT study) and the British Medical Research Council Working Party study.

C. Reimbursement criteria include each of the following
  1. P_{O_2}: ≤ 55 mm Hg (group I)
  2. P_{O_2}: 56 to 59 mm Hg (group II) with
     a. Dependent edema suggestive of congestive heart failure
     b. Pulmonary hypertension or cor pulmonale determined by measurement of the pulmonary artery pressure, gated blood pool scan/echocardiogram, or "P" pulmonale on the electrocardiogram (ECG), or
     c. Erythrocythemia with a hematocrit $\geq 56\%$ (polycythemia)
  3. Hemoglobin saturation: $\leq 88\%$ (group I)
  4. Hemoglobin saturation: 89% (group II), and
     a. Dependent edema suggestive of congestive heart failure
     b. Pulmonary hypertension or cor pulmonale determined by measurement of the pulmonary artery pressure, gated blood pool scan/echocardiogram, or "P' pulmonale on the ECG, or
     c. Erythrocythemia with a hematocrit $\geq 56\%$
  5. Criteria for activity-based oxygen desaturation
     a. P_{O_2} of ≤ 55 mm Hg or hemoglobin saturation of $\leq 88\%$
     b. Taken during activity for a patient who demonstrates an arterial P_{O_2} of ≥ 56 mm Hg or an arterial oxygen saturation of $\geq 89\%$ during the day while at rest
     c. In this case supplemental oxygen is provided for use during exercise if it is documented that the use of oxygen improves the hypoxemia that was demonstrated during exercise when the patient was breathing room air.
  6. Criteria for sleep-induced oxygen desaturation
     a. P_{O_2} of ≤ 55 mm Hg or an arterial saturation of $\leq 88\%$ taken during sleep for a patient who demonstrates an arterial P_{O_2} of ≥ 56 mm Hg or an arterial oxygen saturation of $\geq 89\%$ while awake, or
     b. A greater than normal decrease in oxygen level during sleep (a decrease in arterial P_{O_2} >10 mm Hg or a decrease in arterial oxygen saturation >5%) associated with "P" pulmonale on ECG, documented pulmonary hypertension, and erythrocytosis.
     c. In either of these cases coverage is provided only for nocturnal use of oxygen.

D. Because the relationship between P_{O_2} and hemoglobin saturation is variable and affected by a number of factors, criteria for home oxygen therapy generally should be based on P_{O_2}, not on $HbO_2\%$, as depicted in Figure 32-1, where some nonqualifying $HbO_2\%$ are a result of qualifying P_{O_2}.
  1. Factors affecting P_{O_2} versus $HbO_2\%$ (see Chapter 7)
     a. Temperature
     b. P_{CO_2}
     c. pH
     d. 2,3-Diphosphoglycerate levels

E. Physiologic effects of long-term oxygen therapy
  1. Increased exercise capacity
  2. Decreased work of the myocardium
  3. Decreased work of breathing
  4. Decreased pulmonary hypertension
  5. Normalization of the hemoglobin level
  6. Increased perceived quality of life
  7. Decreased mortality

F. Oxygen containment systems used in the home (see Chapter 34 for details)
  1. System choice is commonly based more on cost versus reimbursement issues than on clinical efficacy; nonetheless the system chosen for a specific patient should satisfy the domiciliary and mobility needs. Each system has major advantages and disadvantages (Table 32-1).

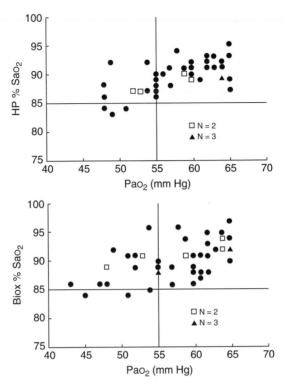

FIG. 32-1 The relationship between resting arterial oxygen tension (Pao_2) and arterial saturation ($Hbo_2\%$) measured by a Hewlett Packard HP47201A *(top)* or a Biox 11A *(bottom)* ear oximeter. Solid lines (Pao_2, 55 mm Hg; $Hbo_2\%$, 85%) represent Medicare criteria for long-term oxygen therapy prescription.

TABLE **32-1**

Advantages Versus Disadvantages of Various Oxygen Delivery Systems

	Advantages	**Disadvantages**
Cylinder oxygen	Fixed finite source of oxygen	Heavy/bulky
	May be stored indefinitely	Represents the smallest content
	Large liter flows transiently available	Requires frequent redeliveries
	100% oxygen source	High pressure 2000-3000 psi
	Quiet oxygen delivery	Represents weight and high-pressure danger
Liquid oxygen	Patient can transfill portable	Evaporation/flash loss
	Large content 860 times compressed	Requires frequent redeliveries
	Liter flow limited to 8-10 L/min	May freeze, interrupting O_2 flow indefinitely
	Low pressure <20 psi	Represents thermal hazard
	100% oxygen source	Requires backup cylinder O_2
	Quiet oxygen delivery	
Concentrator oxygen	Infinite source of oxygen	Consumes patient electricity
	Simplicity of operation	Noisy
	Least supplier intrusion	Potential of mechanical failure
		Requires patient/supplier maintenance
		Liter flow limited to 5-6 L/min
		Requires backup cylinder O_2
		85-98% O_2 dependent on liter flow
		Represents electric shock hazard

2. Oxygen concentrators are most commonly used when the patient is essentially homebound for the majority of time. This system provides an infinite amount of oxygen supply with proper maintenance. However, being electrically powered, concentrators should have a backup source of oxygen for power and/or equipment failures. Oxygen cylinders typically provide backup oxygen in the amount to cover three times the supplier's average response time. With the concentrator there exists the additional cost of electricity, which is incurred by the patient and can be substantial. Specialty concentrators are manufactured that allow the user to slowly transfill aluminum portable cylinders. Portable concentrators with internal battery power and integral oxygen conservers also have recently been introduced. Further a single manufacturer has brought a concentrator capable of delivering 10 L/min to market.

3. Liquid oxygen systems are especially useful for travel, work, and patients with consistent out-of-the-home mobility needs. Liquid oxygen systems represent a large finite source of oxygen with features allowing patient transfilling of portable units. Liquid oxygen units should have a backup source of oxygen for equipment failures or complete depletion of the liquid oxygen contents. Oxygen cylinders typically provide backup oxygen in the amount to cover three times the supplier's average response time. This finite source of oxygen, which is continuously being consumed, requires weekly (or more often) replenishment by the oxygen supplier.

4. Oxygen cylinders are the least commonly used, are the most labor intensive, and are the most expensive. However, cylinders represent a small finite source of oxygen that can be stored indefinitely, hence making them ideal backup sources of oxygen for the home care patient. Smaller cylinders are commonly used to satisfy the periodic mobility needs of patients using an oxygen concentrator for their primary oxygen source. Cylinders made of composite light-weight resin material that may be filled to 150% the normal filling pressure (3000 psi) are available and represent a significant increase in duration and portability (Table 32-2).

5. Some patients use a combination of oxygen concentrator for their stationary oxygen source and a portable liquid oxygen unit (transfilled from a stationary liquid oxygen reservoir) for their portable oxygen needs. Note that third-party payers will only pay for one stationary oxygen source under most circumstances.

G. Oxygen therapy equipment (see Chapter 34)

1. The simple cannula is most common; however, smaller-sized, low-flow cannulas have been used by long-term users of oxygen because of their comfort and inconspicuous appearance. Such cannulas are reserved for liter flows of ≤2 L/min.

2. The simple cannula is usually supplemented with a 25- to 50-foot oxygen extension to provide mobility from the stationary oxygen source. The 50-foot extension is the longest recommended by oxygen equipment manufacturers.

TABLE 32-2

Comparison of Available Portable Oxygen Delivery Systems

Portable Device	Weight	Gas Contents	Duration[†]
Aluminum M-6 or "B" cylinder*	2.2 lb	164 L	42 min
Aluminum M-9 or "C" cylinder*	3.7 lb	255 L	2 hr 7 min
Aluminum M-15 or "D" cylinder*	5.3 lb	425 L	3 hr 30 min
Aluminum M-22 or "E" cylinder*	7.9 lb	680 L	5 hr 40 min
Composite 3000 psi M-9 "B" cylinder size*	1.7 lb	246 L	2 hr 3 min
Composite 3000 psi M-15 "C" cylinder size*	2.6 lb	410 L	3 hr 23 min
Composite 3000 psi M-22 "D" cylinder size*	3.2 lb	640 L	5 hr 20 min
Small representative LOX portable	5.5 lb	542 L	4 hr 31 min
Large representative LOX portable	8.5 lb	1058 L	8 hr 50 min

*Require cylinder valve stem and regulator weighing 1.75 lb.
[†]@ 2 L/min liter flow.

3. Oxygen-conserving devices are used for normal mobility, long-distance travel, or high oxygen demand.
   a. Oxygen reservoir systems function by increasing the anatomic reservoir available for oxygen accumulation.
      (1) Reservoir cannula
      (2) Pendant cannula
   b. Pulse dose or demand systems deliver a predetermined dose of oxygen at the initial portion of inspiration on every- or multiple-breath variations. Such devices are either independent or integral to the oxygen equipment.
      (1) Independent devices are commonly electronically controlled sensors or fluidic switches that are connected in series between the patient and the oxygen source. These may be used with a variety of portable or stationary oxygen sources (e.g., cylinders or liquid oxygen units).
      (2) Integral devices are incorporated directly by the oxygen manufacturer and are typically found on small liquid oxygen portable units that provide for extraordinarily small size and light weight without compromise in duration of oxygen provision.
   c. Transtracheal oxygen is useful in continued work or other activities away from home or for those with hypoxemia refractory to conventional home oxygen system limits.
H. Monitoring home oxygen therapy
   1. Patients who meet the criteria for oxygen therapy at discharge frequently do not require oxygen after a few months as a result of
      a. Complete resolution of the acute precipitating problem
      b. Overall medical care
      c. Use of bronchodilator therapy
      d. Pulmonary rehabilitation programs
   2. Monthly monitoring of status should occur in the home.
      a. Pulse oximetry: After the need is established with Po_2 criteria, $Hbo_2\%$ is concurrently determined with and without oxygen to establish an $Hbo_2\%$ baseline. Oximetry should also be performed with the patient performing the most strenuous activity of his or her normal day to ensure adequacy of the oxygen prescription. These data are to be used as the baseline for future home monitoring.
      b. Sequential monitoring of $Hbo_2\%$ will provide screening for need to assess Po_2 by arterial blood gas.
      c. Adequacy of Po_2 coupled with medical optimization should guide the physician's decision to maintain or discontinue home oxygen.
      d. Vital signs and ventilatory pattern
      e. Chest auscultation
      f. Changes in patient activity levels
   3. Office follow-up evaluation: Frequency depends on the severity of the overall disease process.
I. Complications/safety considerations
   1. Fire hazard is increased in the presence of increased concentrations of oxygen. Generally oxygen should be kept a minimum of 5 feet away from any source of spark and/or flame.
   2. Unsecured cylinders present a physical hazard, as does thermal (cold) burn from mishandling liquid oxygen and electric shock from ungrounded oxygen concentrators.
   3. Fall secondary to oxygen extension tubing clutter.
   4. Complications may occur from the oxygen appliance (e.g., cannula or transtracheal device).

V. Aerosol Therapy
A. Patients with an intact airway and thick, tenacious secretions (e.g., cystic fibrosis, bronchiectasis) may require intermittent administration of aerosol therapy via pneumatic nebulizer.

B. Patients with permanent artificial airways
   1. Most patients are capable of acclimating to artificial airways without the need for continuous aerosol therapy other than the use of artificial noses or heat and moisture exchangers.
   2. Many require nocturnal aerosol therapy. Whether heated or unheated, with or without oxygen, depends on the patient's medical status and tolerance. Note that use of oxygen as a convenient vehicle of aerosol delivery, as is commonly used in the hospital setting, is normally not done in the home care setting. This is a result of home care equipment limitations and third-party payer (reimbursement) constraints.
   3. Occasionally the direct instillation of 3 to 5 ml of sterile 0.9% NaCl into the tracheostomy tube on an intermittent or before suction basis is used to thin secretions and/or induce cough.
   4. *Systemic hydration remains the cornerstone of maintaining normal viscosity of pulmonary secretions.*
C. Small-volume aerosolized drug therapy (see Chapters 17 and 35) is typically delivered via metered dose inhaler (MDI) or small volume nebulizers (SVNs) with a compressor.
   1. Many nontracheostomized, nonmechanically ventilated patients are capable of coordinating the use of an MDI with a spacer, and delivery of medication is best served in that fashion for convenience and cost.
   2. However, in those who have psychomotor and/or cognitive impairments precluding the coordinated ventilatory act required of the MDI, the use of pneumatically operated SVNs is warranted. Young pediatric patients unable to grasp verbal instruction also commonly use such devices. These devices are typically AC powered, but variations with rechargeable self-contained batteries and/or cigarette lighter adapters are manufactured.
   3. Most common drugs delivered by aerosol in the home include
      a. β-Adrenergics (sympathomimetic bronchodilators)
      b. Anticholinergics (parasympatholytic bronchodilators)
      c. Corticosteroids
      d. Prophylactic antihistaminics
      e. Antibiotics (most require specific nebulizers)
      f. Pentamidine (normally requiring specialized nebulizer)
      g. Mucolytics
D. Complications/safety considerations
   1. Aerosol provides the perfect vehicle for droplet nuclei transmission of contaminants to the lower airway; therefore
      a. Proper hand washing should be used before handling equipment.
      b. Equipment should undergo regular mechanical cleaning with liquid detergent and water.
      c. Equipment should be disinfected periodically with weak acetic acid solution, quaternary ammonium compound, glutaraldehyde, or boiled per equipment manufacturer's recommendations.
   2. By ensuring that the patient and/or caregiver understand the prescription dosage, diluent, and frequency and can physically prepare medication for aerosolized delivery, improper medication dosing is minimized. Unit dose preparations often provide the greatest insurance of proper dosing for those experiencing problems.

VI. **Bronchial Hygiene Techniques Used in Home Care (Box 32-1)**
A. Postural drainage, percussion, and vibration (see Chapter 36)
   1. Postural drainage uses bodily positioning along with gravity to drain secretions from specific targeted segments of the lung to larger, central airways.
   2. Chest percussion is used to dislodge secretions and is performed on inspiration and exhalation using the cupped-hand technique, a palm-held, molded rubber cup-shaped device, or alternatively an electric- or pneumatic-powered percussor. Mechanical percussors are generally a nonreimbursed item.

BOX 32-1

Bronchial Hygiene Techniques Used in Home Respiratory Care

Postural drainage
Chest percussion
Chest vibration
Incentive spirometry
IPPB therapy
PEP/flutter valve therapy
Directed cough techniques
Cough assist devices
High frequency chest wall compression
Intrapulmonary percussive ventilation
Oral and lower airway suctioning

IPPB, Intermittent positive pressure breathing; *PEP,* positive expiratory pressure.

3. Chest vibration is used to mobilize secretions to larger airways and is performed by placing one hand on top of the other over the affected area. The therapist performs a vibrating action with the arms and hands by tensing his or her shoulders during the patient's exhalation. This can be delivered via a mechanical vibrating device, which is typically nonreimbursed. Vibration is used alone if the patient cannot tolerate percussion.

B. Incentive spirometry, also referred to as sustained maximal inspiration (SMI), is designed to encourage and reinforce the patient to take protracted, slow, deep breaths. This is accomplished using a device that provides patients with visual positive feedback when they inhale at a predetermined flow rate or volume and sustain the inflation for a predetermined amount of time.

C. Intermittent positive pressure breathing (IPPB) is a technique used to provide short-term or intermittent mechanical ventilation for the purpose of augmenting lung expansion, delivering aerosolized medication, or assisting ventilation. The goal is to deliver a tidal volume (V_T) greater than the patient can initiate on his or her own; therefore, delivered V_T measurement is used to assess the therapeutic efficacy of IPPB in select patient populations. However, it is used infrequently.

D. Flutter valves and positive expiratory pressure (PEP) devices

1. The Flutter device is a small handheld mucus clearance device made of plastic with a pipelike shape. The mouthpiece (or mask) is connected on one end, and an encased steel ball (the flutter device) resting in a plastic circular cone is connected on the other end.
   a. Provides PEP therapy
   b. On exhalation into the device the steel ball rolls and bounces, creating vibrating PEP in the lungs. The vibrations loosen secretions, and the positive backpressure provides improved peripheral air distribution.
   c. The resulting oscillation frequencies range between 6 and 20 Hz.
   d. The vibrations, in conjunction with the increase in expiratory pressure, aid in opening airways and facilitate the clearance of mucus.
   e. The optimal oscillating frequency for a given patient varies and is determined based on the response to therapy.
   f. The oscillation frequencies are adjusted by changing the angle of the tilt of the Flutter device.

2. The PEP device consists of a removable mouthpiece (or mask) and includes a one-way inspiratory valve and an expiratory resistance/frequency adjustable dial with an optional pressure measurement port.
   a. Provides PEP therapy
   b. Exhaled air is directed through an opening, which is periodically closed by a pivoting cone. The result is a vibrating PEP.
   c. The frequency of oscillations ranges from 0 to 30 Hz.

    d.   The vibrations, in conjunction with the increase in expiratory pressure, aid in opening airways and facilitate the clearance of mucus.

    e.   The frequency of the vibrations and the resistance of the opening are adjusted by rotating the dial.

  3. The primary benefit of the Flutter or PEP devices is that after instruction, the need for a professional to oversee its use is only periodically necessary, with the patient typically self-administering therapy.

E. Directed cough techniques

  1. The forced expiratory technique (FET; "huff cough") is performed as follows.

    a.   One or two huffs (forced expirations) from mid to low lung volumes

    b.   Followed by relaxation and then slow, diaphragmatic breathing for 30 to 60 seconds

    c.   Deep inspiration with breath-holding for 2 or 3 seconds

    d.   Forceful cough once or twice while keeping the glottis open

    e.   Repeat as necessary

  2. Manually assisted cough

    a.   Patient takes a deep breath in (or assisted inspiration via manual resuscitation bag).

    b.   Apply external pressure to the thoracic cage or epigastric region coordinated with a forced exhalation

F. Cough assist devices

  1. CoughAssist or in-exsufflator (formerly the Coffilator) by J. H. Emerson Company

    a.   A portable electric device that uses a blower and valve to alternately apply a positive followed by a negative pressure to the patient's airway

    b.   Air is delivered to and from the patient via a breathing circuit with flex tube, bacteria filter, and patient attachment via mask, mouthpiece, or standard artificial airway adapter.

    c.   Indicated for patients with reduced peak expiratory flows, such as those with high spinal cord injury, neuromuscular deficits, or fatigue secondary to intrinsic pulmonary disease. Medicare reimbursement is provided in these cases.

G. High frequency chest wall compression (HFCC)

  1. THAIRapy vest developed by American Biosystems Inc.

    a.   The vest consists of an inflatable jacket and an air-pulse generator.

    b.   The vest fits snugly over the entire thorax and is connected to the front panel of the air-pulse generator by two hoses to create external chest wall oscillations.

    c.   Increasing oscillatory frequencies ranging from 5 to 20 Hz are used during the course of each treatment.

    d.   The device is activated at the patient's full inspiration, and a 5-minute period of oscillation at low frequency is initiated.

    e.   Transient increases in airflow are produced at each stepwise increase in compression and result in mobilization and physical alteration of secretions.

    f.   The patient performs a forced expiratory maneuver before the device is deactivated to allow expectoration of secretions.

    g.   The cycle is repeated five or six times at gradually increasing frequencies.

  2. Hayek Oscillator by Breasy Medical Equipment

    a.   Uses a microprocessor-controlled noninvasive ventilator

    b.   The unit is connected to the patient via a traditional cuirass.

    c.   There is a range of cuirass sizes suitable for preterm infants to adults.

    d.   The cuirass is attached to a piston pump that can provide ventilation up to high frequencies, and baseline negative pressure is produced from a vacuum pump.

    e.   Frequencies of up to 15 Hz can be achieved, and frequency, inspiratory and expiratory pressures, and inspiratory-to expiratory (I:E) ratio are controlled variables for patients.

    f.   Negative and positive pressures are alternately applied during inspiration and exhalation, respectively, with oscillations around a negative baseline followed by an artificial cough.

    g.   The artificial cough has a prolonged inspiratory phase followed by a short expiratory phase.

H. Intrapulmonary percussive ventilation (IPV)
1. Percussionare developed by Dr. Forest Bird
2. IPV is used to mobilize and clear retained secretions, assist in the resolution of atelectasis, and deliver aerosolized medications.
   a. Oscillatory pulsations are delivered that generate high frequency bursts of gas at rates of 100 to 300 cycles/min (2 to 5 Hz).
   b. The minibursts of air are delivered to the patient's airway at pressures of 10 to 45 cm H_2O during inspiration, with the range adjusted to match the compliance and resistance of the lung and chest wall.
3. Three therapeutic results are provided during IPV.
   a. Percussive oscillatory vibrations, which loosen retained secretions
   b. High-density aerosol delivery to hydrate secretions
   c. PEP to recruit alveolar lung units and assist in expiratory flow acceleration during a cough maneuver

I. Home suctioning techniques
1. Clean versus sterile technique
   a. Accepted practice to use a "clean" suction technique in the home
   b. The patient should be instructed in self-care whenever possible.
   c. Patient or caregiver should use proper hand-washing techniques before handling equipment.
   d. Caregivers should use nonsterile (clean) gloves when suctioning a patient with an artificial airway to
      (1) Reduce introduction of contaminants to the lower airway
      (2) Reduce risk of self- and cross-contamination of others
   e. Gloves are not necessary when suctioning the oral pharynx with a hard tonsillar-type (Yankauer) suction catheter.
2. Reuse of suction catheters is commonly used in the home care setting when the catheters are
   a. Externally wiped clean, and the internal lumen is rinsed by aspirating cooled, boiled water (<24 hours old) until clear.
   b. Air is aspirated to remove residual water and dry the internal lumen.
   c. The catheter is then stored on a clean surface to air dry until next use.
   d. Catheters should undergo regular mechanical cleaning with liquid detergent and water followed by daily disinfection with weak acetic acid solution, quaternary ammonium compound, glutaraldehyde, or boiled per equipment manufacturer's recommendations.
   e. Suction catheters handled in this fashion may be used until they lose their integrity.

VII. **Nasal CPAP and Nasal Positive Pressure Ventilation (NPPV)**
A. Nasal CPAP is used to manage obstructive sleep apnea (OSA).
1. Nasal CPAP is achieved by creating a prescribed CPAP from a flow generator via a nasal appliance. This same device may be alternatively used with an oral mask.
2. Medicare reimbursement criteria for nasal CPAP
   a. Diagnosis of OSA documented by an attended, facility-based polysomnogram that meets either of the following criteria.
      (1) The apneic/hypopneic index (AHI) is ≥15 events per hour, or
      (2) The AHI is from 5 to 14 events per hour with documented symptoms of
         (a) Excessive daytime sleepiness, impaired cognition, mood disorders, or insomnia, or
         (b) Hypertension, ischemic heart disease, or history of stroke.
   b. Polysomnographic studies must be performed in a facility-based sleep study laboratory and not in the home or a mobile facility. These laboratories must be qualified providers of Medicare services and comply with all applicable state regulatory requirements.
   c. A home medical equipment (HME) supplier must not perform polysomnographic studies.

      d. Continued coverage of the CPAP device beyond the first 3 months of therapy requires that no sooner than the 61st day after initiating therapy, the supplier ascertain and document from either the patient or the treating physician that the patient is continuing to use the CPAP device.

      e. Noncompliant and/or periodic discontinuation of usage of the device may interrupt the supplier's billing for the equipment and related accessories and supplies.

      f. Other third-party payers follow similar, less stringent criteria.

B. Nasal noninvasive intermittent positive pressure ventilation (NIPPV) is used to manage OSA, restrictive thoracic disease, severe chronic obstructive pulmonary disease (COPD), or central sleep apnea (CSA). Numerous small NPPV units are available from many manufacturers, but all function in a similar manner.

    1. Nasal NPPV is patient sensitive and assists ventilation by creating a prescribed positive inspiratory pressure (IPAP) followed by a less but still positive expiratory pressure (EPAP) via an electronically controlled flow generator applied via a nasal appliance. This same device may alternatively be used with an oral mask. Some units have the feature of setting a backup respiratory rate in the "timed mode," providing for an assist-control mode.

    2. Medicare reimbursement criteria for nasal NPPV

      a. Physician must fully document in the patient's medical record symptoms characteristic of sleep-associated hypoventilation, such as daytime hypersomnolence, excessive fatigue, morning headache, cognitive dysfunction, and dyspnea.

      b. Indicated for those patients with clinical disorder groups characterized as (1) restrictive thoracic disorders (i.e., progressive neuromuscular diseases or severe thoracic cage abnormalities); (2) severe COPD; (3) CSA; or (4) OSA, and who also meet the following criteria.

        (1) Restrictive thoracic disorders

          (a) There is documentation in the patient's medical record of a progressive neuromuscular disease (e.g., amyotrophic lateral sclerosis) or a severe thoracic cage abnormality (e.g., postthoracoplasty for tuberculosis), and

          (b) An arterial blood gas $PaCO_2$, done while awake and breathing the patient's usual F_IO_2 that is ≥ 45 mm Hg, or

          (c) Sleep oximetry demonstrates oxygen saturation $\leq 88\%$ for at least five continuous minutes, done while breathing the patient's usual F_IO_2, or

          (d) For a progressive neuromuscular disease (only), maximal inspiratory pressure <60 cm H_2O or forced vital capacity is <50% predicted, and

          (e) COPD does not contribute significantly to the patient's pulmonary limitation.

          (f) If all the aforementioned criteria are met, nasal NPPV (based on the judgment of the treating physician) will be covered for patients within this group of conditions during the first 3 months of therapy.

        (2) Severe COPD

          (a) An arterial blood gas $PaCO_2$, done while awake and breathing the patient's usual F_IO_2 that is ≥ 52 mm Hg, and

          (b) Sleep oximetry demonstrates oxygen saturation $\leq 88\%$ for at least 5 continuous minutes done while breathing oxygen at 2 L/min or the patient's usual F_IO_2 (whichever is higher), and

          (c) Before initiating therapy, OSA (and treatment with CPAP) has been considered and ruled out.

          (d) If all of the aforementioned criteria for patients with COPD are met, nasal NPPV will be covered for the first 3 months of therapy.

        (3) CSA (i.e., apnea not caused by airway obstruction)

          (a) A complete facility-based, attended polysomnogram must be performed documenting the following.

          (b) The diagnosis of CSA, and

      (c) The exclusion of OSA as the predominant cause of sleep-associated hypoventilation, and

      (d) The ruling out of CPAP as effective therapy if OSA is a component of the sleep-associated hypoventilation, and

      (e) Oxygen saturation ≤88% for at least 5 continuous minutes, done while breathing the patient's usual F_IO_2, and

      (f) Significant improvement of the sleep-associated hypoventilation with the use of nasal NPPV on the settings that will be prescribed for initial use at home, while breathing the patient's usual F_IO_2.

      (g) If all the aforementioned criteria for patients with CSA are met, nasal NPPV (based on the judgment of the treating physician) will be covered for the first 3 months of therapy.

    (4) OSA

      (a) A complete facility-based, attended polysomnogram has established the diagnosis of OSA according to the following criteria:

        (i) The AHI is ≥15 events per hour, or

        (ii) The AHI is from 5 to 14 events per hour with documented symptoms of excessive daytime sleepiness, impaired cognition, mood disorders, or insomnia, hypertension, ischemic heart disease, or history of stroke, and

      (b) A CPAP device has been tried and proven ineffective.

      (c) If the aforementioned criteria for patients with OSA are met, nasal NPPV will be covered for the first 3 months of therapy.

  c. Continued coverage of nasal NPPV therapy beyond the first 3 months of therapy requires that no sooner than the 61st day after initiating therapy the physician ascertain and document progress of relevant symptoms and that the patient continues to use the nasal NPPV device at least an average of 4 hours every 24 hours. The supplier also must obtain such documentation from the physician, as well as a statement from the patient documenting use, benefit, and intention for continued use.

  d. This reimbursement criterion put forth by Medicare is supported by a review of the available science investigating the clinical indications for Noninvasive Positive Pressure Ventilation in Chronic Respiratory Failure Due to Restrictive Lung Disease, COPD, and Nocturnal Hypoventilation consensus report findings, published in 1999.

  e. As with CPAP, other third-party payers follow similar but generally less stringent criteria.

VIII. Mechanical Ventilation

  A. Thousands of individuals in the United States require long-term mechanical ventilatory assistance.

  B. It is likely that this number will increase in the future as a result of

    1. Improved medical care

    2. Cost-effectiveness of elective nocturnal ventilatory support

    3. U.S. population demographics increased health care demands

    4. Improved and simplified technology

  C. Possible solutions to the increased need for long-term invasive ventilatory support in the home

    1. Meticulous consideration before initiation of mechanical ventilation in the acute care setting of the following.

      a. Reversibility of the acute pulmonary disease process

      b. Chronicity of underlying disease

    2. Appropriate elective use of alternative ventilatory assistance

      a. NIPPV

      b. Negative pressure ventilation (NPV)

    3. Use of alternative care sites

      a. Alternative care sites include (listed in order of increasing independence and decreasing cost)

        (1) Long-term care hospitals

        (2) Skilled nursing facilities

        (3) Congregate living center

        (4) Home

    b. The patient may transition from site to site based on changing personal desires, financial factors, medical conditions, and associated care needs.

D. General indications and disease categories requiring long-term ventilatory support

    1. Patients requiring invasive long-term ventilatory support who have demonstrated

        a. An inability to be completely weaned from invasive ventilatory support

        b. Progression of disease etiology that requires increasing ventilatory support

    2. Neuromusculoskeletal disorders: The best candidates have chronic, slowly progressive diseases.

    3. Central hypoventilation: Those with sleep apnea secondary to a dominant central (versus obstructive) component, including patients with obese hypoventilation syndrome (OHS), generally are good candidates.

    4. Obstructive lung disease: Selective patients are good candidates. Many comply poorly, are difficult to treat, and have many other organ system problems and the typical sequelae associated with chronic pulmonary disease.

    5. Restrictive lung disease: Normally such patients are rarely candidates; they generally have the highest respiratory needs.

E. The ideal patient for long-term ventilatory support

    1. Has a neuromuscular or neurologic disorder

    2. Is clinically stable

    3. Is well educated

    4. Is motivated

    5. Is interested in self-care

    6. Has good support systems

    7. Has some ventilatory independence

F. The keys to successful transition to the home are appropriate predischarge planning and a well-coordinated team effort. Key members of the discharge team include

    1. Physician

    2. Patient/family and/or caregivers

    3. Case manager

    4. Respiratory care practitioner

    5. Primary nurse

    6. Social worker

    7. Dietician, physical, occupational, and speech therapist as necessary

    8. Home health agency

    9. Home medical equipment provider

G. Patients requiring *nonelective* mechanical ventilatory assistance generally require approximately 4 weeks of in-hospital training and acclimation to equipment before transitioning into the home. In the instance of elective ventilatory assistance, namely, the use of NIPPV, the equipment and care needs of the patient are typically less extensive. The discharge plan and process will be streamlined and much quicker than for nonelective cases. In either case the discharge timeframe should be accelerated or decelerated based on individual patient and family needs.

H. All respiratory care and other assistive equipment anticipated to be used in the home should be used in the predischarge hospital training to allow mastery of related technique, patient acclimation, and documented medical efficacy. Further home care procedures that may differ from hospital procedures should be adopted by patient and family during the predischarge period as soon as educational mastery is achieved.

I. The need for skilled full-time caregivers in the home is based on numerous factors.

    1. Patient

        a. Adult, adolescent, infant; most infants require at least 8 hr/day of skilled caregiver support.

      b. Ventilatory dependence: Typically the greater the number of hours requiring continuous support, the greater the need for skilled caregivers.

      c. Ability to provide self-care

      d. Rehabilitation potential

  2. Family

      a. Ability to provide care

      b. Ability to direct care

      c. Need for respite care

  3. Third-party coverage

      a. Reimbursement for ventilator and related equipment and supplies varies greatly among payers. Coverage of outside professionals and/or lay care providers varies to an even greater extent.

      b. Many insurers provide minimal home care support.

      c. Others reimburse only registered nurse care, even though the patient requires only a companion or lay sitter.

      d. Most private insurers have a maximum cap (lifetime benefit) on monies available.

  4. Infants generally require more caregiver assistance than adults.

  5. Length of time home on ventilatory assistance is generally inversely related to the need for skilled caregivers as patient and family become accustomed with requisite care provision over time.

J. Invasive positive pressure ventilation

  1. Medical discharge criteria

      a. Absence of severe dyspnea or frequent episodes of dyspnea and/or tachypnea

      b. Acceptable blood gases with F_IO_2 level <0.40

      c. Psychological stability

      d. Stable cardiac function and absence of life-threatening arrhythmia

      e. Manageable pulmonary secretions

      f. Protected airway

      g. Absence of significant nutritional deficit

      h. In general, overall medical optimization and clinical stability with utilization of home care equipment and procedures

  2. Other discharge criteria as modified from AARC clinical practice guidelines: 1995

      a. The caregivers (lay and professional) must clearly demonstrate and have documented the competencies required for caring for the specific patient. *This should include all aspects of the patient's care needs.*

      b. Availability of caregivers for each 24-hour period must be ensured.

      c. The chosen site must be capable of housing, operating, maintaining, and supporting the equipment required by the patient's medical condition. This should include respiratory and ancillary equipment and supplies, such as the ventilator, suction, oxygen, intravenous therapy, nutritional therapy, adaptive equipment, and disposable supplies.

      d. The physical environment must be evaluated for safety and suitability. It should be free of fire, health, and safety hazards; provide adequate heating, cooling, and ventilation; provide adequate electrical service (and backup generator as indicated); and provide for patient access and mobility with adequate patient space (room to house medical and adaptive equipment) and storage facilities.

      e. Financial resources must be identified at the beginning of the discharge process. Lack of or inadequate funding impacts the entire discharge plan and can dictate the discharge care site. Sources and adequacy of funds for alternate-site care, medical equipment and supplies, the required medical personnel, any modifications necessary to environment, and ongoing medical care should be fully evaluated.

      f. Development of a multidisciplinary plan of care is based on the evaluation of the patient's needs and goals. The plan should be consistent with recommended practices and guidelines for the patient's condition. Key elements of the plan should include

     (1) Integration into the community
     (2) Patient self-care as appropriate
     (3) Roles and responsibilities of team members for daily care management
     (4) Documented mechanism for securing and training additional caregivers
     (5) Alternative emergency and contingency plans
     (6) Use, maintenance, and troubleshooting of equipment
     (7) Monitoring and appropriately responding to changes in the patient's medical condition
     (8) Medication administration
     (9) Method for ongoing assessment of outcomes
    (10) Time frame for implementation
    (11) Method to assess growth and development of pediatric patients
    (12) Provision of professional medical follow-up evaluation
    (13) Documented mechanism for recertifying and remediating patient and other caregivers
    (14) Provision of respite care

  g. Some have found a 1- to several-day trial period at home helpful in allowing unanticipated, real day-to-day issues to be identified and then later prepared for in the controlled environment of the hospital before final discharge home. Others view such efforts as laborious and expensive, consuming disproportionate emotional and physical resources for small return. There are no hard and fast rules, and individual consideration of the concept should be given to each discharge situation.

  h. *When all medical and other criteria have been satisfied, the patient is appropriately prepared for discharge. It should be noted that whatever the external demands, fiscal or otherwise, there are no shortcuts to education or planning that will allow safe, successful discharge.*

 3. Home mechanical ventilators (general descriptions)

  a. Today there are essentially five categories of mechanical ventilators specifically designed and manufactured for home use.

    (1) BiPAP ventilators
      (a) Widespread use in noninvasive home ventilation
      (b) New generations continue to be produced; this is the fastest growing segment of home ventilation.
      (c) Flow generators capable of delivering high flows
      (d) Some have a timed mode providing for backup rate.
      (e) Most offer clinician-settable inspiratory rise time and duration.
      (f) Some offer adjustable inspiratory and expiratory triggers.
      (g) Quiet, compact, and lightweight
      (h) Oxygen supplementation can be problematic.
      (i) Lack internal battery backup
      (j) Relatively inexpensive

    (2) Volume-targeted home care ventilators
      (a) Traditional, historical mainstay of home care ventilators
      (b) Typically piston driven
      (c) Limited variety of mode application
      (d) Sufficiently alarmed
      (e) Stable oxygen delivery
      (f) Provide internal battery backup
      (g) Expensive
      (h) Generally used for stable invasive home ventilation

    (3) Pressure/volume-targeted home care ventilators
      (a) Newest generation of home care ventilators
      (b) Typically turbine driven, capable of delivering large flows
      (c) Microprocessor controlled
      (d) Hybrid of bilevel and acute care ventilators

(e) Adjustable inspiratory rise time and duration
(f) Large variety of mode applications
(g) Alarmed and full featured
(h) Stable to precise oxygen delivery
(i) Provide internal battery backup
(j) Expensive
(k) Can be used for invasive and noninvasive home ventilation

(4) Negative pressure ventilators (see Section K-1, a-g, Negative Pressure Ventilators)

(5) High frequency ventilators (HFVs) or oscillators (see Chapter 42)

b. Ventilators designed primarily for hospital use should not be used in the home. With the large variety of commercially available, full-featured, home care ventilators, it is rare to find a justified exception to this axiom.

4. Ideal characteristics of home care ventilators
   a. Designed exclusively with the home care patient in mind
   b. User-friendly operation
   c. Reliable operation
   d. Absence of confusing digital readouts that change on a breath-by-breath basis
   e. Provide ventilatory support of infant, children, and adult populations
   f. Available modes: Assist/control (AC), control, pressure support, synchronized intermittent mandatory ventilation (SIMV), positive end-expiratory pressure (PEEP), and NPPV
   g. Respiratory rate: 1 to 80 breaths/min
   h. VT: 50 to 2000 ml
   i. Peak flow capability: 30 to 140 L/min
   j. Spontaneous demand peak flow provision: ≤180 L/min
   k. Automatic and/or settable leak compensation
   l. Inspiratory time: 0.3 to 3.0 seconds
   m. Assisted breaths triggered by PEEP compensated, proximal patient airway pressure sensing
   n. Direct setting of F_IO_2 or access for titration of oxygen
   o. Integral PEEP feature
   p. Internal battery capable of functioning for >2 hours
   q. Appropriately alarmed
      (1) High/low pressure
      (2) High/low tidal and/or minute volume
      (3) High/low respiratory rate
      (4) Ventilator failure to deliver gas as programmed
      (5) Ventilator inoperable
      (6) Low battery (power)
   r. Remote alarm capability
   s. Remote "nurse" call capability
   t. Compact (fits on wheelchair), light (<35 lb)
   u. Such home care ventilators are manufactured; however, they are the newest, generally most expensive, and not the norm and probably contain features not required in a given patient situation.

5. The internal gas flow pathway of an older simple, piston-operated, volume-targeted, commonly used home care ventilator in the United States is illustrated in Figure 32-2.
   a. Gas enters these units by way of an oxygen-accumulating device with a one-way valve.
   b. A one-way valve is also located just inside the unit's intake filter.
   c. From here gas enters the piston chamber during the piston's back stroke.
   d. During the piston's forward stroke gas exits the piston chamber via a one-way valve, which prevents gas from being drawn into the piston chamber during the piston's back stroke.

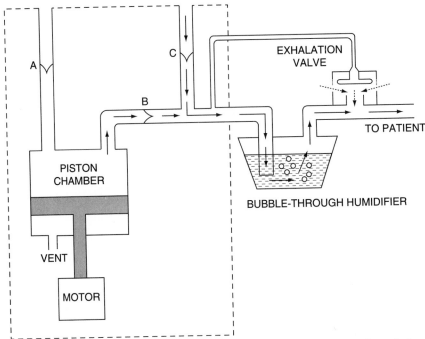

FIG. 32-2 Basic gas flow during spontaneous inspiration with a typical home care ventilator. **A,** One-way check valve allows gas entry into the piston chamber during piston back stroke. **B,** One-way check valve prevents negative ventilatory circuit pressure from developing during back stroke of piston. **C,** One-way check valve allows patient to spontaneously inspire during closure of (B) when piston back stroke is in progress. Some gas may enter the system at the exhalation valve. Arrows depict gas flow during spontaneous inspiration.

  e. A pop-off valve is located in the piston chamber (vent) to prevent excessive chamber pressurization.

  f. Once gas exits the piston chamber it normally passes a pressure limit control adjustable by operator and a one-way inlet valve, allowing inspiration of gas from the unit's circuit during the piston's back stroke.

  g. Not all units include the one-way inlet valve.

  h. No demand or continuous gas flow system is included. During spontaneous breathing or SIMV the patient must draw gas from

    (1) The exhalation valve

    (2) The piston chamber

    (3) The one-way air inlet valve

  i. *Note: Spontaneous demand flow systems are integral on bilevel and pressure/volume-targeted home care ventilators that avoid the aforementioned problems observed with the older volume-targeted ventilators.*

 6. Delivery of oxygen

  a. Some of these units accept a high 50-psi oxygen and/or air source or a low-pressure 0.5- to 10-psi source.

  b. Essentially all units allow an oxygen-accumulating device (reservoir) to be attached to the gas entry port.

  c. The use of the integral F_IO_2 blender is the most accurate when supplied; however, the use of an accumulator produces a suitably consistent F_IO_2 ($\pm3\%$ to 4%) with home care ventilators.

  d. Oxygen may also be bled into the circuit by the use of a T attached between the ventilator and the humidifying device.

  e. In the instance of NPPV, oxygen may be bled directly into the facial appliance within manufacturer-recommended limitations.

7. PEEP
    a. Bilevel and most pressure- and volume-targeted home care ventilators have an integral PEEP feature with manually settable or automatic sensitivity compensation available.
    b. The traditional volume-targeted home care ventilators are not designed for the application of PEEP.
    c. A PEEP valve may be placed at the exhalation valve.
    d. However, the patient's ability to trigger the machine is grossly affected with the work of breathing (WOB) greatly increased (see Chapter 40).
    e. As a result the use of external PEEP devices with these ventilators is discouraged.
8. The SIMV/IMV mode
    a. Spontaneous demand systems are integral on pressure- and volume-targeted home care ventilators and are capable of meeting most patient peak inspiratory flow demands.
    b. Many of the volume-targeted home care ventilators posing a SIMV/IMV mode do not have a demand system or continuous flow setup included in the system's basic design.
    c. When such a unit is set on SIMV/IMV with the use of a bubble-through humidifier, the imposed WOB is excessive (Figure 32-3).
    d. Even the use of passover humidifiers or heat and moisture exchangers does not sufficiently reduce the WOB.
    e. In this situation if the SIMV/IMV mode is to be used, a one-way H-valve system placed before the system's passover humidifier should be used (Figure 32-4).
    f. If an increased F_IO_2 value is needed oxygen can be titrated into the one-way H-valve system as shown in Figure 32-4.

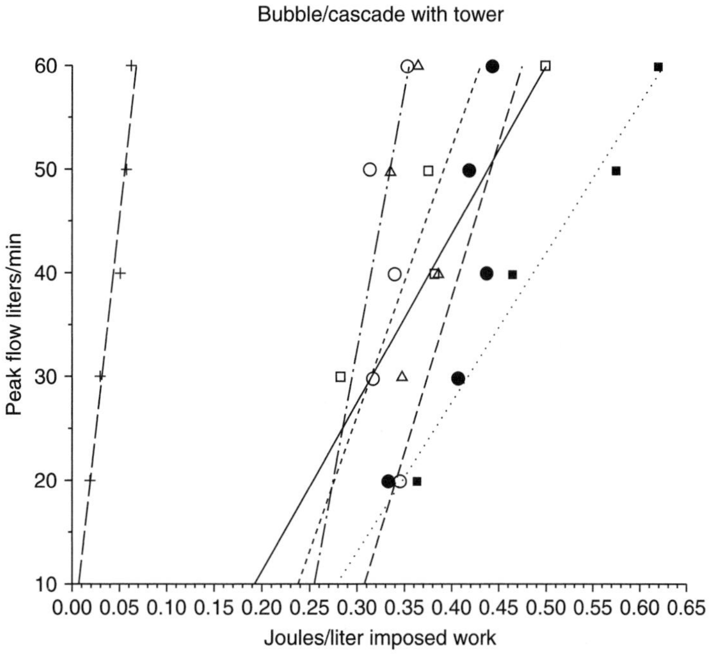

FIG. 32-3 Imposed work of breathing (WOB) versus peak inspiratory flow for five home care ventilators with a normally functioning bubble-through humidifier and an H-valve continuous flow system with a passover humidifier. The H-valve system produced the least imposed WOB. Positive sign and dashes and dots represent the H-valve continuous flow system with the passover humidifier. Open circles and large and small dashes represent the Intermed Bear 33. Open triangles and small dashes represent the Puritan Bennett 2800. Open squares and the solid line represent the Acquitron LP-6. The closed circle and large dashes represent the Medimax ARF 1500E. Closed squares and small dots represent the Life Care PLV-100.

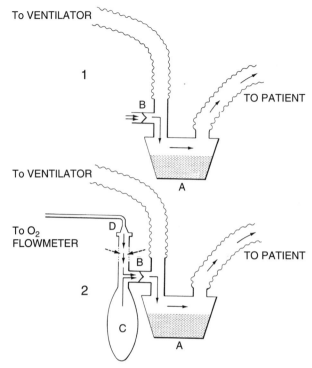

FIG. 32-4 One-way H-valve systems. 1, Valve open to atmosphere. 2, Valve with 3-L reservoir bag attached to 0.28 F_IO_2 Venturi, powered by 4 L of oxygen/min. **A,** Passover humidifier. **B,** One-way valve. **C,** Reservoir; **D,** 0.28 F_IO_2 Venturi. Arrows depict gas flow during spontaneous inspiration.

      g. The use of a one-way valve and a passover humidifier greatly reduces the imposed WOB of these systems in the SIMV/IMV mode.
   9. Selection of ventilator parameters (adults)
      a. Criteria outlined in Chapters 21, 22, and 41 should be followed.
      b. Volume or pressure AC when the ventilator is equipped with a spontaneous demand system; otherwise volume AC
        (1) To decrease imposed WOB
        (2) To improve ventilatory muscle rest
        (3) Because adults normally do not wean from ventilatory support at home
        (4) Muscular capabilities during periods independent of the ventilator are enhanced if rest is maximized.
  10. Selection of ventilator parameters (infants)
      a. Many infants are weaned from mechanical ventilation in the home.
      b. Small, eventually weanable infants may require the use of pressure-limited continuous flow SIMV or PSV.
      c. Accomplished by most of the commercially available home care ventilators or alternatively by the addition of the one-way H-valve reservoir system depicted in Figure 32-4 and the use of a pop-off valve in the ventilator circuit to maintain the pressure plateau.
      d. Criteria outlined in Chapters 28 and 30 should be followed during parameter selection.
  K. Noninvasive nonpositive pressure approaches to mechanical ventilation
   1. NPV
      a. NPV is provided by applying a settable subatmospheric pressure to the thorax and abdomen on an intermittent basis, which causes an increase in thoracic and

abdominal volume and a resultant decrease in respective pressures. These subatmospheric pressures are in turn transmitted to the lungs, creating a pressure gradient from atmosphere to lungs and resulting in inspiratory flow. Exhalation occurs passively when the machine-imposed subatmospheric pressure is intermittently stopped, and the normal elastic recoil of lungs, thorax, and abdomen increases intrapulmonary pressure, creating a pressure gradient from lungs to atmosphere.

   b. NPV can be provided with the use of

     (1) Iron lung

     (2) Negative pressure ventilator, and

        (a) Porta lung (full-body chamber)

        (b) Poncho with chest shell

        (c) Pneumosuit with chest shell

        (d) Mass-produced or customized chest cuirass

   c. The size of the V_T generated by a given negative pressure is a function of the thoracic and abdominal compliance, the airway resistance, and the surface area of negative pressure exposure. Hence NPV functions best on individuals with normal lungs and normal thoracic compliance typical of patients with neuromuscular disease. However, NPV has successfully been used to support other disease entities.

   d. It should not be used for patients with upper airway obstruction because it will exaggerate the obstructive component.

   e. For optimal use, respiratory rates and pressure must be high enough to capture the diaphragm and inhibit spontaneous ventilation. Optimally the diaphragm will work in synchrony with the ventilator.

   f. Most negative pressure units are controllers, with the newly manufactured units featuring a patient-triggered AC mode providing greater synchrony with spontaneous ventilatory effort.

   g. The use of NPV is frequently successful when it is combined with other noninvasive approaches to ventilation.

  2. Pneumobelt (Figure 32-5)

   a. This is a belt with an inflatable bladder designed to compress the abdominal contents and move the diaphragm up to assist exhalation.

   b. Inspiration occurs when the balloon deflates, allowing the abdominal contents and diaphragm to move downward.

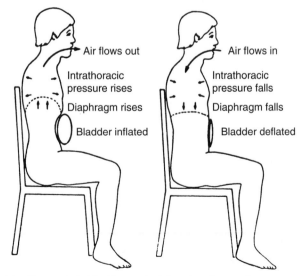

Air flows out
Intrathoracic pressure rises
Diaphragm rises
Bladder inflated

Air flows in
Intrathoracic pressure falls
Diaphragm falls
Bladder deflated

FIG. 32-5 Function of the Pneumobelt. The Pneumobelt functions by exerting pressure on the abdominal contents by inflation of a rubber bladder forcing the diaphragm upward and assisting exhalation *(left)*. When the bladder deflates, gravity pulls the diaphragm back down, assisting inhalation *(right)*.

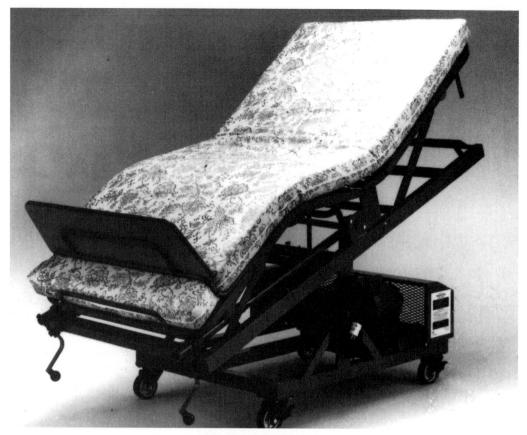

FIG. 32-6 Rocking bed.

    c. It is effective only in the sitting position (at least 30 degrees).

    d. A pressure generator is used to inflate the bladder. Pressures of 50 to 70 cm H_2O are required, with the volume of gas entering the bladder approaching 2000 ml to ensure appropriate movement.

    e. VT of 300 to 500 ml can be achieved.

    f. These units typically function as controllers, with newer devices incorporating an AC mode.

3. Rocking bed (Figure 32-6)

    a. A rocking bed is a hospital-style bed designed to move the head and the foot of the bed in alternating rhythmic, opposite directions.

    b. Thus head up/feet down tilt assists inspiration by moving the abdominal contents downward.

    c. Head down/feet up tilt assists exhalation by moving the abdominal contents upward.

    d. A maximum of a 60-degree arc is available.

    e. The rocking occurs at a rate between 8 and 34/min.

    f. It is most effective for neuromuscular disease patients.

    g. Normally it is ineffective in thin patients.

    h. Frequently it is used with other forms of noninvasive mechanical ventilation.

BIBLIOGRAPHY

AARC: AARC Clinical Practice Guideline Discharge Planning for the Respiratory Care Patient. *Respir Care* 40:1308-1312, 1995.

AARC: AARC Clinical Practice Guideline Long-Term Invasive Mechanical Ventilation in the Home. *Respir Care* 40:1313-1320, 1995.

American Respiratory Care Foundation: Consensus conference: non-invasive positive pressure ventilation. *Respir Care* 42:364-369, 1997.

Bach JR: *Noninvasive Mechanical Ventilation.* Philadelphia, Elsevier Health Sciences Division, 2002.

British Medical Research Council Working Party: Long-term domiciliary oxygen therapy in chronic hypoxic cor pulmonale complicating chronic bronchitis and emphysema. *Lancet* 1:681-686, 1981.

Hill N: Use of negative pressure ventilation, rocking beds, and pneumobelts. *Respir Care* 39:532-549, 1994.

Hill N: Noninvasive ventilation: state of the art. *Am J Respir Crit Care Med* 163:540-577, 2001.

Janssens JP, Derivaz S, Breitenstein E, et al: Changing patterns in long-term noninvasive ventilation: a 7-year prospective study in the Geneva Lakes area. *Chest* 123:67-79, 2003.

Kacmarek R: New ventilator options for the long-term mechanical ventilation in the home. In: Hill N (ed): *Long-Term Mechanical Ventilation.* New York, NY, Marcel Dekker, 2001, p. 375-409.

Kacmarek RM, Hess DR: Equipment required for home mechanical ventilation. In: Tobin MJ (ed): *Principles and Practice of Mechanical Ventilation.* New York, McGraw Hill, 1994, p. 111-115.

Kacmarek RM, Hill NS: Ventilators for noninvasive positive pressure ventilation: technical aspects. *Euro Resp Monograph* 6:76-105, 2001.

Kacmarek RM, Stanek K, McMahon K, et al: Imposed work of breathing during synchronized intermittent mandatory ventilation using home care ventilations. *Respir Care* 35:405-414, 1990.

Make B, Bach JR, Criner CG, et al: ACCP Consensus Conference on mechanical ventilation outside the critical care unit. *Chest* 113:289S-344S, 1998.

NAMDRC: Clinical indications for noninvasive positive pressure ventilation in chronic respiratory failure due to restrictive lung disease, COPD, and nocturnal hypoventilation—A consensus report. *Chest* 116:521-534, 1999.

Nocturnal Oxygen Therapy Trial Group: Continuous or nocturnal oxygen therapy in hypoxemic chronic obstructive lung disease; a clinical trial. *Ann Intern Med* 93:391-398, 1980.

Petty TL, Casaburi R: Recommendations of the fifth oxygen consensus conference. *Respir Care* 45:957-961, 2000.

Chapter 33

Gas Therapy

I. **Medical, Laboratory, and Therapeutic Gases and Mixtures**
   A. Ethylene (C_2H_4)
   B. Nitrous oxide (N_2O)
   C. Cyclopropane [$(CH_2)_3$]
   D. Oxygen (O_2)
   E. Nitrogen (N_2)
   F. Carbon dioxide (CO_2)
   G. Helium (He)
   H. Oxygen/nitrogen (21% O_2/79% N_2)
   I. Oxygen/carbon dioxide (90% to 98% O_2/2% to 10% CO_2)
   J. Helium/oxygen (40% to 80% He/20% to 60% O_2)
   K. Air
   L. Nitric oxide (NO)

II. **Flammable Gases**
   A. Ethylene
   B. Cyclopropane

III. **Nonflammable Gases**
   A. Nitrogen
   B. Carbon dioxide
   C. Helium

IV. **Gases That Support Combustion**
   A. Oxygen
   B. Helium/oxygen
   C. Oxygen/carbon dioxide
   D. Oxygen/nitrogen
   E. Nitrous oxide
   F. Nitric oxide
   G. Air

V. **Gas Cylinders**
   A. Cylinder types and composition
      1. Type 3AA: Seamless, high-quality, heat-treated tempered alloy-steel
      2. Type 3A: Seamless, low carbon, heat-treated steel (no longer produced)

a. Line 1: ICC or DOT, 3A or 3AA, 2015
    (1) ICC or DOT: The organization governing the transport of cylinders
        (a) ICC: Interstate Commerce Commission. The agency that regulated construction, transport, and testing of compressed gas cylinders from 1948 to 1970.
        (b) DOT: Department of Transportation. The federal agency responsible for construction, transport, and testing of compressed gas cylinders since 1970.
    (2) 3A or 3AA: Cylinder type
    (3) 2015: Maximum working pressure in pounds per square inch (psi), which normally can be exceeded by 10% (2200 psi).
b. Line 2: 28300, Serial number
c. Line 3: PCGC
    (1) PCGC: Initial of owner
d. Line 4: Manufacturer's mark
2. Rear: Refer to Figure 33-1.
C. Cylinder size
1. Large cylinders using hexagonal nut connections (see Section VII, B, American Standard Compressed Gas Cylinder Valve Outlet and Inlet Connections Safety System index)
    a. H or K: 9-in. diameter, 55-in. height
    b. G: 8.5-in. diameter, 55-in. height
    c. M: 7.125-in. diameter, 46-in. height
    d. F: 5.5-in. diameter, 55-in. height
2. Small cylinders using yoke connections (see Section VII, A, Pin-Index Safety System)
    a. E: 4.25-in. diameter, 30-in. height
    b. D: 4.25-in. diameter, 20-in. height
    c. B: 3.5-in. diameter, 16-in. height
    d. A: 3-in. diameter, 10-in. height
    e. DD: 3.75-in. diameter, 23.25-in. height
    f. BB: 2.75-in. diameter, 19.75-in. height
    g. AA: 2.75-in. diameter, 11-in. height

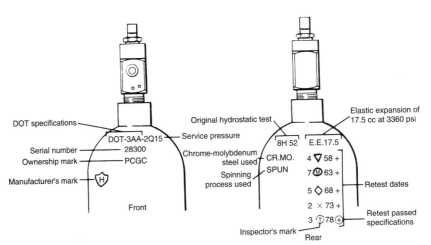

FIG. 33-1 Typical markings for cylinders containing medical gases, front and rear views.

D. Cylinder capacities for oxygen
   1. D: 12.7 ft^3
   2. E: 22 ft^3
   3. G: 187 ft^3
   4. H or K: 244 ft^3
E. Maximum filling pressure of 3AA oxygen cylinders: 2015 psi plus 10% (2200 psi)
F. Calculation of duration of flow from oxygen and compressed air cylinders
   1. One cubic foot of gas = 28.3 L
   2. The volume of gas in liters in a full cylinder = cubic foot volume × 28.3 L/ft^3
   3. Dividing the aforementioned determined value by the maximum filling pressure of 2200 psi results in the calculation of a factor indicating the number of L/psi:

$$\text{Factor for duration of flow} = \frac{(\text{ft}^3 \text{ vol})(28.3 \text{ L/ft}^3)}{2200 \text{ psi}} = \text{L/psi} \qquad (1)$$

   4. For a D-sized cylinder:

$$\frac{(12.7 \text{ ft}^3)(28.3 \text{ L/ft}^3)}{2200 \text{ psi}} = 0.16 \text{ L/psi}$$

   5. L/psi factors for oxygen cylinders
      a. D: 0.16 L/psi
      b. E: 0.28 L/psi
      c. G: 2.41 L/psi
      d. H or K: 3.14 L/psi
   6. Calculation of duration of flow in minutes
      a. Gauge pressure multiplied by duration of flow factor (L/psi) equals the number of liters in the cylinder.
      b. Dividing the result of no. 6a by the flow in L/min results in the time in minutes that the cylinder will last:

$$\begin{array}{c} \text{Time in minutes} \\ \text{cylinder will last} = \\ \dfrac{(\text{Gauge pressure})(\text{Duration of flow factor})}{(\text{Flow in L/min})} \end{array} \qquad (2)$$

      c. Example for E cylinder:

Gauge pressure	1500 psi
Duration of flow factor	0.28 L/psi
Flow in L/min	10 L/min

$$42 \text{ minutes} = \frac{(1500 \text{ psi})(0.28 \text{ L/psi})}{10 \text{ L/min}}$$

   The cylinder will deliver 10 L/min for 42 minutes before it is completely empty.
      d. Clinically it is advisable to subtract 500 psi from the gauge pressure to provide a safety margin before the duration of flow is calculated.
G. Color code for E cylinders (Color coding is mandatory for E-sized cylinders only; other sizes of cylinders are not required to follow any coding system.)
   1. Oxygen: Green (universal code: white)
   2. Helium: Brown
   3. Ethylene: Red

       4. Cyclopropane: Orange

       5. Nitrous oxide: Light blue

       6. Carbon dioxide: Gray

       7. Oxygen and carbon dioxide: Green and gray

       8. Oxygen and helium: Green and brown

       9. Nitrogen: Black

     10. Nitrogen and oxygen: Black and green (other than room air)

     11. Air: Yellow

H. Hydrostatic testing of cylinders

    1. Perform periodic high-pressure testing of gas cylinder integrity.

    2. Cylinder expansion is determined by measuring water displacement of an empty cylinder compared with that cylinder when filled to ⅗ of its maximum pressure.

    3. All cylinders must be retested every 5 to 10 years, depending on elastic expansion of the original testing.

I. Cylinder stem pop-off valves

    1. Large cylinders use a frangible disk designed to rupture at a pressure within 5% of cylinder-bursting pressure.

    2. Small cylinders use a fusible plug designed to melt at a temperature of 65.6° C to 76.7° C (150° F to 170° F).

J. Gas cylinder storage and handling

    1. Storage areas must meet National Fire Protection Association (NFPA) guidelines regarding construction materials, location, and actual structure; the area must be well ventilated, cool, and dry.

    2. Only flame-resistant construction materials should be used in storage areas.

    3. Full and empty cylinder areas must be separated to prevent confusion.

    4. All cylinders should be restrained; usually chains are used for large cylinders, and racks are used for small cylinders.

    5. All storage areas should be locked.

    6. No oil- or petroleum-based lubricants should come in contact with valves, regulators, fittings, or gas hoses.

    7. Soapy water should be used to detect system leaks.

    8. Only regulators designed for a specific cylinder type and content should be used.

    9. Valves on a cylinder should be cracked slowly before attachment of regulator to remove particulate matter from the valve and to dissipate heat of compression.

   10. Damaged or unlabeled cylinders should not be used.

   11. Cylinders should not be exposed to open flames or sparks and should not be subjected to temperatures >51.6° C/125° F.

   12. Cylinder valves should be closed when not in use, and cylinder caps (large cylinders) should be in place during storage and transport.

   13. Cylinders should only be transported in suitable containers or carts.

   14. In some institutions there is a practice of transfilling small cylinders from large cylinders (which is not recommended because of the tremendous energy transfer and the potential for contamination). If this process is performed, labeling and cylinder inspection must conform to DOT standards. The Compressed Gas Association (CGA) also recommends that the supply cylinder be isolated, that calibrated pressure gauges be used on the cylinder being filled, and that the filling rate be limited to 200 L/min.

VI. **Regulation of Gas Flow**

  A. High-pressure gas regulators

    1. Regulators limit flow in a system by reducing maximum working pressure.

    2. Regulators reduce cylinder pressures to a usable working pressure of ≤50 psi.

    3. Single-stage regulators

       a. Cylinder pressure is reduced to a working pressure of ≤50 psi in one step or stage.

       b. One high-pressure pop-off valve is incorporated in the regulator and set at approximately 200 psi.

4. Multistage regulators
  a. Cylinder pressure is reduced to a working pressure of ≤50 psi in a series of steps or stages.
  b. A high-pressure pop-off valve is incorporated into each stage of the regulator, with the final stage pop-off valve set at approximately 200 psi.
5. Preset regulators (Figure 33-2)
  a. Pressure is reduced in one or more stages to a fixed working pressure of 50 psi.
  b. Normally a low-pressure gas-regulating device (e.g., Thorpe tube) is incorporated to reduce flows to working levels.
  c. Preset regulators are used without a Thorpe tube when connected to a system using a 50-psi pressure source (e.g., ventilators).
6. Adjustable regulators (Figure 33-3)
  a. Pressure is reduced in one or more stages to a final working pressure adjustable to between 0 and 50 psi.
  b. Normally a Bourdon pressure gauge calibrated in L/min indicates flow leaving the final stage of the adjustable regulator.
B. Low-pressure gas regulators (flowmeters)
  1. Bourdon gauge (Figure 33-4)
    a. The Bourdon gauge is a pressure-sensitive gauge that uses an expandable copper coil to indicate pressure readings.
    b. Bourdon gauges can be calibrated to indicate flow and are used as flow-measuring devices.
    c. If backpressure is applied distal to the gauge, it will indicate a flow higher than actual flow (Figure 33-5).

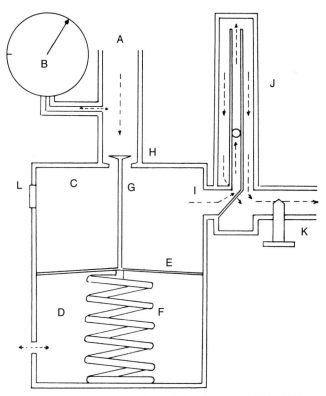

FIG. 33-2 Diagram of preset, high-pressure gas regulator. **A,** Attachment to cylinder. **B,** Pressure gauge. **C,** Pressure chamber. **D,** Ambient pressure chamber. **E,** Flexible diaphragm. **F,** Spring. **G,** Valve stem. **H,** Gas entry valve. **I,** Outflow port. **J,** Thorpe tube flowmeter. **K,** Needle valve. **L,** Pop-off valve.

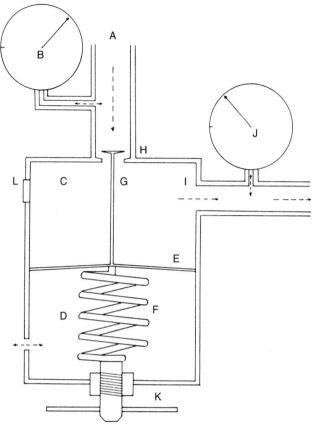

FIG. 33-3 Diagram of an adjustable, high-pressure gas regulator. **A,** Attachment to cylinder. **B,** Pressure gauge. **C,** Pressure chamber. **D,** Ambient pressure chamber. **E,** Flexible diaphragm. **F,** Spring. **G,** Valve stem. **H,** Gas entry valve. **I,** Outflow port. **J,** Bourdon flow gauge. **K,** Threaded gas flow control. **L,** Pop-off valve.

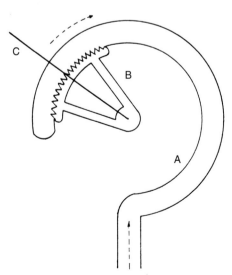

FIG. 33-4 Internal function of a Bourdon gauge. **A,** Curved, flexible, closed tube. **B,** Gear mechanism. **C,** Indicator needle, reflecting flow or pressure on face of valve.

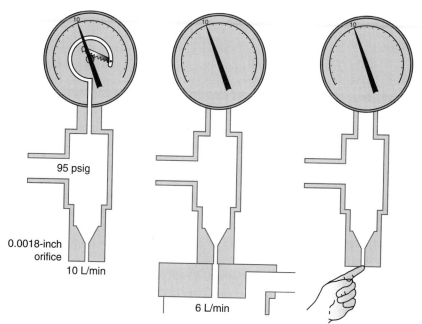

95 psig

0.0018-inch
orifice

10 L/min

6 L/min

FIG. 33-5 Bourdon gauge performance when downstream pressures increase as a result of high-resistance equipment or blockage. *Left,* Normal state with fixed orifice and no downstream resistance results in an accurate flow reading. *Center,* High-resistance nebulizers increase downstream pressure, or backpressure. The result is a falsely high reading (10 L/min versus actual flow of 6 L/min). *Right,* Complete blockage (zero flow) results in flow reading on gauge but no gas delivered.

2. Orificial resistor-type flowmeters use variously sized orifices to regulate flow.
   a. Currently used on small-sized cylinders to regulate gas flow
   b. Only allow precise flows (i.e., 1, 2, 3, and so on) but no flows in between actual settings
   c. Can be used in any orientation or position and do not affect output of gas flow
   d. Actual flow through the orifice is based on the law of flow or resistance. With the driving pressure constant the size of the orifice determines the exact flow exiting the orifice.
3. Thorpe tube flowmeters (Figure 33-6): Gas flow is measured by the vertical displacement of a float in an increasing diameter tube. Flow is regulated by a needle valve placed proximal or distal to the float.
   a. Compensated Thorpe tubes are designed to function accurately at a working pressure of 50 psi at 21.1° C (70° F).
      (1) The needle valve is always located distal to the float.
      (2) If backpressure is applied distal to the needle valve, the float will indicate the actual flow delivered.
   b. Uncompensated Thorpe tubes are designed to function at variable working pressures.
      (1) The needle valve is always located proximal to the float.
      (2) If backpressure is applied distal to the float, the float will always indicate a flow lower than the actual flow delivered.

VII. **Safety Systems Incorporated in Gas Flow Systems and Cylinders**
   A. Pin-Index Safety System (PISS) (Figure 33-7)
      1. This system is used only on *E-sized cylinders or smaller.*
      2. It is used on connections for which the maximum working pressure is >200 psig (pounds per square inch gauge).

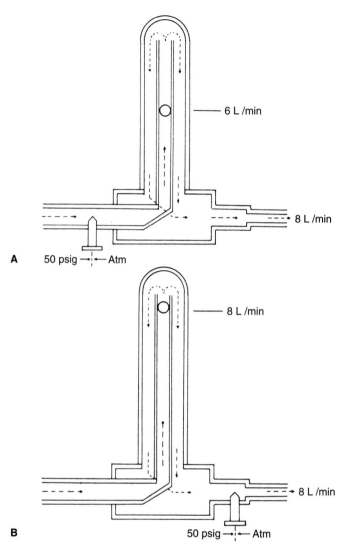

FIG. 33-6 Comparison of pressure-uncompensated **(A)** and pressure-compensated **(B)** flowmeters. In the former the flow-control valve is proximal to the meter, and the gauge records less than the actual output. In the latter location of the valve distal to the meter correlates the gauge reading with the output.

3. It incorporates a yoke-type of connection where two pins on the regulator connection (yoke) are matched to holes on the cylinder stem (Figure 33-8).
4. Ten possible combinations are available; nine currently are in use.
5. Pin positions 2 and 5 are used for oxygen.
B. American Standard Compressed Gas Cylinder Valve Outlet and Inlet Connections Safety System (Figure 33-9)
1. This system is only used on cylinders *larger than E size*.
2. It is used on connections for which the maximum working pressure is >200 psig.
3. It incorporates a hexagonal nut and specific nipple on the regulator fitted to an externally threaded cylinder connection.
4. For oxygen the connection is CGA-540, 0.903-14 NGO, RH-Ext, which indicates a CGA connection no. 540 is used with a 0.903-in. threaded outlet diameter and 14 threads/in. of the National Gas Outlet type, and the threads are external and right handed.

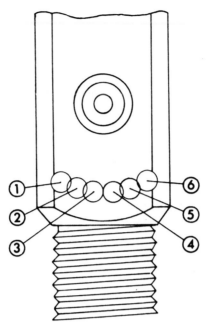

FIG. 33-7 Location of the Pin-Index Safety System holes in the cylinder valve face, various pairs of which constitute indices for different gases. See text for complete pairings.

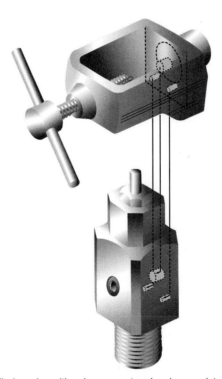

FIG. 33-8 Yoke-type cylinder valve with yoke connector showing regulator inlet and pin placements.

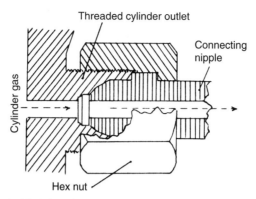

FIG. 33-9 Structure of a typical American Standard connection such as may be used to attach a reducing valve to a large high-pressure cylinder. The hexagonal nut is held onto the nipple of the reducing valve by a circular collar, seen as a cross-sectional projection on the nipple. As the hexagonal nut is tightened on the threaded cylinder outlet, the end of the nipple is snugly seated into the conical outlet.

    C. Diameter-Index Safety System (DISS) (Figure 33-10)
        1. Used on all connections distal to the regulator for which maximum working pressures are <200 psig.
        2. Used for connections of flowmeters to regulators or other connections where frequent equipment changes are made.
        3. It incorporates a hexagonal nut and a nipple designed with two shoulders fitted into a body and externally threaded with two concentric borings.
        4. The DISS connection for oxygen is no. 1240 with a 0.5625-in. diameter and 18 threads/in.

VIII. Agencies Regulating Medical Gases
    A. Food and Drug Administration (FDA): Determines purity standards and labeling for all medical gases listed in the United States Pharmacopeia (USP).
    B. Compressed Gas Association (CGA): Sets standards and makes recommendations to manufacturers and municipal authorities on manufacture of gases and safety standards for cylinders.
    C. National Fire Prevention Agency (NFPA): Sets standards and makes recommendations to manufacturers and municipal authorities on storage and handling of cylinders.
    D. Department of Transportation (DOT): The federal agency responsible for construction, transport, and testing of compressed gas cylinders since 1970.

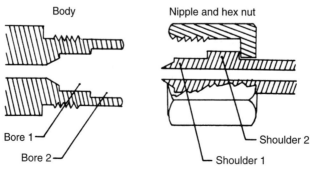

FIG. 33-10 Components of a representative Diameter-Index Safety System connection. The two shoulders of the nipple allow the nipple to unite only with a body having corresponding borings. If the match is incorrect, the hexagonal nut will not engage the body threads.

IX. **Fractional Distillation of Air**
   A. The gas is filtered to remove all dust and impurities.
   B. The gas is dried to remove all water vapor.
   C. The gas is compressed to 200 atm pressure.
   D. The heat of compression is removed by heat exchangers until the temperature returns to ambient.
   E. By decreasing the pressure 5 atm the gas is then rapidly and repeatedly decompressed. The reduction in pressure allows tremendous cooling by expansion to occur, bringing the temperature below the boiling point and liquifying all gases in the air.
   F. The temperature of the liquid is then increased, and the various gases are evaporated and collected at their respective boiling points.

X. **Bulk Gas Oxygen Systems**
   A. There are three types of centrally located systems.
      1. Alternating gas supply system (Figure 33-11).
         a. Consists of large cylinders of oxygen banked together in two separate series
         b. These two banks are called the primary and reserve bank.

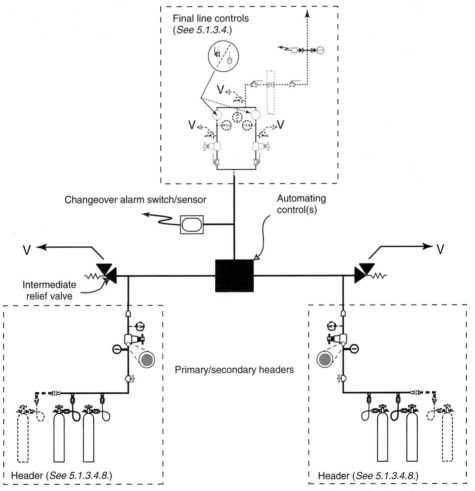

FIG. 33-11 Alternating supply system is composed of primary and secondary supplies that alternate to charge the piping system.

    c. When the pressure of the primary bank reaches a certain level a control valve switches to the reserve supply.

    d. Because the primary bank is now empty, the reserve bank becomes the primary bank. The empty cylinders are filled, and this bank is now called the reserve.

2. Gas cylinder supply system with reserve supply

    a. Consists of a primary, secondary, and reserve supply system

    b. Once the primary supply is empty of gas, a valve automatically switches to the secondary supply, similar to the alternating system.

    c. Alarms signal when changeovers have occurred and refilling the primary and/or secondary systems is needed.

3. Bulk gas system with a reserve

    a. These are usually liquid oxygen containers backed up by a gas cylinder supply system.

XI. Bulk Liquid Oxygen Systems (Figure 33-12)

    A. These systems are more efficient than the gaseous systems because 1 ft^3 of liquid O_2 is equal to 860.6 ft^3 of gaseous O_2, or 24,354.98 L of O_2.

    B. Liquid O_2 must be stored below its critical temperature of –181.1° F and prevented from exerting a pressure >250 psi.

    C. The storage unit is composed of an inner and outer steel shell separated by an insulating vacuum to prevent transfer of heat to the liquid; the inner shell is coated with silver to aid in repelling heat. The unit is also vented to allow vaporized O_2 to exit, maintaining internal pressure <250 psi. This is essentially a large thermos bottle (see Figure 33-12).

    D. Liquid O_2 leaving the storage unit is converted to a gaseous state by a vaporizer, after which it is reduced to 50 psi for delivery into the central piping system.

    E. Storage areas must meet NFPA guidelines regarding construction, design, and location. Among key provisions in these standards is the requirement for a reserve or backup gas supply to equal the average daily usage of the hospital. To meet this demand, hospitals may use either a smaller liquid O_2 storage tank or a bulk gas oxygen system as a backup measure.

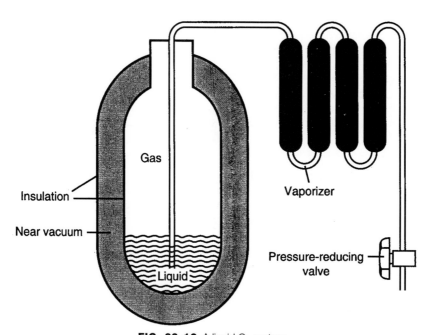

FIG. 33-12 A liquid O_2 system.

XII. Portable Liquid Oxygen Systems
   A. These systems are used primarily for home oxygen therapy or intrahospital transport.
   B. Because a larger volume of oxygen (860.6 L gas/L liquid) can be stored more easily as a liquid than as a gas, these systems are most useful for home care.
   C. During storage there is evaporative loss of oxygen because of the continual conversion of the liquid to a gas.
   D. Available oxygen flow rates are up to 8 L/min.
   E. These units do not provide the 50-psi power source needed to drive other respiratory care equipment.
   F. These units are generally stationary and can provide oxygen therapy for 4 to 12 days at 2 L/min.
   G. Many companies also manufacture portable liquid oxygen systems.
      1. These systems contain approximately 0.5 to 1.5 L of liquid oxygen.
      2. They are generally lightweight (5 to 13.5 lb).
      3. Provision of oxygen at 1 L/min can be maintained for up to 24 hours with some units.
   H. Cylinders of liquid gases are filled to a specified filling density. Weighing a liquid-filled cylinder is the only accurate method to determine the contents of the cylinder.
   I. Calculating the duration of flow in minutes for liquid oxygen
      1. One liter of liquid oxygen weighs 2.5 lb = 860 L of oxygen in a gaseous state.
      2. Amount of gas in cylinder = (Liquid O_2 weight [lb])(860)/2.5 lb/L
      3. Duration of gas in minutes = Amount of gas in cylinder (L)/Flow (L/min)
         a. Example of duration of flow

$$\text{Amount of gas in cylinder} = \frac{(1.5 \text{ lb})(860)}{2.5/\text{L}} = 516 \text{ L}$$

$$\text{Duration of the gas in minutes} = \frac{516 \text{ L}}{3 \text{ L/min}} = 172 \text{ minutes}$$

The cylinder will deliver 3 L/min for 172 minutes before it runs out.

XIII. Oxygen Concentrators
   A. These systems incorporate molecular sieves of permeable membranes to purify entrained ambient air.
   B. Concentrations of 80% to 95% oxygen are generally available. The higher the delivered flow, the lower the F_1O_2 *level.*
   C. Maximum delivered flow is approximately 5 L/min.
   D. These units are stationary and are designed for home use.

XIV. Air Compressors
   A. Large medical air compressors (Figure 33-13)
      1. Used to provide high flow rates at working pressures of 50 psig
      2. A motor drives a piston in a compression cylinder, which draws air in through a filtered valve into a reservoir tank. The pressure in the reservoir tank is higher than line pressure.
      3. The gas leaves the reservoir and then goes through a dryer to remove the moisture and then goes through a reducing valve to bring it to line pressure.
   B. Small compressors
      1. Used for home and bedside for operating small volume nebulizers (most models operate at 6 L/min).
      2. These compressors have a diaphragm or turbine that compresses air and generally do not have a reservoir.

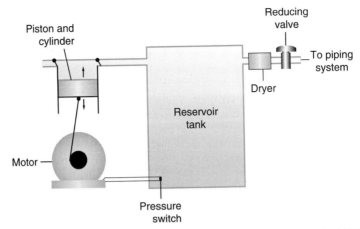

FIG. 33-13 Large medical air compressor: The compressor sends gas to the reservoir at higher than line pressure. When the preset pressure level is reached, the pressure switch shuts off the compressor. Gas leaves the reservoir and passes through the dryer to remove moisture, and the reducing valve reduces gas to the desired line pressure. When reservoir pressure has decreased to near line pressure, the pressure switch turns the compressor back on.

BIBLIOGRAPHY

Branson RD, Hess DR, Chaptburn RL: *Respiratory Care Equipment*, ed 2. Philadelphia, Lippincott Williams & Wilkins, 1999.

Burton GG, Hodgkin JE, Ward JJ: *Respiratory Care: A Guide to Clinical Practice*, ed 4. Philadelphia, JB Lippincott, 1997.

Christopher KL: At home administration of oxygen. In Kacmarek RM, Stoller JK, (eds): *Current Respiratory Care*. Toronto, BC Decker, 1988.

Compressed Gas Association: *Handbook of Compressed Gases*. New York, Compressed Gas Association, 1990.

Compressed Gas Association: *Pamphlet V-1: American Standard Compressed Gas Cylinder Valve Outlet and Inlet Connections*. New York, Compressed Gas Association, 1997.

Compressed Gas Association: *Pamphlet V-5: Diameter Index Safety System*. New York, Compressed Gas Association, 1989

Deshpande VM, Pilbeam SP, Dixon RJ: *A Comprehensive Review in Respiratory Care*. East Warwick, CT, Appleton & Lange, 1988.

Hess DR, MacIntyre N, Mishoe S, et al: *Respiratory Care Principles and Practice*. St. Louis, Mosby, 2002.

McPherson SP: *Respiratory Therapy Equipment*, ed 3. St. Louis, Mosby, 1988.

Pierson DJ, Kacmarek RM: *Foundations of Respiratory Care*. New York, Churchill Livingstone, 1992.

Wilkins RL, Stoller JK, Scanlon CG: *Egan's Fundamentals of Respiratory Care*, ed 8. St. Louis, Mosby, 2003.

Chapter 34

Oxygen, Helium, and Nitric Oxide Therapy

I. **General Characteristics of Oxygen**
   A. Colorless
   B. Odorless
   C. Tasteless
   D. Molecular weight: 32 g
   E. Density at standard temperature and pressure: 1.43 g/L
   F. Boiling point at 1 atm: −183° C (−297.4° F)
   G. Melting point at 1 atm: −216.6° C (−361.1° F)
   H. Critical temperature: −118.4° C (−181.1° F)
   I. Critical pressure: 736.9 pounds per square inch absolute (psia)
   J. Triple point: −218.7° C (−361.89° F) at 0.2321 psia
   K. Forms oxides with all elements except inert gases
   L. Constitutes approximately 20.95% of atmosphere
   M. Used at the cellular level as the final electron acceptor in electron transport chain located in mitochondria of cell

II. **Hypoxia: Inadequate Quantities of Oxygen at the Tissue Level**
   A. Decreased carrying capacity of blood for oxygen (anemic hypoxia)
      1. Anemia or hemorrhage
      2. Carbon monoxide poisoning
      3. Methemoglobinemia
      4. Shift of the oxyhemoglobin dissociation curve to the right
      5. Hypoxemia may or may not be present
   B. Decreased cardiac output, resulting in increased systemic transit time (stagnant hypoxia)
      1. Shock
      2. Cardiovascular instability
      3. Regional vasoconstriction
   C. Inability of tissue to use available oxygen (histotoxic hypoxia)
      1. Cyanide poisoning
      2. Rarely accompanied by hypoxemia
   D. Decrease in diffusion of oxygen across alveolar capillary membrane (hypoxemic hypoxia)
      1. Low inspired F_IO_2
      2. Ventilation/perfusion inequalities
      3. Increased true shunt
      4. Cardiac anomalies
      5. Diffusion defects

III. Hypoxemia: Inadequate Quantities of Oxygen in the Blood

A. Evaluation of hypoxemia

1. Normal: Pao_2 80 to 100 mm Hg
2. Mild hypoxemia: Pao_2 <80 mm Hg
3. Severe hypoxemia: Pao_2 <60 mm Hg
4. The lower level of acceptable Pao_2 decreases with age because the normal aging process of the lung affects respiratory functions (Table 34-1).
   a. The lower limit of "normal" Pao_2 is decreased approximately 4 mm Hg per decade in later life.
      (1) Pao_2 <60 mm Hg is always considered hypoxemia.
   b. Because the lung changes with age there is a progressive increase in the alveolar-arterial O_2 partial pressure difference (Figure 34-1).
   c. Acceptable lower limits of Pao_2 for older adults can be estimated using the following formula.

$$Pao_2 = 100.1 - (0.323 \times age) \text{ mm Hg} \tag{1}$$

B. Causes of hypoxemia (see Chapters 8 and 15)

1. True shunting
2. Ventilation/perfusion mismatch
3. Hypoventilation
4. Impaired diffusion
5. Decreased ambient O_2 tension

TABLE 34-1

Changes in Respiratory Function with Aging

Function	Mechanism	Clinical Manifestation
Mechanics of ventilation	Loss of lung elastic recoil; decreased chest wall compliance	↓ VC; ↑ RV; no change in TLC; ↓ expiratory flow rates
	Decreased respiratory muscle mass and strength	↓ Maximal inspiratory and expiratory force
Perfusion, ventilation, and gas exchange	Decreased uniformity of ventilation, with small airway closure during tidal breathing, especially while supine	↑ $P(A\text{-}a)o_2$; ↓ Pao_2; no change in $Paco_2$ or pH ↓ cardiac output; ↓ $C\bar{v}o_2$
	Increased physiologic deadspace	None (slightly ↑ $\dot{V}E$)
	Decreased alveolar surface area	↓ D_{LCO}
Exercise capacity	Decreased aerobic work capacity of skeletal muscle; deconditioning	↓ Maximum $\dot{V}o_2$
	Decreased efficiency of ventilation	↑ $\dot{V}E/L \dot{V}o_2$
Regulation of ventilation	Decreased responsiveness of central and peripheral chemoreceptors	↓ $\dot{V}E$ and $P_{0.1}$ responses to hypoxia and hypercapnia
Sleep and breathing	Decreased ventilatory drive	↑ Frequency of apneas, hypopneas, and desaturation episodes during sleep
	Decreased upper airway muscle tone	Snoring; ↑ incidence of obstructive sleep apnea
	Decreased arousal and cough reflexes	↑ Susceptibility to aspiration and pneumonia
Lung defense mechanisms	Decreased upper airway function; decreased mucociliary clearance	↑ Susceptibility to aspiration and pneumonia
	Decreased humoral and cellular immunity	↑ Susceptibility to infection; ↓ clinical response to infection

$\dot{V}E$, Expired minute ventilation; D_{LCO}, diffusing capacity for carbon monoxide; $\dot{V}o_2$, O_2 consumption; $P_{0.1}$, mouth occlusion pressure; $C\bar{v}o_2$, mixed venous O_2 content; $P(A\text{-}a)o_2$, alveolar-arterial Po_2 difference.
From Pierson DJ, Kacmarek RM: *Foundations of Respiratory Care*. New York, Churchill Livingstone, 1993.

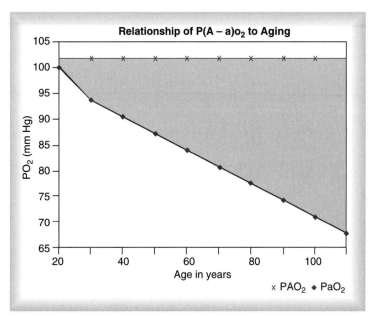

FIG. 34-1 The relationship between P(A–a)o$_2$ and aging. Because Pao$_2$ naturally decreases with age, P(A–a)o$_2$ increases at the rate of approximately 3 mm Hg each decade beyond 20 years.

    C. Responsive versus refractory hypoxemia
        1. Refractory hypoxemia is hypoxemia demonstrating a negligible increase in the Pao$_2$ with the application of an acceptable level of oxygen.
            a. If the F$_I$O$_2$ is >0.40 to 0.50 and the Pao$_2$ is <60 mm Hg (Sao$_2$ <90%), the hypoxemia is refractory.
            b. If a 0.20 increase in the F$_I$O$_2$ results in a <10-mm Hg increase in the Pao$_2$, the hypoxemia is refractory.
            c. Refractory hypoxemia is a result of true shunting.
        2. Responsive hypoxemia is hypoxemia that demonstrates a significant response to an increase in the F$_I$O$_2$.
            a. A 0.20 increase in the F$_I$O$_2$ results in a >10-mm Hg increase in the Pao$_2$.
            b. Responsive hypoxemia is a result of ventilation/perfusion inequalities.
    D. Clinical manifestations of hypoxemia
        1. Rapid respiratory rate and/or large tidal volume (V$_T$)
        2. Dyspnea
        3. Tachycardia and hypertension
            a. If cardiovascular status is poor or hypoxemia is severe, bradycardia and hypotension may result.
        4. Peripheral vasoconstriction with moderate to severe hypoxemia
        5. Constriction of pulmonary vascular bed leading to pulmonary hypertension
        6. Development of cyanosis if hypoxemia is severe
        7. Headache, restlessness
        8. Confusion, disorientation, or both
        9. Secondary polycythemia (with chronic hypoxemia)

IV. Indications for Oxygen Therapy, Modified from AARC Clinical Practice Guidelines on Oxygen Therapy, 2002.
    A. Documented hypoxemia: Pao$_2$ is <60 mm Hg or Sao$_2$ is <90%
    B. Acute care situations in which hypoxemia is suspected

1. Severe trauma
2. Acute myocardial infarction
3. Short-term therapy (e.g., postanesthesia recovery)

V. **General Goals of Oxygen Therapy**
   A. Maintain adequate tissue oxygenation and minimize cardiopulmonary work
      1. Increasing alveolar P_{O_2} increases pressure gradient for oxygen diffusion into blood-stream. This may increase Pa_{O_2}.
      2. An increase in Pa_{O_2} may reduce stimulation of peripheral chemoreceptors and reduce work of breathing.
      3. Oxygen therapy may correct hypoxemia and decrease the stimulus to increase cardiac output.

VI. **Hazards of Oxygen Therapy**
   A. Retinopathy of prematurity (ROP) (see Chapter 27)
      1. Occurs primarily in premature infants (<34 weeks gestation) with incomplete vascularization of the retina
         a. Incidence of ROP is inversely proportional to birth weight and gestational age.
      2. Increased oxygen exposure (Sa_{O_2} 96% to 99%) is just one of many factors involved in the pathogenesis of ROP.
      3. Maintaining Sa_{O_2} ≤96% may reduce the risk of ROP.
   B. Oxygen toxicity
      1. A series of reversible pathophysiologic inflammatory changes of lung tissue that can produce a progressive and lethal form of lung injury similar to acute respiratory distress syndrome (ARDS)
      2. Free radical theory of oxygen toxicity
         a. The following free radicals of oxygen can be produced at the cellular level.
            (1) Hydrogen peroxide: H_2O_2
            (2) Superoxide radical: O_2^-
            (3) Hydroxyl radical: $OH\cdot$
            (4) Singlet excited oxygen: $^1O_2$
         b. The following enzymes are important cellular defenses against oxygen free radicals.
            (1) Superoxide dismutase (SOD), which converts O_2^- to O_2
            (2) Catalase (CAT), which converts H_2O_2 to H_2O and O_2
            (3) Additional intracellular antioxidants that provide defense against oxygen free radicals include
               (a) Glutathione peroxide
               (b) Glutathione
               (c) N-acetyl-L-cysteine
               (d) Cysteamine
               (e) Vitamin E in lipid membrane
               (f) Vitamin C (intracellular)
               (g) Selenium
               (h) Ceruloplasmin
               (i) Transferrin
         c. The quantity of oxygen free radicals depends on Pa_{O_2}. The greater the Pa_{O_2}, the greater the quantity of free radicals.
         d. Effects of oxygen free radicals
            (1) Inhibition of glycolysis
            (2) Interference with surfactant transport and production
            (3) Nucleic acid (DNA) damage
            (4) Cross-linkage of DNA molecules
            (5) Cell and organelle membrane disruption
            (6) Enzyme inhibition

   3. Pathophysiology of oxygen toxicity
       a. Cellular susceptibility to hyperoxia (100% O_2)
           (1) Pulmonary capillary endothelium (most susceptible)
           (2) Alveolar type I epithelial cells
           (3) Alveolar type II epithelial cells
           (4) Alveolar type III epithelial cells (least susceptible)
       b. With continued exposure to 100% O_2, type I alveolar cells are destroyed and replaced by type II cells.
       c. Early or acute exudative phase is characterized by perivascular, interstitial, and intraalveolar edema with destruction and necrosis of endothelial cells. Alveolar congestion and fibrinous exudation (hyaline membrane) develop.
       d. Late or chronic proliferative phase is characterized by a progressive reabsorption of the exudate and a thickening of the alveolar septa.
       e. Clinical manifestations
           (1) Tracheobronchitis
           (2) Cough
           (3) Substernal pain
           (4) Nausea and vomiting
           (5) Anorexia
           (6) Paresthesia
           (7) Refractory hypoxemia
           (8) Diffuse patchy bilateral infiltrates
           (9) Alveolar atelectasis
          (10) Decreased compliance
   4. Susceptibility and risk factors associated with the development of oxygen toxicity
       a. The balance between oxidant and antioxidant activity determines the severity of tissue injury.
       b. Exposure to F_IO_2 levels >0.40 for lengthy periods
       c. Previous development of severe acute pulmonary disease, which decreases the risk of toxicity. The acute disease is believed to induce the production of SOD and glutathione, thus reducing the oxygen free radical levels.
   5. Prevention: Judicious use of oxygen therapy. Use only enough to maintain adequate tissue oxygenation.
       a. When possible limit exposure to 100% oxygen to <24 hours. Decrease to level maintaining acceptable PaO_2 >60 mm Hg as soon as possible.
   6. Treatment: Appropriate use of positive end-expiratory pressure therapy, diuretics, and fluids while reducing the F_IO_2 as soon as possible.
C. Oxygen-induced hypoventilation
   1. This is infrequently observed in patients with chronic CO_2 retention or central nervous system depression (see Chapter 20).
   2. The increased PaO_2 decreases or eliminates the hypoxic drive, inducing greater levels of hypoventilation. Although rare it can be potentially life threatening.
   3. Intermittent use of oxygen therapy may cause arterial PO_2 to decrease below pretreatment levels.
   4. If oxygen is indicated it should never be withheld because of the risk of ventilatory depression.
D. Absorption atelectasis (Figure 34-2)
   1. Nitrogen is metabolically inactive and constitutes 80% of alveolar gas. Nitrogen is essential to maintain alveolar stability.
   2. Administration of high F_IO_2 (>0.50) washes out nitrogen.
   3. In poorly ventilated alveoli more oxygen is removed per unit time by the perfused blood than can be replaced by normal ventilation.
   4. This results in a decrease in alveolar size.
   5. As alveoli reach their critical volume, collapse and atelectasis occur.

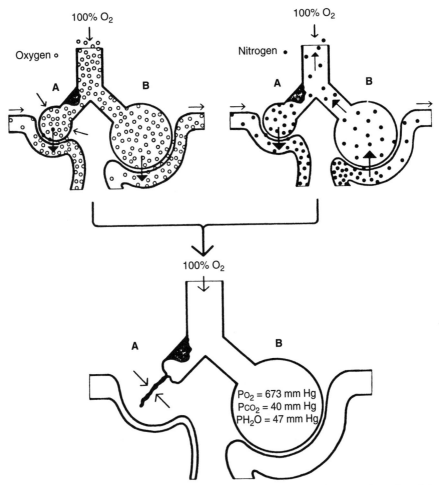

FIG. 34-2 Schematic representation of primary mechanisms causing denitrogenation absorption atelectasis. Top drawings represent the alveolar-capillary units shortly after administration of 100% inspired oxygen. White circles represent oxygen molecules that have increased in concentration in both units. **A** and **B,** The ablation of alveolar hypoxia in unit A results in loss of vasoconstriction with considerably increased blood flow. The increased blood flow to this still poorly ventilated alveolus results in significantly increased oxygen extraction, which results in decreased gas volume. Black circles represent nitrogen, which is rapidly depleted from all units secondary to the fact that inspired nitrogen concentration is now zero. Initially more nitrogen leaves the blood and the body via unit B because it is better ventilated. However, as the blood PN_2 level progressively decreases, nitrogen will start to leave alveolus A via the blood. This results in further loss of gas volume from alveolus A because it remains poorly ventilated but well perfused. Thus nitrogen is depleted from all units within 5 to 15 minutes. The bottom drawing represents the final steady state in which increased oxygen and nitrogen extraction has caused the alveolus to collapse. Thus a poorly ventilated, poorly perfused unit A becomes a nonventilated, poorly perfused unit after administration of 100% inspired oxygen.

> 6. This commonly occurs in patients with low VT or poor distribution of ventilation because of partial airway obstruction.

VII. **Oxygen Delivery Systems**
 A. Delivery systems generally are divided into two categories: high flow and low flow (Table 34-2).
 B. High-flow systems
  1. The patient's entire inspired gas volume is consistently and predictably delivered by the system.

TABLE **34-2**

Classification of Oxygen Delivery System

Low-flow systems	Cannula
	Simple mask
	Partial rebreathing mask
	Nonrebreathing mask*
High-flow systems†	Venturi masks
	Aerosol systems
	Large-volume humidifier systems

*The disposable nonrebreathing mask is not tight fitting; thus entrainment of room air normally occurs.
†For a system to be considered high flow, it must provide ≥40 L/min flow.

2. To maintain a consistent F_IO_2 the apparatus flow must exceed the peak inspiratory flow of the patient.
3. Peak inspiratory flows are difficult to measure but may be approximated by delivering a total flow at least *four times* the patient's measured minute volume (V_E).
   a. Normal peak inspiratory flows are approximately four times the patient's measured V_E.
   b. This flow usually will provide adequate volume in the face of a changing ventilatory pattern.
4. Typical high-flow systems
   a. Air entrainment masks: Deliver a specific F_IO_2 level up to 0.50 (Table 34-3; Figure 34-3).
      (1) Care should be taken to ensure the air entrainment mask provides sufficient flow to meet a patient's need. This is especially true with masks delivering higher F_IO_2 levels.
   b. Large-volume mechanical aerosol systems: Set up singly or in tandem to deliver high humidity along with a specific F_IO_2 level (see Table 34-3; Figure 34-4).
      (1) F_IO_2 varies by amount of gas entrainment.
      (2) Most nondisposable units have fixed air entrainment ports, whereas most disposable units offer a wide spectrum of available F_IO_2 levels.
      (3) Some units adapt to heaters and provide temperature control and extra humidification.
      (4) Always ensure sufficient flow, and if heated, unit should be monitored for temperature.

TABLE **34-3**

Entrainment Ratios and Outputs of Specific Air Entrainment Systems*

System	F_IO_2	Entrainment Ratio	Flow at which Operated	Total Flow (L/min)
Ventimasks	0.24	1-25	4	104
	0.28	1-10	4	44
	0.31	1-7	6	48
	0.35	1-5	8	48
	0.40	1-3	8	32
	0.50	1-1.7	12	32
Mechanical aerosol generators	0.60	1-1	12	24
	0.70	1-0.6	12	19

*Clinical trials indicate some variation in F_IO_2 levels provided by air entrainment masks.

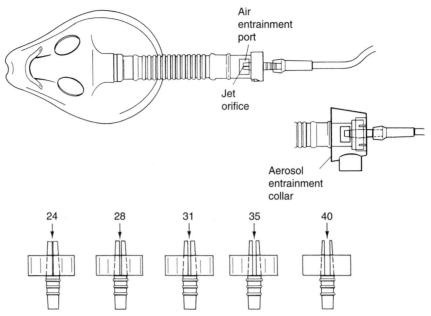

FIG. 34-3 Air entrainment mask with various jet orifices. Each orifice provides a specific delivered F_IO_2.

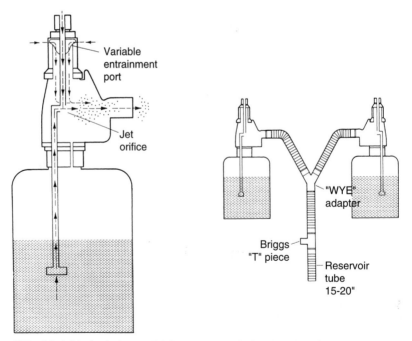

FIG. 34-4 Mechanical aerosol delivery system: single unit and tandem arrangement.

c. Wick-type passover humidification systems
(1) Volume and concentration of gas are determined by titration of compressed air and oxygen or the use of an oxygen blender (Figure 34-5).
(2) Virtually any F_IO_2 level is available.
(3) Virtually any flow is available.

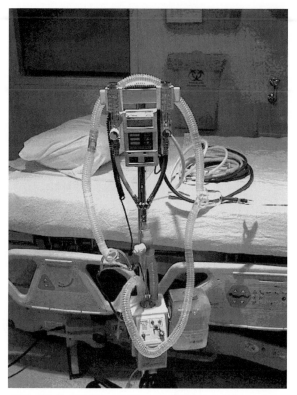

FIG. 34-5 High-flow wick type passover humidifier system.

    (4) Systems are extremely versatile and may be applied to a patient via an aerosol mask, continuous positive airway pressure (CPAP)-type mask, or standard artificial airway attachment.

    (5) Most systems are able to deliver controlled heated humidification for a wide range of flow rates.

  d. Determinations of F_IO_2 with any system combining gas flows

$$F_IO_2 = \frac{(F_IO_2 \text{ of A}) \text{ (Flow of A)} + (F_IO_2 \text{ of B}) \text{ (Flow of B)} + \text{etc.}}{\text{Total flow of combined systems}} \qquad (2)$$

  e. High-flow systems can be attached to patients by a variety of devices in addition to the typical air entrainment mask (Figure 34-6).

    (1) Aerosol mask

    (2) Face hood

    (3) Tracheostomy collar

    (4) Briggs T piece

    (5) CPAP mask

C. Low-flow systems

  1. The apparatus does not deliver the total $\dot{V}E$.

  2. The F_IO_2 delivered to the patient depends on

    a. Flow of gas from equipment

    b. Patient anatomic reservoir (oral and nasal cavity)

      (1) Normal anatomic reservoir in adults is approximately 50 ml.

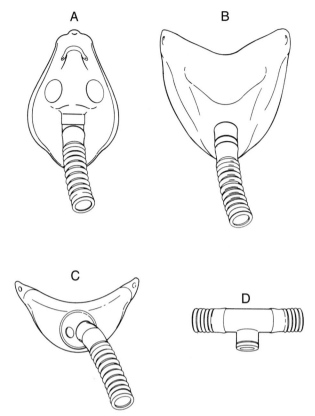

FIG. 34-6 Various appliances used to apply high-flow system. **A**, Aerosol mask. **B**, Face hood. **C**, Tracheostomy collar. **D**, Briggs T piece.

      (2)   Normal end-expiratory pause may allow for filling of anatomic reservoir with 100% oxygen.

   c. Reservoir of equipment

   d. Patient respiratory rate, V_T, and $\dot{V}_E$

      (1)   *The F_IO_2 delivered with any low-flow system is extremely variable and unpredictable.*

      (2)   If the patient's $\dot{V}_E$ were to increase on a particular low-flow system, the F_IO_2 would *decrease*. The patient would entrain a larger percentage of room air in the $\dot{V}_E$.

      (3)   If the patient's $\dot{V}_E$ were to decrease on a particular low-flow system, the F_IO_2 would *increase*. The patient would entrain a smaller percentage of room air in the $\dot{V}_E$.

   e. An example of the calculations used to estimate the F_IO_2 delivered by a low-flow oxygen therapy system and the effect on the F_IO_2 when there is a change in the respiratory pattern can be seen in Table 34-4.

   f. *It must be kept in mind that the F_IO_2 listed for each low-flow system is purely speculative and that the F_IO_2 is totally dependent on the patient's ventilatory pattern. The values provided should be used only as gross guidelines rather than as the exact F_IO_2 delivered.*

      (1)   Calculations similar to those in Table 34-4 have been used to determine the approximate F_IO_2 levels for various low-flow systems (Figure 34-7). The approximate F_IO_2 at specific flows with an oxygen cannula are:

(a)   1 L/min F_IO_2: 0.24
(b)   2 L/min F_IO_2: 0.28
(c)   3 L/min F_IO_2: 0.32
(d)   4 L/min F_IO_2: 0.36
(e)   5 L/min F_IO_2: 0.40
(f)   6 L/min F_IO_2: 0.44

3. Simple oxygen mask: Generally a minimum flow of 5 L/min should be used to flush the mask of carbon dioxide and prevent rebreathing. F_IO_2 levels vary greatly depending on the ventilatory pattern. Flows between 5 and 12 L/min will generally provide an F_IO_2 between 0.3 and 0.6 (see Figure 34-7).

4. *Partial rebreathing mask uses a simple mask connected to a bag reservoir with no valve between the bag and mask* (Figure 34-8).

    a. Called a partial rebreathing mask because the first one third of exhalation enters the bag, mixes with source oxygen, and is consumed during the next inhalation. Because it comes from anatomic deadspace it is primarily oxygen with a negligible amount of carbon dioxide.

    b. Flow must be sufficient to prevent the bag from deflating no more than one third to one half during inspiration to ensure that no CO_2 accumulates during exhalation. This is usually a minimum of 8 L/min flow.

    c. Flows of 8 to 15 L/min will deliver an F_IO_2 concentration between 0.35 and 0.60 or more, depending on the patient's ventilatory pattern.

TABLE 34-4

Estimation of F_IO_2 from Low-Flow Systems

Cannula		6 L/min	VT	500 ml
Mechanical reservoir		None	I:E ratio	1:2
Anatomic reservoir		50 ml	Rate	20/min
100% O_2 provided per sec		100 ml	Inspiratory time	1 sec
Volume inspired O_2*				
Automatic reservoir		50 ml		
Flow/sec		100 ml		
Inspired room air*		70 ml		
O_2 inspired		220 ml		

$$F_IO_2 = \frac{220\ ml\ O_2}{500\ ml\ VT} = 0.44$$

If VT is decreased to 250 ml		
Volume inspired O_2		
Anatomic reservoir		50 ml
Flow/sec		100 ml
Inspired room air†		20 ml
O_2 inspired		170 ml

$$F_IO_2 = \frac{170\ ml\ O_2}{250\ ml\ VT} = 0.64$$

If VT increased to 1000 ml		
Volume inspired O_2		
Anatomic reservoir		50 ml
Flow/sec		100 ml
Inspired room air‡		170 ml
O_2 inspired		320 ml

$$F_IO_2 = \frac{320\ ml\ O_2}{1000\ ml\ VT} = 0.32$$

---

*Because 150 ml of 100% O_2 is inspired, the remainder of VT is room air (350 ml), 20% of 350 ml = 70 ml – amount of O_2 in room air that is inspired.
†20% of 250 – 150.
‡20% of 1000 – 150.

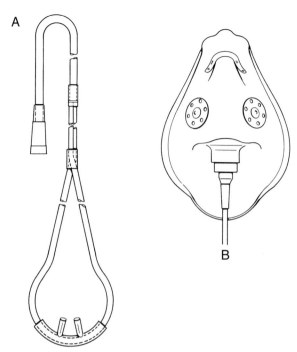

FIG. 34-7 A, Nasal cannula. **B,** Simple oxygen mask.

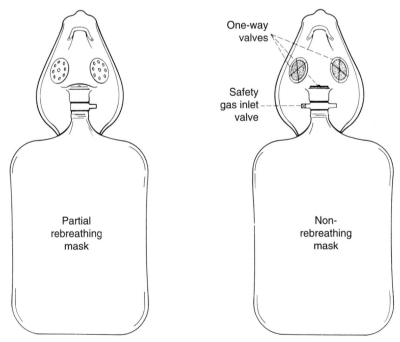

FIG. 34-8 Partial rebreathing and nonbreathing masks.

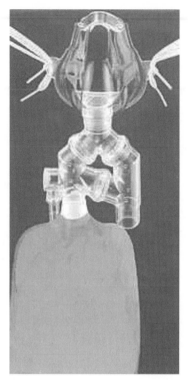

FIG. 34-9 Hi-Ox 80 oxygen mask.

5. Nonrebreathing mask: Variation of a partial rebreathing mask with a one-way valve between the mask and the reservoir bag, as well as a one-way valve over one or both exhalation ports on the mask body (see Figure 34-8).
   a. Must have sufficient flow to *prevent* the reservoir bag from collapsing on inspiration.
   b. If functioning properly, flows of 10 to 15 L/min will produce an F_IO_2 of 0.6 to 0.8 or more, depending on the patient's ventilatory pattern.
6. Hi-Ox oxygen mask (Respironics Inc., Merryville, PA) is a variation of a nonrebreathing mask using a manifold and valve system to connect the reservoir bag and mask (Figure 34-9).
   a. According to the manufacturer an F_IO_2 of ≥0.80 can be achieved at a flow of 8 L/min, depending on the patient's ventilatory pattern (VT cannot exceed 0.75 L).
   b. As with other nonrebreathing masks the flow must be sufficient to prevent the bag from collapsing.
7. Vapotherm humidification device (Vapotherm Inc., Annapolis, MD) is a mechanical unit that provides high flow (up to 40 L/min) of heated humidified oxygen via nasal cannula, simple mask, or partial rebreathing mask (Figure 34-10).
   a. There is some evidence to suggest that this device can provide F_IO_2 ≥0.7 at flow rates of 10 to 25 L/min with a partial rebreathing mask.
   b. This device can also be used to provide heated humidified Heliox mixture via nasal cannula or mask.
D. Criteria for use of high- and low-flow oxygen delivery systems
   1. *Whenever a consistent and predictable F_IO_2 is required, a high-flow system should be used.*

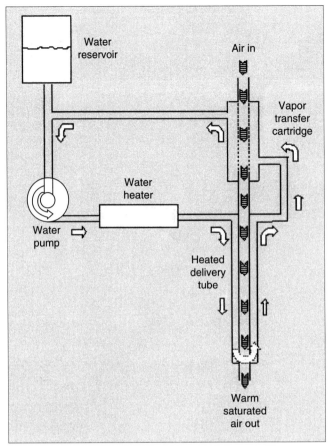

FIG. 34-10 Vapotherm 2000i humidification and oxygen delivery system (see text for details).

2. A low-flow system provides relatively stable F_IO_2 levels if the patient's
   a. Ventilatory pattern is consistent and regular.
   b. VT is between 300 and 700 ml.
   c. Respiratory rate is <25 breaths/min.
E. Oxygen-conserving devices
   1. These devices either use a reservoir designed into an oxygen cannula system or provide pulsed flow of oxygen based on the patient demand.
   2. Reservoir cannula (Figure 34-11)
      a. This device incorporates two reservoir bags in the body of the cannula.
      b. On exhalation the reservoir bags fill with oxygen.
      c. Thus a larger volume of 100% oxygen is available on the next inspiration.
      d. Oxygen use may be decreased up to 50% with this unit.
      e. Major problems
         (1) Size of the unit
         (2) Weight of the unit
         (3) Aesthetics of the unit
      f. It is designed for home oxygen delivery.
   3. Pendant cannula (Figure 34-12)
      a. It functions on the same principle as the reservoir cannula.

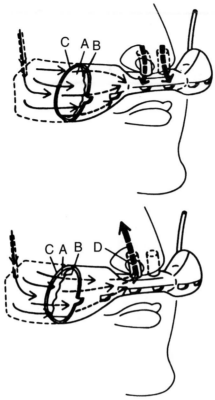

FIG. 34-11 Reservoir cannula. While the patient is exhaling *(top)*, oxygen is accumulating in the reservoir **(A)** formed by the inflated diaphragm **(B)** and the back wall of the conserver **(C)**. While the patient inhales *(bottom)*, the diaphragm **(B)** collapses, and the oxygen-enriched gas from the reservoir **(A)** is released to the patient **(D)**.

    b.   Its reservoir is located in the pendant setting on the patient's chest.

    c.   It may reduce oxygen use from 50% to 75%.

    d.   Major problems are size, weight, and aesthetics.

    e.   It is designed for home oxygen delivery.

  4. Pulse dose oxygen or demand oxygen delivery system

    a.   These systems provide delivery of oxygen only during inspiration.

    b.   Negative pressure generated by the patient triggers gas delivery.

    c.   Two general types exist: Variable pulsed volume and variable ratio of pulsed breaths to no oxygen delivery breaths.

       (1) Variable pulsed volume devices alter the volume of oxygen from approximately 10 to 40 ml/breath.

       (2) Variable ratio devices vary delivery of a fixed volume every breath to a fixed volume every fourth breath.

    d.   Adequate oxygenation is maintained because only that gas at the lung parenchymal level participates in gas exchange.

    e.   Only the first one third of inspiration reaches the lung parenchyma.

    f.   These devices may conserve 50% to 75% of the oxygen used.

    g.   They are designed primarily for home use.

    h.   Their function with every patient should be carefully evaluated.

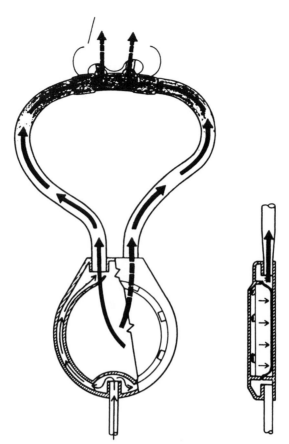

FIG. 34-12 Pendant cannula. Frontal view and cross-sectional view *(right)* of the pendant during inspiration. Negative pressure in the tubing causes the membrane to rapidly move posteriorly, thus providing a burst of oxygen-rich gas. During exhalation the first part of exhalation enters the pendant (100% oxygen). Once it is filled (40 ml) exhaled gas enters the room.

    5. Transtracheal oxygen catheter (Figure 34-13)
        a. With this system an 8-French catheter is inserted between the second and third tracheal rings and extended to approximately 2 cm above the carina.
        b. Continuous delivery of oxygen is provided via the catheter.
        c. Because oxygen is directly delivered into the trachea, oxygen use can be decreased by 50%.
        d. In some patients refractory to oxygen therapy because of severe pulmonary fibrosis, transtracheal oxygen therapy has improved arterial oxygenation.
        e. General indications
            (1) Need for improved mobility
            (2) Compliance with nasal cannula (poor)
            (3) Complications with nasal cannula (high)
            (4) Hypoxemia refractory to nasal oxygen
            (5) Patient preference because of comfort or cosmesis
        f. Generally it is used for long-term oxygen therapy in the home.
        g. Complications
            (1) Bronchospasm
            (2) Subcutaneous emphysema
            (3) Keloids at site of insertion
            (4) Pneumothorax
            (5) Infection

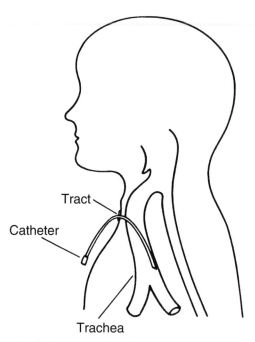

Tract

Catheter

Trachea

FIG. 34-13 Schematic of transtracheal oxygen catheter in place. It is inserted between the second and third tracheal rings and extended to approximately 2 cm above the carina.

(6) Bleeding

(7) Obstruction from mucous balls on the catheter

VIII. **Selection of Oxygen System for Adults (see Chapters 26, 27, and 29 for guidance regarding infants and children)**
   A. Patients with artificial airways
      1. Only high-flow systems are adaptable to artificial airways.
      2. With an endotracheal tube a Briggs T piece can be used.
      3. With a tracheotomy tube
         a. A Briggs T piece is used if a consistent F_IO_2 level is essential.
         b. If humidity is the primary concern a tracheotomy mask or tracheotomy collar is more comfortable and produces less torque on the trachea.
         c. At lower F_IO_2 levels (≤ 0.40) aerosol generators provide sufficient flow.
         d. If the F_IO_2 level needed is >0.40, a wick-type large-volume passover humidifier system may be necessary, which can deliver high flows at high F_IO_2.
   B. Patients without artificial airways
      1. Any system discussed may be used.
      2. The low-flow system, especially the O_2 cannula, is normally the best tolerated of all systems and has the best compliance. If it can provide adequate oxygenation it should be the first choice.
      3. In the emergency room a simple oxygen mask or partial rebreathing mask should be used if the cannula does not provide sufficient F_IO_2.
      4. In the recovery room an aerosol generator, normally unheated, with a face mask is usually sufficient.

IX. **Use of 100% Oxygen**
   A. The use of 100% oxygen may result in
      1. Oxygen toxicity
      2. Absorption atelectasis
      3. Oxygen-induced hypoventilation (rare)

    B. Despite these possibilities short-term 100% oxygen should always be used during
        1. Cardiac arrest
        2. Transport
        3. Acute cardiopulmonary instability
        4. Carbon monoxide poisoning, whenever carboxyhemoglobin levels are >10%

X. Monitoring of Oxygen Therapy
    A. Pulse oximetry
    B. Arterial blood gas analysis
    C. V_T and respiratory rate
    D. Pulse and blood pressure
    E. It is important to evaluate the work of breathing and the work of the myocardium to determine the overall effectiveness of an increase in the F_IO_2. A minor change in the P_{O_2} may be accompanied by a decrease in the work of breathing and the work of the myocardium, indicating the effectiveness of the F_IO_2 increase.

XI. Nitric Oxide
    A. General characteristics of nitric oxide (NO·)
        1. Colorless
        2. Metallic odor
        3. Tasteless
        4. Nonflammable
        5. Supports combustion
        6. Highly soluble
        7. Highly reactive
        8. Gaseous diatomic free radical
        9. Universally present in nature
       10. Short acting: Biologic half-life <5 seconds
           a. Rapidly oxidizes to nitrites and nitrates
       11. Atmospheric concentration: 10 to 100 parts per billion (ppb); as by-product of combustion (Box 34-1)
       12. NO· in the atmosphere rapidly changes to nitrogen dioxide, a toxic substance.
       13. NO· binds to the iron atoms of the hemoglobin molecule.
       14. NO· causes vascular smooth muscle relaxation.
       15. NO· is present in cigarette smoke, 400 to 1000 parts per million (ppm).
    B. Nitric oxide production
        1. Commercial manufacture
           a. Reaction of sulfur dioxide with nitric acid
           b. Ammonia oxidized at high temperatures
           c. After manufacture NO· is purified and mixed with nitrogen.
        2. Biologic synthesis: Naturally produced in many human tissues
           a. In endothelial cells NO· is produced from L-arginine in the presence of nitric oxide synthase (NOS) (Figure 34-14).

BOX 34-1

Relationship Among Parts per Million (ppm), Parts Per Billion (ppb), and Percent

```
1% = a part per 100
1 part per 100 = 10,000 ppm
10,000 ppm = 10,000,000 ppb
0.0001% = 1 ppm
1 ppm = 1000 ppb
0.0000001% = 1 ppb
```

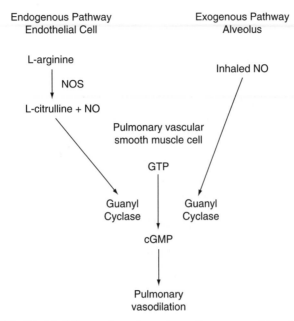

FIG. 34-14 Pathways for endogenous and exogenous nitric oxide.

C. Biologic action
 1. NO· diffuses into pulmonary vascular smooth muscle, where it activates guanyl cyclase, which converts guanosine triphosphate (GTP) to cyclic guanosine monophosphate (cGMP), resulting in smooth muscle relaxation (see Figure 34-14).
 2. Inhaled NO· is considered a selective pulmonary vascular dilation (Figure 34-15).
    a. NO· inhaled in low concentrations (5 to 80 ppm) is a selective pulmonary vasodilator only in ventilated areas of the lung because of the high affinity of hemoglobin for NO·.
    b. Systemic vasodilatation does not occur because NO· is rapidly inactivated by hemoglobin to produce methemoglobin (met-Hb).

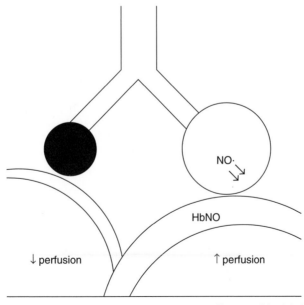

FIG. 34-15 Depiction of inhaled nitric oxide selective pulmonary vasodilatory activity. Inhaled NO only dilates blood vessels adjacent to ventilated alveoli.

c. Inhaled NO· improves blood flow to ventilated alveoli.
d. Reduces intrapulmonary shunt, thus improving $\dot{V}/\dot{Q}$
e. Improves arterial oxygenation
f. Decreases pulmonary artery pressure

D. Indications
1. Food and Drug Administration–approved indication
a. Hypoxic respiratory failure of the newborn
(1) >34 weeks gestation
(2) Mechanically ventilated
(3) Oxygenation index >25
(4) Clinical evidence of pulmonary hypertension
2. Inhaled NO· is used off label in many centers for the treatment of
a. Adult/pediatric ARDS patients considered for extracorporeal life support
b. Postpulmonary resection
c. Postoperative heart and lung transplant recipients
d. Severe inhalation injury
e. Acute right ventricular failure
f. Assessment of pulmonary vasoreactivity

E. Delivery systems
1. INOvent nitric oxide delivery system (INOtherapeutics, Clinton, NJ) (Figure 34-16)

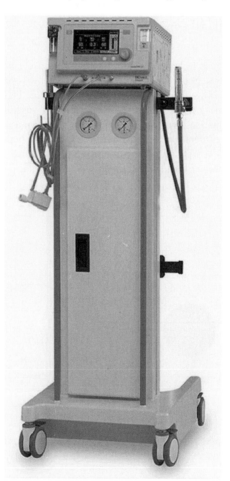

FIG. 34-16 INOvent nitric oxide delivery system.

      a. Universal use

        (1) Neonatal ventilators

        (2) Adult ventilators

        (3) Anesthesia machines

        (4) Spontaneously breathing patients

      b. Delivers 0 to 80 ppm inhaled $NO\cdot$

      c. 800 ppm $NO\cdot$ in large cylinders

      d. Injection module measures flow and injects $NO\cdot$ proportional to changes in flow.

      e. Gas monitoring unit for O_2, $NO\cdot$, and NO_2

      f. Continuous analysis is mandatory because of potential toxic effect of $NO\cdot$ and NO_2.

  2. Electrochemical nitric oxide analyzer affected by humidity

      a. Sample gas should be dry.

      b. $NO\cdot$ analyzer is pressure sensitive; should use side-stream sample techniques.

  F. Complications/precautions of $NO\cdot$ therapy

    1. NO_2 is produced when $NO\cdot$ reacts with oxygen.

      a. Conversion rate is determined by $NO\cdot$ concentration, oxygen concentration, and residence time.

      b. The Occupational Safety and Health Administration has set safety limits for NO_2 at 5 ppm and $NO\cdot$ at 25 ppm for 8 hours (time-weighted average).

      c. Airway and parenchymal lung injury has been reported with inhalation of NO_2 as low as 2 ppm.

      d. Ventilator exhaust does not need to be scavenged because environmental contamination does not exceed 150 ppb when delivering $NO\cdot$ concentrations ≤ 80 ppm at a minute ventilation of 15 L/min.

      e. The INOvent delivery system should be flushed before each use to ensure no residual NO_2 remains in the system.

    2. Met-Hb is produced when $NO\cdot$ binds to hemoglobin.

      a. Decreases oxygen-carrying capacity of blood

      b. Toxic levels (>5%) are rare at $NO\cdot$ doses used therapeutically (≤ 20 ppm).

XII. Helium

  A. General characteristics of helium

    1. Colorless

    2. Odorless

    3. Transparent

    4. Tasteless

    5. Nonflammable

    6. Non–life-supporting

    7. Chemically and physically inert

    8. Second lightest element

    9. Density: 0.179 g/L

   10. Specific gravity: 0.126

  B. Heliox

    1. Mixture of oxygen and helium

      a. Need at least 20% oxygen in mixture

      b. Gas mixture has a density less than that of air or oxygen.

      c. Used to decrease the turbulence of gas flow

    2. Low density produces greater tendency for laminar flow

      a. Turbulent flow is density dependent.

      b. Lower density of Heliox has a greater tendency for laminar flow.

      c. Laminar flow is more energy efficient; thus less pressure is needed to move gas through constricted airways, resulting in decreased work of breathing.

    3. Heliox (80% helium/20% oxygen) diffuses at a rate 1.8 times faster than oxygen.

C. Clinical applications
   1. Partial upper airway obstruction
      a. Post-extubation stridor
   2. Used for patients with acute asthma to decrease turbulent flow in constricted airways
      a. Pressure required to produce flow is decreased, decreasing energy expenditure.
         (1) Decreases work of breathing
         (2) Decreases $Paco_2$
         (3) Improves oxygenation
         (4) Increases peak flow
   3. Diagnostic: Pulmonary function test
      a. Measures lung volumes
      b. Diffusing capacity

D. Relative contraindications
   1. F_IO_2 needs >0.6
      a. Heliox not effective at concentrations <50%.
   2. Disease of small airways (chronic obstructive pulmonary disease)
      a. In small airways flow is not density dependent; thus Heliox has limited effect.
      b. Some data indicated beneficial results using Heliox with noninvasive positive pressure ventilation (NPPV).
         (1) Reduced $Paco_2$, dyspnea, and work of breathing to a greater extent than oxygen alone

E. Delivery mechanisms
   1. Mix with oxygen to provide adequate F_IO_2.
      a. F_IO_2 >0.5 limits clinical benefit of helium.
      b. Oxygenation should be monitored to ensure adequate F_IO_2 is delivered.
   2. Heliox delivery to spontaneous breathing patients (Figure 34-17)
      a. Face mask with reservoir bag
         (1) Bag must be kept inflated (12 to 15 L/min).
         (2) Helium flow is 1.8 times greater than indicated on an oxygen-calibrated flowmeter.
         (3) Y piece allows simultaneous delivery of aerosolized medication.
   3. Mechanical ventilation: Use with caution; many ventilators do not function with Heliox.
      a. Measurement problems: Low density
         (1) Affects delivered V_T

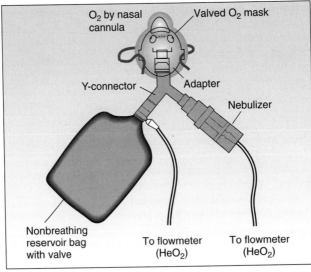

FIG. 34-17 Modified nonrebreathing mask used to delivery Heliox and aerosol therapy.

(2) Affects measurement of exhaled VT
(3) Partial solution: Using pressure ventilation
    (a) Pressure sensors not affected by gas composition
  b. Exhaled volume needed to be corrected
    (1) Ventilators using screen pneumotachometers are less affected by density of gas.
    (2) Servo 900c, 300c (Siemens Corp., Danvers, MA), and Avea (Viaysis Healthcare, Palm Springs, CA) most capable of delivering Heliox.
4. Aerosol delivery
  a. Heliox can affect nebulizer function.
    (1) Smaller particle size
    (2) Reduced output
    (3) Longer nebulization time
  b. Increase Heliox flow 50% to 100% when powering nebulizer to ensure adequate output.
  c. Heliox may improve aerosol penetration.
  d. Heliox may improve aerosol delivery during mechanical ventilation.

BIBLIOGRAPHY

AARC clinical guidelines. *Oxygen Ther Respir Care* 47:717-720, 2002.

Barnes TA: Equipment for mixed gas and oxygen therapy. *Respir Care Clin N Am* 6:545-595, 2000.

Branson RD: The nuts and bolts of increasing arterial oxygenation: devices and techniques. *Respir Care* 38:672-686, 1993.

Branson RD, Hess DR, Charburn RL: *Respiratory Care Equipment*, ed 2. Philadelphia, Lippincott Williams & Wilkins, 1999.

Cairo JM, Pilbeam SP: *Mosby's Respiratory Care Equipment*, ed 6. St. Louis, Mosby, 1999.

Hess DR, MacIntyre NR, Mishoe S, et al: *Respiratory Care Principles and Practices*. Philadelphia, WB Saunders, 2002.

Hurford WE: The biological basis for inhaled nitric oxide. *Respir Care Clin N Am* 3:357-369, 1997.

Kemper KJ, Ritz RH, Benson MS, et al: Helium-oxygen mixture in the treatment of postextubation stridor in pediatric trauma patients. *Crit Care Med* 19:356-359, 1991.

Kinsella JP, Truog WE, Walsh WF, et al: Randomized, multicenter trial of inhaled nitric oxide and high-frequency oscillatory ventilation in severe, persist-ent pulmonary hypertension of the newborn. *J Pediatr* 131:55-62, 1997.

Manthous CA, Hall JB, Caputo MA, et al: Heliox improves pulsus paradoxus and peak expiratory flow in nonintubated patients with severe asthma. *Am J Respir Crit Care Med* 151:310-314, 1995.

Neonatal Inhaled Nitric Oxide Study Group: Inhaled nitric oxide in full-term and nearly full-term infants with hypoxic respiratory failure. *N Engl J Med* 336:597-604, 1997.

NIOSH recommendations for occupational safety and health standards 1988. *MMWR Morb Mortal Wkly Rep* 37:1-29, 1988.

Pierson DJ, Kacmarek RM: *Fundamentals of Respiratory Care*. New York, Churchill Livingstone, 1993.

Tassaux D, Jolliet P, Roeseler J, et al: Effects of helium-oxygen on intrinsic positive end-expiratory pressure in intubated and mechanically ventilated patients with severe chronic obstructive pulmonary disease. *Crit Care Med* 28:2721-2728, 2000.

Wilkins RL, Stoller JK, Scanlan CL: *Egan's Fundamentals of Respiratory Care*, ed 8. St. Louis, Mosby, 2003.

Chapter 35

Aerosol and Humidity Therapy

An aerosol is a suspension of liquid or solid particles in a gas such as smoke or fog. Humidity refers to the addition of water vapor to a gas (i.e., water in molecular form only).

I. **Stability: Stability is the tendency of aerosol particles to remain in suspension. The following factors affect the stability of an aerosol.**
   A. Size: The smaller the aerosol particle, the greater the tendency toward stability. The larger the particle, the greater its tendency to rain out of suspension.
   B. Concentration: The greater the concentration of particles, the greater the tendency for individual particles to coalesce into larger particles and rain out of suspension.
   C. Humidity: The greater the relative humidity of the gas carrying the aerosol, the greater the stability of the aerosol.

II. **Penetration and Deposition of an Aerosol in the Respiratory Tract**
   A. Penetration refers to the depth within the respiratory tract that an aerosol reaches.
   B. Deposition is the rain-out of aerosol particles within the respiratory tract.
   C. Depth of penetration and volume of deposition depend on
      1. Gravity: Gravity decreases penetration and increases premature deposition but has minimal effect on aerosol particles in the therapeutic range of 1 to 5 μm (Table 35-1).
      2. Kinetic energy: The greater the kinetic energy of the gas carrying the particles, the greater the tendency for premature deposition. This is because coalescence and impaction are increased.
      3. Inertial impaction: Deposition of particles is increased at any point of directional change or increased airway resistance. Thus the smaller the airway diameter, the greater the tendency for deposition.

III. **Ventilatory Pattern for Optimal Penetration and Deposition**
   A. The patient's ventilatory pattern is the most important variable that can be controlled to ensure maximum penetration and deposition of aerosol particles during aerosol treatments.
   B. Ideal ventilatory pattern
      1. Large, slowly inspired tidal volume (V_T) over 3 to 4 seconds except with dry powder aerosols. Dry powder aerosols require a fast inspiratory flow rate.
      2. After inhalation a 3- to 4-second breath-holding period is advisable to ensure maximum deposition.
      3. With large-volume aerosols (ultrasonic nebulizers) a face mask should be used.
      4. Exhalation should be relaxed and normal.
      5. Coughing should be encouraged if secretion mobilization occurs and at the completion of treatment.

TABLE **35-1**	

Penetration and Deposition Versus Particle Size

Particle Size (μm)	Deposition in Respiratory Tract
>100	Do not enter respiratory tract
100-10	Trapped in mouth
100-5	Trapped in nose
5-2	Deposited proximal to alveoli
2-1	Can enter alveoli, 95-100% of particles 1 μm in size settling
<1-0.25	Stable, with minimal settling

    C. Attempts should be made to have all patients receiving aerosol therapy assume the described ventilatory pattern.

IV. Clearance of Aerosols
    Inhaled particles are removed from the respiratory tract by three mechanisms.
    A. Primary mechanism: Mucociliary escalator, which moves approximately 100 ml of secretions to the oropharynx per day.
    B. Normal cough mechanism
    C. Phagocytosis by type III alveolar cells

V. Indications for Aerosol Therapy
    A. Bland aerosol administration is the delivery of aerosolized sterile water and isotonic or hypertonic saline.
        1. Indications (Modified from AARC Clinical Practice Guideline: Bland aerosol administration, 2003)
            a. Presence of upper airway edema
            b. Laryngotracheobronchitis
            c. Subglottic edema
            d. Postextubation edema
            e. Postoperative management of the upper airway
            f. Presence of a bypassed upper airway-heated bland aerosol
            g. Need for sputum specimens or mobilization of secretions
        2. Contraindications
            a. Bronchoconstriction
            b. History of airway hyperresponsiveness
        3. Hazards and complications
            a. Wheezing or bronchospasm
                (1) Most common in asthmatic patients
                (2) May result in hypoxemia
            b. Bronchoconstriction when artificial airway is used
            c. Infection
            d. Overhydration
                (1) May be a problem primarily with neonates and infants
                (2) Associated more frequently with the use of ultrasonic nebulizers than with the use of jet nebulizers
            e. Patient discomfort
            f. Edema of the airway wall
            g. Edema is associated with decreased compliance and gas exchange and with increased airway resistance
            h. Caregiver exposure to droplet nuclei
            i. Bronchoconstriction with hypertonic saline

B. Indications for medicated aerosol administration are the need to deliver bronchodilators, antibiotics, or other pharmacologic agents in aerosol form to the lung parenchyma.

VI. **General Goals of Aerosol Therapy**
   A. Improve bronchial hygiene
      1. Improve efficiency of cough mechanism
      2. Restore and maintain normal function of mucociliary escalator
   B. Humidify gases delivered to patients with artificial airways (large volume nebulizer; Figure 35-1). Aerosol delivered to patients with artificial airways should be heated.
   C. Deliver medications by small volume nebulizer (SVN), metered dose inhaler (MDI), or dry powder inhaler (DPI)
      1. When administering inhaled medications, one should be cautious of the side effects associated with each medication.

VII. **Jet Aerosol Generators (Gas Powered)**
   A. These generators use jet mixing to produce an aerosol and entrain a second gas.
   B. A system of baffles is used to impact large particles out of suspension.
   C. These generators are commonly used for delivery of medications (SVNs) and for humidification of inspired gases (large volume nebulizers).
   D. Heating increases water content of delivered gas.

VIII. **Aerosol Generators to Deliver Medications**
   A. Small volume (jet) nebulizer (Figure 35-2)
      1. Does not require patient coordination
      2. A mouthpiece or face mask may be used.
      3. Able to deliver high doses of medication

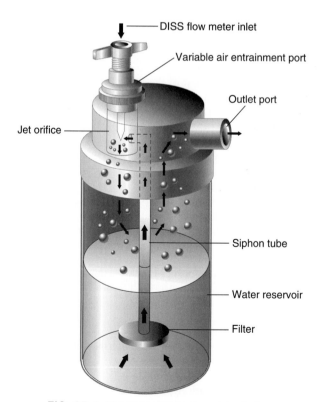

FIG. 35-1 All-purpose large volume jet nebulizer.

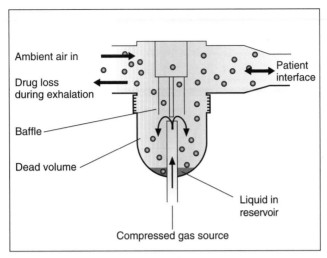

FIG. 35-2 Schematic drawing of a small volume jet nebulizer.

4. The amount of drug nebulized increases as the fill volume increases. A fill volume of 4 ml is recommended.
5. Generally the higher the flow to the nebulizer, the smaller the particle size generated; 6 to 8 L/min is recommended.
6. May be powered by oxygen or compressed air
7. SVNs are inconvenient to use outside the hospital environment and not portable.
8. Bacterial contamination of the SVN is common.
9. SVNs are usually used to administer aerosolized medications to infants and young children or to administer medications not available in MDIs.
10. SVNs may be used to deliver aerosolized medications during mechanical ventilation.
   a. Proper technique for aerosol delivery by SVN during mechanical ventilation
      (1) Fill the nebulizer with the drug and diluent to the optimal fill volume, 4 to 6 ml.
      (2) Place the nebulizer in the inspiratory limb of the circuit at least 30 cm from the patient's Y piece.
      (3) Attach the nebulizer tubing to the nebulizer outlet on the ventilator or to an external source of gas flow.
      (4) Ensure that the flow through the nebulizer is 6 to 8 L/min.
      (5) Ensure that the VT is sufficient (≥500 ml in adults).
      (6) If necessary adjust the delivered minute volume, trigger sensitivity, flow, and alarms to compensate for the additional flow through the nebulizer. In pediatric ventilators the additional flow may cause an increase in airway pressure or positive end-expiratory pressure and/or expiratory retard.
      (7) Turn off the continuous flow on the ventilator, and remove or bypass the heat and moisture exchanger (HME) if present.
      (8) Check the nebulizer for adequate aerosol generation.
      (9) Disconnect the nebulizer when no more aerosol is produced.
      (10) Reconnect the ventilator circuit, and reset to the original ventilator and alarm settings.
      (11) Rinse the nebulizer with sterile water, let air dry, and store aseptically. To minimize bacterial contamination it is recommended that SVNs be changed *at least* every 24 hours.
B. Metered dose inhaler (Figure 35-3)
   1. The MDI is the most common method used to deliver medication aerosols because it is convenient, portable, and less expensive.

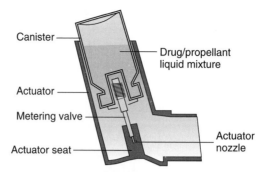

FIG. 35-3 Schematic drawing of a metered dose inhaler.

2. The MDI is used to administer bronchodilators, anticholinergics, antiinflammatory agents, and steroids.
3. Proper use requires patient coordination.
4. It consists of a canister containing the drug, propellants, and an actuator.
5. Chlorofluorocarbon propellants have been used. More recently hydrofluoroalkene propellants are used because they are less harmful to the environment.
6. Effective use of the MDI depends on patient technique and coordination. Depending on technique, lung deposition in adults may vary between 10% and 25% of the nominal dose.
   a. Proper technique for use of the MDI
      (1) Warm the MDI canister to hand or body temperature.
      (2) Insert canister into actuator, shake vigorously, and uncap the mouthpiece.
      (3) When the MDI is new or has not been used recently, prime the metering chamber by actuating the MDI several times before use.
      (4) Open mouth wide so tongue does not obstruct the mouthpiece.
      (5) Hold the MDI vertically with the outlet aimed at the mouth.
      (6) Breathe out normally.
      (7) Place outlet either between the lips or approximately 4 cm (two fingers' width) from the mouth.
      (8) Breathe in slowly, and actuate the MDI just after the beginning of inspiration.
      (9) Continue to inhale to total lung capacity (TLC).
      (10) Hold breath for 4 to 10 seconds.
      (11) Wait 30 seconds between actuations, and repeat until prescribed dose is administered.
      (12) Recap mouthpiece.
7. An MDI may be used with a spacer or valved holding chamber to reduce oropharyngeal deposition of the drug, decrease the bad taste of some medications, and aid the patient with poor hand-breath coordination.
   a. Spacers with masks may be used to administer aerosolized medications to small children.
   b. Proper technique for use of an MDI with a spacer
      (1) Warm the MDI canister to hand or body temperature.
      (2) Shake vigorously, insert canister into actuator, and insert the actuator into the spacer.
      (3) Place the spacer between lips and teeth, and close mouth around the mouthpiece of the spacer.
      (4) Actuate MDI into spacer.
      (5) One second later begin to inhale completely to TLC.
      (6) Hold breath for 4 to 10 seconds.
      (7) Repeat inhalation if V_T is small.
      (8) Wait 30 seconds, and then repeat the process until prescribed dose is delivered.
   c. A spacer should always be used with MDIs delivering steroids.

8. Bacterial contamination of the MDI is uncommon.
9. It is difficult to deliver high doses of medication with the MDI.
10. MDIs with an appropriate spacer can be used to administer aerosolized drugs into the inspiratory limb of a ventilator circuit.
    a. Proper technique for use of an MDI during mechanical ventilation
        (1) Decrease the inspiratory flow rate or extend the inspiratory time during administration.
        (2) Ensure the ventilator breath is synchronous with the patient's inspiration.
        (3) Shake the MDI canister vigorously.
        (4) Place the canister in the actuator of a cylindrical spacer placed in the inspiratory limb of the ventilator circuit.
        (5) Actuate the MDI at the beginning of inspiration of a ventilator breath.
        (6) Remove the canister, and shake between actuations.
        (7) Wait 20 to 30 seconds between actuations, and repeat until prescribed dose is delivered.
        (8) Remove canister from actuator in spacer, and close opening in spacer as indicated.

C. Dry powder inhaler (Figure 35-4)
    1. DPI is breath activated and requires some patient coordination.
    2. DPI produces drug particles in the respirable range, 1 to 5 μm.
    3. A fast inspiratory flow rate (>30 to 60 L/min) is required to deliver an effective dose.
    4. There are four different types of DPIs: rotahaler, turbuhaler, diskus, and diskhaler.
    5. DPIs should not be used for patients with acute bronchospasm or children aged <6 years.
    6. It is difficult to deliver high doses with a DPI.

D. There are several types of special jet nebulizers commonly used for specific applications.
    1. A vented breath-enhanced nebulizer is used to administer aerosolized antibiotics.
    2. A valved nebulizer with an expiratory filter is used to administer pentamidine.
    3. Nebulizers specifically made to provide continuous infusion of medications into the nebulizer are used for continuous aerosolized bronchodilator administration.
    4. The small particle aerosol generator (SPAG) is only used to administer the drug ribavirin.

IX. **Ultrasonic Aerosol Generators (Electrically Powered)**
    A. Ultrasonic nebulizers function by transforming standard household current into ultrasonic sound waves (Figure 35-5).

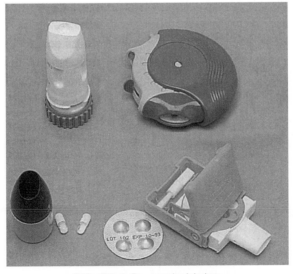

FIG. 35-4 Dry powder inhalers.

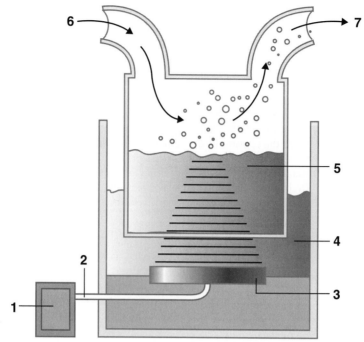

FIG. 35-5 Functional schematic of a typical large volume ultrasonic nebulizer (USN). *1,* Radiofrequency generator. *2,* Shielded cable. *3,* Piezoelectric crystal transducer. *4,* Water-filled couplant reservoir. *5,* Solution chamber. *6,* Chamber inlet. *7,* Chamber outlet.

    B. The Federal Commerce Commission governs the frequency range (1 to 2 megacycles/sec) for ultrasonic sound waves of ultrasonic nebulizers. All ultrasonic nebulizers produced and sold in the United States have preset frequencies in this range.

    C. The ultrasonic sound waves are applied to a quartz crystal or ceramic disk, causing it to vibrate at the same frequency as the ultrasonic waves. This is referred to as the *piezoelectric quality of the disk.*

    D. The crystal or disk transfers its vibratory energy to the fluid to be nebulized, creating an aerosol.

    E. These nebulizers incorporate an amplitude control that varies the intensity of ultrasonic waves, allowing varying aerosol outputs.

    F. Ultrasonic nebulizers are used principally to deliver bland aerosols for sputum induction.

 X. **Comparison of Nebulizer Output**
    A. Jet nebulizers: Up to 1 to 1.5 ml/min
    B. Ultrasonic nebulizers: Up to 6 ml/min

 XI. **Comparison of Nebulizer Particle Size**
    A. Jet nebulizers: 55% of aerosol particles produced fall in the therapeutic range of 1 to 5 μm.
    B. Ultrasonic nebulizers: 97% of aerosol particles produced fall in the therapeutic range of 1 to 5 μm.

 XII. **Humidifiers**
    A. A humidifier is designed to increase the water vapor content of a dry gas.
    B. There are two types of humidifiers.
       1. Active humidifiers add water vapor to the inspired gas.
       2. Passive humidifiers are HMEs.
    C. Generally three types of active humidifiers are used.

      1. Bubble
      2. Passover
      3. Wick
  D. Humidifiers also are either heated or unheated.
  E. Unheated bubble humidifiers may be used with simple oxygen therapy appliances.
      1. These units are intended to bring dry gas to approximately 40% relative humidity at body temperature.
      2. The humidification capacity of these units depends on
        a. Temperature of atmosphere
        b. Gas flow, most efficient at flows ≤5 L/min
        c. Size of the bubble formed
        d. Volume of water in the humidifier
  F. Heated humidifiers are normally used during mechanical ventilation.
      1. Bubble, passover, and wick humidifiers are available (Figure 35-6).
      2. Systems are usually heated to achieve 34° C to 37° C and 100% relative humidity at the patient's airway.
      3. As a result of the temperature decrease as a gas moves from the humidifier to the patient, excess water vapor condenses in the tubing.
      4. The use of heated ventilator circuits with some humidifier systems has greatly reduced condensate in circuits.
      5. Hazards and complications of heated humidifiers (Modified from AARC Clinical Practice Guideline: Humidification During Mechanical Ventilation, 1992)
        a. Potential for electrical shock
        b. Hypothermia
        c. Hyperthermia
        d. Thermal injury to the airway
        e. Burns to the patient and tubing meltdown if heated-wire circuits are covered or circuits and humidifiers are incompatible
        f. Underhydration and impaction of mucous secretions
        g. Hypoventilation and/or alveolar gas trapping caused by mucous plugging of airways

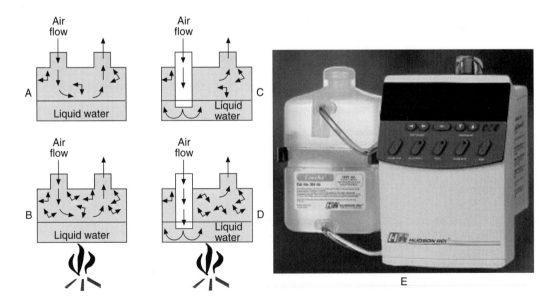

⋏⋏ = Water vapor

FIG. 35-6 A, Passover humidifier. **B,** Heated passover humidifier. **C,** Bubble humidifier. **D,** Heated bubble humidifier. **E,** Commercially available heated wick humidifier.

h.   Possible increased resistive work of breathing through the humidifier or because of mucous plugging of airways
i.   Inadvertent overfilling resulting in unintentional tracheal lavage–heated reservoir humidifiers
j.   When disconnected from the patient some ventilators generate a high flow through the patient circuit that may aerosolize contaminated condensate, putting the patient and clinician at risk for nosocomial infection.
k.   Potential for burns to caregivers from hot metal
l.   Inadvertent tracheal lavage from pooled condensate in patient circuit
m.   Elevated airway pressures caused by pooled condensation
n.   Patient-ventilator dyssynchrony and improper ventilator performance caused by pooled condensation in the circuit
G.   Humidifiers, either unheated or heated, may be used with noninvasive ventilators (bilevel positive airway pressure or continuous positive airway pressure) for patient comfort and to prevent drying of secretions.

XIII.   **Heat and Moisture Exchangers (Artificial Noses)**
A.   These devices sequester some or most of the water vapor exhaled by the patient. On the subsequent inspiration, the sequestered water is used to humidify the next inspiration.
B.   Three types: Condenser humidifiers, hygroscopic condenser humidifiers (Figure 35-7), and hydrophobic condenser humidifiers.
C.   Condenser humidifiers usually are only 50% efficient.
D.   Hygroscopic condenser humidifiers are up to 70% efficient.
E.   Hydrophobic condenser humidifiers are approximately 70% efficient and are capable of filtering bacteria (Figure 35-8).
F.   HMEs are capable of maintaining adequate humidification for short-term (up to 72 hours) and periodic use (16 to 20 hr/day) in patients with chronic disease.
G.   Contraindications for HME use (Modified from AARC Clinical Practice Guideline: Humidification During Mechanical Ventilation, 1992)
1.   Patients with thick, copious, or bloody secretions
2.   Patients with an expired V_T <70% of the delivered V_T (e.g., those with large bronchopleurocutaneous fistulas or incompetent or absent endotracheal tube cuffs)
3.   Patients with body temperature <32° C

Hygroscopic Condenser

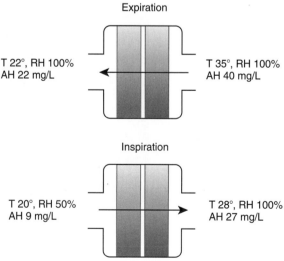

Expiration

T 22°, RH 100%   T 35°, RH 100%
AH 22 mg/L   AH 40 mg/L

Inspiration

T 20°, RH 50%   T 28°, RH 100%
AH 9 mg/L   AH 27 mg/L

FIG. 35-7 Process of humidification with a hygroscopic condenser humidifier. *AH,* Absolute humidity; *RH,* relative humidity; *T,* temperature.

Hydrophobic Condenser

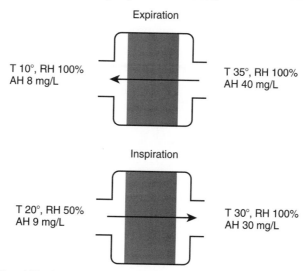

FIG. 35-8 Process of humidification with a hydrophobic condenser humidifier. *AH,* Absolute humidity; *RH,* relative humidity; *T,* temperature.

  4. Patients with high spontaneous minute volume (>10 L/min)
  5. An HME must be removed from the patient circuit during aerosol treatments when the nebulizer is placed in the patient circuit.
H. Hazards and complications of HME
  1. Underhydration and impaction of mucous secretions
  2. Hypoventilation and/or alveolar gas trapping caused by mucous plugging of airways
  3. Possible increased resistive work of breathing through the HME or because of mucous plugging of airways
  4. Possible hypoventilation caused by increased deadspace
  5. Ineffective low pressure alarm during disconnection because of resistance through HME

BIBLIOGRAPHY

American Association for Respiratory Care: Clinical practice guideline: humidification during mechanical ventilation. *Respir Care* 37:887-890, 1992.

American Association for Respiratory Care: Clinical practice guideline: bland aerosol administration, 2003 revision and update. *Respir Care* 48:529-533, 2003.

American Association for Respiratory Care: Consensus statement: aerosols and delivery devices. *Respir Care* 45:589-596, 2000.

Branson RD, Davis K: Evaluation of 21 passive humidifiers according to the ISO 9360 standard: moisture output, deadspace, and flow resistance. *Respir Care* 41:736, 1996.

Burton GG, Hodgkin JE, Ward JJ: *Respiratory Care: A Guide to Clinical Practice,* ed 4. Philadelphia, JB Lippincott, 1997.

Deshpande VM, Pilbeam SP, Dixon RJ: *A Comprehensive Review in Respiratory Care.* Norwalk, CT, Appleton & Lange, 1988.

Fink JB: Metered dose inhalers, dry powder inhalers, and transitions. *Respir Care* 45:623-625, 2000.

Hess DR: Nebulizers: principles and performance. *Respir Care* 45:609-622, 2000.

Hess D, Fisher D, Williams P, et al: Medication nebulizer performance: effects of diluent volume, nebulizer flow, and nebulizer brand. *Chest* 110:498-505, 1996.

Hess DR, MacIntyre NR, Mishoe SC, Galvin WF, Adams AB, Saposnick AB: *Respiratory Care Principles and Practice.* Philadelphia, WB Saunders, 2002.

Holt T: Aerosol generators and humidifiers. In Barnes TA (ed): *Respiratory Care Practice.* Chicago, Year Book Medical Publishers, 1988.

McPherson SP: *Respiratory Therapy Equipment,* ed 3. St. Louis, Mosby, 1989.

Miyao H, Hirokawa T, Miyasaka K, et al: Relative humidity, not absolute humidity, is of great importance when using a humidifier with a heating wire. *Crit Care Med* 20:674-679, 1992.

Nishida T, et al: Performance of heated humidifiers with a heated wire according to ventilatory settings. *J Aerosol Med* 14:43, 2001.

Peterson BD: Heated humidifiers. *Respir Care Clin North Am* 4:243-260, 1998.

Pierson DJ, Kacmarek RM: *Foundations of Respiratory Care.* New York, Churchill Livingstone, 1993.

Shapiro BA, Harrison RA, Kacmarek RM, et al: *Clinical Application of Respiratory Care,* ed 4. Chicago, Year Book Medical Publishers, 1990.

Wilkes AR: Heat and moisture exchangers: structure and function. *Respir Care Clin N Am* 4:261-279, 1998.

Wilkins RL, Stoller JK, Scanlon CL: *Egan's Fundamentals of Respiratory Therapy,* ed 8. St. Louis, Mosby, 2003.

Chapter 36

Airway Clearance Techniques

I.   Definition: Airway clearance techniques include the use of invasive and noninvasive therapy to help mobilize and remove secretions and improve gas exchange.

II. Airway Clearance Physiology
   A.   Normal airway clearance (see Chapter 4)
       1.   Normal clearance of the airway depends on a patent airway, a functional mucociliary transport system, and an effective cough.
       2.   The mucociliary transport system functions from the larynx down to the respiratory bronchioles.
       3.   Goblet cells and submucosal glands are responsible for the majority of secretions in the central airways.
       4.   Ciliated epithelial cells in a coordinated wavelike motion move mucus toward the trachea and larynx where it can be swallowed or expectorated.
       5.   The normal respiratory tract produces approximately 100 ml of mucus per day.
   B.   Four phases of normal cough reflex (Figure 36-1)
       1.   Irritation
           a.   Inflammatory, mechanical, chemical, or thermal stimulus trigger airway sensory receptors, sending impulses to the brain's medullary cough center.
       2.   Inspiration
           a.   In response to these afferent impulses the cough center reflexively stimulates the inspiratory muscles to initiate a deep inspiration.
       3.   Compression
           a.   Reflex nerve impulses cause the glottis to close and the expiratory muscles to contract.
           b.   Pleural and alveolar pressures increase rapidly.
       4.   Expulsion
           a.   The glottis opens, causing a large pressure gradient between the alveoli and the airway opening.
           b.   Expiratory muscles continue to contract.
           c.   The pressure gradient causes a high-velocity gas flow that displaces the mucus from the airway walls and into the air stream.
   C.   Abnormal airway clearance
       1.   Airway abnormalities that alter airway patency, mucociliary transport, or cough reflex may impede airway clearance and cause retention of secretions.
       2.   Mucous plugging can cause complete obstruction of the airway, resulting in atelectasis and impaired gas exchange because of shunting.
       3.   Partial obstruction from retained secretions restricts airflow, causing increased work of breathing, air trapping, overdistention, and ventilation/perfusion ($\dot{V}/\dot{Q}$) mismatch.

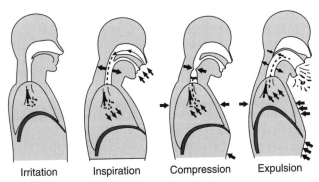

Irritation   Inspiration   Compression   Expulsion

FIG. 36-1 The cough reflex.

4. Infectious processes caused by microorganisms in retained secretions cause an inflammatory response and the release of chemical mediators, resulting in increased mucus production.
5. Causes of impaired mucociliary transport in intubated patients
    a. Endotracheal or tracheostomy tube
    b. Tracheobronchial suction
    c. Inadequate humidification
    d. High F_IO_2
    e. Drugs: General anesthetics, opiates, and narcotics
    f. Underlying pulmonary disease
6. Diseases that affect normal airway clearance
    a. Cystic fibrosis
    b. Bronchiectasis
    c. Ciliary dyskinetic syndromes
    d. Chronic bronchitis
    e. Neuromuscular disease

III. **Methods to Manage Thick Secretions**
   A. Bland aerosol therapy
      1. Bland aerosol therapy can be used for the management of thick, tenacious secretions in patients who have intact upper airways.
      2. However, no studies have reported a benefit from external humidification in improving the character or mobilization of thick secretions.
      3. Systemic hydration is the most effective method to improve the character of pulmonary secretions.
      4. Indications
         a. The presence of upper airway edema (cool bland aerosol): laryngotracheobronchitis, subglottic edema, postextubation edema, and postoperative management of the upper airway
         b. The presence of a bypassed upper airway
         c. The need for sputum specimens
      5. Contraindications
         a. Bronchoconstriction
         b. History of airway hyperresponsiveness
      6. Hazards and complications
         a. Bronchospasm
         b. Infection
         c. Overhydration
         d. Patient discomfort
         e. Caregiver exposure to droplet nuclei of *Mycobacterium tuberculosis* or other airborne contagions produced as a consequence of coughing, particularly during sputum induction

B. Mucolytic agents
  1. Dornase alfa (Pulmozyme)
     a. Approved for the management of cystic fibrosis
     b. Delivered to the airway via small volume nebulizer
     c. Efficacy not proven for acute exacerbations of cystic fibrosis or for the management of other chronic airway diseases
  2. Acetylcysteine
     a. Delivered to the airway via small volume nebulizer or instillation into artificial airway
     b. Has never been approved for inhalation
     c. Few or no data to support its efficacy when nebulized
     d. Can irritate the airway and induce bronchospasm
     e. Effective when instilled into specific lung segments during bronchoscopy

IV. **Invasive Bronchial Hygiene**
  A. Suctioning through an artificial airway
     1. Indications
        a. Secretions seen in airway
        b. Wheezing, rhonchi, or rales or decreased breath sounds
        c. Unexplained increases in ventilator pressure during volume ventilation or decreases in tidal volume during pressure control ventilation
        d. Unexplained deterioration of arterial blood gases
     2. Sterile technique must be used when suctioning an artificial airway, except when an in-line suction catheter is used.
     3. Preoxygenation can help minimize hypoxemia caused by suctioning.
     4. The suction catheter should not remain in the airway for >15 seconds.
     5. Sterile saline should not routinely be instilled into the airway. There is no evidence that this practice increases the amount of secretions removed from the airway, and it may worsen oxygenation. Sterile saline should only be used to help loosen exceptionally thick and tenacious secretions encountered during suctioning.
  B. Nasotracheal suctioning
     1. Patients with excessive secretions and a poor cough reflex may benefit from nasotracheal suctioning.
     2. Placement of a nasopharyngeal airway may help to reduce trauma to the nasal passage from repeated suctioning.
     3. Indications
        a. Inability to clear secretions
        b. Audible evidence of secretions in the large/central airways that persist despite patient's best cough effort
     4. Contraindications
        a. Occluded nasal passages
        b. Nasal bleeding
        c. Epiglottitis or croup
        d. Acute injury of head or facial or neck injury
        e. Coagulopathy or bleeding disorder
        f. Laryngospasm
        g. Irritable airway
        h. Upper respiratory tract infection
     5. Hazards and complications
        a. Mechanical trauma to upper airway
        b. Hypoxemia/hypoxia
        c. Cardiac dysrhythmias/arrest
        d. Bradycardia
        e. Hypertension
        f. Hypotension

g. Respiratory arrest
h. Uncontrolled coughing
i. Gagging/vomiting
j. Laryngospasm
k. Bronchospasm
l. Pain
m. Nosocomial infection
n. Atelectasis
o. Misdirection of catheter
p. Increased intracranial pressure (ICP)

C. Bronchoscopy
1. Therapeutic bronchoscopy is used for the removal of foreign bodies from the airway, management of focal atelectasis, and airway occlusion caused by retained secretions.
2. There is limited evidence that routine bronchoscopy for removal of retained secretions provides any greater benefit than suctioning and chest physiotherapy techniques.
3. Bronchoscopy is beneficial for the removal of secretions from the airway for diagnostic testing purposes.

V. **Noninvasive Bronchial Hygiene**
A. Postural drainage
1. Postural drainage is a method of removing pooled secretions by positioning the patient to allow gravity to assist in movement of secretions. The patient should be positioned so that the affected lung segments are superior to the carina, with each position maintained for 3 to 15 minutes.
2. Indications (Modified from AARC Clinical Practice Guideline: Postural Drainage, 1991)
a. Inability or reluctance of patient to change body position
b. Poor oxygenation associated with position (e.g., unilateral lung disease)
c. Potential for or presence of atelectasis
d. Presence of artificial airway
e. Evidence or suggestion of difficulty with secretion clearance
f. Difficulty clearing secretions, with expectorated sputum production >25 to 30 ml/day (for an adult)
g. Evidence or suggestion of retained secretions in the presence of an artificial airway
h. Presence of atelectasis caused by or suspected of being caused by mucous plugging
i. Diagnosis of diseases such as cystic fibrosis, bronchiectasis, or cavitating lung disease
j. Presence of foreign body in airway
k. External manipulation of the thorax: Sputum volume or consistency suggesting a need for additional manipulation
3. Contraindications (Modified from AARC Clinical Practice Guideline: Postural Drainage, 1991)
a. The decision to use postural drainage therapy requires assessment of potential benefits versus potential risks. Therapy should be provided for no longer than necessary to obtain the desired therapeutic results. Listed contraindications are relative unless marked as absolute (A).
b. Positioning: All positions are contraindicated for
(1) Head and neck injury until stabilized (A)
(2) Active hemorrhage with hemodynamic instability (A)
(3) ICP >20 mm Hg
(4) Recent spinal surgery or acute spinal injury
(5) Active hemoptysis
(6) Empyema
(7) Bronchopleural fistula
(8) Pulmonary edema associated with congestive heart failure
(9) Aged, confused, or anxious patients who do not tolerate position changes

        (10)   Pulmonary embolism
        (11)   Rib fracture, with or without flail chest
        (12)   Surgical wound or healing tissue
        (13)   Large pleural effusions
   c.   Trendelenburg position is contraindicated for
        (1)   Recent gross hemoptysis related to recent lung carcinoma managed surgically or with radiation therapy
        (2)   ICP >20 mm Hg
        (3)   Uncontrolled hypertension
        (4)   Distended abdomen
        (5)   Patients in whom increased ICP is to be avoided (e.g., neurosurgery, aneurysms, or eye surgery)
        (6)   Uncontrolled airway at risk for aspiration (e.g., tube feeding or recent meal)
        (7)   Esophageal surgery
   d.   External manipulation of the thorax (in addition to contraindications previously listed)
        (1)   Subcutaneous emphysema
        (2)   Recent epidural, spinal fusion or spinal anesthesia
        (3)   Recently placed transvenous pacemaker or subcutaneous pacemaker
        (4)   Lung contusion
        (5)   Osteomyelitis of the ribs
        (6)   Coagulopathy
        (7)   Recent skin grafts or flaps on the thorax
        (8)   Burns, open wounds, and skin infections of the thorax
        (9)   Suspected pulmonary tuberculosis
        (10)   Bronchospasm
        (11)   Osteoporosis
        (12)   Complaint of chest-wall pain

4.   Hazards and complications (Modified from AARC Clinical Practice Guideline: Postural Drainage, 1991)
   a.   Hypoxemia
   b.   Increased ICP
   c.   Acute hypotension during procedure
   d.   Pulmonary hemorrhage
   e.   Pain or injury to muscles, ribs, or spine
   f.   Vomiting and aspiration
   g.   Bronchospasm
   h.   Dysrhythmias

5.   Standard postural drainage positions for each of the lung segments
   a.   *Apical segments of right and left upper lobes*: Patient in semi-Fowler's position with head of the bed raised 45 degrees (Figure 36-2).
   b.   *Anterior segments of both upper lobes*: Patient supine with the bed flat (Figure 36-3).
   c.   *Posterior segments of right upper lobe*: Patient one-quarter turn from prone with the right side up, supported by pillows, and with head of the bed flat (Figure 36-4).
   d.   *Apical-posterior segment of left upper lobe*: Patient one-quarter turn from prone with the left side up, supported by pillows, and with head of the bed elevated 30 degrees (Figure 36-5).
   e.   *Medial and lateral segments of right middle lobe*: Patient one-quarter turn from supine with right side up and foot of the bed elevated 12 in. (Figure 36-6).
   f.   *Superior and inferior segments of lingula*: Patient one-quarter turn from supine with left side up and foot of the bed elevated 12 in. (Figure 36-7).
   g.   *Superior segments of both lower lobes*: Patient prone with head of the bed flat and pillow under the abdominal area (Figure 36-8).
   h.   *Anteromedial segment of left lower lobe and anterior segment of right lower lobe*: Patient supine, with foot of the bed elevated 20 in. (Figure 36-9).

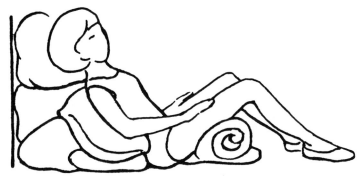

FIG. 36-2 Position for drainage of apical segments of upper lobes.

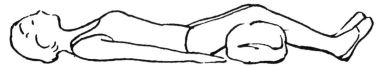

FIG. 36-3 Position for drainage of anterior segments of upper lobes.

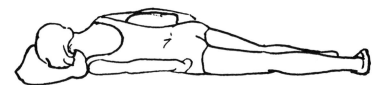

FIG. 36-4 Position for drainage of posterior segment of right upper lobe.

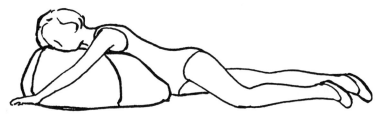

FIG. 36-5 Position for drainage of apical-posterior segment of left upper lobe.

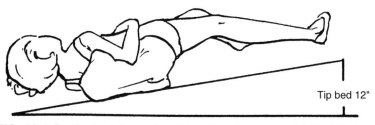

Tip bed 12"

FIG. 36-6 Position for drainage of medial and lateral segments of right middle lobe.

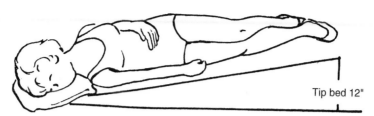

FIG. 36-7 Position for drainage of superior and inferior segments of lingula.

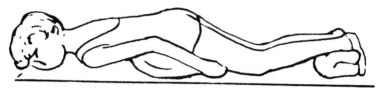

FIG. 36-8 Position for drainage of superior segments of both lower lobes.

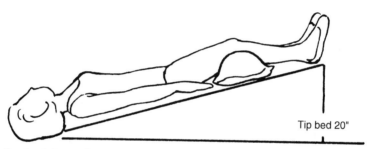

FIG. 36-9 Position for drainage of anteromedial segment of left lower lobe and anterior segment of right lower lobe.

    i. *Lateral segment of right lower lobe*: Patient directly on left side with right side up and foot of the bed elevated 20 in. (Figure 36-10).

    j. *Lateral segment of left lower lobe and medial (cardiac) segment of right lower lobe*: Patient directly on right side, with left side up and foot of the bed elevated 20 in. (Figure 36-11).

    k. *Posterior segment of both lower lobes*: Patient prone with foot of the bed elevated 20 in. (Figure 36-12).

  B. Percussion

    1. Percussion is a technique of rhythmically tapping the chest wall with cupped hands or mechanical device. No convincing evidence demonstrates the superiority of one method

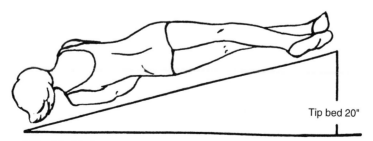

FIG. 36-10 Position for drainage of lateral segment of right lower lobe.

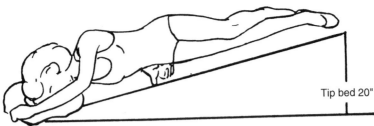

FIG. 36-11 Position for drainage of lateral segment of left lower lobe and medial segment of right lower lobe.

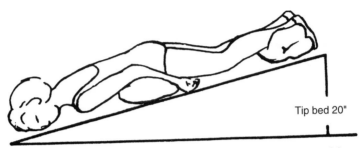

FIG. 36-12 Position for drainage of posterior segments of both lower lobes.

over the other. It is designed to loosen secretions in the area underlying the percussion by the air pressure that is generated by the cupped hand on the chest wall. Percussion is performed during inspiration and expiration (Figure 36-13).

2. There is no evidence that percussion alone increases the amount of secretions removed from the airway. Select patients may benefit if percussion is added to postural drainage therapy.

3. If percussion is performed care must be taken to carefully monitor the patient's cardiopulmonary status throughout the procedure.

4. Indications (same as those for postural drainage)

5. Percussion may be contraindicated in patients with the following conditions.
   a. Cancer with known metastatic changes
   b. Anticoagulant therapy
   c. Tuberculosis
   d. Petechiae
   e. Osteoporotic changes
   f. Empyema
   g. Pulmonary embolus
   h. Wounds, skin grafts, and burns

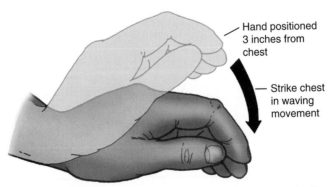

Hand positioned 3 inches from chest

Strike chest in waving movement

FIG. 36-13 Movement of cupped hand at wrist to percuss chest.

      i. Untreated tension pneumothorax
      j. Flail chest
      k. Frank hemoptysis
      l. Acute spinal cord injuries
     m. Limited patient tolerance
      n. Chest tubes
      o. Unstable cardiac status
      p. Thoracic surgery
      q. Increased ICP >20 mm Hg
      r. Risk for aspiration
      s. Distended abdomen
      t. Recent esophageal surgery
   6. Hazards and complications (same as those for postural drainage)

C. Vibration

   1. Vibration involves the application of a fine tremorous action (manually performed by pressing in the direction that the ribs and soft tissue of the chest move during expiration) over the draining area. Vibrations are intended to move secretions into the larger airways. No conclusive evidence supports the efficacy of vibration, the superiority of either manual or mechanical methods, or an optimum frequency.

   2. Indications, possible contraindications, hazards, and complications are the same as postural drainage and percussion.

D. Directed cough

   1. Directed cough (DC) to clear or mobilize secretions is a component of bronchial hygiene therapy when spontaneous cough is inadequate.

   2. DC is a deliberate maneuver that is taught, supervised, and monitored. It attempts to mimic an effective spontaneous cough, to assist in voluntary control of the cough reflex, and to compensate for physical limitations that impair this reflex.

   3. Forced expiratory technique (FET), or huff coughing, and manually assisted cough are examples of DC.

   4. Indications (Modified from AARC Clinical Practice Guideline: Directed Cough, 1993)
      a. The need to aid in the removal of retained secretions from central airways
      b. The presence of atelectasis
      c. Prophylaxis against postoperative pulmonary complications
      d. Routine part of bronchial hygiene in patients with cystic fibrosis, bronchiectasis, chronic bronchitis, necrotizing pulmonary infection, or spinal cord injury
      e. Integral part of other bronchial hygiene therapies, such as postural drainage therapy (PDT), positive expiratory pressure therapy (PEP), and incentive spirometry (IS)
      f. To obtain sputum specimens for diagnostic analysis

   5. Contraindications (Modified from AARC Clinical Practice Guideline: Directed Cough, 1993)
      a. DC is rarely contraindicated. The contraindications listed must be weighed against potential benefit in deciding to eliminate cough from the care of the patient. Listed contraindications are relative.
         (1) Inability to control possible transmission of infection from patients suspected or known to have pathogens transmittable by droplet nuclei (e.g., *M. tuberculosis*)
         (2) Presence of an elevated ICP or known intracranial aneurysm
         (3) Presence of reduced coronary artery perfusion, such as in acute myocardial infarction
         (4) Acute unstable head, neck, or spine injury
      b. Manually assisted DC with pressure to the epigastrium may be contraindicated in the presence of
         (1) Increased potential for regurgitation/aspiration (e.g., unconscious patient with unprotected airway)
         (2) Acute abdominal pathology, abdominal aortic aneurysm, hiatal hernia, or pregnancy

        (3)   A bleeding diathesis

        (4)   Untreated pneumothorax

   c.   Manually assisted DC with pressure to the thoracic cage may be contraindicated in the presence of

        (1)   Osteoporosis

        (2)   Flail chest

6.   Hazards/complications (Modified from AARC Clinical Practice Guideline: Directed Cough, 1993)

   a.   Reduced coronary artery perfusion

   b.   Reduced cerebral perfusion leading to syncope or alterations in consciousness, such as lightheadedness or confusion and vertebral artery dissection

   c.   Incontinence

   d.   Fatigue

   e.   Headache

   f.   Paresthesia or numbness

   g.   Bronchospasm

   h.   Muscular damage or discomfort

   i.   Spontaneous pneumothorax, pneumomediastinum, and subcutaneous emphysema

   j.   Cough paroxysms

   k.   Chest pain

   l.   Rib or costochondral juncture fracture

   m.   Incisional pain, evisceration

   n.   Anorexia, vomiting, and retching

   o.   Visual disturbances, including retinal hemorrhage

   p.   Central line displacement

   q.   Gastroesophageal reflux

7.   DC is of limited value in the obtunded, paralyzed, or uncooperative patient.

8.   The following clinical entities may compromise the effectiveness of a DC maneuver.

   a.   The presence of severe obstructive airway disease

   b.   Severe restrictive disease

   c.   Pain exacerbated by coughing

   d.   Fear of pain

   e.   Neurologic, muscular, or skeletal abnormalities

   f.   Systemic dehydration

   g.   Antitussives

9.   In patients with a bypassed upper airway or other conditions that preclude the ability to effectively close the glottis, the effectiveness of the cough may be limited.

10.   Thick, tenacious sputum may limit the effectiveness of the techniques and may require other supplemental strategies to optimize clearance of secretions.

11.   Directed force technique

   a.   Instruct patient to take three to five slow deep breaths, inhaling through the nose, exhaling through pursed lips, and using diaphragmatic breathing.

   b.   Ask the patient to take a deep breath and hold for 1 to 3 seconds.

   c.   Exhale rapidly from mid lung volumes to low lung volumes to clear secretions from periphery.

   d.   Take in normal breath, and contract the abdominal and chest wall muscles with the mouth (and glottis) open while whispering the word "huff." Repeat several times.

   e.   As secretions enter the larger airways, exhale rapidly from high to mid lung volumes to clear secretions from the more proximal airways. Repeat maneuver two or three times.

   f.   Take several relaxed diaphragmatic breaths before the next cough.

   g.   Manually assisted cough can be used by applying mechanical pressure to the epigastric region or thoracic cage with a forced exhalation.

E. Active cycle of breathing
   1. The active cycle of breathing (ACB) is a modification of the FET maneuver. It has three stages: breathing control, thoracic expansion control, and FET.
   2. Indications, contraindications, hazards, and complications are similar to those of DC.
   3. ACB technique
      a. Position patient properly, either relaxed sitting or reclined position.
      b. Breathing control: Several minutes of relaxed diaphragmatic breathing
      c. Thoracic expansion: Three or four active deep inspirations with passive relaxed exhalation
      d. Relaxed diaphragmatic breathing
      e. FETs: As the patient feels secretions enter the larger central airway, two or three huffs followed by relaxed breathing control are performed.
      f. Repeat the cycle two to four times, as tolerated.

F. Autogenic drainage
   1. Autogenic drainage is another modification of DC. Three phases of staged breathing at different lung volumes are performed until secretions are felt in the central airway. Several huff coughs at this point help to remove the secretions.
   2. Indications, contraindications, hazards, and complications are similar to those of DC.
   3. This technique requires a great deal of patient cooperation. It is recommended for patients aged ≥8 years.

G. Exercise
   1. Exercise has been shown to increase sputum production compared with rest. Exercise should be encouraged, as tolerated, to augment bronchial hygiene.

H. Cough assistance
   1. Cough assistance is indicated for the patient who cannot develop a forceful cough.
   2. Cough assistance can be performed by
      a. Applying pressure to the upper abdominal area during the compression and expiratory phase of the cough.
      b. For patients with an artificial airway this is done by hyperinflating the lung with a manual ventilator, holding gas volume in the lung at end of inspiration, and then rapidly releasing pressure, allowing exhalation, while an associate applies vigorous chest wall compression in an inward and downward fashion. Care should be taken to follow the normal anatomic movement of the chest.

I. Breathing instruction and retaining
   1. These techniques are designed to assist patients with muscular weakness, postoperative pain, or chronic pulmonary disease to assume an efficient ventilatory pattern and effective cough.
   2. Goals
      a. To increase and improve ventilation
      b. To strengthen respiratory musculature
      c. To prevent development of atelectasis
      d. To decrease work of breathing
      e. To improve the effectiveness of cough
   3. Specific techniques
      a. Diaphragmatic breathing exercises
         (1) The therapist and patient locate the xiphoid process. The patient is instructed to "sniff" to determine the location of the diaphragm.
         (2) The patient is relaxed, supported with a pillow, and directed to inspire by contracting the diaphragm slowly and completely to allow a normal inspiratory pattern.
            (a) Abdominal expansion
            (b) Lateral chest expansion
            (c) Upper chest expansion
         (3) The patient is encouraged to exhale slowly, passively, and completely. The therapist may assist exhalation by exerting a slight inward and upward pressure below the xiphoid process.

    b. Lateral costal expansion exercises

       (1) The therapist places his or her hands over the patient's lower rib cage with the thumbs just above the xiphoid process.

       (2) The patient is encouraged to relax and inspire against a slight pressure exerted by the therapist's hands. The patient is instructed to try to expand the area located under the therapist's hands.

       (3) Exhalation should be passive but complete. The therapist can assist exhalation by applying an inward and downward pressure during exhalation.

    c. Localized expansion exercises designed to direct the gas flow to a specific area of the lung

       (1) The therapist places his or her hands over the problem area and instructs the patient to inspire against a slight pressure exerted by the therapist.

       (2) Exhalation should be passive, complete, and assisted by the therapist. The therapist exerts an inward and downward force during exhalation, following the natural movement of the rib cage.

VI. Mechanical Aids to Bronchial Hygiene and Lung Expansion

  A. Intermittent positive pressure breathing (IPPB)

    1. IPPB is a technique used to provide short-term or intermittent mechanical ventilation for the purpose of augmenting lung expansion, delivering aerosol medication, clearing retained secretions, or assisting ventilation.

    2. IPPB is usually administered using a pneumatically driven, pressure-triggered, and pressure-cycled ventilator (Figure 36-14).

    3. IPPB may be delivered to artificial airways and nonintubated patients.

    4. IPPB should not be the first choice to deliver aerosol or as a method of lung expansion in spontaneously breathing patients who are capable of using other less expensive but clinically comparative methods.

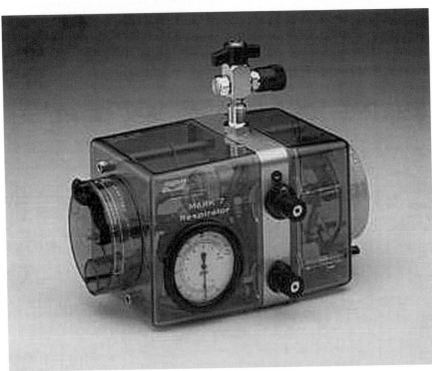

FIG. 36-14 Bird Mark 7 intermittent positive pressure breathing machine.

5. Indications (Modified from AARC Clinical Practice Guideline: Intermittent Positive Pressure Breathing, 2003)
   a. The need to improve lung expansion
      (1) The presence of clinically significant pulmonary atelectasis when other forms of therapy have been unsuccessful (e.g., IS, chest physiotherapy, deep breathing exercises, or positive airway pressure) or the patient cannot cooperate
      (2) Inability to clear secretions adequately because of pathology that severely limits the ability to ventilate or cough effectively and failure to respond to other modes of treatment
   b. The need for short-term ventilatory support for patients who are hypoventilating as an alternative to tracheal intubation and continuous mechanical ventilation. Devices specifically designed to deliver noninvasive positive pressure ventilation (NPPV) should be considered first (see Chapter 43).
   c. The need to deliver aerosol medication. (This is a highly controversial indication. The data indicate that IPPB adds no additional benefit to the spontaneous inhalation of aerosolized medication.)
      (1) Some clinicians oppose the use of IPPB for the management of severe bronchospasm (e.g., acute asthma or status asthmaticus and exacerbated chronic obstructive pulmonary disease [COPD]); however, a careful, closely supervised trial of IPPB as a medication-delivery device when treatment using other techniques (e.g., metered dose inhaler or nebulizer) has been unsuccessful may be warranted.
      (2) IPPB may be used to deliver aerosol medications to patients with fatigue as a result of ventilatory muscle weakness (e.g., failure to wean from mechanical ventilation, neuromuscular disease, kyphoscoliosis, or spinal injury) or chronic conditions in which intermittent ventilatory support is indicated (e.g., ventilatory support for home care patients and the more recent use of nasal positive pressure ventilation for respiratory insufficiency).
      (3) For patients with severe hyperinflation IPPB may decrease dyspnea and discomfort during nebulized therapy.
6. Contraindications (Modified from AARC Clinical Practice Guideline: Intermittent Positive Pressure Breathing, 2003)
   a. There are several clinical situations in which IPPB should not be used. With the exception of untreated tension pneumothorax, most of these contraindications are relative.
      (1) Tension pneumothorax (untreated)
      (2) ICP >15 mm Hg
      (3) Hemodynamic instability
      (4) Recent facial, oral, or skull surgery
      (5) Tracheoesophageal fistula
      (6) Recent esophageal surgery
      (7) Active hemoptysis
      (8) Nausea
      (9) Air swallowing
      (10) Active untreated tuberculosis
      (11) Radiographic evidence of bleb
      (12) Singulation (i.e., hiccups)
7. Hazards/complications (Modified from AARC Clinical Practice Guideline: Intermittent Positive Pressure Breathing, 2003)
   a. Increased airway resistance and work of breathing
   b. Barotrauma, pneumothorax
   c. Nosocomial infection
   d. Hypocarbia
   e. Hemoptysis
   f. Hyperoxia when oxygen is the gas source

g. Gastric distention
h. Impaction of secretions (associated with inadequately humidified gas mixture)
i. Psychological dependence
j. Impedance of venous return
k. Exacerbation of hypoxemia
l. Hypoventilation or hyperventilation
m. Increased mismatch of ventilation and perfusion
n. Air trapping, auto-positive end-expiratory pressure, or overdistended alveoli

B. Incentive spirometry (IS)
1. IS is designed to mimic natural sighing or yawning by encouraging the patient to take long, slow, deep breaths.
2. The apparatus acts purely as a visual motivator encouraging patient effort and compliance.
3. The IS maneuver consists of a sustained, maximal inspiration (SMI), followed by a 5- to 10-second breath-hold. Patients should be encouraged to take 5-10 breaths every hour.
4. The goals of IS are to increase transpulmonary pressure and inspiratory volumes, improving inspiratory muscle performance, and reestablishing or simulating the normal pattern of pulmonary hyperinflation.
5. Indications (Modified from AARC Clinical Practice Guideline: Incentive Spirometry, 1991)
    a. Presence of conditions predisposing to the development of pulmonary atelectasis
        (1) Upper abdominal surgery
        (2) Thoracic surgery
        (3) Surgery in patients with COPD
    b. Presence of pulmonary atelectasis
    c. Presence of a restrictive lung defect associated with quadriplegia and/or dysfunctional diaphragm
6. Contraindications (Modified from AARC Clinical Practice Guideline: Incentive Spirometry, 1991)
    a. Patient cannot be instructed or supervised to ensure appropriate use of the device.
    b. Patient cooperation is absent, or patient is unable to understand or demonstrate proper use of the device.
    c. Patients unable to deep breathe effectively (e.g., with vital capacity less than approximately 10 ml/kg or inspiratory capacity less than approximately one third of predicted)
    d. Presence of an open tracheal stoma is not a contraindication but requires adaptation of the spirometer.
7. Hazards and complications (Modified from AARC Clinical Practice Guideline: Incentive Spirometry, 1991)
    a. Ineffective unless closely supervised or performed as ordered
    b. Inappropriate as sole therapy for major lung collapse or consolidation
    c. Hyperventilation
    d. Barotrauma
    e. Discomfort secondary to inadequate pain control
    f. Hypoxia secondary to interruption of prescribed oxygen therapy if face mask or shield is used
    g. Exacerbation of bronchospasm
    h. Fatigue
8. Types of ISs
    a. Flow oriented (Figure 36-15, *B*)
        (1) The patient's inspiratory flow rate causes a float or ball to rise in a canister. The float or ball remains suspended for a sustained period.
        (2) The patient should maintain an inspiratory flow that slowly elevates the float.
        (3) A rapid inspiration will cause the float to rise quickly but will not maintain it in a suspended position.
        (4) Slow inspirations do not generate sufficient flow to raise the float.

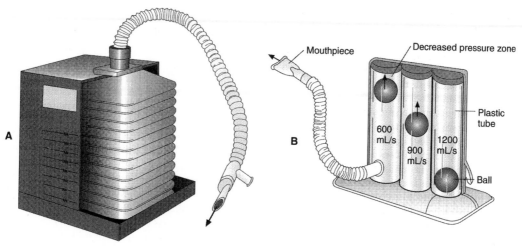

FIG. 36-15 A, Volume-oriented incentive spirometer. **B,** Flow-oriented incentive spirometer.

    b. Volume oriented (Figure 36-15, *A*)
        (1) The patient inspires until a preset volume of gas is inhaled.
        (2) Indicators are used to motivate patients and indicate when desired volume is achieved.
        (3) Most systems are designed to require a sustained inspiration before the achieved volume indicator is activated.

VII. Positive Airway Pressure
    A. Positive airway pressure therapy (PAP) is used to mobilize secretions and manage atelectasis. The three adjuncts to PAP are continuous positive airway pressure (CPAP), positive expiratory pressure (PEP), and expiratory positive airway pressure (EPAP).
    B. Studies have shown that PAP therapy is most effective when combined with cough or other airway clearance techniques.
    C. CPAP therapy requires the patient to breathe from a pressurized circuit against a threshold resistor that maintains consistent preset airway pressures from 5 to 20 cm H_2O (Figure 36-16).
    D. PEP therapy requires the patient to exhale against a fixed-orifice resistor, generating pressures during expiration that usually range from 10 to 20 cm H_2O (Figure 36-17).
    E. EPAP therapy requires the patient to exhale against a threshold resistor, generating preset pressures of 10 to 20 cm H_2O.
    F. Indications (Modified from AARC Clinical Practice Guideline: Use of Positive Airway Pressure Adjuncts to Bronchial Hygiene Therapy, 1993)
        1. To reduce air trapping in patients with asthma and COPD
        2. To aid in mobilization of retained secretions in those with cystic fibrosis and chronic bronchitis
        3. To prevent or reverse atelectasis
        4. To optimize delivery of bronchodilators in patients receiving bronchial hygiene therapy
    G. Contraindications (Modified from AARC Clinical Practice Guideline: Use of Positive Airway Pressure Adjuncts to Bronchial Hygiene Therapy, 1993)
        1. Patients unable to tolerate the increased work of breathing (e.g., those with acute asthma or COPD)
        2. ICP >20 mm Hg
        3. Hemodynamic instability
        4. Recent facial, oral, or skull surgeries or trauma
        5. Acute sinusitis
        6. Epistaxis
        7. Esophageal surgery

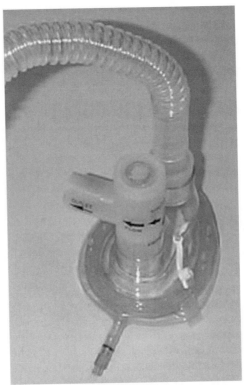

FIG. 36-16 Continuous positive airway pressure mask with fixed positive end-expiratory pressure exhalation valve.

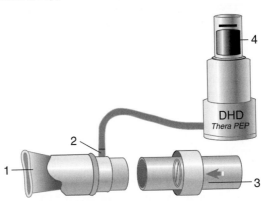

FIG. 36-17 Example of commercial single-use positive expiratory pressure device (DHD TheraPEP). *1,* Mouthpiece. *2,* Pressure tap. *3,* One-way inlet valve. *4,* Pressure generator.

    8. Active hemoptysis
    9. Nausea
   10. Known or suspected tympanic membrane rupture or other middle ear pathology
   11. Untreated pneumothorax
  H. Hazards and complications (Modified from AARC Clinical Practice Guideline: Use of Positive Airway Pressure Adjuncts to Bronchial Hygiene Therapy, 1993)
    1. Increased work of breathing that may lead to hypoventilation and hypercarbia
    2. Increased ICP
    3. Cardiovascular compromise
      a. Myocardial ischemia
      b. Decreased venous return

4. Air swallowing, with increased likelihood of vomiting and aspiration
5. Claustrophobia
6. Skin breakdown and discomfort from mask
7. Pulmonary barotrauma

VIII. **Mechanical Insufflation/Exsufflation (MIE)**
   A. MIE is indicated for patients with decreased cough ability (e.g., those with neuromuscular disorders). Its purpose is to simulate a spontaneous cough (Figure 36-18).
   B. A positive pressure breath is delivered at 30 to 50 cm H_2O for 1 to 3 seconds via an oronasal mask or artificial tracheal airway. A negative pressure of −30 to −50 cm H_2O follows this for 2 or 3 seconds to stimulate a cough.
   C. This process is repeated with breaks for spontaneous or assisted breathing until secretions are cleared from the airway.
   D. The expiratory flow remains high immediately after exsufflation, indicating that MIE does not promote airway collapse.
   E. Although studies have found this to be a useful adjunct for patients with neuromuscular disease, there is no evidence of its effectiveness in critically ill patients.

IX. **High Frequency Oscillation of the Airway**
   A. High frequency oscillation of the airway (HFOA) is the rapid vibratory movement of small volumes of air produced by either a mechanical device or the patient's own expiration with an oscillatory device.

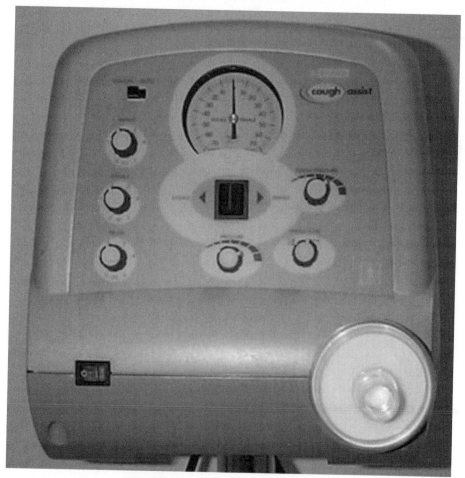

FIG. 36-18 Mechanical insufflator/exsufflator.

  B. HFOA has been shown to increase mucous clearance by altering mucous rheology and enhancing mucous-airflow interaction and reflex mechanisms.

  C. HFOA methods include the flutter valve and intrapulmonary percussive ventilation (IPV).

    1. The flutter valve

      a. The flutter valve is a mucous clearance device that combines the technique of PEP with high frequency oscillations at the airway opening.

      b. It is pipe shaped with a steel ball in the bowl covered by a cap. When the patient exhales actively into the device, the ball creates a positive pressure between 10 and 25 cm H_2O and generates oscillations of approximately 15 Hz (Figure 36-19).

      c. It may decrease mucous viscoelasticity within the airways, thus modifying mucus and allowing it to be cleared.

      d. To use the flutter valve, instruct the patient to sit comfortably and take in a breath slightly larger than normal. Place the flutter in the mouth, seal lips, and the patient exhales actively but not forcefully. Do this for 10 to 20 breaths.

      e. There are few data on its efficacy, but it has been shown to be of benefit for patients with cystic fibrosis.

    2. IPV

      a. IPV is a form of chest physiotherapy (CPT) that uses a pneumatic device to deliver pressurized gas minibursts at rates of 100 to 225 cycles/min to the respiratory tract via a mouthpiece. Normal treatment time is 20 minutes.

      b. IPV can be used to manage atelectasis, enhance the mobilization and clearance of retained secretions, and deliver nebulized medications to the distal airways.

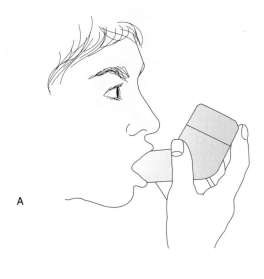

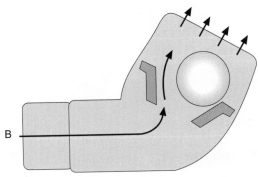

FIG. 36-19 A, Position of flutter valve in patient's mouth. **B,** Internal mechanics of flutter valve.

    c. Limited data reported show that IPV may be comparable with the results of standard CPT.

X. High Frequency Chest Wall Oscillation

  A. High frequency chest wall oscillation (HFCWO) is a noninvasive form of oscillation that uses an air-pulse generator and a nonstretch inflatable vest that covers the patient's torso.

  B. HFCWO methods include the ThAIRapy Vest and the Hayek oscillator.

    1. ThAIRapy Vest

      a. The ThAIRapy Vest is an airway clearance device that consists of an inflatable vest connected to an air-pulse generator. The generator rapidly inflates and deflates the vest, which helps move mucus toward the large airways, where it can be cleared by coughing.

      b. The frequency of oscillations and flow bias are variable and it is important to determine optimal settings for maximal effectiveness.

      c. The data show the ThAIRapy Vest is effective for secretion clearance in patients with cystic fibrosis.

    2. Hayek oscillator

      a. The Hayek oscillator is an electrically powered, noninvasive ventilator that uses a chest cuirass to apply negative and positive pressure to the chest wall, which delivers oscillations to the lungs.

      b. Frequency, inspiration/expiration ratio, inspiratory pressure, and expiratory pressure are variable settings and it is important to determine optimal settings for maximal effectiveness.

      c. Limited data on the efficacy of the Hayek oscillator are available.

      d. At best it is no better than traditional CPT techniques.

BIBLIOGRAPHY

American Association for Respiratory Care: Clinical practice guideline: IS. *Respir Care* 36:1402, 1991.

American Association for Respiratory Care: The pros and cons of IPPB: AARC provides an assessment on its effectiveness. *AARC Times* 10:48, 1986.

American Association for Respiratory Care: Clinical practice guideline: intermittent positive pressure breathing—2003 revision and update. *Respir Care* 48:540, 2003.

American Association for Respiratory Care: Clinical practice guideline: use of positive airway pressure adjuncts to bronchial hygiene therapy. *Respir Care* 38:516, 1993.

American Association for Respiratory Care: Clinical practice guideline: postural drainage therapy. *Respir Care* 36:1418, 1991.

American Association for Respiratory Care: Clinical practice guideline: directed cough. *Respir Care* 38:495, 1993.

Arens R, Gozal D, Omlin KJ, et al: Comparison of high frequency chest compression and conventional chest physiotherapy in hospitalized patients with cystic fibrosis. *Am J Respir Crit Care Med* 150:1154-1157, 1994.

Fink JB, Mahlmeister MJ: High-frequency oscillation of the airway and chest wall. *Respir Care* 47:797-807, 2002.

Fink JB: Positioning versus postural drainage. *Respir Care* 47:769-777, 2002.

Hess D, MacIntyre N, Mishoe S, et al: *Respiratory Care: Principles and Practice.* St. Louis, Mosby, 2002.

Hess DR: The evidence for secretion clearance techniques. *Respir Care* 46:1276-1293, 2001.

Langenderfer B: Alternatives to percussion and postural drainage. A review of mucus clearance therapies: percussion and postural drainage, autogenic drainage, positive expiratory pressure, flutter valve, intrapulmonary percussive ventilation, and high-frequency chest compression with ThAIRapy Vest. *J Cardiopulm Rehabil* 18:283-289, 1998.

Natale JE, Pfeifle J, Homnick DN: Comparison of intrapulmonary percussive ventilation and chest physiotherapy. *Chest* 105:1789-1793, 1994.

Pasquina P, Tramer MR, Walder B: Prophylactic respiratory physiotherapy after cardiac surgery: systematic review. *BMJ* 327:1379, 2003.

Sancho J, Servera E, Vergara P, Marin J: Mechanical insufflation-exsufflation vs. tracheal suctioning via tracheostomy tubes for patients with amyotrophic lateral sclerosis: a pilot study. *Am J Phys Med Rehabil* 82:750-753, 2003.

Sivasothy P, Brown L, Smith IE, Shneerson JM: Effect of manually assisted cough and mechanical insufflation on cough flow of normal subjects, patients with chronic obstructive pulmonary disease (COPD), and patients with respiratory muscle weakness. *Thorax* 56:438-444, 2001.

Sorenson HM: Managing secretions in dying patient. *Respir Care* 45:1355-1362, 2000.

Varekojis, SM, Douce FH, Flucke RL, et al: A comparison of the therapeutic effectiveness of and preference for postural drainage and percussion, intrapulmonary percussive ventilation, and high-frequency chest wall compression in hospitalized cystic fibrosis patients. *Respir Care* 48:24-28, 2003.

Wilkins R, Stoller J, Scanlan CL: *Egan's Fundamentals of Respiratory Therapy*, ed 8. St. Louis, Mosby, 2003.

Chapter 37

Analyzers

I. **Oxygen Analyzers**
  A. Analyzers operating on the polarographic principle (Clark electrode) (Figures 37-1 and 37-2)
    1. The basic overall chemical reaction occurring in electrode system is

$$O_2 + 2\ H_2O + 4\ electrons \rightarrow 4\ OH^-$$

    2. The analyzer is composed of two electrodes immersed in a potassium chloride electrolyte solution.
      a. At the silver anode, oxidation of chloride ion to silver chloride takes place. This reaction releases electrons, developing a current.
      b. At the platinum cathode, oxygen is reduced to form OH^- ions, thus consuming electrons produced from the anode.
    3. In solution the greater the partial pressure of oxygen, the greater the current produced and used.
    4. A -0.6 volt (V) polarizing voltage is applied to the anode.
    5. This voltage is needed to maintain direction of current from anode to cathode through the electrolyte solution.
    6. At -0.6 V oxygen is the only respiratory gas that will be readily reduced.
    7. The tip of the Clark electrode is covered with a polypropylene membrane that allows slow diffusion of oxygen from blood or gas being analyzed.
    8. This analyzer type directly measures partial pressure of the gas. For this reason the analyzer must be carefully calibrated at varying altitudes and to changing atmospheric pressures.
    9. The analyzer is used in all respiratory gas mixtures and is the type incorporated into most blood gas analyzer systems.
    10. Measurement of flow of electrons is referred to as an *amperometric measurement.*
    11. Response times for Clark electrode oxygen analyzers range between 10 and 30 seconds.
  B. Analyzers operating using a galvanic cell
    1. The galvanic cell is similar to a battery cell that uses oxygen to create a current between its electrodes.
    2. Current is continually produced if the cell is exposed to oxygen; thus the life of the cell depends on duration and frequency of use.
    3. The analyzer is composed of two electrodes immersed in an alkali metal hydroxide solution. Generally the electrolyte is potassium hydroxide, but some models use cesium hydroxide.
      a. A lead anode, in the presence of oxygen, produces a current as a result of an oxidation reaction with the hydroxide compound.
      b. A gold cathode, in the presence of oxygen, produces the following reaction.

$$O_2 + 2\ H_2O + 4\ electrons \rightarrow 4\ OH^-$$

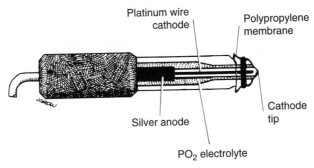

FIG. 37-1 The Clark electrode. See Figure 37-2 for specifics.

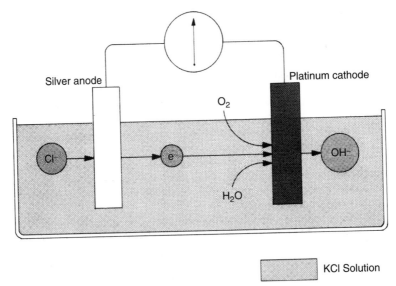

FIG. 37-2 The basic principle of the polarographic electrode. The chloride ion will react with the silver anode to form silver chloride, an oxidation reaction that produces electrons. Oxygen will react with platinum and water, using electrons (a reduction reaction). The flow of electrons can be measured as a current. The greater the concentration of oxygen in solution, the greater the current used.

   c. The overall reactions for galvanic cell and polarographic analyzers are the same.
4. The current is measured from anode to cathode, which allows completion of an electric circuit.
5. The greater the partial pressure of oxygen, the greater the measured current.
6. As with the polarographic analyzer the galvanic cell measures the partial pressure of oxygen and consequently must be carefully calibrated at varying altitudes and atmospheric pressure.
7. The response time for galvanic cell analyzers is longer, sometimes taking as long as 60 seconds.

II. **pH (Sanz) Electrode (Figures 37-3 and 37-4)**
  A. The electrode is composed of two half-cells connected via a potassium chloride electrolyte bridge.
    1. A reference half-cell composed of mercury/mercurous chloride (calomel)
    2. A measuring half-cell composed of silver/silver chloride
  B. The measuring half-cell has two chambers separated by pH-sensitive glass, which allows measurement of voltage differences across the glass.

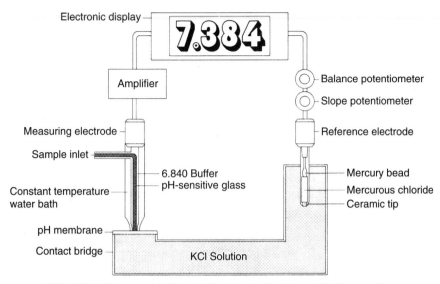

FIG. 37-3 The complete Sanz (pH) electrode. See Figure 37-4 for specifics.

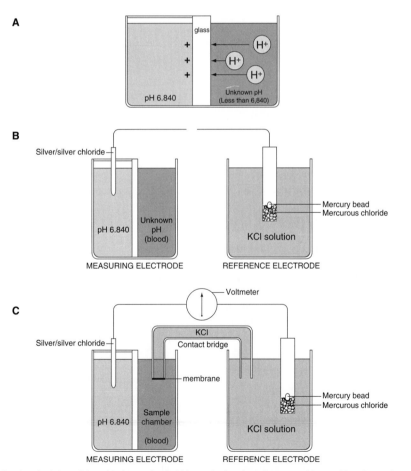

FIG. 37-4 Basic principles of the pH electrode. **A,** Voltage is developed across pH-sensitive glass when the hydrogen ion concentration is unequal in the two solutions. **B,** Chemical half-cell is used as the measuring electrode, and another half-cell is the reference electrode. **C,** The basic principle of the modern pH electrode.

1. The enclosed buffer chamber with a buffer of a constant pH surrounds the pH-sensitive glass capillary tube.
        2. The sample chamber capillary tube allows blood to be in contact with the pH-sensitive glass.
    C. The reference half-cell is immersed in potassium chloride solution, which allows completion of the basic electrical circuit while providing constant reference voltage.
    D. As a result of electric activity on the pH-sensitive glass, a potential difference can be measured.
    E. The potential difference is measured on a voltmeter calibrated in pH units.
    F. This type of system comparing voltage measurements is termed *potentiometer*.

III. **Pco_2 (Severinghaus) Electrode (Figure 37-5)**
    A. The Pco_2 electrode is a modified pH electrode.
    B. The Pco_2 is measured indirectly by determining the change in pH of an $NaHCO_3$ solution.
    C. The electrode is composed of two half-cells, each composed of silver/silver chloride.
    D. Functioning of electrode
        1. Carbon dioxide diffuses across a silicon membrane into an $NaHCO_3$ electrolyte solution.
        2. After the solution is entered carbon dioxide reacts with water to form hydrogen and bicarbonate ions:

$$CO_2 + H_2O \rightarrow H_2CO_3 \rightarrow H^+ + HCO_3^-$$

3. The H^+ formed sets up a potential difference across the pH-sensitive glass in the measuring half-cell.
    E. All other aspects of the electrode are consistent with the pH electrode.
    F. The potential difference is measured on a voltmeter and reflected as millimeters of mercury of carbon dioxide. (*Note:* The Po_2 (Clark) electrode for blood gas analyzers is covered in Section I, A.)

IV. **Point of Care Testing**
    A. Bedside arterial blood gas (ABG) analysis (Figure 37-6)
        1. Bedside ABG analysis can be cost effective.
        2. Some models can measure several additional chemistry and hematology parameters, including
            a. Serum electrolytes
            b. Blood glucose levels
            c. Blood urea nitrogen
            d. Hematocrit
            e. Prothrombin times
    B. Some are portable roll-about or handheld and operate via alternating current (AC) or direct current (DC).
    C. Analysis of blood takes place in a disposable, self-calibrating cartridge (Figure 37-7).
        1. Each cartridge contains
            a. Necessary calibration solution
            b. Sample handling system

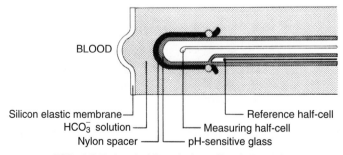

BLOOD

Silicon elastic membrane
HCO$_3^-$ solution
Nylon spacer

Reference half-cell
Measuring half-cell
pH-sensitive glass

FIG. 37-5 A typical Severinghaus (Pco_2) electrode.

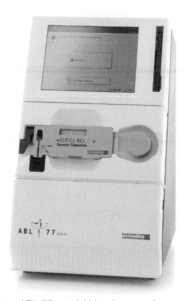

FIG. 37-6 Radiometer ABL 77 arterial blood gas analyzer and electrolyte system.

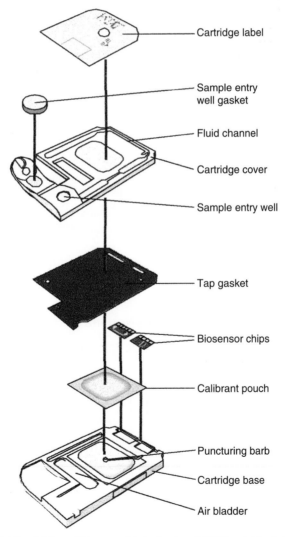

FIG. 37-7 Microfluidic and bisensor chip technology I-STAT portable clinical analyzer.

  c. Waste chamber
  d. Miniaturized electrochemical or photochemical sensor
 2. Test results are available within 90 seconds.
 3. Proven to be as accurate as laboratory-based blood gas analyzers

V. **Indwelling (Intraarterial) Continuous Blood Gas Monitoring (Figure 37-8)**
 A. Current technology using fiberoptic photochemical sensors or optodes
  1. Optodes measure blood gas parameters using photochemical reactions through the following.
   a. Optode contains photosensitive dye at distal end of the optic fiber.
   b. Light transmitted to this dye can be absorbed, reflected, or reemitted.
   c. Measuring the changes in light transmission, the concentration of these substances can be measured.

VI. **Transcutaneous Po_2 ($TcPo_2$) and Pco_2 ($TcPco_2$) Monitoring**
 A. Both of these techniques make use of miniaturized blood gas (Clark and Severinghaus) electrodes (Figure 37-9).
  1. $TcPo_2$ monitoring
   a. Oxygen molecules diffusing through the skin diffuse through the semipermeable membrane covering the Clark electrode.
   b. The skin surface under the electrode is heated to approximately 42° C to facilitate diffusion and to arterialize the blood.
   c. Normally electrodes are placed on flat surfaces of the chest and abdomen.
   d. This electrode is reasonably accurate if perfusion is normal and the skin over which it is placed is thin.
   e. As a result it is used almost exclusively for infants.

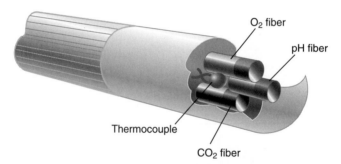

FIG. 37-8 A diagram of an indwelling optode-based arterial blood gas catheter with O_2, CO_2, pH, and thermocouple fibers.

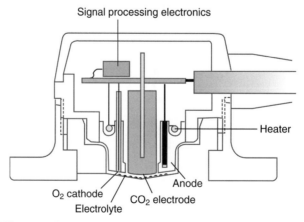

FIG. 37-9 Schematic diagram of the oxygen-carbon dioxide sensor.

2. TcPCO₂ monitoring
   a. The skin under the electrode is heated to approximately 44° C.
   b. Heating of the skin increases diffusion, allowing more carbon dioxide to diffuse, but may increase local metabolism and carbon dioxide production.
   c. Electrodes are placed on the chest and abdomen.
   d. As long as perfusion is adequate and diffusion is normal, TcPCO₂ accurately tracks PCO₂.
   e. TcPO₂ and TcPCO₂ electrodes should be changed every 2 to 6 hours to prevent thermal injury.

VII. **Spectrophotometric Analyzers: Oximetry**
   A. A spectrophotometer is an apparatus that determines the light absorbance of matter in solution by the quantity of light absorbed in passing through the fluid.
      1. Molecules of a substance in solution can absorb light waves. Various substances absorb differing spectra.
      2. Spectrophotometers create light waves specific to the substance to be measured.
      3. Light waves of specific spectra are passed through a sample and measured.
      4. Because the amount of input light waves is constant, measuring the output waves allows determination of the amount of light absorption by the sample.
      5. Finally, according to the Lambert-Beer law, the absorption of light by a solution is a function of the concentration of the solute and the absorption depth of the solution. The greater the sample absorption, the greater the concentration of the substance measured because the absorption depth is a constant determined by the sample chamber.
   B. Functional components of spectrophotometers
      1. Light source of known intensity
      2. Sample chamber of known depth
      3. Light collector (photo multiplier)
      4. Readout display
   C. Types of spectrophotometers commonly used
      1. Pulse oximeters (Figure 37-10)
         a. These units use two wavelengths of light: red and infrared.
         b. The absorption of light by oxyhemoglobin and reduced hemoglobin is compared.
         c. Both require a pulsating arterial bed for operation. Typical measurement sites are
            (1) Finger
            (2) Earlobe
            (3) Bridge of the nose
            (4) Toe
         d. The emitter and detector are placed on each side of the capillary bed.
         e. Most units fail to function if a pulse is not noticeable.
         f. These units measure oxyhemoglobin saturation with an accuracy of ±2% to ±5% within the 80% to 100% saturation range.

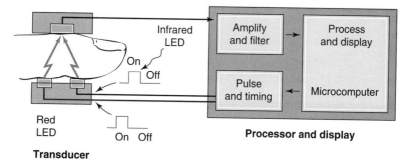

FIG. 37-10 Schematic block diagram of a pulse oximeter.

g. They are frequently used on all sizes of patients in all clinical settings to monitor oxyhemoglobin saturation.

h. Factors that may affect accuracy of pulse oximeters
   (1) Motion artifact
   (2) Dark skin pigmentation
   (3) Nail polish
   (4) Ambient light interference
   (5) Poor peripheral perfusion
   (6) Anemia (low hematocrit)

2. CO-oximeter
   a. It uses light wave spectra specific to
      (1) Oxyhemoglobin
      (2) Reduced hemoglobin
      (3) Carboxyhemoglobin
      (4) Methemoglobin
   b. Total hemoglobin readout also is provided.

3. Capnography (end-tidal CO_2 monitoring) (Figure 37-11)
   a. Infrared capnometer is the most common technology used.
   b. This device uses the radio absorptive quality of CO_2.
   c. Filtered infrared light source passes through a sample chamber.
   d. A lens focuses the remaining unabsorbed radiation onto a photo detector.
   e. The greater the concentration of CO_2, the less infrared light will arrive at the photo detector, which alters the electrical output signal.
   f. There are advantages and disadvantages to using a mainstream sampling and a side-stream sampling method.
   g. End-tidal CO_2 readings also are altered by any factor affecting deadspace.
   h. The greater the deadspace, the poorer the correlation of end-tidal CO_2 with Pa_{CO_2}.
      (1) A normal capnogram tracing is depicted in Figure 37-12.
      (2) From point a to b, gas is exhaled from the anatomic deadspace; no CO_2 is present.
      (3) From point b to c, there is a changeover from deadspace to alveolar gas, and the amount of exhaled CO_2 rapidly increases.
      (4) From point c to d, gas is exhaled entirely from alveoli. In this stage a gently sloping plateau should be established.
      (5) From point d to e, inspiration begins, which continues into point a.
   i. Many variations in the normal capnogram are noticed clinically (Figure 37-13).

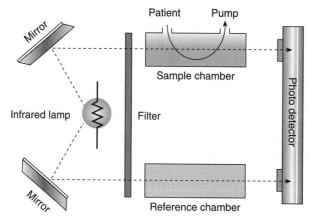

FIG. 37-11 Schematic representation of an infrared capnometer.

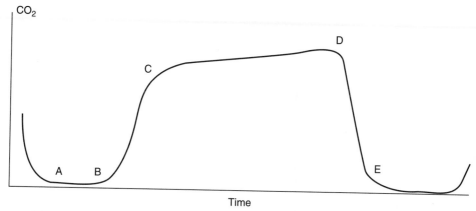

FIG. 37-12 Normal capnogram end-tidal CO_2 percentage tracing (see text for discussion).

(1) Pulsing of exhaled gas caused by cardiac oscillations is noted in Figure 37-13, *A.*

(2) Hyperventilation is noted in Figure 37-13, *B.* The percentage of exhaled CO_2 is normally decreased.

(3) The beginning of hypoventilation is noted in Figure 37-13, *C.* Carbon dioxide levels start to increase.

(4) Rebreathing of CO_2 results in the baseline CO_2 level increasing above zero (see Figure 37-13, *D*).

(5) A disconnected mechanical ventilator or apnea in spontaneous ventilation is indicated by a sudden loss of the capnogram tracing (see Figure 37-13, *E*).

(6) A rapid progressive decay in the plateau is noted during cardiac arrest or severely developing hypotension. Because of loss of perfusion, deadspace markedly increases and CO_2 decreases (see Figure 37-13, *F*).

(7) Spasmodic contraction of the diaphragm or the interruption of exhalation by an incomplete breath is illustrated in Figure 37-13, *G.*

(8) A periodic decrease in CO_2 level and a loss of plateau are associated with same ineffective tidal breaths or poor sampling (see Figure 37-13, *H*).

VIII. Nitric Oxide and Nitrogen Dioxide Analyzers (Figures 37-14 and 37-15)
   A. Nitric oxide and nitrogen dioxide analyzers
      1. Two types of analyzers
         a. Chemiluminescence monitoring
           (1) Available in single- or dual-reaction chambers
           (2) Measures gas concentration by stimulated photoemission
           (3) Sample gas reacts with ozone (O_3) to produce NO_2 (nitrogen dioxide).
           (4) $NO + O_3 \rightarrow NO_2^* + O_2$ (7%)
           (5) $NO + O_3 \rightarrow NO_2 + O_2$ (93%)
           (6) The NO_2^* releases a photon $NO_2^* \rightarrow +$ (photon).
           (7) Measured by a photomultiplier tube that proportionately converts the intensity of the luminescence into an electrical signal for display.
           (8) NO_2 is measured indirectly by converting NO_2 to NO and measures total NO concentrations in either a thermal catalytic converter (600 to 800° C) or chemical converter (using molybdenum or carbon).
           (9) $2\,NO_2 \rightarrow 2\,NO + O_2$ (thermal catalytic converter)
          (10) $3\,NO_2 + Mo \rightarrow MoO_3 + 3\,NO$ (chemical converter)
          (11) NO_2 concentration is the difference between total nitrogen oxides measured (NOx) and the NO concentration.
          (12) Advantages: Chemical converters are more stable.

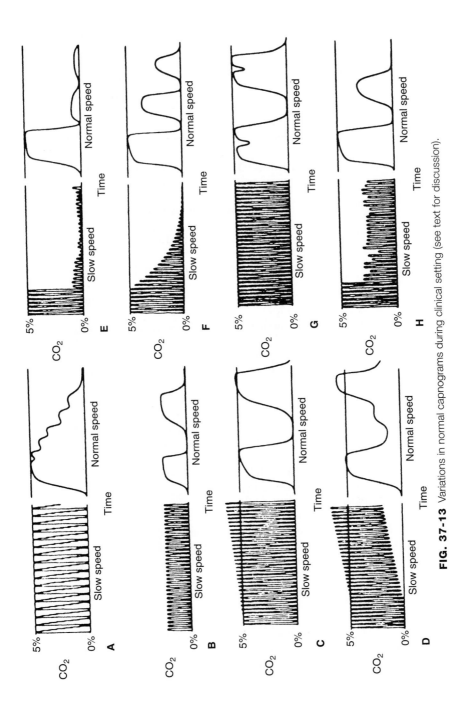

FIG. 37-13 Variations in normal capnograms during clinical setting (see text for discussion).

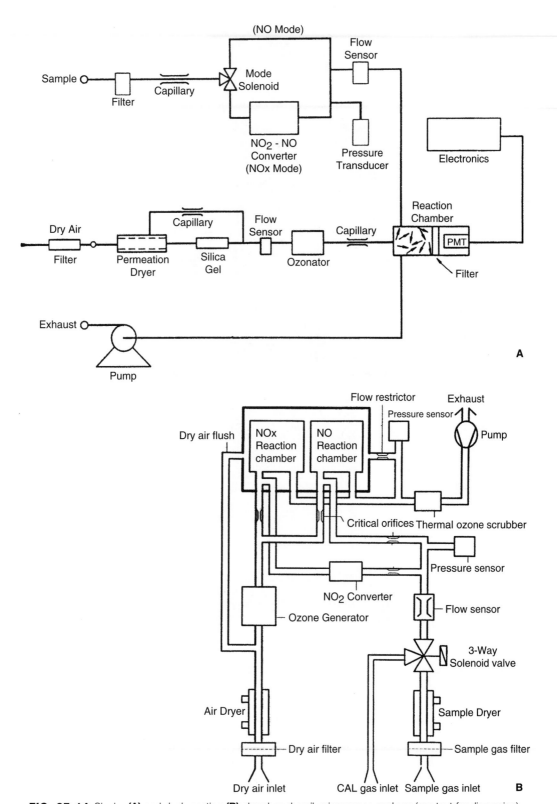

FIG. 37-14 Single- **(A)** and dual-reaction **(B)** chamber chemiluminescence analyzer (see text for discussion).

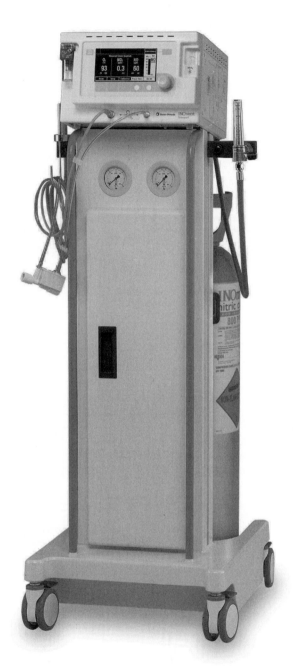

FIG. 37-15 INOvent delivery system for administration of nitric oxide to mechanically ventilated patients.

      (13)   Disadvantages: Chemical must be replenished.

      (14)   Oxygen concentrations near 100% decrease the NO reading between 7% and 15% and the NOx by between 15% and 26%.

   b. Electrochemical monitoring

      (1)   Based on the principle these gases react with an electrolyte solution

      (2)   Electrons are liberated and generate a current between two polarized electrodes.

      (3)   Reactions occurring to measure NO

      (a) $NO + 2 H_2O \rightarrow HNO_3 + 3 H^+ + 3 e^-$

      (b) $O_2 + 4 H^+ + 4e^- \rightarrow 2 H_2O$

      (c) $4 NO + 2 H_2O + 3 O_2 \rightarrow 4 HNO_3$

  (4) Reactions occurring to measure NO_2

      (a) $NO_2 + 2 H^+ + 2e^- \rightarrow NO + H_2O$

      (b) $2 H_2O \rightarrow 4H^+ + 4e^- + O_2$

      (c) $2 NO_2 \rightarrow 2 NO + O_2$

  (5) Accuracy can be affected by direct pressure from mechanical ventilators but can be minimized by using a side-stream sampling technique.

2. Calibration

    a. Calibration of NO is performed with calibrated gas cylinders of NO in the 20- to 100-ppm range.

    b. Calibration of NO_2 is performed with calibrated gas cylinders of NO_2 in the 5- to 10-ppm range.

BIBLIOGRAPHY

Betit P, Grenier B, Thompson JE, et al: Evaluation of four analyzers used to monitor nitric oxide and nitrogen dioxide concentrations during inhaled nitric oxide administration. *Respir Care* 41: 817-825, 1996.

Body S, Hartigan P, Sherman S., et al: Nitric oxide: delivery, measurement, and clinical application. *J Cardiothoracic Vasc Anesth* 9:748-763, 1995.

Branson RD, Hess DR, Chatburn RL: *Respiratory Care Equipment*, ed 2. Philadelphia, Lippincott, Williams & Wilkins, 1999.

Burton G, Hodgkin JE, Ward JJ: *Respiratory Care: A Guide to Clinical Practice*, ed 4. Philadelphia, Lippincott, Williams & Wilkins, 1997.

Cairo JM, Pilbeam SP: *Mosby's Respiratory Care Equipment*, ed 7. St. Louis, Mosby, 2004.

Hess D: Capnometry and capnography: technical aspects, physiologic aspects, and clinical applications. *Respir Care* 35:557-576, 1990.

Hess D, Macintyre NR, Mishoe SC, Galvin WF, Adams AB, Saposnick AB: *Respiratory Care: Principles and Practice*. Philadelphia, WB Saunders, 2002.

Kacmarek RM: *Monitoring in Respiratory Care*. St. Louis, Mosby, 1993.

Kacmarek RM, Mack CW, Dimas S: *The Essentials of Respiratory Care*, ed 3. St. Louis, Mosby, 1990.

Martin RJ: Transcutaneous monitoring: instrumentation and clinical applications. *Respir Care* 35: 577-583, 1990.

Nishimura M, Imanaka H, Uchiyama A, et al: Nitric oxide (NO) measurement accuracy. *J Clin Monit* 13:241-248, 1997.

Pierson DJ, Kacmarek RM: *Foundations of Respiratory Care*. New York, Churchill Livingstone, 1992.

Purtz E, Hess D, Kacmarek R: Evaluation of electrochemical nitric oxide and nitrogen dioxide analyzers suitable for use during mechanical ventilation. *J Clin Monit* 13:25-34, 1997.

Severinghaus JW: History and recent developments in pulse oximetry. *Scand J Clin Lab Invest Suppl* 214:105-111, 1993.

Shapiro BAD, Peruzzi WT, Kozlowski-Templin R: *Clinical Application of Blood Gases*, ed 3. Chicago, Mosby Yearbook, 1982.

Swedlow DB: Capnometry and capnography: the anesthesia disaster early warning system. *Semin Anesth* 5:194-202, 1986.

Volsko TA, Chatburn RL, Kallstrom TJ: Evaluation of a commercial standard for checking pulse oximeter performance. *Respir Care* 41:100-104, 1996.

Wilkins RL, Stoller JK: *Egan's Fundamentals of Respiratory Care*, ed 8. St. Louis, Mosby, 2003.

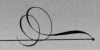

Chapter 38

Airway Care

I. Use of Artificial Airways (Modified from AARC Clinical Practice Guideline: Management of Airway Emergencies, 1995)
    A. Indications
        1. Conditions requiring management of the airway generally are impending or actual
            a. Airway obstruction
            b. Need to ventilate
            c. Inability to protect the airway
            d. Need to remove secretions
        2. Specific conditions include but are not limited to
            a. Airway emergency before endotracheal intubation
            b. Obstruction of the artificial airway
            c. Apnea
            d. Acute traumatic coma
            e. Penetrating neck trauma
            f. Cardiopulmonary arrest and unstable dysrhythmia
            g. Severe bronchospasm
            h. Severe allergic reactions with cardiopulmonary compromise
            i. Pulmonary edema
            j. Sedative or narcotic drug effect
            k. Foreign body airway obstruction
            l. Choanal atresia in neonates
            m. Aspiration
            n. Risk of aspiration
            o. Severe laryngospasm
            p. Self-extubation
        3. Conditions requiring *emergency tracheal* intubation include, but are not limited to
            a. Persistent apnea
            b. Traumatic upper airway obstruction (partial or complete)
            c. Accidental extubation of the patient unable to maintain adequate spontaneous ventilation
            d. Obstructive angioedema (edema involving the deeper layers of the skin, subcutaneous tissue, and mucosa)
            e. Massive uncontrolled upper airway bleeding
            f. Coma with potential for increased intracranial pressure
            g. Infection-related upper airway obstruction (partial or complete)
            h. Epiglottitis in children or adults
            i. Acute uvular edema
            j. Tonsillopharyngitis or retropharyngeal abscess
            k. Suppurative parotitis
            l. Laryngeal and upper airway edema

4. Neonatal or pediatric specific
    a. Perinatal asphyxia
    b. Severe adenotonsillar hypertrophy
    c. Severe laryngomalacia
    d. Bacterial tracheitis
    e. Neonatal epignathus
    f. Obstruction from abnormal laryngeal closure caused by arytenoid masses
    g. Mediastinal tumors
    h. Congenital diaphragmatic hernia
    i. Presence of thick and/or particulate meconium in amniotic fluid
    j. Absence of airway protective reflexes
    k. Cardiopulmonary arrest
    l. Massive hemoptysis
5. Conditions in which endotracheal intubation may not be possible and in which alternative techniques may be used include, but are not limited to
    a. Restriction of endotracheal intubation by policy or statute
    b. Difficult or failed intubation in the presence of risk factors associated with difficult tracheal intubations
    c. When endotracheal intubation is not immediately possible
B. Contraindication
    1. Patient's desire not to be resuscitated
C. Hazards and complications
    1. Failure to establish a patent airway
    2. Failure to intubate the trachea
    3. Failure to recognize esophageal intubation
    4. Unrecognized bronchial intubation
    5. Upper airway trauma, laryngeal and esophageal damage
    6. Eye injury
    7. Dental accidents
    8. Vocal cord paralysis
    9. Cervical spine trauma
    10. Aspiration
    11. Pneumonia
    12. Endotracheal tube (ETT) problems (e.g., cuff perforation, cuff herniation, pilot tube-valve incompetence, tube kinking during biting, tube occlusion, and inadvertent extubation)
    13. Inappropriate tube size
    14. Bronchospasm
    15. Laryngospasm
    16. Dysrhythmias
    17. Hypotension and bradycardia caused by vagal stimulation
    18. Hypertension and tachycardia
    19. Bleeding
    20. Mouth ulceration
    21. Tongue ulceration
    22. Specific problems resulting from nasal intubation (e.g., nasal damage including epistaxis, tube kinking in the pharynx, sinusitis, and otitis media)
    23. Tracheal damage (e.g., tracheoesophageal fistula, tracheal innominate fistula, tracheal stenosis, and tracheomalacia)
    24. Laryngeal damage with consequent laryngeal stenosis, laryngeal ulcer, granuloma, polyps, or synechiae
    25. Specific problems resulting from surgical cricothyrotomy or tracheostomy (e.g., stomal stenosis, innominate erosion)
    26. Specific problems resulting from needle cricothyrotomy (e.g., bleeding at the insertion site with hematoma formation, subcutaneous and mediastinal emphysema, and esophageal perforation)

II. **General Classification of Artificial Airways**
   A. Oropharyngeal airway (Figure 38-1)
      1. Used to relieve upper airway obstruction by maintaining the base of the tongue off the posterior wall of the oral pharynx
      2. Used to prevent inadvertent laceration of the tongue in the incoherent or seizuring patient
      3. May be used as a bite block with oral ETTs
      4. To insert the oropharyngeal airway, turn the airway 180 degrees from its normal position, insert it into the patient's mouth, and when it is at the back of the tongue rotate it 180 degrees to its normal position so that the tip is behind the tongue and facing the larynx. A tongue depressor may be used to facilitate insertion of the airway.
      5. Poorly tolerated in alert patient because of stimulation of gag reflex
   B. Nasopharyngeal airway
      1. It is used to relieve upper airway obstruction caused by the tongue or soft palate falling against the posterior wall of the pharynx.
      2. To insert the nasal airway lubricate the outside of the nasal airway with water-soluble lubricant, insert it into the nares, and advance gently until the tip is behind the tongue just above the epiglottis.
         a. If resistance is met try the other nares or a smaller size airway.
         b. Laryngospasm may occur if the airway is too long.
      3. Suctioning via this airway is less traumatic than nasal suctioning.
      4. It is better tolerated than an oropharyngeal airway.
      5. It should be alternated every 24 hours between right and left nares to minimize complications.
      6. Sinusitis, otitis media, and nasal necrosis are possible complications of its use.
   C. Laryngeal mask airway (LMA)
      1. The LMA may be used to manage the airway during anesthesia or as an emergency airway when the airway is difficult to intubate.
      2. The LMA is a tube with a small, inflatable mask at the distal end.
      3. The LMA is inserted deep into the oropharynx with the tip of the mask just above the esophageal sphincter. After insertion the cuff of the mask is inflated. The opening in the mask should face the laryngeal opening when inserted properly (Figure 38-2).
      4. Available in sizes 3, 4, and 5 for adults
      5. Advantages of the LMA include
         a. Easy to insert and requires no special equipment
         b. Maintains patent upper airway
         c. Better ventilation delivered than with bag-mask
         d. May use a special intubating LMA to intubate a difficult airway without removing the LMA
         e. No risk of trauma to the larynx and trachea

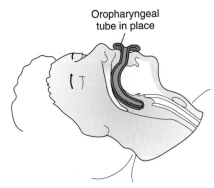

Oropharyngeal tube in place

FIG. 38-1 Oropharyngeal airway in place.

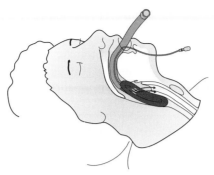

FIG. 38-2 Laryngeal mask airway placed in the upper airway.

6. Disadvantages of the LMA include
   a. Some risk of regurgitation and aspiration
   b. Should be used only short term
   c. Applying high ventilation pressures may cause gastric insufflation.
   d. Because it will stimulate a gag reflex it cannot be used for a conscious or semi-conscious patient.

D. Orotracheal tube
   1. Advantages when compared with nasotracheal tubes
      a. It is easy to insert and is the airway of choice in an emergency.
      b. A larger-diameter tube can be inserted orally than by the nasal route.
         (1) Men: 8 to 9 mm inside diameter (ID)
         (2) Women: 7 to 8 mm ID
      c. Sinusitis and otitis media are not problems.
      d. The angle of curvature is less acute than with nasal tubes; it is easier to suction.
      e. Generally there is less resistance to gas flow, and less work of breathing is imposed.
   2. Problems associated with orotracheal tubes
      a. They are poorly tolerated in conscious and semiconscious patients.
      b. They are difficult to stabilize and may be easily dislodged.
      c. Inadvertent extubation is common.
      d. A bite block may be necessary to prevent biting of tube.
      e. Vagal stimulation may cause bradycardia and hypotension.
      f. Oral hygiene is difficult.
      g. They require a laryngoscopy during insertion.
      h. Patients are unable to mouth words.
      i. Lips may be lacerated.
      j. There is a potential for laryngeal pathology.
      k. The tip of the tube moves when the patient's head position changes.
         (1) Extension of the head moves the tip toward the oropharynx (possible extubation).
         (2) Flexion of the head moves the tip toward the carina (possible right endobronchial intubation).
      l. Oral feeding is difficult.

E. Nasotracheal tube
   1. Advantages over orotracheal tube for long-term intubation
      a. Easier to stabilize
      b. May be better tolerated by some patients
      c. May be inserted blindly (laryngoscopy is unnecessary in most cases)
      d. Oral hygiene is easily accomplished.
      e. The patient is able to mouth words.
      f. Attachment of equipment is easier and safer; there is less torque on the trachea.

2. Problems associated with nasotracheal tubes
   a. The tip of the tube moves when the patient's head position changes.
   b. Pressure necrosis in area of the alae nasi may occur.
   c. Sinus drainage may be obstructed, and acute sinusitis may result.
   d. Eustachian tube drainage may be obstructed, and otitis media may result.
   e. The incidence of vocal cord damage after 3 to 7 days (also seen with oral ETTs) increases.
   f. Vagal stimulation is possible, but it occurs less frequently than with the oral ETT.
   g. Skilled personnel are necessary for placement.
   h. The nasal passage limits the tube size; a tube at least 0.5 mm ID smaller than the oral route is required.
      (1) Men: 7.5 to 8.5 mm ID
      (2) Women: 6.5 to 7.5 mm ID
   i. The angle of curvature is acute; the resistance to gas flow is increased; there is difficulty in suctioning; and the work of breathing is increased when compared with an orotracheal tube in the same patient.
   j. There is a potential for laryngeal pathology.

F. Tracheostomy tube
   1. The size, length, and shape of a tracheostomy tube vary depending on the manufacturer and style of the tube.
   2. Tracheostomy tube shapes are curved, angled, or extra long (Figure 38-3).

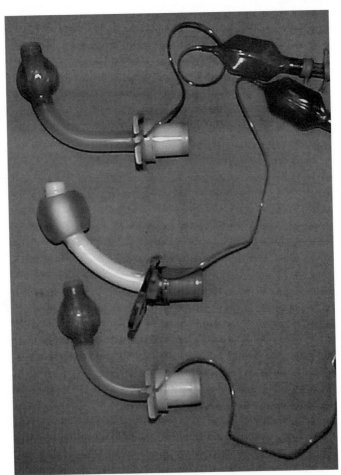

FIG. 38-3 Examples of curved *(top)*, angled *(center)*, and extra-long *(bottom)* tracheostomy tubes.

3. Careful consideration of the anatomy of each patient when choosing the brand and size of a tracheostomy tube may aid in preventing future complications.
4. Most tracheostomy tubes are sized according to ID in millimeters.
5. Advantages over ETTs
   a. There are no complications with the upper airway or glottis.
   b. It is easier to suction.
   c. It is easier to stabilize.
   d. The tracheostomy tube is the best tolerated of all airways.
   e. The patient is able to mouth words, and talking or fenestrated tubes are available.
   f. A speaking valve may be applied to either a fenestrated or a standard tracheostomy tube with the cuff deflated and the inner cannula removed (if present) so the patient can speak.
   g. The patient has the ability to swallow.
   h. With a mature stoma reinsertion is easy.
6. Problems associated with tracheostomy tubes
   a. Surgery is required.
   b. There may be immediate complications.
      (1) Bleeding
      (2) Pneumothorax or pneumomediastinum
      (3) Air embolism
      (4) Subcutaneous emphysema
   c. There may be late complications.
      (1) Infection of surgical wound
      (2) False passage into subcutaneous tissue
      (3) Hemorrhage may occur.
      (4) Granulomas may form.
      (5) Tracheal malacia or stenosis may occur.
      (6) Tracheal-esophageal or tracheal-innominate artery fistulas are less common occurrences but are more serious.
7. Frequent and routine changing of tracheostomy tubes is unnecessary if the airway is functioning properly and is properly humidified.
8. If a stomal infection develops frequent tracheostomy care using aseptic technique and changing of soiled dressings is recommended. Changing the tracheostomy tube may also be necessary.

G. Percutaneous dilational tracheostomy (PDT) tubes are inserted by a relatively new procedure performed at the bedside.
   1. A small incision is made in the neck and trachea, and the opening is dilated with special dilators until the desired size tube fits into the incision.
   2. Advantages when performed properly as compared with surgical tracheostomy are
      a. No operating room required
      b. No need to move high-risk patients
      c. General anesthesia not required
      d. Decreased incidence of pneumothorax, bleeding, and stenosis
      e. Stoma closes quickly after decannulation with less scar tissue formed
   3. Disadvantages are
      a. If inadvertent decannulation occurs before maturation of tracheostomy tract (2 weeks), reinsertion may lead to complications such as bleeding and tracheal trauma. Oral intubation is recommended in this case.
      b. Should not be performed on patients who are morbidly obese, have burns to the neck, have bleeding disorders, have anatomic abnormalities of the trachea or cervical region, or had a previous tracheostomy

H. Uncuffed tracheostomy tubes
   1. Routinely used for infants and small children
   2. In adults primarily used for patients who require frequent suctioning but do not require mechanical ventilation

3. Should not be used for patients who are unable to protect their airways and prevent aspiration.

I. Fenestrated tracheostomy tube (Figure 38-4)
   1. Fenestration(s) may be located in the outer cannula only or in both cannulas, depending on the brand of tube.
   2. The inner cannula is similar in design to the inner cannula of a nonfenestrated tracheostomy tube.
   3. Proper procedure when capping the tube to allow a patient to speak includes
      a. Suctioning the trachea and oropharynx
      b. Removal of inner cannula
      c. Deflation of cuff while positive pressure is applied to direct any pooled secretions above the cuff up and out of the airway into the oropharynx
      d. Suction the oropharynx again.
      e. Cap the outer cannula with the cap or a speaking valve such as the Passy-Muir valve (PMV) (Figure 38-5).
      f. Assess patient for adequate flow through upper airway with no stridor present.
   4. The patient must ventilate via the upper airway through the fenestration(s) in the cannula of the tracheostomy tube and around the tube.
   5. Problems associated with the fenestrated tube include
      a. Possible formation of granular tissue at site of fenestration when fenestration(s) is improperly positioned
      b. Increased resistance to gas flow and work of breathing
   6. Commercial fenestrated tubes are available from several manufacturers; however, these do not always fit properly.
   7. Patients may require the fitting of a customized tube.

J. Talking tracheostomy tube (Figure 38-6)
   1. Is designed to allow the patient to verbalize when the cuff is inflated
   2. It functions by directing secondary gas flow through ports in the tube above the patient's cuff, allowing gas to move past the vocal cords while maintaining ventilation via the airway.
   3. The ID of the airway is smaller than the standard tube of the same size.

K. Tracheal button (Figure 38-7)
   1. Used to maintain patency of the tracheal stoma
   2. The inner lip of the button lies on the internal anterior tracheal wall, and the outer lip lies on the tissue of the neck.

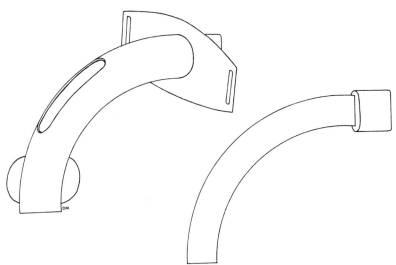

FIG. 38-4 Fenestrated tracheostomy tube. Inner and outer cannulas are depicted.

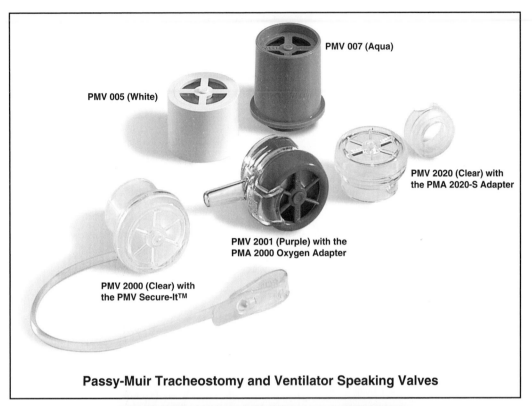

Passy-Muir Tracheostomy and Ventilator Speaking Valves

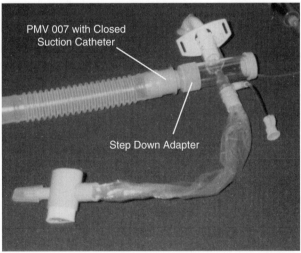

FIG. 38-5 *Top*, Passy-Muir speaking valves. *Bottom*, Passy-Muir valve in-line during mechanical ventilation.

    3. The tracheal button allows the patient to ventilate completely from the upper airway without tracheal obstruction.

    4. In an emergency the patient may be suctioned via the tracheal button.

  L. Cricothyroidotomy

    1. Incision through the cricothyroid membrane located between the cricoid and thyroid cartilages

    2. Used as an emergency airway if upper airway obstruction prevents orotracheal intubation and ventilation

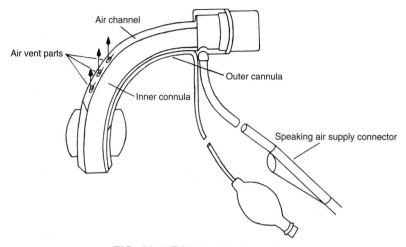

FIG. 38-6 Talking tracheostomy tube.

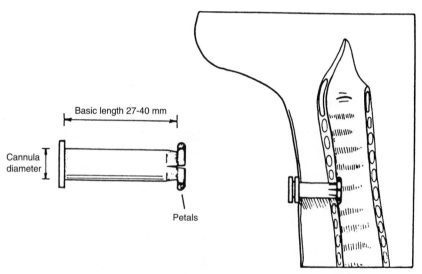

FIG. 38-7 Dimensions and actual positioning of an Olympic tracheostomy button.

   3. Advantages
       a. Rapid establishment of airway
       b. Easily accomplished during cardiopulmonary resuscitation
   4. Possible complications include
       a. Perforation of thyroid gland
       b. Perforation of esophagus
       c. Mediastinal or subcutaneous emphysema
       d. Pneumothorax
       e. Hemorrhage
       f. Vocal cord damage if performed too high
       g. Increased airway resistance because of the small ID of the tube

III. **Extubation or Decannulation**
   A. Indications for extubation (Modified from AARC Clinical Practice Guideline: Removal of the Endotracheal Tube, 1999)

1. When the airway control afforded by the ETT is deemed to be no longer necessary for the continued care of the patient, the tube should be removed.
2. The patient generally should be capable of maintaining a patent airway and adequate spontaneous ventilation and should not require high levels of positive airway pressure to maintain normal arterial blood oxygenation.
3. Patients in whom further medical care is considered (and explicitly declared) futile may have the ETT removed despite continuing indications for the artificial airway.
4. Acute artificial airway obstruction mandates immediate ETT removal if the obstruction cannot be cleared rapidly. Reintubation or other appropriate techniques to reestablish the airway must be used to maintain effective gas exchange (i.e., surgical airway management).

B. Contraindications
  1. There are no absolute contraindications to extubation.
    a. However, some patients may require reintubation, positive pressure ventilation, continuous positive airway pressure, noninvasive ventilation, or high inspired oxygen fraction to maintain acceptable gas exchange after extubation.
    b. Airway protective reflexes are usually depressed immediately and for some time after extubation; therefore measures to prevent aspiration should be considered.

C. Hazards and complications
  1. Hypoxemia after extubation may result from, but is not limited to
    a. Failure to deliver adequate inspired oxygen fraction through the natural upper airway
    b. Acute upper airway obstruction
    c. Development of postobstruction pulmonary edema
    d. Bronchospasm
    e. Development of atelectasis or lung collapse
    f. Pulmonary aspiration
    g. Hypoventilation
  2. Hypercapnia after extubation may be caused by, but is not limited to
    a. Upper airway obstruction resulting from edema of the trachea, vocal cords, or larynx
    b. Respiratory muscle weakness
    c. Excessive work of breathing
    d. Bronchospasm
  3. Death may occur when medical futility is the reason for removing the ETT.

D. Procedure for extubation includes
  1. Suctioning the trachea and oropharynx
  2. Deflation of cuff while positive pressure is applied to direct any pooled secretions above the cuff up and out of the airway into the oropharynx
  3. Suctioning the oropharynx again
  4. Listening for an audible leak around the tube with the cuff fully deflated
  5. Removing the tube, preferably as the patient takes a deep breath
  6. Administer supplemental oxygen as needed.

E. Decannulation is the removal of a tracheostomy tube.
  1. Indications
    a. The patient generally should be capable of maintaining a patent airway and adequate spontaneous ventilation and should not require high levels of positive airway pressure to maintain normal arterial blood oxygenation.
  2. Before decannulation the patient's ability to swallow and protect the airway should be assessed.
  3. A simple swallowing test may be done at the bedside using food coloring.
    a. With the tracheostomy tube cuff deflated, have the patient swallow a small amount of ice chips or water colored with food coloring.
    b. Tracheal suction the patient, and inspect the secretions for any coloration.
    c. The test is useful if positive (coloration is present) because it demonstrates that the patient is unable to protect the airway and should not be decannulated. However, false-negative results can occur.

    4. Procedure for decannulation is the same as for extubation.

    5. A sterile, occlusive dressing should be applied over the stoma.

IV. **Laryngotracheal Complications of Endotracheal Intubation**
    A. Sore throat and/or hoarse voice
    B. Glottic or subglottic edema as evidenced by stridor
    C. Tracheal injury: Ulceration, granuloma, malacia, or stenosis
    D. Vocal cord ulceration, granuloma, or polyp formation
    E. Vocal cord paralysis (less common)

V. **Postextubation Therapy**
    A. Administration of racemic epinephrine or dexamethasone may reverse or prevent glottic or subglottic edema.
    B. Until the edema decreases administration of Heliox may decrease the work of breathing and improve oxygenation when there is partial airway obstruction caused by glottic or subglottic edema.
    C. If symptoms of glottic or subglottic edema persist, reintubation may be necessary.

VI. **Airway Cuffs**
    A. Uses
        1. Mechanically ventilate patient
        2. Protect airway from aspiration
    B. Tracheal wall pressures
        1. Intraarterial pressure, approximately 30 mm Hg (42 cm H_2O)
        2. Venous pressures, approximately 18 mm Hg (24 cm H_2O)
    C. Lateral tracheal wall pressures
        1. Greater than 30 mm Hg causes cessation of arterial blood flow.
        2. Greater than 18 mm Hg obstructs venous flow.
        3. Greater than 5 mm Hg inhibits lymphatic flow.
    D. Cuff pressures ideally should be maintained at 20 to 25 mm Hg to maintain tracheal capillary blood flow and prevent aspiration.
    E. Effects of high lateral tracheal wall pressures and sequence of tracheal changes
        1. Mucosal ischemia
        2. Mucosal inflammation, hemorrhage, and/or ulceration
            a. Tracheal granuloma formation
        3. Exposure of cartilage
        4. Tracheal ring destruction
            a. Tracheomalacia
            b. Tracheal stenosis
                (1) At cuff site
                (2) At tip of airway
                (3) At stoma in tracheostomies
    F. Additional factors predisposing to tracheal damage
        1. High peak airway pressure or positive end-expiratory pressure (PEEP) requiring higher cuff pressures
        2. Too small or too large a cuff in relation to tracheal size
        3. Noncircular cross-sectional tracheal shape
        4. Cuff material
            a. Silicon: Requires least inflation pressure
            b. Polyvinyl chloride
            c. Latex: Requires greatest inflation pressure
    G. High-volume, low-pressure vs. low-volume, high-pressure cuffs (Figure 38-8)
        1. High-volume, low-pressure cuffs are the cuffs of choice for long-term airway maintenance.
            a. Advantages

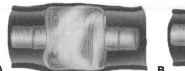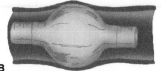

FIG. 38-8 Comparison of shapes of high-volume, low-pressure cuff **(A)** and low-volume, high-pressure cuff **(B)**.

        (1)   Intracuff pressures are lower than with high-pressure cuffs.

        (2)   Lateral tracheal wall pressure is dissipated over a large surface area.

    b. Disadvantage: May form folds when inflated, allowing aspiration of liquids or entrapment of secretions that cause infection

  2. Most modern cuffs are high-volume, low-pressure cuffs.

H. Special cuffs

  1. Bivona foam cuff (Kamen-Wilkinson cuff)

    a. Made of polyurethane foam with a silicone covering

    b. Inflated by atmospheric pressure

    c. No positive pressure is added to cuff.

    d. Minimum pressures normally are applied to the tracheal wall.

    e. Deflation of the cuff with a syringe before insertion allows reexpansion by atmospheric pressure.

    f. This cuff may not form a complete seal in the trachea of some patients.

  2. Tight-to-shaft (TTS) cuff

    a. A silicone cuff

    b. Facilitates insertion of the tube through a tight stoma

    c. When deflated it collapses tight to the shaft of the tube; therefore it functions like an uncuffed tube, allowing the use of the upper airway for speaking and/or easier swallowing.

    d. May be inflated for short periods to protect the airway from aspiration and/or provide an airway seal for ventilatory support

    e. Available in neonatal, pediatric, and adult sizes

I. Cuff inflation techniques

  1. Minimal leak technique: Cuff volume maintains the seal except at maximum inspiratory pressure.

    a. Insert enough air into the cuff until no leak is present.

    b. While positive pressure is applied to the airway, withdraw air from the cuff until a slight leak develops. The leak should not be so great as to overcome the purpose of the cuff.

    c. Aspiration of pharyngeal secretions may occur.

  2. Minimal occluding volume technique: A minimal volume of gas is required to maintain the airway seal at peak positive pressure during inspiration.

    a. Insert enough air to prevent any leak.

    b. Withdraw gas during inspiration until a leak occurs.

    c. Carefully inflate until the gas leak is stopped at peak inspiratory pressure.

    d. There is less risk of aspiration of pharyngeal secretions than with the minimal leak technique.

  3. Monitoring of cuff pressures and volumes

    a. A pressure monitor is used to evaluate actual intracuff pressure (Figure 38-9).

    b. It is important to monitor intracuff pressures routinely and especially if high peak airway pressures are necessary or if high levels of PEEP are used.

    c. If the minimal occluding volume technique is used, cuff pressures should be monitored frequently. A 1- to 2-ml increase in cuff volume can cause a precipitous increase in intracuff pressure.

    d. Actual cuff pressures should be monitored and recorded routinely with ventilator checks or oxygen therapy equipment checks.

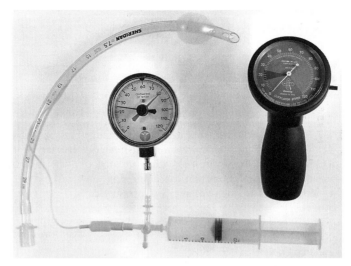

FIG. 38-9 Equipment for measuring cuff pressure.

    e. Cuff volumes should be monitored less frequently. Frequent deflation and inflation of a cuff increase the likelihood of improper maintenance.
    f. Steadily increasing cuff volume necessary to maintain a specific cuff pressure may indicate
        (1) An overdistended cuff
        (2) Tracheomalacia

VII. Cuff Deflation Technique
    A. Complete suctioning of lower airway
    B. Complete suctioning of upper airway above the cuff
    C. Deflation of cuff while positive pressure is applied to direct any pooled secretions above the cuff up and out of the airway into the oropharynx
    D. Suction oropharynx again.

VIII. Artificial Airway Emergencies
    A. Inadvertent extubation
    B. Airway obstruction
        1. Mucous plug
        2. Granuloma tissue
        3. Herniation of the cuff over the end of the tube
    C. Endobronchial intubation
    D. Kinking of the airway

IX. Management of Acute Obstruction of Artificial Airway
    A. Manipulate tube (check for kinks).
    B. Attempt to suction airway.
    C. Deflate cuff.
    D. If all of these fail and tension pneumothorax is ruled out, remove the tube and ventilate with bag and mask.

X. Artificial Airway Suctioning (Modified from AARC Clinical Practice Guideline: Endotracheal Suctioning of Mechanically Ventilated Adults and Children with Artificial Airways, 1993)
    A. Indications
        1. The need to remove accumulated pulmonary secretions as evidenced by one of the following

      a. Coarse breath sounds or "noisy" breathing
      b. Patient's inability to generate an effective spontaneous cough
      c. Radiograph changes consistent with retained secretions
      d. Changes in monitored flow/pressure graphics
      e. Increased peak inspiratory pressure on volume control ventilation; decreased tidal volume on pressure control ventilation
      f. Visible secretions in the airway
      g. Suspected aspiration of gastric or upper airway secretions
      h. Clinically apparent increased work of breathing
      i. Deterioration of arterial blood gas values
      j. The need to obtain a sputum specimen to rule out or identify pneumonia or other pulmonary infection or for sputum cytology
      k. The need to maintain the patency and integrity of the artificial airway
      l. The need to stimulate a cough in patients unable to cough effectively secondary to changes in mental status or the influence of medication
      m. Presence of pulmonary atelectasis or consolidation, presumed to be associated with secretion retention

B. Contraindications
    1. No absolute contraindication

C. Hazards and complications
    1. Hypoxia/hypoxemia
    2. Tissue trauma to the tracheal and/or bronchial mucosa
    3. Cardiac arrest
    4. Respiratory arrest
    5. Cardiac dysrhythmias
    6. Pulmonary atelectasis
    7. Bronchoconstriction/bronchospasm
    8. Infection (patient and/or caregiver)
    9. Pulmonary hemorrhage/bleeding
   10. Elevated intracranial pressure
   11. Interruption of mechanical ventilation
   12. Hypertension
   13. Hypotension

D. Ways to minimize risk of complications
    1. Hyperoxygenation, when indicated, should minimize the risk of hypoxemia, arrhythmias, and cardiac arrest.
    2. Use of appropriate suction pressure should minimize the risk of tracheal or bronchial trauma and pulmonary hemorrhage.

E. Requisites of suction catheters
    1. They should be constructed of a material that will cause minimal irritation and trauma to tracheal mucosa.
    2. Minimal frictional resistance when passing through the artificial airway is essential.
    3. They should be sufficiently long to easily pass the tip of the artificial airway.
    4. They should have smooth, molded ends and side holes to prevent mucosal trauma.
    5. The catheter outer diameter (OD) should be less than one half to two thirds the ID of the artificial airway.
      a. Catheter size is the OD of the catheter in French (Fr) units, which refers to the circumference of the tube.
      b. To convert French size to size in millimeters (approximation):

$$mm = \frac{Fr - 2}{4} \tag{1}$$

      c. To convert the size in millimeters to French size (approximation):

$$Fr = (4)(mm) + 2 \tag{2}$$

   6. To minimize airway trauma use the following suction pressures.
      a. Infants: 75 to 100 mm Hg
      b. Children: 100 to 125 mm Hg
      c. Adults: 125 to 150 mm Hg
F. Suctioning of an artificial airway with open technique
   1. Use completely sterile technique to prevent infection.
   2. Assess SpO_2 and vital signs of the patient for the need of hyperoxygenation.
   3. Hyperoxygenate the patient, if indicated, by increasing the F_IO_2 delivered to the patient. Hyperinflation/hyperventilation with manual ventilator is usually not necessary and may be harmful to some patients.
   4. Insert the catheter without applying suction until an obstruction is met, and then slightly retract the catheter.
   5. Apply suction only during removal of the catheter.
   6. The suction catheter should remain in the airway no longer than 10 to 15 seconds to minimize risk of hypoxemia and/or airway trauma.
   7. Oxygenate and ventilate the patient as indicated.
   8. In the event of catheter adherence to the wall of the airway, release suction, withdraw the catheter, and reapply suction.
G. Suctioning an artificial airway with closed suctioning system (Figure 38-10)
   1. This system is permanently affixed to the airway-ventilator tubing system.
   2. During suctioning mechanical ventilation is still maintained.
   3. The suction catheter is located in the plastic sleeve and is advanced into the airway at the time of suctioning.
   4. This system is useful if
      a. Disconnection from the ventilator, even for short periods, results in desaturation, bradycardia, and hypotension.
      b. Patients require isolation because of highly communicable diseases.
   5. This system generally reduces the risk of contamination of practitioners during suctioning.
   6. The F_IO_2 with these systems generally does not require adjustment during suctioning. However, each patient's tolerance of the system should be evaluated with a pulse oximeter before the decision to maintain the F_IO_2 level during suctioning is made.

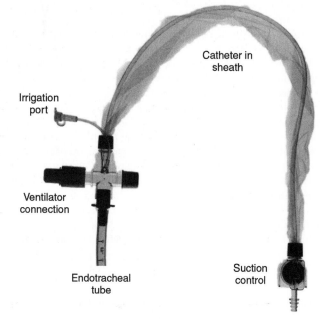

FIG. 38-10 Closed suction catheter.

H. Instillation of normal saline
   1. The instillation of normal saline into the airway at the time of suctioning is normally unnecessary if
      a. Proper systemic hydration is maintained.
      b. Proper bronchial hygiene is provided.
      c. Proper humidification of inspired gases is ensured.
      d. However, if these criteria are not maintained, the instillation of 3 to 5 ml of sterile, normal saline solution before suctioning may help to mobilize thick, retained, difficult-to-suction secretions.

BIBLIOGRAPHY

American Association for Respiratory Care: Clinical Practice Guideline. Endotracheal suctioning of mechanically ventilated adults and children with artificial airways. *Respir Care* 38:500, 1993.

American Association for Respiratory Care: Clinical Practice Guideline. Management of airway emergencies. *Respir Care* 40:749, 1995.

American Association for Respiratory Care: Clinical Practice Guideline. Removal of the endotracheal tube. *Respir Care* 44:85, 1999.

Asai T, Morris S: The laryngeal mask airway; its features, effects, and roles. *Can J Anaesth* 41:930-960, 1994.

Burton GG, Hodgkin JE, Ward J: *Respiratory Care: A Guide to Clinical Practice*, ed 4. Philadelphia, JB Lippincott, 1997.

Freeman BD, Isabella K, Lin N, et al: A metaanalysis of prospective trials comparing percutaneous and surgical tracheostomy in critically ill patients. *Chest* 118:1412-1418, 2000.

Hess DR: Managing the artificial airway, *Respir Care* 44:759-772, 1999.

Hess DR, MacIntyre NR, Mishoe SC, Galvin WF, Adams AB, Saposnick AB: *Respiratory Care Principles and Practice*. Philadelphia, WB Saunders, 2002.

Johnson KL, Kearney PA, Johnson SB, et al: Closed versus open endotracheal suctioning: costs and physiologic consequences. *Crit Care Med* 22:658, 1994.

Pierson DJ, Kacmarek RM: *Foundation of Respiratory Care*. New York, Churchill Livingstone, 1993.

Shapiro BA, Harrison RA, Kacmarek RM, et al: *Clinical Application of Respiratory Care*, ed 4. Chicago, Year Book Medical Publishers, 1990.

Stauffer JL: Complications of endotracheal intubation and tracheostomy. *Respir Care* 44:828, 1999.

Wilkins RL: Suctioning and airway care. In Kacmarek RM, Stoller JK (eds): *Current Respiratory Care*. Toronto, BC Decker, 1988.

Wilkins RL, Stoller JK, Scanlon CL: *Egan's Fundamentals of Respiratory Therapy*, ed 8. St. Louis, Mosby, 2003.

Wilson DJ: Airway appliances and management. In Kacmarek RM, Stoller JK (eds): *Current Respiratory Care*. Toronto, BC Decker, 1988.

Chapter 39

Modes of Mechanical Ventilation

I. **Pressure and Volume Targeting (Table 39-1)**
   A. Regardless of terminology used to identify a mode of ventilation, all modes operate by targeting pressure, volume, or both of these variables.
   B. With volume targeting, a specific volume of gas is delivered each tidal volume (V_T). As a result
      1. V_T is consistent.
      2. Peak flow or inspiratory time must be selected.
      3. A gas flow pattern must be set.
         a. Square wave and decelerating wave flow patterns are available on current generation ventilators (Figure 39-1).
         b. With square wave flow, the set flow is constant throughout inspiration.
         c. With a decelerating wave flow pattern, the flow decreases from the maximum set flow to a minimal end-inspiratory flow.
         d. The minimal flow in decelerating wave is variable from ventilator to ventilator and in some ventilators can be adjusted.
         e. The flow waveform affects peak flow and the inspiratory time required to deliver a given V_T.
         f. If the peak flow is constant, inspiratory time must be longer with a decelerating flow pattern than with a square wave flow pattern.
         g. If inspiratory time is constant, peak inspiratory flow must be higher with a decelerating flow pattern than with a square wave flow pattern.
         h. When changing flow pattern care must be exercised to ensure that proper peak flow or inspiratory time is set.
      4. Pressure is the resultant variable, and it can vary considerably from breath to breath.
   C. With pressure targeting, maximum preset peak airway pressure is set, and this limits peak alveolar pressure to the set level. As a result
      1. Maximum airway and alveolar pressures are targeted.
      2. V_T can vary from breath to breath.
      3. Gas flow delivery is variable (Figure 39-2).
         a. A high initial flow is delivered. The rate of initial flow delivery is based on set peak pressure, the patient's lung mechanics, and patient demand.
         b. Peak flow must rapidly decrease as the target pressure is reached to prevent pressure from exceeding the target level.
            (1) The higher the set pressure, the higher the initial flow.

689

	Pressure	Volume
Peak airway pressure	Constant	Variable
Peak alveolar pressure	Constant	Variable
Tidal volume	Variable	Constant
Peak flow	Variable	Constant
Flow pattern	Decelerating	Preset
Inspiratory time	Preset	Preset
Minimum rate	Preset	Preset

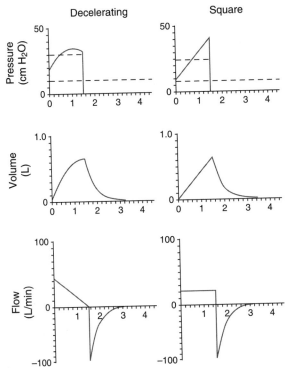

FIG. 39-1 Volume, pressure, and flow waveforms during decelerating and constant flow wave patterns in volume-targeted ventilation. Note peak flow is constant; as a result inspiratory time is longer with a decelerating flow. Peak pressure also is less because the impact of airway resistance is reduced by the end of the breath because flow rate is minimal.

    (2) The higher the patient demand, the greater the initial flow.
    (3) The higher the resistance and the lower the compliance, the lower the initial flow.
  c. To prevent pressure from exceeding the target, flow may decrease to zero before the end of inspiration.
  d. Inspiratory time may be set or the breath may end when inspiratory flow decreases to a predetermined level.
  D. With pressure and volume combined targeting modes, the ventilator attempts to ensure a preselected maximum pressure is never exceeded and a preselected VT is delivered.
    1. Gas delivery is usually in a pressure-targeting format but may change to a volume format during the breath in some modes.

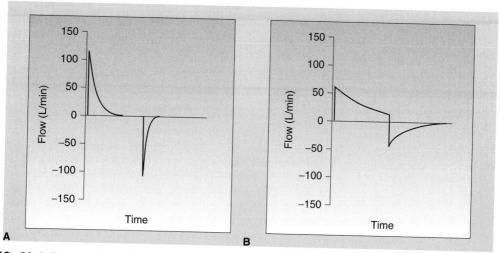

FIG. 39-2 Flow waveforms during pressure-assist/control ventilation. **A,** High resistance or low compliance; the flow has returned to zero before the end of the breath. In this setting the end-inspiratory airway pressure is equal to the plateau pressure. **B,** Low resistance or high compliance: in this setting end-inspiratory flow is still high; as a result end-inspiratory pressure does not equal plateau pressure.

  2. A high initial flow is delivered that rapidly decelerates over time.
  3. System pressure is maintained below the maximum selected but may change on a breath-to-breath basis to ensure that the V_T selected is delivered.
E. In all of these different gas delivery formats
  1. A preset minimum rate can be set.
  2. Patients are able to trigger each breath.
  3. Positive end-expiratory pressure (PEEP) can be added.
F. Pressure- and volume-targeted breaths respond differently to changes in compliance and resistance of the respiratory system (Table 39-2).
  1. Any factor that increases resistance or decreases compliance during volume ventilation causes the *peak airway* and *peak alveolar* pressure to increase.
  2. Any factor that decreases resistance or increases compliance during volume ventilation causes the *peak airway* and *peak alveolar* pressure to decrease.
  3. Any factor that increases resistance or decreases compliance during pressure ventilation causes V_T to decrease.

TABLE 39-2

Effect of Changing Compliance and Resistance During Pressure and Volume Ventilation

	Pressure	Volume
Decreased compliance	↓ Volume	↑ Pressure
Increased compliance	↑ Volume	↓ Pressure
Increased auto-PEEP	↓ Volume	↑ Pressure
Decreased auto-PEEP	↑ Volume	↓ Pressure
Pneumothorax	↓ Volume	↑ Pressure
Bronchospasm	↓ Volume	↑ Pressure
Mucosal edema	↓ Volume	↑ Pressure
Secretions	↓ Volume	↑ Pressure
Pleural effusion	↓ Volume	↑ Pressure
Increased patient effort	↑ Volume	↓ Pressure
Decreased patient effort	↓ Volume	↑ Pressure

PEEP, Positive end-expiratory pressure.

4. Any factor that decreases resistance or increases compliance during pressure ventilation causes V_T to increase.

G. During pressure and volume ventilation, effective static compliance can be measured if a static condition is achieved (Figure 39-3).

1. With volume ventilation an end-inspiratory pause is set, allowing all airflow to cease. Effective total respiratory system compliance is calculated by:

$$\text{Compliance} = \frac{\text{Plateau Pressure} - \text{Total PEEP}}{\text{Actual } V_T \text{ Delivered}} \quad (1)$$

a. Volume compressed in the ventilator circuit must be subtracted from the ventilator set volume to identify the actual V_T entering the airway. Some ventilators automatically correct for compressed volume in the ventilator circuit. Normally approximately 1 to 2 ml/cm H_2O plateau pressure minus total PEEP is compressed in the ventilator circuit.

b. Total PEEP (applied plus any additional auto-PEEP) is subtracted from the plateau pressure to ensure that only the actual pressure needed to maintain the V_T in the lung is identified.

2. During pressure ventilation, compliance can be calculated if the flow rate returns to zero 200 to 300 msec before the end of the breath (see Figure 39-2, *A*). If this occurs the set pressure level is equal to the plateau pressure, which is equal to the average peak alveolar pressure.

$$\text{Compliance} = \frac{\text{Set Peak Pressure}}{\text{Actual } V_T \text{ Delivered}} \quad (2)$$

H. Estimation of airway resistance can be determined during volume ventilation but not pressure ventilation (see Figure 39-3).

1. To calculate airway resistance during mechanical ventilation, a constant gas flow rate must be provided.

2. Constant flow (square wave) is only possible during volume ventilation.

3. When flow is constant the pressure difference between the peak pressure and the plateau pressure is the pressure required to overcome airway resistance.

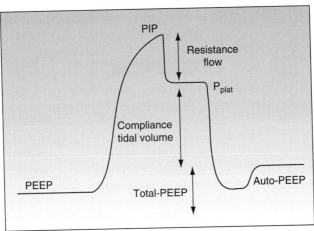

FIG. 39-3 Airway pressure waveform during volume-control ventilation with a constant flow. An end-inspiratory and end-expiratory breath-hold is applied to measure the plateau pressure (P_{plat}) and auto-positive end-expiratory pressure (PEEP). The difference between the peak inspiratory pressure (PIP) and P_{plat} is the pressure needed to overcome airway resistance. The higher the flow, the greater the difference. P_{plat} minus total PEEP is the pressure to overcome compliance. The greater the tidal volume, the greater this pressure difference.

$$\text{Airway Resistance} = \frac{\text{Peak} - \text{Plateau Pressure}}{\text{Peak Flow}} \tag{3}$$

II. **Triggering the Breath**
   A. All modes of ventilation on current generation ventilators allow the patient to trigger (activate) gas delivery.
   B. Controlled ventilation, the absence of patient active interaction with the ventilator, can only truly be established by sedating the patient to apnea.
   C. The sensitivity control on ventilators allows the clinician to determine the amount of patient effort required to trigger a ventilator-assisted breath.
   D. Even at sensitivity settings requiring large inspiratory efforts, patients with strong ventilatory demands can trigger a breath.
   E. Ventilator triggering can occur by two mechanisms: change in pressure or flow (Figure 39-4).
      1. Traditionally all ventilator modes were pressure triggered.
      2. To activate a breath the patient had to decompress the ventilator circuit a sufficient level to overcome the sensitivity setting.
      3. The major problem with pressure triggering is the location of pressure sensing.
         a. If pressure is sensed at the ventilator, pressure at the wye of the ventilator circuit must be less than that measured at the ventilator.
         b. If the sensitivity is set at -2 cm H_2O the patient may have to establish a -4 cm H_2O pressure at the wye.
         c. If pressure is measured at the circuit wye this concern is eliminated.

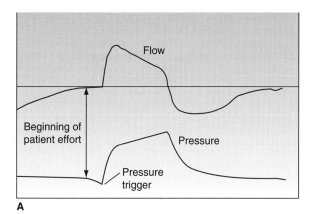

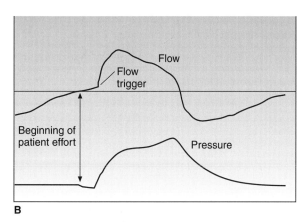

FIG. 39-4 Effect of trigger type on flow and airway pressure. **A,** A pressure-triggered breath. **B,** A flow-triggered breath.

    d.   With pressure triggering pressure changes before flow is provided.

    e.   During flow triggering either the patient must divert a set flow from a low continuous flow or generate a specific flow through a pneumotachograph placed at the airway.

    f.   As a result of the design of flow-triggered systems they tend to minimize effort to a greater extent than pressure triggering.

    g.   With flow triggering flow is established before the ventilator generates airway pressure.

    h.   Less effect is required to trigger a ventilator set at 2 L/min flow triggering versus −2 cm H_2O pressure triggering.

    i.   Regardless of the trigger available on a given ventilator, trigger sensitivity should always be set as sensitive as possible to avoid auto-triggering and to minimize patient effort.

    j.   With pressure triggering, water in the ventilator circuit tends to increase auto-triggering.

    k.   With flow triggering, leaks in the system tend to increase auto-triggering. This also occurs in pressure triggering when PEEP is set.

    l.   All factors being equal, flow triggering seems to be the most efficient method of triggering a breath.

III. Assist/Control Mode

    A. This mode of ventilation can be provided in pressure and volume targeting (Figures 39-5 and 39-6).

    B. The basic operation is that every breath is a positive-pressure breath triggered by the patient.

    C. If the patient does not trigger the breath, the ventilator automatically delivers a back-up breath (controlled breath).

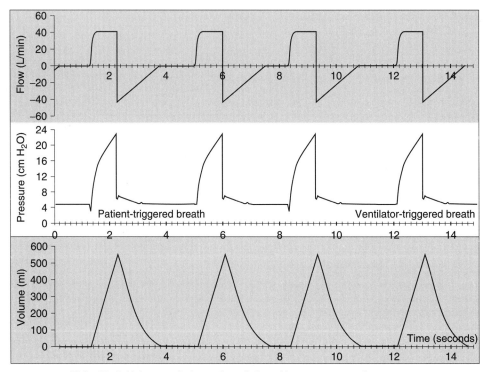

FIG. 39-5 Volume-assist/control ventilation with a square wave flow pattern.

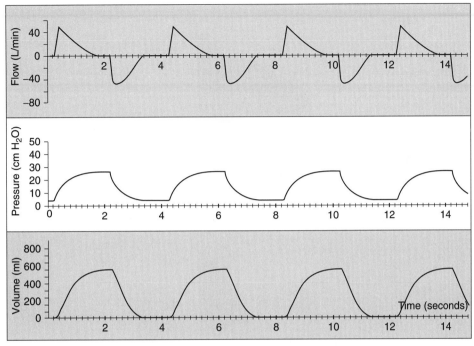

FIG. 39-6 Pressure-assist/control ventilation.

D. Volume-targeted assist/control (AC) mode is the most common mode of ventilation used worldwide.

E. During volume AC the following variables must be set.

1. VT

2. Flow waveform

3. Peak flow

   a. Setting of peak flow along with VT and flow waveform determines the inspiratory time.

   b. Peak flow in assisted ventilation is set to meet patient's inspiratory flow demand (Figure 39-7). If peak flow is set too low, patients may be required to perform a large amount of the work of breathing.

   c. Figure 39-7 depicts the airway pressure waveforms during controlled and assisted ventilation in a patient with all ventilator settings constant.

   d. During controlled ventilation the area under the airway pressure curve is equal to the total work required to ventilate a patient.

   e. During assisted ventilation the same amount of work must be done, but the patient now shares the work.

   f. As a result the area in Figure 39-7 (bottom) identified as subject work can be high if the peak flow is inadequate.

   g. Figure 39-8 indicates an airway pressure waveform in which the peak flow is grossly inadequate, indicating excessive patient work.

   h. The more the actual airway pressure waveform deviates from the expected airway pressure waveform (see Figure 39-8), the greater the work performed by the patient.

   i. Peak flow frequently needs to be set ≥80 L/min to meet patient peak inspiratory demands and minimize the work of breathing.

4. Inspiratory time (set on some ventilators)

   a. During assisted ventilation patients usually require an inspiratory time ≤1.0 seconds.

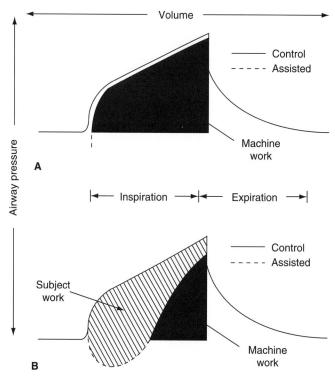

FIG. 39-7 *Top*, Depiction of an actual pressure-time curve *(dotted line)* superimposed on the ideal curve. *Bottom*, Note the scooped-out actual pressure waveform when the patient's demand increases. The hatched area reflects the work performed by the patient during assisted volume-targeted ventilation.

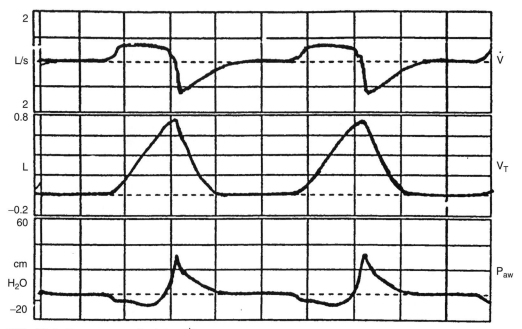

FIG. 39-8 Airway pressure (P_{aw}), flow ($\dot{V}$), and volume (V_T) waveforms during volume-targeted ventilation. The P_{aw} grossly illustrates inadequate peak inspiratory flow. This patient's work of breathing is excessive despite ventilatory assistance. The peak flow needs to be markedly increased.

  b. It is unusual for spontaneously breathing patients to desire an inspiratory time >1.0 second.

  c. During controlled ventilation inspiratory time can be lengthened (see inverse ratio ventilation).

  5. Rate or expiratory time

  6. In some ventilators the inspiratory to expiratory (I:E) ratio is set.

   a. The I:E ratio is the relationship between inspiratory and expiratory time.

   b. During normal breathing I:E ratios are approximately 1:2.

   c. In patients with obstructive lung disease I:E ratios are smaller, 1:3 to 1:6 or more.

   d. Most do not set I:E ratio, preferring to set inspiratory time directly or indirectly by setting peak flow and rate.

  7. PEEP

  8. Sensitivity

  9. F_1O_2

 F. Pressure AC essentially functions the same as volume AC except by pressure targeting.

 G. During pressure AC the following variables must be set.

  1. Pressure level

  2. Inspiratory time

  3. Rate

  4. With some units I:E can be set.

  5. PEEP

  6. Sensitivity

  7. F_1O_2

  8. Rise time (see later section)

   a. Inspiratory time is usually ≤1.0 seconds in patients actively triggering the ventilator.

   b. It is unusual for patients to desire an inspiratory time >1.0 second when spontaneously breathing.

   c. During control ventilation inspiratory time can be lengthened; however, it is questionable whether this is beneficial (see inverse ratio ventilation).

IV. Synchronized Intermittent Mandatory Ventilation

 A. Figure 39-9 illustrates a typical volume-targeted square wave flow synchronized intermittent mandatory ventilation (SIMV) breath.

 B. With this mode of ventilation a mixture of spontaneous and mechanically assisted breaths is provided.

 C. SIMV can be provided using volume- or pressure-targeted ventilation for the mandatory breaths.

 D. During the spontaneous breaths pressure support (PS; see Section VI, Pressure Support) can be added (Figure 39-10).

 E. In SIMV a mandatory rate is set and provided in an AC format. However, only the set number of mandatory breaths is provided.

 F. In between these breaths spontaneous effort by the patient does not trigger a mandatory breath.

 G. However, as noted previously PS may be added to provide assistance between the mandatory breaths.

 H. If a mandatory rate of 10 is set every 6 seconds, the ventilator will apply a mandatory breath. The breath is an assisted (patient-triggered) breath if the patient makes an inspiratory effort within the 1- to 2-second window of time set aside to allow patient triggering.

 I. If the breath is not triggered in the allotted time a controlled breath is delivered.

 J. The goal is to only provide partial ventilatory support, allowing the patient to perform a varying level of breathing effort.

 K. As noted in Figure 39-11 there is a difference in the distribution of ventilation during unassisted breaths and mechanical breaths that favors improved ventilation to perfusion matching during unassisted spontaneous breathing.

 L. Spontaneous breathing also improves venous return and, as a result, cardiac output.

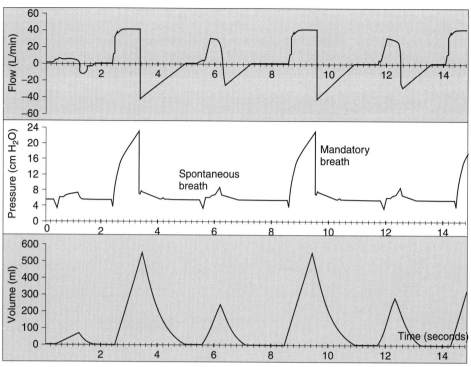

FIG. 39-9 Synchronized intermittent mandatory ventilation (SIMV) provided by volume-targeted square wave flow. Mandatory and spontaneous breaths are illustrated.

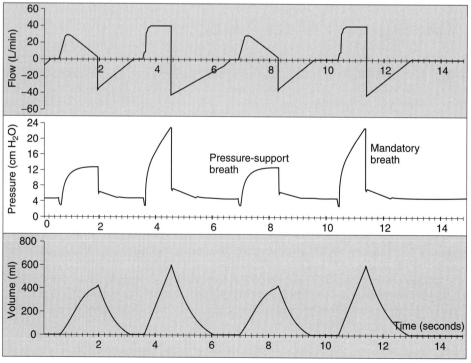

FIG. 39-10 Synchronized intermittent mandatory ventilation using volume-targeted square wave flow mandatory breaths with pressure support applied to the spontaneous breath.

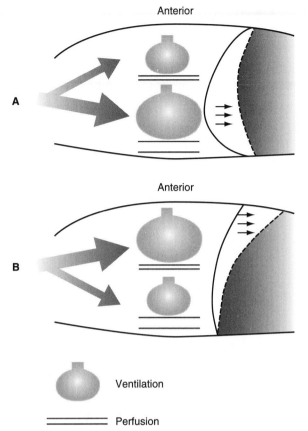

FIG. 39-11 Effect of spontaneous ventilation and positive-pressure ventilation on gas distribution in a supine subject. During spontaneous ventilation **(A)** diaphragmatic action distributes most ventilation to the dependent zones of the lungs, where perfusion is greatest. The result is good matching of ventilation to perfusion. During positive-pressure ventilation **(B)** because the diaphragm is doing little to no contraction, ventilation is primarily distributed to nondependent lung, increasing the level of ventilation to perfusion mismatch.

    M. Many believe patients also are less likely to hyperventilate to alkalosis with SIMV than AC.
    N. Increased work of breathing is of major concern with SIMV at moderate and lower mandatory rates.
        1. Figure 39-12 depicts the impact of decreasing the mandatory rate on patient work of breathing.
        2. As noted when the mandatory rate is decreased, work of breathing increases for the spontaneous and mandatory breaths.
        3. The work of breathing during the mandatory breath can be high at moderate and lower mandatory rates.
        4. Figure 39-13 illustrates the change in esophageal pressure during moderate rate SIMV, demonstrating equal pressure change with spontaneous and mandatory breaths and thus equal patient effort.
        5. When the SIMV mandatory rate is <70% to 80% of the total respiratory rate, concern about patient effect should be raised.
    O. In the United States SIMV is as popular a mode as AC. However, the rest of the world rarely uses the SIMV mode in adults.
    P. During SIMV the following variables should be set.
        1. V_T (volume targeted only)

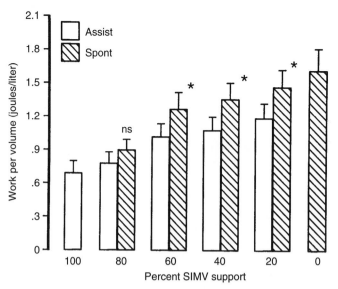

FIG. 39-12 Inspiratory work per unit volume (work per liter, Wp/L) done by the patient during assisted cycles *(open bars)* and spontaneous cycles *(reverse cross-hatched bars)*. Wp/L increased with decreasing synchronized intermittent mandatory ventilation percentage for both types of breath. Wp/L for spontaneous breaths tended to exceed Wp/L for machine-assisted breaths. Asterisk indicates p<0.01.

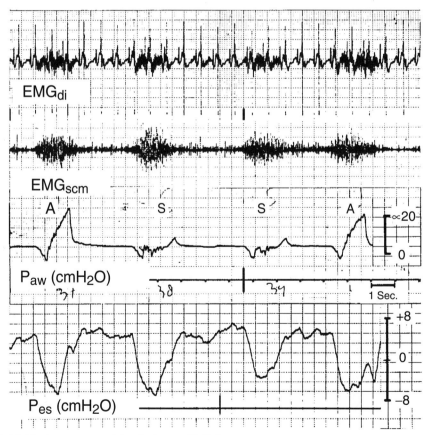

FIG. 39-13 Electromyograms of the diaphragm (EMG_{di}) and of the sternocleidomastoid muscles (EMG_{scm}) in a representative patient, showing similar intensity and the duration of electrical activity in successive assisted (A) and spontaneous (S) breaths during synchronized intermittent mandatory ventilation. Also note that esophageal (P_{es}) pressure changes are equal (equal effort) during A and S breaths. P_{aw}, Airway pressure.

    2. Peak flow (volume targeted only)
    3. Flow waveform (volume targeted only)
    4. Pressure level (pressure targeted only)
    5. Inspiratory time (always with pressure targeted and on some ventilators with volume targeting)
    6. Rate
    7. Sensitivity
    8. F_IO_2
    9. PEEP
   10. PS level if desired
   11. Rise time (pressure targeted only)
   12. Inspiratory termination criteria (pressure-supported breaths only, see Section VI, G, Inspiratory Termination Criteria)

V. Intermittent Mandatory Ventilation
    A. This is similar to SIMV except all mandatory breaths are control breaths, and PS cannot be added to the spontaneous breaths.
    B. During spontaneous breathing a continuous flow of gas is provided.
    C. Intermittent mandatory ventilation (IMV) is not available on modern ventilators.
    D. In addition to the problems with SIMV, during IMV the mandatory breath could be stacked on top of the spontaneous breath, increasing dyssynchrony and increasing intrathoracic and intracranial pressure.
    E. Similar to SIMV all the described variables are set except
        1. Sensitivity
        2. PS
    F. A continuous flow also must be set.

VI. Pressure Support
    A. PS is one of the modes of ventilation that allow the patient a significant level of control over the application of ventilatory support.
    B. The pressure, flow, and volume waveforms (Figure 39-14) during PS are the same as during pressure AC.
    C. The only variable that differs is the mechanism that terminates the breath.
        1. In pressure AC the breath ends when the set inspiratory time is reached; with PS the primary mechanism ending the breath is flow (Table 39-3).
        2. A PS breath ends when flow has decreased to a predetermined percentage of the peak flow.
        3. With most ventilators the termination flow percentage is fixed at 25%.
        4. Some ventilators allow the inspiratory terminating flow to be adjusted (see Section VI, G, Inspiratory Termination Criteria).
        5. The secondary terminating criterion is pressure. With all ventilations if the pressure exceeds the set level after the first 200 to 300 ms of inspiration, the breath is ended. The magnitude of the pressure increase varies from ventilator to ventilator but is usually 2 to 5 cm H_2O above set level.
        6. The third factor that will terminate a PS breath is time. After 2 to 3 seconds of inspiratory time, all ventilators will automatically end the breath.
    D. A backup rate is not set in most ventilators during PS; however, all new generation ventilators allow the setting of apnea ventilation, a controlled gas delivery pattern that takes over in the presence of apnea.
    E. During PS the following variables are set.
        1. Pressure level
        2. Sensitivity
        3. F_IO_2
        4. PEEP
        5. Rise time (most ventilators)
        6. Inspiratory termination criteria (some ventilators)

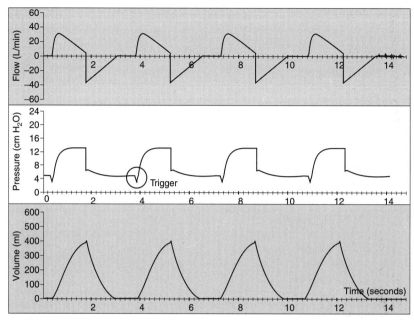

FIG. 39-14 Pressure support mode flow, airway pressure, and volume waveform.

	TABLE **39-3**

Criteria for Terminating a Pressure Support Breath

1° Mechanism	• A decrease in flow to a % of peak flow
	• 25% most common
	• A number of ventilators allow adjustment of this percentage
2° Mechanism	• An increase in pressure above the set level 200-300 msec after the start of the breath
	• With most ventilators this is 2-5 cm H$_2$O above set level
3° Mechanism	• Lengthy inspiratory time
	• Most ventilators will end the breath if inspiratory time is >2 to 3 sec

  F. Rise time (Table 39-4)

    1. Figure 39-15 illustrates the potential problems with gas delivery that can cause dyssynchrony during PS.

      a. At the onset of a pressure-targeted breath, gas can be delivered too rapidly or too slowly compared with patient demand. Either can cause dyssynchrony.

      b. At the termination of the breath, the breath can end before the patient is ready to end the breath or the patient can desire to exhale before the ventilator is ready to allow the patient to exhale.

    2. The effect of changing rise time is illustrated in Figure 39-16.

      a. Essentially rise time alters the slope of the airway pressure rise by changing the time needed for flow to increase to its maximum level.

      b. A rapid rise time ensures that flow will be delivered quickly at the start of the breath, causing pressure to almost immediately rise to the set level.

      c. A slow rise time decreases the rise in flow to its maximum level, and as a result pressure may not reach the set level until late in the breath.

      d. As illustrated in Figure 39-15, rise time should be set to ensure pressure rises rapidly in a linear manner but does not exceed the set level at the beginning of inspiration.

      e. An inadequate rise time can result in a concave airway pressure curve similar to that in Figures 39-7 and 39-8.

TABLE **39-4**	
Rise Time and Inspiratory Termination Criteria	

Rise time	• Available during pressure AC and PS (potentially other pressure-targeted modes)
	• Affects the initial flow delivery
	• Set to avoid
	• A pressure spike above set level
	• A concave inspiratory airway pressure curve
	• Normally set between maximum and middle settings
Inspiratory termination criteria	• Available during PS only
	• Affects the % of peak flow terminating the breath
	• Set to avoid
	• A spike above set level at the end of the breath
	• The appearance of two quick breaths in a row
	• When unavailable use pressure AC mode
	• Normally start with the 20-25% setting

AC, Assist/control; *PS*, pressure support.

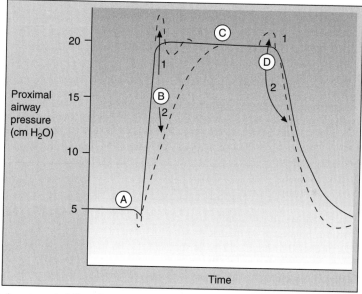

FIG. 39-15 Design characteristics of a pressure-supported breath. In this example, the baseline pressure (i.e., continuous positive airway pressure [CPAP]) is set at 5 cm H_2O (**A**), and pressure support is set at 15 cm H_2O (a peak inspiratory pressure [PIP] of 20 cm H_2O) (**B**). The inspiratory pressure is triggered at point A by a patient effort that results in a decrease in airway pressure. Demand valve sensitivity and responsiveness are characterized by the depth and duration of this negative pressure. The increase to pressure *(line B)* is provided by a fixed high initial flow delivery into the airway. Note that if flows exceed patient demand, the initial pressure exceeds the set level (*B1*), and if flow falls short of patient demand, a slow increase in pressure can occur (*B2*). The plateau of pressure support *(line C)* is maintained by servo control of flow. A smooth plateau reflects appropriate responsiveness to patient demand, whereas fluctuations reflect less responsiveness of the servo mechanisms. Termination of pressure support occurs at point D and should coincide with the end of the spontaneous inspiratory effort. If termination is delayed, the patient actively exhales (the bump in pressure above the plateau) *(D1)*; if termination occurs prematurely, the patient continues his or her inspiratory effort *(D2)*.

    f. Too rapid a rise time causes pressure to exceed the set level at the onset of the breath.

    g. With a rapid rise time, peak flow increases and inspiratory time tends to shorten (see Figure 39-16).

  3. Rise time is operable on most ventilators during pressure AC and PS but could be functional on any mode that uses a pressure-targeted gas delivery format.

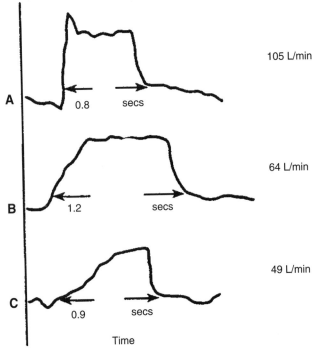

FIG. 39-16 Effect of changing rise time in a lung model preferring a midrange rise time. **A,** Flow is in excess of demand, and a pressure spike is seen. **B,** As flow rate is decreased, inspiratory time (T_I) lengthens, and the pressure spike is absent: machine output matches demand. **C,** When flow rate is further reduced, demand exceeds machine flow rate, and T_I decreases. Deformation of the pressure waveform during the increase to the set pressure support ventilation level is also seen in C.

G. Inspiratory termination criteria, inspiratory cycling criteria, or expiratory sensitivity (see Table 39-4)
1. As noted previously terminology regarding this control *only available on* PS varies from ventilator to ventilator.
2. As discussed in Figure 39-15 at the end of a PS breath, pressure should decrease linearly from the set level to PEEP.
3. When the patient's desire to end a breath and the ventilator settings to end the breath do not match, dyssynchrony occurs.
4. Figure 39-17 illustrates the patient desiring to end the breath before the ventilator flow has decreased to the terminating level.
5. The increase in pressure at the end of the breath above set level (see Figure 39-17) is a result of activation of accessory muscles of exhalation during the end of the ventilator's inspiratory phase.
6. This causes the pressure to increase above set level cycling to expiration by the 2nd degree cycling mechanism, an increase in end-inspiratory airway pressure.
7. When this happens the patient's ventilatory drive is increased, and his or her respiratory rate increases.
8. Adjustment of the inspiratory cycling criteria can correct this problem.
9. A higher percent cycling criteria should be set by slowly increasing the setting and observing the response. When the pressure spike is eliminated the termination criteria are set correctly.
10. Figure 39-18 illustrates the opposite problem, the patient desiring to continue inspiration after the ventilator has cycled to exhalation.
11. Note the second bump in the airway pressure and flow waveform on Figure 39-18, *bottom*. These indicate continued inspiratory effort before the patient begins exhalation after the ventilator ends the breath.

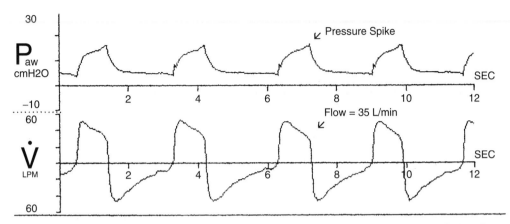

FIG. 39-17 Pressure and flow tracings during pressure support ventilation with the Nellcor Puritan Bennett 7200ae demonstrating pressure cycling in pressure support. The patient desires to end the breath before the ventilator will allow exhalation.

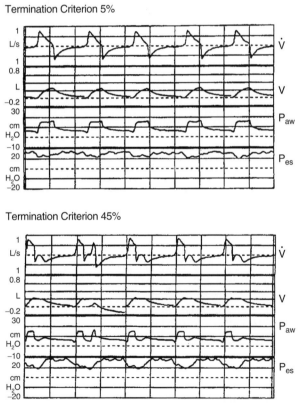

FIG. 39-18 Flow ($\dot{V}$), volume (V), airway pressure (P_{aw}), and esophageal pressure (P_{es}) curves with termination criterion (TC) 5% and TC 45% during 10 cm H_2O of pressure support ventilation. With TC 5%, inspiratory flow terminated simultaneously with the cessation of the patient's inspiratory effort estimated by P_{es}. In contrast, premature termination with double breathing occurred with TC 45%. Work of breathing also increased from 0.42 J/L with TC 5% to 0.64 J/L with TC 45%.

12. In this setting the termination criteria should be set at a lower percentage to lengthen the ventilator inspiratory time (see Figure 39-18, *top*).
13. Inspiratory termination criteria should be initially set at 20% to 25% and then adjusted to meet the patient's needs.
14. If inspiratory termination criteria is not available on a particular ventilator and problems with cycling to exhalation exist, change the patient to pressure AC.
    a. In pressure AC all gas-delivery features are the same as with PS except the ending of the breath.
    b. Set the inspiratory time equal to the patient's desired inspiratory time; remember this will most likely be <1.0 second.
    c. Set the backup rate at a level that will not affect the patient's control of the rate; usually 10 breaths/min is adequate.
15. When correct termination criteria are set, patient-ventilator dyssynchrony is eliminated, and respiratory rate frequently decreases.
16. The two ventilators in which inspiratory termination dyssynchrony during PS is most common are the Puritan Bennett 7200 (cycling criteria, 5 L/min) and the Servo 300 (cycling criteria, 5%) because of their low and nonadjustable cycling criteria.
17. Patients with chronic obstructive pulmonary disease (COPD) are most likely to experience problems with inspiratory termination during PS because they tend to desire to end inspiration with a flow that is relatively high. Adjustment of the termination criteria has the greatest impact on COPD patients.

H. PS is a useful mode in many clinical settings. Of primary concern is the patient's ventilatory drive. If it is intact, PS may be used to provide ventilatory support to most spontaneously breathing patients.

VII. **New Modes of Mechanical Ventilation**
    A. Box 39-1 lists the six modes of ventilation that are considered by most as new modes of ventilatory support.
    B. AC, SIMV, and PS have been available for >20 years on most mechanical ventilators and have a large database of information from which to draw material about their use.
    C. The new modes have only been available for a short period, and for many only limited information on their use is available except from the manufacturer.
    D. All of these modes in the broadest sense incorporate some level of computerized control of ventilation.
        1. A range of variables is set, but the ventilator is able to change gas delivery based on evaluation of changes in various measured variables.
        2. In some modes ventilatory support can go from near controlled ventilation to continuous positive airway pressure (CPAP).
    E. Most of these modes use a pressure-targeted ventilation format to delivery gas during at least part of the inspiratory cycle.
    F. As indicated in Box 39-1 these modes can be divided into two groups, depending on how adjustment to gas delivery is accomplished.
        1. *Within-breath adjustments:* As the patient is ventilated the ventilator assesses gas delivery and adjusts delivery during the breath.
        2. *Between-breath adjustments:* The ventilator evaluates gas delivery during the current breath and makes adjustments to delivery on the next breath.

BOX 39-1

New Modes of Mechanical Ventilation

Within-Breath Adjustment	Between-Breath Adjustment
Automatic tube compensation (ATC)	Volume support (VS)
Volume-assured pressure support (VAPS)	Pressure-regulated volume control (PRVC)
Proportional support ventilation (PAV)	Adaptive support ventilation (ASV)

G. Pressure-regulated volume control (PRVC), pressure control plus, auto flow, and so on
   1. Many terms are used by various manufacturers to indicate this between-breath adjustment mode.
   2. The airway pressure, flow, and volume waveforms on a given breath are exactly the same as with pressure AC.
   3. This mode differs from pressure AC by adjusting the pressure level on a breath-to-breath basis to ensure a targeted V_T is delivered.
   4. With this mode the following must be set.
      a. Maximum pressure level
      b. Target V_T
      c. Inspiratory time
      d. Backup rate
      e. Rise time (on most ventilators)
      f. F_IO_2
      g. PEEP
      h. Sensitivity
   5. When applied to a patient the ventilator gives a few test breaths at a low-pressure level and calculates the pressure setting required to delivery the V_T.
   6. The ventilator then applies a higher-pressure setting near 60% to 80% of the required level to achieve the targeted V_T, reassessing its calculation.
   7. The ventilator then will deliver the pressure level required to deliver the V_T.
   8. For each breath the ventilator assesses the V_T delivered.
   9. If V_T is low, on the next breath the pressure is increased, usually between 1 and 3 cm H_2O, and the V_T is reassessed.
   10. If V_T is high, on the next breath the pressure level is decreased usually between 1 and 3 cm H_2O, and the V_T is reassessed.
   11. The pressure level may be adjusted for every breath if there is a lot of variability in the V_T.
   12. Pressure can be increased to the maximum target set and can be decreased in some ventilators to PEEP level.
   13. In no ventilator is there currently the ability to set a lower pressure limit.
   14. This mode is capable of ensuring the target V_T is delivered using a pressure ventilation format.
   15. It is used by many in settings in which variation in V_T is large, and concerns exist about the patient being allowed to inhale a large V_T during a pressure-targeted breath.
   16. This mode works best in patients who are apneic or have a weak ventilatory drive.
   17. Significant concern should be exercised for patients with a high ventilatory demand because any stimulus that would increase ventilatory demand causing an increased V_T results in a decrease in inspiratory pressure.
      a. If this stimulus is sufficient, pressure could decrease all the way to the PEEP level.
      b. A patient markedly stressed with a high ventilatory drive may not receive any ventilatory support.
   18. The addition of a minimum pressure limit adjustable by the clinician would greatly improve the safety of this mode.
H. Volume support and volume guarantee
   1. This mode operates the same as PRVC except on a PS format.
   2. All comments related to PRVC are also accurate for volume support.
   3. During volume support the following variables must be set.
      a. Maximum pressure
      b. V_T target
      c. Sensitivity
      d. PEEP
      e. F_IO_2
      f. Rise time (most ventilators)
      g. Inspiratory termination criteria (some ventilators)

I. Adaptive support ventilation
   1. This mode of ventilation is only available on Hamilton ventilators.
   2. This is a *between-breath adjustment* mode that is used in conjunction with other modes of pressure-targeted ventilation: pressure AC, PS, and SIMV.
   3. It is a mode designed to ensure that the ventilatory pattern is one that results in the least work of breathing.
   4. This is accomplished by the setting of the following variables.
      a. Patient ideal weight
      b. Percent of ideal minute volume to be delivered
      c. Maximum peak inspiratory pressure
      d. Backup rate
   5. The ventilator calculates ideal minute volume as 0.1 L/min/kg.
   6. The percentage of ideal minute volume to be ensured can be any valve ≤200%.
   7. Five test breaths are delivered to define dynamic compliance and the expiratory time constant.
   8. The ventilator then calculates the V$_T$ and rate that will result in *the least work of breathing*.
   9. The ventilators follow an algorithm essentially with four gradients designed to adjust the respiratory rate and peak inspiratory pressure to move the respiratory pattern to the ideal V$_T$ and rate.
      a. Measure V$_T$ increased, rate decreased
         (1) Decrease peak pressure
         (2) Increase respiratory rate
      b. Measured V$_T$ decreased, rate decreased
         (1) Increase peak pressure
         (2) Increase respiratory rate
      c. Measured V$_T$ increased, rate increased
         (1) Decrease peak pressure
         (2) Decrease respiratory rate
      d. Measured V$_T$ decreased, rate increased
         (1) Increase peak pressure
         (2) Decrease respiratory rate
   10. Few data are available to evaluate the effect of this mode.
   11. From a theoretical perspective it seems an interesting approach to maintaining a ventilatory pattern that minimizes work of breathing.
J. Automatic tube compensation (ATC)
   1. This *within-breath adjustment* mode of ventilation can be used by itself or during the spontaneous breaths of SIMV and bilevel pressure ventilation (see Section X, Bilevel Pressure Ventilation).
   2. It is designed to apply sufficient pressure to eliminate the flow-resistant work of breathing imposed by the endotracheal tube.
   3. Essentially it attempts to maintain the pressure at the tip of the endotracheal tube equal to the end-expiratory baseline pressure.
   4. This is accomplished by applying a varying level of positive pressure during inspiration and a varying level of negative pressure during exhalation.
   5. The level of pressure applied is based on the ventilator knowing the exact airway size (tracheostomy or endotracheal) and instantaneous changes in flow.
   6. As noted in Figure 39-19 with this information the pressure at the tracheal level can be calculated, and as a result the correct pressure is applied to minimize tracheal pressure change.
   7. Figure 39-20 illustrates the effect of ATC in a COPD patient with a high demand and a postoperative patient with a low ventilatory demand.
   8. ATC is most effective in reducing resistive effort in COPD patients because of their high demand, requiring greater pressure than originally applied with PS (see Figure 39-19).

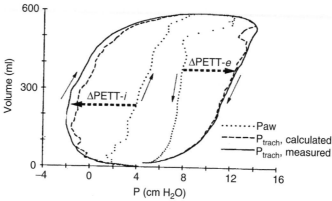

FIG. 39-19 Volume/pressure diagram in a tracheally intubated patient during inspiratory pressure support (PEEP = 5 cm H_2O; IPS = 5 cm H_2O). P_{trach} is calculated using the same endotracheal tube (ETT) coefficients for resistance. The pressure decrease across the ETT (ΔPETT) is indicated in inspiration and in expiration by a broken arrow. The direction of the arrow points from airway pressure to tracheal pressure.

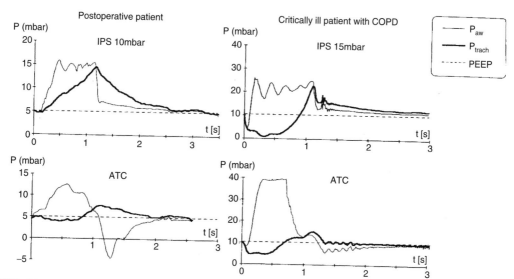

FIG. 39-20 Airway pressure and tracheal pressure curves under inspiratory pressure support (IPS; *top*) and automatic tube compensation (ATC; *bottom*) in a patient after open heart surgery *(left)* and a critically ill patient with chronic obstructive pulmonary disease (COPD; *right*). Note although the ventilator decreases airway pressure (P_{aw}) during expiration to subatmospheric pressure *(bottom left)*, controlling the expiratory valve ensures that tracheal pressure (P_{trach}) is above or equal to positive end-expiratory pressure (PEEP). The patient with acute respiratory insufficiency under ATC generates an inspiratory gas flow of >2 L/sec *(bottom right)*, which accounts for part of the deviation between P_{trach} and PEEP.

9. As noted in the example of the postoperative patient (see Figure 39-20), the applied pressure peaks at the onset of the breath but decreases at the end of the breath because ventilatory demand decreases.

10. Ventilators with this mode may allow ATC to be used only during inspiration or during inspiration and expiration.

11. Use during expiration is a concern for patients with airway obstruction (e.g., COPD, asthma) because the negative airway pressure may increase air trapping.

12. There are no specific indications for the use of ATC, but it appears it may be useful to identify the PS level needed to overcome the resistance of the endotracheal tube.

13. Others have proposed the use of ATC during weaning. When patients are able to adequately ventilate with a low ATC level, they are considered ready to be extubated.

14. However, there are no outcome data indicating more rapid weaning.

K. Volume assured PS (VAPS) or pressure augmentation

1. Similar to ACT, VAPS is a *within-breath adjustment* mode that can be considered a dual mode of ventilatory support.

2. This mode is designed to reduce the work of breathing while maintaining a minimum minute volume and a minimum V_T.

3. This mode combines the high initial flow of a pressure-targeted breath with the constant volume delivery of a volume-targeted breath.

4. With VAPS the following variables are set.

  a. PS level

  b. V_T target

  c. Peak flow setting

  d. Sensitivity

  e. PEEP

  f. F_IO_2

5. When the ventilator is triggered, the initial pressure target is the PS level (Figure 39-21).

6. However, if the targeted volume is not delivered before flow is decreased to the inspiratory cycling criteria, the breath changes from a pressure-targeted to a volume-targeted breath.

7. The remainder of the breath becomes a volume-targeted breath.

8. If the patient's demand is high and the targeted V_T can be delivered before the PS termination criteria are met, the breath continues as a PS breath only.

9. If the targeted V_T cannot be delivered (e.g., a patient with a weak ventilatory drive), the breath rapidly converts to a volume-targeted breath, ensuring the minimal V_T delivery.

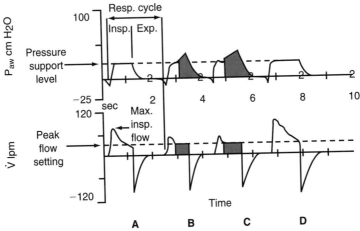

FIG. 39-21 The possible breath types during volume-assured pressure support (VAPS). In breath *A*, the set tidal volume and delivered tidal volume are equal. This is a pressure support breath (patient triggered, pressure limited, and flow cycled). Breath *B* represents a reduction in patient effort. As flow decelerates, the ventilator determines that delivered tidal volume will be less than the minimum set volume. At the shaded portion of the graph, the breath changes from a pressure- to a volume-limited (constant flow) breath. Breath *C* demonstrates a worsening of the compliance and the possibility of extending inspiratory time to ensure the minimum tidal volume delivery. Breath *D* represents a pressure support breath in which the tidal volume is greater than the set tidal volume. This kind of breath allowed during VAPS may aid in reducing work of breathing and dyspnea.

10. Essentially gas delivery always begins as a PS breath but changes to a volume-targeted breath if the target VT is not reached before the PS inspiratory termination criteria are met.
11. This mode ensures a minimum VT is delivered in a partial PS format. It also allows access to additional volume and flow if a patient's ventilatory demand is high.

L. Proportional assist ventilation (PAV)
1. This is the most unique *within-breath adjustment* mode of ventilatory support available.
2. With PAV there are no controls over gas delivery.
3. Airway pressure is provided based on patient demand. The higher the demand, the higher the level of pressure applied; the lower the demand, the lower the level of pressure applied.
4. The level of support provided is determined by setting the percentage of elastic and resistive work that will be unloaded.
5. A schematic of the operation of PAV is depicted in Figure 39-22.
6. As noted the percentage of flow unloading and volume unloading is set by adjusting gain controls affecting volume and flow response.
7. A comparison of the impact of PAV versus other modes is illustrated in Figure 39-23.
8. With PAV, support increases as demand increases, whereas with volume-targeted ventilation (e.g., SIMV), support decreases as demand increases, and with pressure targeting, support stays constant regardless of demand.
9. A major problem with PAV is runaway, an unlimited application of airway pressure.
10. To avoid runaway requires precise measurement of compliance and resistance on an ongoing basis.
11. It is important to remember with PAV a patient may chose a ventilatory rate of 50 breaths/min and a VT of 100 ml or a rate of 5 breaths/min with a VT of 1.0 L.
12. Currently there are no established indications for PAV, but it does seem to provide ventilatory support during noninvasive positive pressure ventilation as well as PS.

VIII. **Inverse Ratio Ventilation**
A. This approach is just what the title implies: exhalation is longer than inspiration.
B. Ideally exhalation is short enough to cause air trapping and auto-PEEP, whereas inspiration is long enough to allow uniform distribution of inspiration.
C. Typically this approach is applied using pressure AC; however, volume ventilation may also be used.
D. Because of the inverse ratio and the design of ventilators, at the time of the introduction of the mode patients required heavy sedation, and frequently neuromuscular paralysis is needed for the mode to be applied.

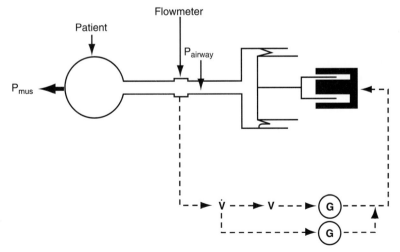

FIG. 39-22 Simple proportional assist ventilation (PAV) delivery system. P_{mus}, Patient inspiratory effort. $\dot{V}$, Instantaneous flow. V, Instantaneous volume. G, Gain control.

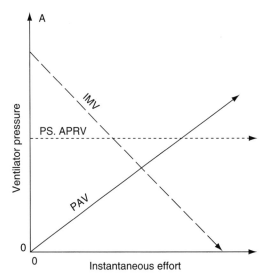

FIG. 39-23 Relation between instantaneous patient effort and pressure delivered by the ventilator with different ventilatory support modalities. *IMV*, Volume-cycled breath. *PS*, Pressure support. *APRV*, Airway pressure release ventilation. *PAV*, Proportional assist ventilation. Note that with all modalities other than PAV, the relation between effort and ventilatory consequences is normal at only one level of effort (intersection between dashed diagonal line and the line representing the particular method used). With PAV the relation is normalized at all levels of effort, within each breath, and as effort changes from breath to breath. See text for additional details.

    E. Inverse ratio ventilation (IRV) does improve oxygenation but does not have any advantages over normal I:E ventilation with appropriately applied PEEP.

    F. IRV has the disadvantage of markedly increasing mean airway pressure, which frequently results in hemodynamic compromise.

    G. IRV is only useful for patients with severe acute respiratory distress syndrome.

  IX. **Airway Pressure Release Ventilation**

    A. Airway pressure release ventilation (APRV) is similar to IRV and SIMV except the patient is allowed to inspire and exhale at the high-pressure setting and low-pressure setting (Figure 39-24).

    B. This mode is frequently considered as the application of two levels of CPAP because spontaneous ventilation is never impaired (i.e., the exhalation valve is active all the time).

    C. The set I:E ratio can be normal (1:2) or inverse (3:1 or 4:1).

    D. Because spontaneous ventilation is not impaired, sedation to apnea or paralysis is unnecessary regardless of the I:E ratio.

    E. Proponents of the mode cite the following advantages.

       1. Minimal sedation

       2. Improved $\dot{V}/\dot{Q}$ matching (see Figure 39-11)

       3. Improved cardiovascular function

    F. However, as noted in Figure 39-25, the work of breathing or ventilatory effort can be excessive, especially at the high CPAP level.

    G. At CPAP levels of 25 or 30 cm H_2O, the diaphragm is essentially flat, requiring large pleural pressure changes to cause further gas movement.

    H. No data indicating APRV is superior to conventional ventilation are available.

  X. **Bilevel Pressure Ventilation**

    A. Bilevel pressure ventilation is similar to APRV except that PS can be applied to all or some spontaneous breaths (Figure 39-26).

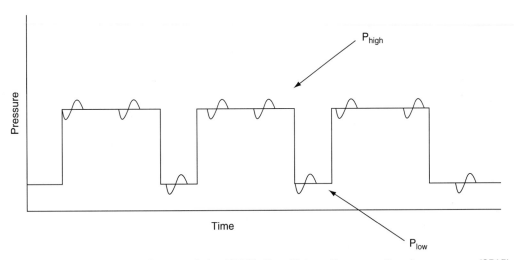

FIG. 39-24 Airway pressure release ventilation (APRV). P_{high}, High continuous positive airway pressure (CPAP) level. P_{low}, Low CPAP level. Note spontaneous breaths at both levels of CPAP.

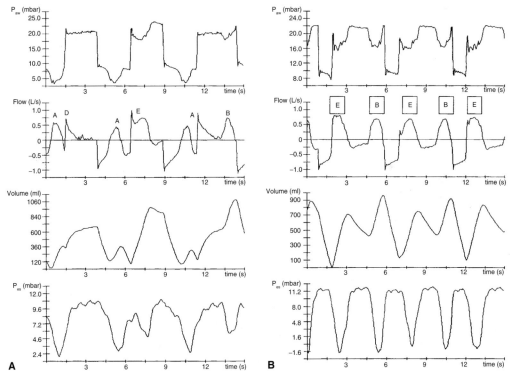

FIG. 39-25 Airway pressure release ventilation original tracings. A synopsis of airway pressure (P_{aw}), flow, volume, and esophageal pressure (P_{es}) is shown for **(A)** time intervals of the upper (P_{high}) and lower airway pressure (P_{low}) set to 2.5 seconds each, and for **(B)** time intervals of P_{high} = 4.0 seconds and P_{low} = 1.0 second in the same patient. Note that spontaneous breathing occurred on the upper and lower airway pressure in *A* and that tidal volumes varied considerably, depending on the pressure level from which an inspiration was started. When P_{low} was decreased to 1.0 second, as shown in B, spontaneous breaths occurred almost exclusively during P_{high}. This resulted in a more regular breathing pattern as compared with A. Note, however, the large esophageal pressure swings (10 to 12 mbar or cm H_2O) per breath, indicating high patient effort on each spontaneous breath. Breaths were classified as type A, spontaneous breath on the lower pressure level; type B, spontaneous breath on the upper pressure level; type C, the pressure increase from the lower to the upper pressure level was triggered by an inspiratory effort of the patient; type D, mechanical breath; and type E, combined mechanical and spontaneous inspiration without a triggered pressure increase from P_{low} to P_{high}.

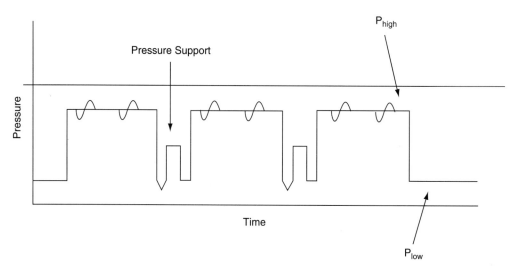

FIG. 39-26 Bilevel ventilation. P_{high}, High continuous positive airway pressure (CPAP) level. P_{low}, Low CPAP level. Note spontaneous breaths at both levels of CPAP, but in this case pressure support is applied to the breaths at the P_{low}. Pressure support could also be applied to P_{high}.

    B. In this approach the I:E ratio is usually normal, and most spontaneous breathing occurs at the low CPAP level .

    C. APRV and bilevel pressure ventilation are indicated in patients with severe acute respiratory failure and acute respiratory distress syndrome.

    D. There are no data to indicate that APRV or bilevel pressure ventilation affects outcome differently than conventional modes of ventilation.

XI. Continuous Positive Airway Pressure

    A. CPAP is not truly a mode of ventilation because no support of inspiration is applied.

    B. CPAP is simply the increasing of the system pressure above atmospheric and allowing spontaneous breathing.

    C. In CPAP the demand valve is activated during inspiration, adding additional flow to the circuit.

    D. CPAP is used

        1. To manage hypoxemia that is related to true shunting

          a. Atelectasis

          b. Acute lung injury

        2. To manage cardiogenic pulmonary edema

        3. To manage sleep apnea

    E. When CPAP is used the following variables are set.

        1. Pressure level

        2. Sensitivity

        3. F_IO_2

BIBLIOGRAPHY

Branson RD, Hess DR, Chalburn RL: *Respiratory Care Equipment*, ed 2. Philadelphia, Lippincott Williams & Wilkins, 1999.

Hess DR, Kacmarek RM: *Essentials of Mechanical Ventilation*, ed 2. New York, McGraw Hill, 2003.

Hess DR, MacIntyre NR, Mishoe SC, et al: *Respiratory Care Principles and Practice*. Philadelphia, WB Saunders, 2002.

Higgins TL, Stemgrub JS, Kacmarek RM, Stoller JK: *Cardiopulmonary Critical Care*. London, Bios Scientific Publications, 2002.

Iotti GA: Closed loop control mechanical ventilation. *Respir Care Clin N Am* 7:341-518, 2001.

Kacmarek RM, Hess DR, Stoller JK: *Monitoring in Respiratory Care*. St. Louis, Mosby, 1993.

Pierson DJ, Kacmarek K: *Foundations of Respiratory Care*. New York, Churchill Livingstone, 1992.

Shapiro BA, Kacmarek RM, Cane RD, et al: *Clinical Application of Respiratory Care*, ed 4. St. Louis, Mosby, 1991.

Tobin MJ: *Principles and Practice of Mechanical Ventilation*. New York, McGraw Hill, 1994.

Wilkins RL, Stoller JK, Scanlon CL: *Egan's Fundamentals of Respiratory Care*, ed 8. St. Louis, Mosby, 2003.

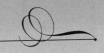

Chapter 40

Positive End-Expiratory Pressure

I. **Definition of Terms**
   A. Positive end-expiratory pressure (PEEP): The establishment and maintenance of a preset airway pressure greater than ambient at end-exhalation.
   B. Continuous positive airway pressure (CPAP): The application of PEEP to the spontaneously breathing patient. Inspiratory and expiratory airway pressures are supraatmospheric, but no inspiratory assistance is provided.
   C. Continuous positive pressure ventilation (CPPV): The application of PEEP to a patient receiving positive pressure ventilation.

II. **Physiologic Effects of PEEP**
   A. Effects on intrapulmonary pressures
      1. When only the end-expiratory pressure is maintained above atmospheric in a spontaneously breathing patient, the shape of the intrapulmonary pressure curve is not altered; only the baseline pressure from which the patient ventilates changes. Therefore, the dynamics of air movement are not directly affected.
      2. As illustrated in Chapter 5, intrapulmonary pressure decreases approximately 3 cm H_2O during inspiration and increases approximately 3 cm H_2O during expiration from the set CPAP level.
      3. During ventilatory support, regardless of mode, PEEP simply increases the baseline about which mechanical ventilation is initiated.
   B. Effects on intrapleural (intrathoracic) pressures
      1. PEEP increases intrapleural pressures.
      2. The extent of the increase is determined by
         a. The amount of PEEP applied
         b. The stiffness of the individual's lung
            (1) The greater the pulmonary compliance, the greater the transmission of PEEP to the intrapleural space and the greater the increase in intrapleural pressure.
            (2) In patients with normal lungs and chest wall approximately 50% of the PEEP applied is transmitted to the intrathoracic space, increasing the intrapleural pressure.
            (3) In patients with acute respiratory distress syndrome (ARDS; stiff lungs) only approximately 25% of the applied PEEP is transmitted to the intrathoracic space, increasing intrapleural pressure.
            (4) Patients with localized pulmonary disease (e.g., pneumonia, atelectasis) demonstrate an increase in overall intrapleural pressure similar to patients with normal pulmonary compliance; however, transmission of pressure may be reduced in the area of concern.
            (5) The effects of PEEP on intrapleural pressure are most marked in patients with chronic obstructive pulmonary disease (COPD) because of their increased pulmonary compliance.

    c.   Changes in thoracic compliance
       (1)   If thoracic compliance is decreased more pressure than normal will be transmitted to the intrapleural space because overall expansion of the lung-thorax system is inhibited. *It is in this setting that hemodynamic compromise is most likely.*
       (2)   An increase in thoracic compliance will allow the system to expand and usually results in less of an increase in intrapleural pressure when compared with normal. *Hemodynamic compromise is minimal in this setting.*

C. Effect on functional residual capacity (FRC) (Figure 40-1)
    1. Regardless of the condition of the lung at the time of application, PEEP increases FRC.
    2. FRC is increased by two primary mechanisms.
      a. Because the lungs are elastic any increase in end-expiratory pressure increases overall lung volume. The diameter of conducting airways can increase 1 to 2 mm as PEEP is applied.
      b. In patients with a decreased FRC as a result of alveolar collapse caused by surfactant instability, PEEP maintains alveoli inflated after they are recruited by the peak airway pressure.
       (1)   This is accomplished by PEEP maintaining a backpressure exceeding the force of surface tension and lung elastance, which tend to collapse alveoli.
       (2)   The actual reexpansion of alveoli is accomplished by the force of normal inspiration or the application of positive inspiratory airway pressure. PEEP simply maintains the alveoli open once they are reexpanded.

D. Effect on pulmonary compliance
    1. Because PEEP increases FRC, it alters pulmonary compliance.
    2. The compliance curve of the normal total respiratory system is depicted in Figure 40-2. Note that the curve is only linear above the FRC level and again becomes alinear at some pressure and volume well beyond FRC.
    3. In the normal lung the increased FRC caused by excessive PEEP levels may move alveoli from the steep portion to the flat portion of the compliance curve, thus decreasing compliance.

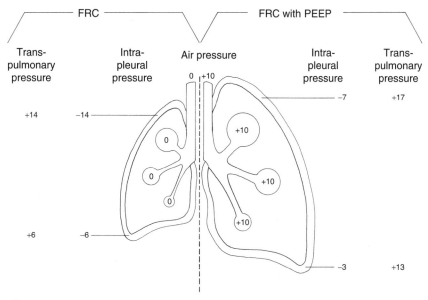

FIG. 40-1 Transpulmonary pressure gradients vary from the apex to the base of the lung. In adult respiratory distress syndrome the magnitude of these gradients increases because of the increased elastance of the lung. Applying positive end-expiratory pressure increases the functional residual capacity by increasing the transpulmonary pressure gradient.

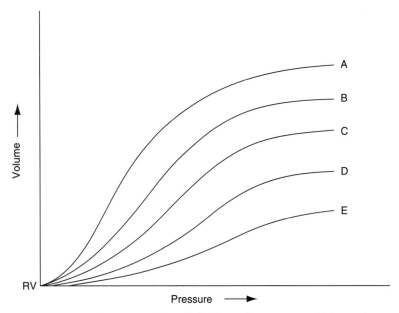

FIG. 40-2 A, Normal total compliance curve. **B** to **E,** Total compliance curves with increasing acute respiratory distress syndrome (ARDS). The application of positive end-expiratory pressure, by maintaining alveoli recruited and increasing transpulmonary pressure gradients, can alter the compliance curve, moving the curve from E to D or from D to B and ideally returning the pressure-volume relationship closer to normal (**A**).

4. In patients with acute lung injury (ALI) or ARDS, the application of PEEP increases compliance (see Figure 40-2).
   a. As ARDS develops the compliance curve shifts to the right and downward.
   b. As PEEP is applied the compliance curve shifts upward and to the left.
   c. With appropriate application of PEEP compliance in ALI/ARDS normally improves.
5. The monitoring of effective static compliance (see Chapter 41) can be used to help to determine the "optimal" or most appropriate PEEP level.
   a. The best compliance is thought to coincide with the most appropriate PEEP level; however, changes in tidal volume (VT) will change the PEEP level considered appropriate. VT should always be constant during PEEP titration.
   b. The major problem associated with the use of compliance as a means to determine optimal PEEP is the difficulty in determining compliance in patients ventilated in anything but the control mode. With other modes a reliable measurement of effective static compliance is often difficult because of active movement of the chest wall, preventing correct determination of the static end-inspiratory plateau pressure.
E. Effect of PEEP on deadspace
   1. Because PEEP increases FRC by distending alveoli, deadspace is usually *increased* in
      a. Patients with normal lungs
      b. Patients with COPD
      c. Patients with a nonhomogeneously distributed disease process
   2. Because of stabilization of recruited alveoli, appropriate PEEP levels usually *decrease deadspace* in patients with ALI/ARDS. Some have proposed monitoring deadspace or change in CO_2 at a constant minute ventilation as an indication of appropriate PEEP level.
F. Effect of PEEP on the cardiovascular system (Table 40-1)
   1. The primary effect of PEEP on the cardiovascular system is a reduction in cardiac output (CO) as a result of increased impedance to venous return by an increase in intrathoracic pressure.

TABLE **40-1**		

Potential Physiologic Effects of Appropriately and Excessively Applied PEEP

	Appropriate Level	Excessive Level
Intrapulmonary pressure	Increased	Increased
Intrathoracic pressure	Increased	Increased
FRC	Increased	Increased
Respiratory system compliance	Increased	Increased or decreased
Closing volume	Decreased	Decreased
Pa_{O_2}	Increased	Increased or decreased
Sa_{O_2}	Increased	Increased or decreased
Pa_{CO_2}	No change or decreased	Increased
$\dot{Q}s/\dot{Q}t$	Decreased	Decreased or increased
$P(A-a)_{O_2}$	Decreased	Decreased or increased
$C(a-\bar{v})_{O_2}$	Decreased	Decreased or increased
$P\bar{v}_{O_2}$	Increased	Increased or decreased
Pa_{CO_2}-P_{ETCO_2}	Decreased	Increased
V_D/V_T	Decreased	Increased
Work of breathing	Decreased	Increased
Extravascular lung water	No change or increased	No change or increased
Pulmonary vascular resistance	Increased	Increased
Total pulmonary perfusion	No change or decreased	Decreased
Cardiac output	No change or decreased	Decreased
Pulmonary artery pressure	No change or increased or decreased	Decreased
Pulmonary capillary wedge pressure	No change or increased or decreased	Decreased
Central venous pressure	No change or increased or decreased	Decreased
Arterial pressure	No change or increased or decreased	Decreased
Intracranial pressure	No change or increased	Increased
Urinary output	No change or decreased	Decreased

FRC, Functional residual capacity; $\dot{Q}s/\dot{Q}_T$, shunt fraction; $P(A-a)_{O_2}$, alveolar-arterial O_2 pressure difference; $C(a-\bar{v})_{O_2}$, arterial-mixed venous O_2 content difference; $P\bar{v}_{O_2}$, mixed venous O_2 pressure; P_{ETCO_2}, end-tidal CO_2 pressure; V_D/V_T, dead space/tidal volume ratio.

2. This increase in pressure decreases cardiac transmural pressure, potentially decreasing the end-diastolic volume and stroke volume of both ventricles.
3. Low-level PEEP reduces right ventricular end-diastolic volume, but right ventricular ejection fraction normally remains constant, provided no previous right ventricular dysfunction exists.
4. Higher levels of PEEP markedly increase right ventricular afterload, increasing end-diastolic volume and decreasing ejection fraction.
5. Increased right ventricular end-diastolic volume with high levels of PEEP causes right ventricular distention and a leftward shift of the interventricular septa.
   a. This reduces left ventricular distensibility.
   b. This results in a decrease in left ventricular end-diastolic volume and stroke volume.
6. Actual changes in pulmonary hemodynamics after the application of PEEP depend on many factors.
   a. PEEP level
   b. Pulmonary compliance
   c. Thoracic compliance
   d. Vascular volume
   e. Myocardial contractility
7. Provided that pulmonary blood flow is not markedly reduced, PEEP generally results in
   a. An increase in right ventricular preload (central venous pressure [CVP])
   b. An increase in right ventricular afterload (pulmonary artery pressure [PAP])
   c. An increase in left ventricular preload (pulmonary capillary wedge pressure [PWP])
   d. Generally the higher the PEEP, the less likely the wedge pressure will reflect left atrial pressure.

e. Because CO is usually decreased with PEEP, left ventricular afterload may also decrease as PEEP is applied.

8. If pulmonary blood flow is markedly reduced by the application of PEEP, the preload and afterload of left and right ventricles decrease. As a result it is difficult to predict the precise effect that PEEP will have on hemodynamics.

9. Any of the hemodynamic pressures measured may increase, decrease, or stay the same, depending on the maintenance of pulmonary blood flow.

10. When the effect of PEEP on CO is evaluated, it is important to place the decreased CO into proper perspective. The following are two examples of the effect of PEEP on CO. In example A the patient is young and has excellent cardiovascular reserves, whereas in example B the patient is older and has limited cardiovascular reserves.

Example A:

A 25-year-old man with ARDS

Pa_{O_2}	48 mm Hg	Pulse	130 beats/min
pH	7.53	Blood pressure (BP)	160/100 mm Hg
Pa_{CO_2}	27 mm Hg	CO	10.5 L/min
HCO_3^-	22 mEq/L	CI	5.7 L/min/m^2
Spontaneous respiration rate (RR)	35 breaths/min	F_IO_2	0.8
V_T	350 ml	No mechanical ventilatory support	

With the application of PEEP the following data are obtained.

Pa_{O_2}	75 mm Hg	Pulse	85 beats/min
pH	7.43	BP	130/80 mm Hg
Pa_{CO_2}	38 mm Hg	CO	6.6 L/min
HCO_3^-	24 mEq/L	CI	3.7 L/min/m^2
Spontaneous RR	20 breaths/min	F_IO_2	0.5
V_T	350 ml	CPAP at 10 cm H_2O by mask	

In this example the patient's CO decreased 4 L, but his cardiac index (CI) returned to normal. This occurred because the original CO of 10.5 L/min was a result of cardiopulmonary stress. With the application of PEEP, oxygenation improved (F_IO_2 was decreased), and cardiopulmonary stress decreased. Thus the CO and CI returned to normal. This reduction in CO and CI was desirable.

Example B:

A 60-year-old man with ARDS

Pa_{O_2}	48 mm Hg	Pulse	130 beats/min
pH	7.48	BP	140/90 mm Hg
Pa_{CO_2}	32 mm Hg	CO	5.5 L/min
HCO_3^-	23 mEq/L	CI	3.6 L/min/m^2
Spontaneous RR	35 breaths/min	F_IO_2	0.6
V_T	300 ml	No mechanical ventilation support	

With the application of PEEP the following data are obtained.

Pa_{O_2}	68 mm Hg	Pulse	150 beats/min
pH	7.47	BP	90/60 mm Hg
Pa_{CO_2}	33 mm Hg	CO	3.5 L/min
HCO_3^-	23 mEq/L	CI	2.3 L/min/m^2
Spontaneous RR	28 breaths/min	F_IO_2	0.6
V_T	300 ml	CPAP at 10 cm H_2O by mask	

In this example the patient's CO decreased only 2 L/min, but the CI is now below normal. A CO of 3.5 L/min is clearly inappropriately low for this patient, and either fluid therapy or pharmacologic support is required to return the CO to an acceptable level. The reduction in CO is small but places the patient at increased risk. The patient's complete clinical presentation must be evaluated to determine whether PEEP had a detrimental effect on CO.

11. The following example is designed to illustrate the effect of PEEP on hemodynamic values.

No PEEP

Pulse	160 beats/min	CVP	12 cm H_2O
BP	150/100 mm Hg	PAP	26 mm Hg
		PWP	10 mm Hg

5 cm H_2O PEEP

Pulse	158 beats/min	CVP	13 cm H_2O
BP	148/92 mm Hg	PAP	27 mm Hg
		PWP	11 mm Hg

10 cm H_2O PEEP

Pulse	140 beats/min	CVP	15 cm H_2O
BP	142/96 mm Hg	PAP	29 mm Hg
		PWP	13 mm Hg

12 cm H_2O PEEP

Pulse	126 beats/min	CVP	16 cm H_2O
BP	130/84 mm Hg	PAP	30 mm Hg
		PWP	14 mm Hg

15 cm H_2O PEEP

Pulse	154 beats/min	CVP	6 cm H_2O
BP	90/60 mm Hg	PAP	22 mm Hg
		PWP	5 mm Hg

The application of 5, 10, and 12 cm H_2O PEEP was appropriately tolerated from a hemodynamic perspective. However, with the application of 15 cm H_2O PEEP, the hemodynamic values decreased sharply, indicating inability of the cardiovascular system to tolerate 15 cm H_2O PEEP at its present status. If this patient receives proper fluid therapy, pharmacologic support, or both, the following profile *may be achieved.*

15 cm H_2O PEEP

Pulse	124 beats/min	CVP	18 cm H_2O
BP	120/84 mm Hg	PAP	32 mm Hg
		PWP	16 mm Hg

Note: In actual clinical practice hemodynamic values should also be correlated with the patient's clinical presentation, signs of adequate tissue perfusion (e.g., urinary output, sensorium, and skin temperature), and CO.

G. Effects of PEEP on lung water (Figure 40-3)
   1. PEEP does not decrease overall pulmonary vascular volume.
   2. Normally PEEP causes a redistribution of lung water and may increase overall lung water.
   3. Fluid generally moves from the intraalveolar to the perivascular interstitial space; extraalveolar and corner vessels are expanded with PEEP.
   4. This movement assists in improving oxygenation, increasing compliance, and decreasing shunting.

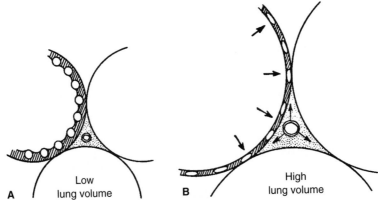

FIG. 40-3 A and **B,** As a result of positive end-expiratory pressure (PEEP) increasing lung volume **(B),** the alveolar capillaries are stretched and compressed, potentially decreasing flow. However, the extraalveolar and corner vessels between alveoli are expanded, which increases the flux of fluid into the interstitial space. At low lung volume (without PEEP) **(A)** these changes are reversed.

   5. PEEP may result in greater transudation of fluid from the pulmonary vasculature into the peribronchial and hilar areas of the lung.
H. Effect of PEEP therapy on PaO_2
   1. Because PEEP therapy causes a minor increase in the partial pressure of oxygen in the lung, a small increase in PaO_2 may be noted even in the healthy lung.
   2. In the patient with ALI/ARDS, PaO_2 levels also demonstrate only a small increase as the PEEP level is increased and will not markedly increase until PEEP sufficient to avoid derecruitment of recruited alveoli has been set. When appropriate PEEP is set, PaO_2 values may increase markedly. The following examples illustrate how PaO_2 may change as PEEP is applied.

PEEP (cm H_2O)	PaO_2 (mm Hg)
0	45
5	48
10	53
12	56
15	110

   3. If higher levels of PEEP are applied, PaO_2 values may continue to increase slightly, remain the same, or decrease, depending on the effect of PEEP on CO.
      a. A continual increase in PEEP will eventually affect CO. However, the blood that is capable of perfusing the lung will still be oxygenated, and its oxygenation state may continue to improve slightly as CO decreases.
      b. When appropriateness of PEEP is monitored, PaO_2 must be evaluated; however, PaO_2 provides no indication of the adequacy of cardiovascular function or of systemic oxygen delivery.
I. Effects on intrapulmonary shunt
   1. Increasing PEEP levels result in a decrease in intrapulmonary shunt.
   2. As recruited alveoli are maintained open with PEEP, ventilation/perfusion matching improves, and shunting decreases.
   3. As with PaO_2 intrapulmonary shunt may continue to decrease even when CO is significantly decreased.
      a. This occurs because any blood that is presented to the lung may be better oxygenated.

   b. When the appropriateness of PEEP is monitored, intrapulmonary shunt should be evaluated; however, the intrapulmonary shunt provides no indication of adequacy of cardiovascular function or systemic oxygen delivery.

J. Mixed venous P_{O_2} ($P\bar{v}_{O_2}$)
   1. $P\bar{v}_{O_2}$ is a variable affected by
      a. CO
      b. Tissue perfusion
      c. Oxygen content
      d. Metabolic rate
   2. A decreased CO, a decrease in oxygen content, a decrease in tissue perfusion, or an increase in metabolic rate can cause a decrease in $P\bar{v}_{O_2}$.
   3. In cardiopulmonary-stressed patients with ALI/ARDS, the $P\bar{v}_{O_2}$ is normally decreased.
      a. The extent of this decrease depends most on the cardiovascular reserves of the patient.
      b. For patients with good cardiovascular reserves, the $P\bar{v}_{O_2}$ will be decreased only slightly (35 to 40 mm Hg) because these patients can increase their COs significantly in response to stress.
      c. However, in patients with limited cardiovascular reserves, the $P\bar{v}_{O_2}$ may be significantly decreased (≤ 30 to 35 mm Hg) because these patients cannot increase their COs in response to stress.
   4. As PEEP is applied the $P\bar{v}_{O_2}$ should increase if the CO is not adversely affected. This occurs because oxygen delivery increases.
   5. If excessive PEEP is applied the $P\bar{v}_{O_2}$ will decrease because of the effect of PEEP on CO, thus decreasing oxygen delivery.

PEEP (cm H_2O)	$P\bar{v}_{O_2}$ (mm Hg)	CO (L/min)
0	36	12.5
5	36	12.3
10	38	9.6
12	40	8.9
15	43	7.2
18	35	4.8

   At PEEP levels from 5 to 15 cm H_2O the $P\bar{v}_{O_2}$ increased appropriately, but at 18 cm H_2O PEEP inhibited CO significantly, resulting in a decrease in the $P\bar{v}_{O_2}$. Fluid therapy, pharmacologic support, or a decrease in PEEP level is indicated to support cardiovascular function and optimize $P\bar{v}_{O_2}$.

K. Arteriovenous oxygen content difference (a-vD_{O_2})
   1. a-vD_{O_2} depends on
      a. Arterial oxygen content
      b. Venous oxygen content
      c. Metabolic rate
      d. CO
   2. In patients with ARDS, a-vD_{O_2} varies from normal, depending on the cardiovascular reserves of the patient.
   3. In patients with good cardiovascular reserves, decreased arterial oxygen content results in an increase in CO.
      a. If the patient's metabolic rate is constant and CO is increased, the volume of oxygen extracted per volume of blood decreases.
         (1) As a result the venous oxygen content of the patient will not be significantly decreased, and
         (2) a-vD_{O_2} will decrease
         (3) Because the tissue is extracting less oxygen per given volume of blood, the difference between the arterial and venous oxygen contents becomes smaller, regardless of the actual content of each.

4. In patients with poor cardiovascular reserves, a decrease in arterial oxygen content may not affect CO.
    a. If the patient's metabolic rate and CO are constant but arterial oxygen content is decreased, then a-vDo$_2$ will increase.
    b. If the patient's metabolic rate is constant and the CO and arterial oxygen content are decreased, then a-vDo$_2$ will also increase.
5. With the appropriate application of PEEP the a-vDo$_2$ should return toward normal levels.
    a. If PEEP is applied and the a-vDo$_2$ levels increase beyond acceptable limits, cardiovascular reserves are questionable. Fluid therapy or pharmacologic support may be indicated.
    b. If, with the application of PEEP, a-vDo$_2$ values increase appropriately but then exceed upper limits, PEEP is beginning to adversely affect CO. Fluid therapy, pharmacologic support, or a decrease in PEEP level may be indicated.

PEEP (cm H$_2$O)	a-vDo$_2$ (vol%)	CO (L/min)
0	2.8	12.2
5	3.0	10.5
10	3.3	9.0
12	3.6	7.5
15	4.0	6.0
18	5.6	3.5

In this table it is assumed the patient's cardiovascular reserves are good. The application of 5 to 15 cm H$_2$O PEEP results in appropriate increases in a-vDo$_2$. However, with the application of 18 cm H$_2$O PEEP, CO was adversely affected, causing a-vDo$_2$ to increase significantly toward the upper limits of normal. Fluid therapy, pharmacologic support, or decreasing PEEP is indicated.

L. Effect of PEEP on oxygen transport
    1. Oxygen transport is defined as CO times arterial oxygen content (CaO$_2$).

$$O_2 \text{ transport} = CO \times CaO_2 \tag{1}$$

    2. With the development of ARDS, oxygen transport normally decreases because of the decrease in CaO$_2$.
    3. As PEEP is applied and CaO$_2$ is increased oxygen transport improves.
    4. With excessive application of PEEP, oxygen transport may decrease because of the effect of PEEP on CO. If this occurs, fluid therapy, pharmacologic support, or decreasing PEEP is indicated.
M. Work of breathing
    1. The appropriate application of PEEP, should decrease the work of breathing by
        a. Maintaining alveoli expanded
        b. Increasing compliance
        c. Improving oxygenation
        d. Reducing ventilatory drive
        e. Minimizing the effects of auto-PEEP (see Section VI, Auto-PEEP or Intrinsic PEEP)
    2. However, if PEEP causes overdistention work of breathing will increase.
    3. The potential for PEEP to increase the work of breathing is greatest when PEEP is applied to the lung without recruitable volume and at levels >10 cm H$_2$O.
    4. The addition of pressure support to the applied PEEP may reduce the work of breathing to pre-PEEP levels.
N. Effects of PEEP on closing volume
    1. Closing volume is that point in a forced vital capacity (FVC) maneuver at which gravity-dependent airways close.

2. The point at which gravity-dependent airways close may become a larger percentage of the FVC and exceed FRC in anesthetized individuals, postoperative patients, and obese patients.
3. PEEP may have the effect of decreasing closing volume and improving oxygenation in the above-defined patients; however, no conclusive data supporting this are available.
O. Effect on intracranial pressure
   1. Because PEEP impedes venous return, it may increase intracranial pressure by causing blood to pool in the cranium.
   2. However, because a Starling resistor located between the sagittal sinus and the cerebral veins controls cerebral blood flow, cerebral blood flow is not markedly affected unless PEEP levels are high.
   3. The effect of PEEP is greatest if cerebral autoregulation is impaired by closed head injury or other factors compromising central nervous system function.
   4. If the head of the bed is elevated 30 degrees, PEEP levels equal to or greater than 10 cm H_2O may be applied without an effect on intracranial pressure.
P. Barotrauma and PEEP
   1. Any time positive pressure is applied to the lung, the likelihood of barotrauma is increased.
   2. However, barotrauma normally occurs with high peak alveolar pressure and marked lung disease or when patients fight the ventilator or engage in any activity that markedly increases intrapulmonary pressure, producing a high peak alveolar pressure.
   3. When high levels of PEEP are applied careful monitoring for barotrauma must be maintained. This is necessary because the lung requiring high levels of PEEP is significantly diseased, and any increase in peak alveolar pressures may result in barotrauma.

III. **Indications for PEEP Therapy (Box 40-1)**
   A. The primary indication for PEEP therapy is ALI/ARDS.
      1. ALI/ARDS (see Chapter 23) is characterized by
         a. Atelectasis and consolidation
         b. Decreased pulmonary compliance
         c. Decreased FRC
         d. Refractory hypoxemia
         e. Increased intrapulmonary shunting
         f. Altered surfactant function
      2. For PEEP to be most effective it should be applied early after diagnosis as part of a lung protective ventilation strategy.
      3. A number of approaches have been used to apply optimal PEEP.
         a. An increasing PEEP trial
         b. The use of a PEEP/F_IO_2 algorithm that is either written or empirical

---

BOX 40-1

Indications for PEEP/CPAP

Primary indication
ALI/ARDS

Secondary indications
Acute cardiogenic pulmonary edema
Chest trauma
Apnea of prematurity
Obstructive sleep apnea
Postoperative atelectasis
Chronic obstructive pulmonary disease
Asthma
Artificial airway placement

    c. The use of the inflation limb of the pressure-volume (P-V) curve of the total respiratory system

    d. The use of the deflation limb of the P-V curve of the total respiratory system

4. Increasing PEEP trial

    a. This approach starts at a PEEP level less than needed and increases PEEP in a stepwise manner (2 to 3 cm H_2O/step) to a PEEP level higher than required.

    b. Various physiologic variables (see Table 40-1) are monitored at each PEEP step. Most commonly the following variables are measured.

        (1) PaO_2 or SpO_2

        (2) $PaCO_2$

        (3) BP

        (4) Heart rate

        (5) Respiratory system compliance

        (6) Arterial BP

        (7) When available pulmonary hemodynamics and cardiac output should be monitored.

    c. The optimal PEEP level using this approach is the level that results in the best overall response from all of these variables.

    d. Ideally an increased PaO_2 (SpO_2), unchanged or decreased $PaCO_2$, and increased compliance without hemodynamic compromise (Table 40-2) identifies the optimal setting.

    e. Normally in patients with severe ARDS an increasing PEEP trial results in a PEEP level of approximately 12 to 16 cm H_2O; however, in some patients PEEP levels of ≥ 20 cm H_2O may be indicated, and in others 8 to 12 cm H_2O PEEP may be indicated.

    f. In patients with ALI, PEEP levels of 8 to 12 cm H_2O are the most commonly required.

    g. An increasing PEEP trial is not the most useful approach to set PEEP after lung recruitment maneuver because it starts at a PEEP level less than required, which may result in derecruitment of unstable lung units.

    h. Once the PEEP level is set the F_IO_2 is reduced to the lowest level maintaining the target PaO_2.

5. PEEP/F_IO_2 table

    a. The most widely used table for setting PEEP is that established by the ARDSnet (Table 40-3).

    b. This table sequentially increases PEEP and then F_IO_2 until the desired PaO_2 is established.

    c. The F_IO_2 and PEEP are sequentially decreased in a similar manner if the PaO_2 is above target level.

    d. This table is difficult to use after lung recruitment because it tends to start at a PEEP level lower than required, allowing for derecruitment of lung units.

    e. This approach does not consider the lung mechanics of the individual patient.

TABLE 40-2

Increasing PEEP Trial

PEEP cm H_2O	PaO_2 mm Hg	$PaCO_2$ mm Hg	Compliance ml/cm H_2O	Cardiac Output L/min	Mean Arterial Pressure mm Hg	Mean Pulmonary Artery Pressure mm Hg
8	50	48	26	7.2	98	32
10	56	48	26	6.6	96	33
12	62	46	28	6.0	92	30
14	73	48	28	6.2	92	29
16	**130**	**42**	**32**	**4.8**	**88**	**28**
18	132	42	30	4.0	80	26
20	128	52	28	3.6	70	24

16 cm H_2O PEEP is the optimal level in this example. Once identified F_IO_2 is decreased until the PaO_2 is in the target range.

TABLE 40-3

ARDSnet PEEP/F$_I$O$_2$ Table

F$_I$O$_2$	0.3	0.4	0.4	0.5	0.5	0.6	0.7	0.7	0.7	0.8	0.9	0.9	1.0
PEEP	5	5	8	8	10	10	10	12	14	14	14	16	18-24

From ARDSnet: Ventilation with lower tidal volumes as compared with traditional tidal volumes for acute lung injury and the acute respiratory distress syndrome. *N Engl J Med* 342:1301-1308, 2000.

6. P-V curve of the inflation limb of the respiratory system
   a. Figure 40-4 illustrates the inflation and deflation limbs of the P-V curve of the respiratory system.
   b. Note on the inflation limb the P$_{flex}$ or lower inflation point. This is an area of the curve where lung compliance increases and is considered the pressure where lung recruitment begins.
   c. The actual P$_{flex}$ is determined by drawing tangents to the slopes of the curve above and below this point of curvature.
   d. The meeting of these tangents is the lower inflection point (P$_{flex}$).
   e. Setting PEEP using the inflation P-V curve calls for PEEP to be set at P$_{flex}$ + 2 cm H$_2$O.
   f. This level of PEEP is believed to avoid significant derecruitment at end exhalation and maintain lung open after lung recruitment maneuver.
   g. This is the only approach to setting PEEP that has shown outcome improvement in animal and clinical trials.
   h. In at least two randomized controlled clinical trials of severe ARDS patients, PEEP at P$_{flex}$ + 2 cm H$_2$O was associated with improved survival or reduced systemic inflammatory mediator response.
   i. However, performing a P-V curve is difficult at the bedside of critically ill patients.
   j. Widespread use of this approach will not occur until the P-V curve and P$_{flex}$ can be automatically determined by mechanical ventilators.
   k. This approach identifies a PEEP level of approximately 14 to 16 cm H$_2$O in most severe ARDS patients but may result in a PEEP of 10 to 20 cm H$_2$O.

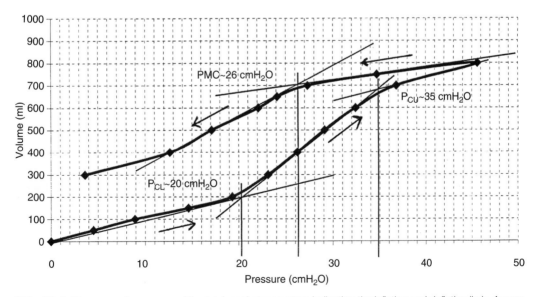

FIG. 40-4 Pressure-volume curve of the total respiratory system indicating the inflation and deflation limb. Arrows indicate direction of flow. *P$_{CL}$*, Lower inflection point-P$_{flex}$; *P$_{CU}$*, upper inflection point; *PMC*, point of maximum compliance change.

l. In some ARDS patients it is impossible to identify a P_{flex} from the inflation P-V curve.

7. P-V curve deflation limb
   a. In Figure 40-4 the deflation limb of the P-V curve of the respiratory system is illustrated.
   b. The use of the deflation limb of the P-V curve requires that the lung be first recruited before PEEP is set (see Chapter 41).
   c. After lung recruitment PEEP is set at approximately 18 to 20 cm H_2O, higher than the level normally required.
   d. Once PEEP is set at this level the F_IO_2 is decreased until PaO_2 is in target range.
   e. Then PEEP is decreased in small steps (1 to 2 cm H_2O), and PaO_2 is reassessed at each step.
   f. As PEEP is decreased the PaO_2 will begin to increase because in most patients a PEEP of 20 cm H_2O is excessive, causing cardiovascular compromise.
   g. PaO_2 will then begin to decrease. When the PaO_2 decreases to approximately 90% of the maximum PaO_2 the trial is stopped.
   h. The PEEP level preceding the PEEP level causing the decrease in PaO_2 is the optimal PEEP.
   i. After completing the decremental PEEP trial the lung is again recruited, and PEEP and F_IO_2 are set at the identified levels.
   j. SpO_2 may be substituted for PaO_2, but one must ensure that the F_IO_2 is initially decreased to ensure the SpO_2 is 90% to 95% so that a change in PEEP will identify a change in SpO_2.
   k. This appears to be the best method to determine the minimum PEEP that maintains the oxygenation benefit of a lung recruitment maneuver.
   l. An example of a decremental PEEP trial is illustrated in Table 40-4.

8. PEEP trials and hemodynamics
   a. Systemic and pulmonary hemodynamics ideally should be carefully monitored during any PEEP trial.
   b. Before a PEEP trial is started hemodynamic stability should be ensured.
   c. During the trial if the patient becomes hemodynamically unstable, the trial should be stopped.
   d. The optimal PEEP level should always be determined with the patient's hemodynamic status as part of the decision.

9. Withdrawal or decreasing PEEP levels
   a. As indicated already PEEP is intended to maintain unstable lung units open.
   b. As a general rule F_IO_2 should be decreased before PEEP.
   c. Once F_IO_2 is <50% PEEP should be slowly decreased.
   d. Ideally PEEP is decreased in 2-cm H_2O steps, one step if tolerated, every 2 to 4 hours.

TABLE 40-4

Decremental PEEP Trial

PEEP cm H_2O	PaO_2 mm Hg	Cardiac Output L/min	Mean Arterial Blood Pressure mm Hg	Mean Pulmonary Artery Pressure mm Hg	Compliance ml/cm H_2O
20	68	3.2	72	20	22
18	72	3.8	76	22	23
16	76	4.2	80	26	25
14	78	4.4	82	28	26
12	**70**	**4.4**	**82**	**28**	**30**
10	68	5.0	88	30	25
8	66	5.2	92	32	23

12 cm H_2O is the optimal PEEP is this example. Before PEEP was decreased F_IO_2 was adjusted to place PaO_2 in the target range.

     e.   The decrease is slow because some lung units may derecruit slowly over hours as PEEP is decreased.

     f.   If after decreasing PEEP the PaO_2 decreases, the PEEP should be reestablished.

     g.   When this occurs it indicates that the lung is still unstable and requires the PEEP level previously set be reestablished.

B. Cardiogenic pulmonary edema

    1. The use of PEEP (CPAP) in acute cardiogenic pulmonary edema has a direct impact on the preload of the left ventricle.

    2. The increased intrathoracic pressure resulting from the application of PEEP (CPAP) reduces venous return, decreasing preload, and as a result decreases fluid movement into the intrapulmonary space.

    3. PEEP (CPAP) also improves oxygenation and decreases the work of breathing.

    4. Essentially PEEP (CPAP) buys time for pharmacologic treatment to improve the patient's cardiovascular status.

    5. Patients with acute cardiogenic pulmonary edema can usually be treated with 8 to 12 cm H_2O mask CPAP provided they can still maintain a normal $PaCO_2$.

    6. In patients with hypoxemic and hypercarbic respiratory failure, noninvasive ventilation by mask (BiPAP) is indicated. Five to 8 cm H_2O CPAP with ventilating pressure of 8 to 12 cm H_2O should be applied.

    7. Patients with myocardial infarction normally require intubation and ventilation.

    8. In many patients 2 to 4 hours of mask CPAP is sufficient to reverse the hypoxemic respiratory failure and allow the pharmacologic action of drug therapy to take effect.

    9. One hundred percent O_2 should initially be administered regardless of the approach to support ventilation.

C. Chest trauma

    1. Chest trauma frequently leads to ALI/ARDS and as a result the use of PEEP.

    2. On initial presentation the use of mask CPAP may help to reduce the work of breathing, improve oxygenation, and stabilize the chest wall.

    3. However, care should be noted because many trauma victims are hemodynamically unstable and may not tolerate the 8 to 12 cm H_2O CPAP required.

D. Apnea of prematurity

    1. PEEP (CPAP) splints the pharynx open in neonates, preventing obstruction and some apnea.

    2. The increased pressure in the pharynx also stimulates respiration.

    3. Usually applied by nasal prongs, CPAP of approximately 2 to 4 cm H_2O reduces the frequency of apnea.

E. Obstructive sleep apnea (OSA)

    1. Nasal CPAP of approximately 8 to 12 cm H_2O is used extensively to manage OSA in adults.

    2. As with neonates PEEP (CPAP) splints open the upper airway, preventing obstruction by the soft palate and base of the tongue.

    3. CPAP is also effective for some patients with central sleep apnea.

    4. A nocturnal sleep study is necessary to determine whether CPAP will be effective and at which level.

    5. CPAP also has been increasingly used for patients with chronic congestive heart failure.

    6. Many of these patients also have OSA.

    7. In some patients the OSA results in the development of heart failure because of the chronic periods of nocturnal hypoxemia.

F. Postoperative atelectasis

    1. Some data indicate that the use of mask CPAP treatments (20 to 60 minutes) reduces postoperative atelectasis.

    2. In this setting normally 10 cm H_2O CPAP is used.

    3. However, simple mobilization of the patient accomplishes the same goals. Most agree that CPAP is unnecessary in this setting.

G. COPD

    1. In COPD patients PEEP and CPAP are generally used to offset the effects of auto-PEEP (see Section VI, Auto-PEEP or Intrinsic PEEP).

2. During assisted ventilation PEEP levels from 5 to 15 cm H_2O are commonly used to balance auto-PEEP levels.
3. This improves trigger synchrony and overall patient-ventilator synchrony.
H. Asthma
1. Similar to COPD, asthma is associated with significant levels of auto-PEEP.
2. As a result some have used mask CPAP to offset auto-PEEP and decrease the work of breathing.
3. However, in many patients auto-PEEP is not a result of dynamic airway obstruction and applied PEEP only adds to the total PEEP level in asthma (see Section VI, Auto-PEEP or Intrinsic PEEP).
4. As a result the use of mask CPAP for patients with acute asthma is controversial.
I. Physiologic PEEP
1. This is the application of 3 to 5 cm H_2O PEEP to replace the glottic mechanism.
2. The placement of an artificial airway results in a reflexive decrease in FRC.
3. This occurs in all individuals but has been demonstrated to be clinically significant in only two populations.
   a. Neonatal and small pediatric patients: This group should not have a short-term artificial airway in place without 3 to 5 cm H_2O PEEP. If extubation is indicated, they are extubated from 3 to 5 cm H_2O PEEP rather than from atmospheric pressure.
   b. Patients with severe COPD: Establishment of an artificial airway under acute conditions again results in a significant decrease in the FRC, causing hypoxemia. It is advisable to maintain 5 cm H_2O PEEP in these patients until extubation.
   c. PEEP of 3 to 5 cm H_2O is often used in all patients requiring a short-term artificial airway. The efficacy of such treatment has not been established, nor have any adverse reactions been documented.

IV. **Monitoring PEEP Therapy**
A. With the application of PEEP or the alteration of PEEP levels, extensive monitoring of the patient's cardiopulmonary status must be performed.
B. Monitoring should be done after each PEEP adjustment and periodically thereafter.
C. Gas exchange should be monitored.
1. Arterial blood gases
2. Oxyhemoglobin percent saturation
D. Pulmonary mechanics should be monitored.
1. Evaluation of V_T, RR, and work of breathing if appropriate
2. Effective static compliance if patient is in control mode or not spontaneously ventilating
E. Cardiovascular function should be monitored.
1. Pulse and BP
2. Skin color
3. Skin turgor
4. Skin temperature
5. Urinary output
6. Sensorium
7. CO
8. CI
9. PAP
10. CVP
11. PWP
12. $P\bar{v}o_2$
13. a-vDo_2
14. Oxygen transport

V. **Periodic Discontinuation of PEEP**
A. The periodic discontinuation of PEEP should be avoided. This is particularly true when higher levels of PEEP are used.

    B. Discontinuation of PEEP on a periodic basis results in
1. Decreased FRC (derecruitment)
2. Significant decreases in Pa_{O_2}
3. Increase in intrapulmonary shunt
4. Possible increased venous return
5. Decreased pulmonary compliance
6. A complete reversal of the changes accomplished with the application of PEEP

    C. PEEP should not be discontinued when hemodynamic monitoring is performed.

    D. Inline suction catheters should be used when PEEP is applied to avoid discontinuation of PEEP during suctioning.

VI. Auto-PEEP or Intrinsic PEEP

    A. Auto-PEEP also referred to as intrinsic PEEP, unidentified PEEP, endogenous PEEP, or occult PEEP is a result of incomplete emptying of the lung at end-exhalation or air trapping.

    B. It is termed unidentified PEEP because auto-PEEP is not identified on the pressure manometer of the ventilator unless an end-expiratory hold is applied (Figure 40-5).

    C. Auto-PEEP develops because of a number of factors.
1. Inadequate expiratory time: As noted in Figure 40-6 it takes approximately four expiratory time constants for passive exhalation to be complete.

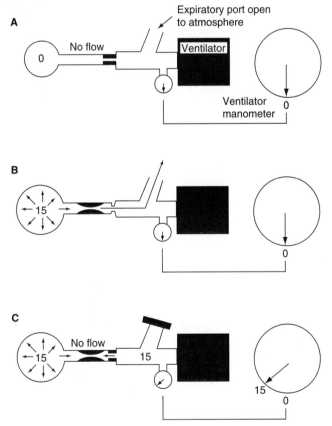

FIG. 40-5 Relationship between alveolar, central airway, and ventilator circuit pressure under **(A)** normal conditions and in the presence of severe dynamic airway obstruction, **(B)** with expiratory port open, and **(C)** with expiratory port occluded. Auto-positive end-expiratory pressure (PEEP) level is identified by creating an end-expiratory hold, allowing alveolar, central airway, and ventilator circuit pressure to equilibrate. Note that during equilibration auto-PEEP level can be read on the system manometer.

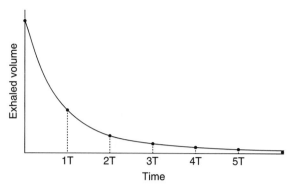

FIG. 40-6 Relationship between volume passively exhaled and number of elapsed time constants (RCs): 63%, 86.5%, 95%, 98.2%, and 99.3% of tidal volume is exhaled in one, two, three, four, and five RCs, respectively.

    a. In normal adults the expiratory time constant is approximately 0.3 to 0.4 second. As a result approximately 1.5 to 2.0 seconds is sufficient expiratory time for complete passive exhalation.

    b. In those with obstructive lung disease expiratory time constants can be as long as 1 to 2 seconds, making air trapping and auto-PEEP impossible to prevent.

    c. Auto-PEEP developed as a result of inadequate expiratory time can occur in any individual simply by sufficiently increasing minute ventilation or decreasing expiratory time.

  2. Increased airway obstruction increases the expiratory time constants.

    a. This occurs in patients with asthma or COPD.

    b. However, the mechanism and as a result the response to applied PEEP are different.

    c. In patients with COPD airway obstruction, producing auto-PEEP is primarily a result of unstable bronchial or bronchiolar walls.

    d. The lumen of the airway in those with COPD is grossly affected by intrathoracic pressure.

      (1) During inspiration the walls of the airway in patients with COPD are dilated by inspiratory efforts.

      (2) As a result airway obstruction decreases during inspiration.

      (3) The exact opposite occurs during exhalation: the increased intrathoracic pressure decreases the lumen of the airway causing obstruction.

      (4) In patients with COPD the obstruction is dynamic. This type of airway obstruction benefits from the application of PEEP during assisted ventilation.

    e. In patients with asthma, airway obstruction is caused by

      (1) Secretions

      (2) Bronchoconstriction

      (3) Mucosal edema

    f. As a result the obstruction is generally fixed and does not vary greatly from inspiration to expiration.

    g. Inspiration is as difficult as expiration because resistance is increased in both.

    h. Applied PEEP in this setting does not usually minimize patient trigger effort; it simply increases overall total PEEP level.

  3. It is impossible to clearly define the exact mechanism responsible for auto-PEEP in a given patient; as a result many believe a trial of applied PEEP to reduce the work of breathing associated with auto-PEEP is indicated in all patients with airway obstruction requiring assisted ventilation.

D. Physiologic effects of auto-PEEP

  1. Auto-PEEP essentially causes the same physiologic effects as applied PEEP.

  2. However, it occurs in a lung with normal or increased compliance.

  3. As a result the effect of auto-PEEP on hemodynamics in COPD patients is greater than applied PEEP in patients with ALI/ARDS.

4. Auto-PEEP markedly increases the work of breathing.
   a. This occurs because the auto-PEEP level must be decompressed on each breath to establish a pressure gradient for gas to flow into the airway (Table 40-5).
   b. As a result if auto-PEEP is 10 cm H_2O, the patient must decrease alveolar pressure >10 cm H_2O for air to flow into the alveoli.
   c. In those with COPD, applying PEEP generally offsets the auto-PEEP level, decreasing work of breathing.
   d. In patients with asthma, applied PEEP is usually additive to auto-PEEP, increasing the work of breathing.

E. Determination of auto-PEEP
   1. As illustrated in Figure 40-5 clinically the best method to assess the level of auto-PEEP in the passively ventilated patient is to perform an end-expiratory hold.
      a. Most modern intensive care unit ventilators incorporate an end-expiratory hold or auto-PEEP measurement control. When activated the increased end-expiratory pressure is the auto-PEEP level (Figure 40-7).
      b. If patients have spontaneous inspiratory efforts it is difficult to make this measurement because an end-expiratory plateau is not achievable.
   2. In spontaneously breathing patients or patients on assisted ventilation the best method to measure auto-PEEP is by evaluating esophageal pressure change at the same time airway pressure or flow is assessed.
      a. As noted in Figure 40-8, if auto-PEEP is present esophageal pressure (a reflection of pleural pressure) decreases before airway pressure or flow is affected.
      b. The magnitude of the change in airway pressure from baseline to the level causing a change in airway pressure or flow is equal to the auto-PEEP level.
   3. Evaluation of expiratory flow provides an indication of the presence of auto-PEEP but not the precise level of auto-PEEP.
      a. Figure 40-9 is an illustration of airway pressure, flow, and volume waveforms in a patient with normal lungs receiving mechanical ventilation.
      b. Note that expiratory flow does not return to zero before the beginning of the next breath. When this occurs there is still a pressure gradient from the alveoli to the airway causing expiratory flow.
      c. Note also that expiratory flow decreases in a linear manner from peak expiratory flow, indicating the absence of dynamic airway obstruction.
      d. Figure 40-10 is from a patient with COPD who has auto-PEEP. As with Figure 40-9, flow does not return to zero before the end of the breath.
      e. The expiratory flow pattern in Figure 40-10 is different from that in Figure 40-9 because in COPD there is marked dynamic airflow obstruction.
      f. With COPD the peak expiratory flow decreases in an exponential manner with a low flow throughout much of the breath.
      g. The level of end-expiratory flow does not indicate the level of auto-PEEP. In Figure 40-9 the auto-PEEP level *could be* 3 cm H_2O, and in Figure 40-10 *it could be* 10 cm H_2O.

TABLE 40-5

Pressure Change Necessary to Inspire with Auto-PEEP

	Asthma/COPD *No* PEEP	COPD PEEP 8 cm H_2O	Asthma PEEP 8 cm H_2O
Auto-PEEP level, cm H_2O	10	10	10
Airway pressure, cm H_2O	0	8	8
Pressure gradient, cm H_2O required to trigger ventilator	>10	>2	>18

In COPD, applied PEEP normally offsets auto-PEEP; in asthma, applied PEEP is normally additive to auto-PEEP.

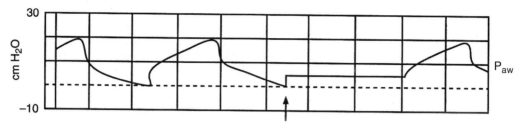

FIG. 40-7 Measurement of auto-positive end-expiratory pressure (PEEP) (arrow) using an end-expiratory hold on the Servo 900C ventilator. Note that peak airway pressure is not affected on the inspiration after measurement because auto-PEEP is present even though unnoticed on every breath.

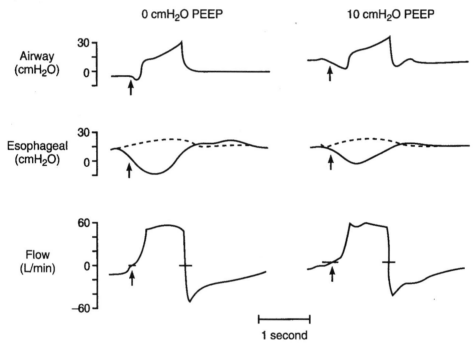

FIG. 40-8 Assessment of the level of auto-positive end-expiratory pressure (PEEP) in spontaneously breathing patients by evaluation of esophageal pressure change relative to either airway opening pressure or flow at airway opening. Arrows indicate pressure and flow change at airway opening. The change in esophageal pressure between baseline and the level that allows change in airway opening pressure or in flow is equal to the auto-PEEP level. Note effect of 10 cm H_2O applied PEEP on the level of auto-PEEP *(right)*.

  4. Patient RR and ventilator response rate
     a. If no auto-PEEP is present every patient inspiratory effort should trigger a mechanical breath.
     b. As noted in Figure 40-11, in patients with auto-PEEP the ventilator does not sense many inspiratory efforts.
     c. As a result the ventilator responds at a rate much slower than the patient's actual RR.
     d. Thus any time the patient's RR is counted and it is higher than the ventilator response rate, auto-PEEP is present, provided the ventilator is functioning properly.
  F. Application of auto-PEEP in COPD
     1. PEEP should be slowly increased in one to two cm H_2O increments until the patient rate and ventilator response rate are equal.

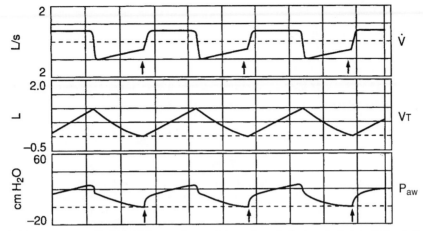

FIG. 40-9 Airway pressure (P_{aw}) and flow waveforms during volume-limited controlled ventilation in the presence of auto-positive end-expiratory pressure (PEEP). The initial airway pressure demonstrates a rapid initial increase *(arrow)*, approximating the auto-PEEP level and then gradually increasing to peak P_{aw}. Expiratory gas flow does not return to zero *(arrow)* in the presence of auto-PEEP.

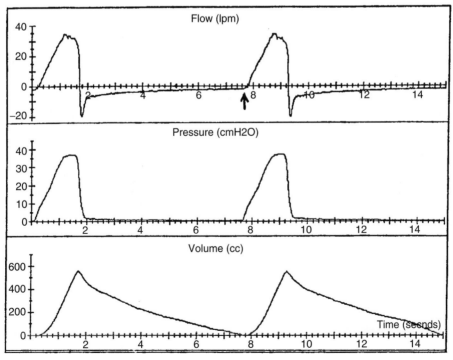

FIG. 40-10 Airway pressure, flow, and volume waveforms during volume-targeted control ventilation in the presence of auto-positive end-expiratory pressure (PEEP). Expiratory gas flow shows an initial spike that rapidly decreases to a low level throughout the prolonged expiratory phase. Note that expiratory gas flow does not return to zero, indicating the presence of auto-PEEP.

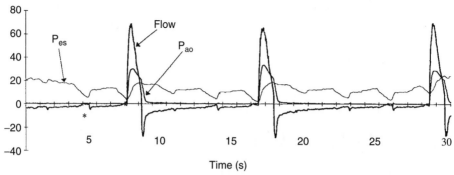

FIG. 40-11 Esophageal pressure (P_{es}), airway opening pressure (P_{ao}), and flow in a patient with auto-positive end-expiratory pressure (PEEP) and air trapping on volume assist/control mode. The units are cm H_2O for the pressure tracing and L/min for flow. The patient's inspiratory efforts are identified by the negative P_{es} swings. The PEEP is set at zero. P_{ao} appropriately decreases to zero during expiration, demonstrating little circuit or valve resistance. Auto-PEEP is evident, with one triggered breath every three to four efforts. Prolonged expiratory flow is caused by airflow limitation. P_{es} swings have little effect in retarding the expiratory flow and even less effect on P_{ao}, depending on the phase of ventilation.

2. The application of PEEP to approximately 80% of the measured auto-PEEP level does not affect lung mechanics in COPD patients.
3. If applied to the appropriate level the patient's work of breathing decreases, the patient's ventilatory pattern improves, and patient-ventilatory synchrony improves.

G. Effect of auto-PEEP on ventilator pressures and flows
1. In volume ventilation any adjustment that results in an increase in auto-PEEP causes peak airway pressure and plateau pressure to increase.
    a. If when applying PEEP plateau pressure increases, either the PEEP application is excessive or the obstruction is *not* dynamic.
2. In pressure ventilation the development of auto-PEEP causes the VT to decrease because ventilating pressure is the variable that is set.

BIBLIOGRAPHY

Albert RK: Non-respiratory effects of positive end-expiratory pressure. *Respir Care* 33:464-471, 1988.

Amato MBP, Barbas CSV, Medeiros DM, et al: Effect of a protective-ventilation strategy on mortality in the acute respiratory distress syndrome. *N Engl J Med* 338:347-354, 1998.

Benson MS, Pierson DJ: Auto-PEEP during mechanical ventilation of adults. *Respir Care* 33:557-568, 1988.

Burton GC, Hodgkin JE, Ward JJ: *Respiratory Care*, ed 4. Philadelphia, JB Lippincott, 1997.

Hess DJ, Kacmarek RM: *Essentials of Mechanical Ventilation*, ed 2. New York, McGraw Hill, 2002.

Hess DJ, MacIntyre NR, Mishoc SC, Galvin WF, Adams AB, Saposnick AB: *Respiratory Care Principles and Practice*. Philadelphia, WB Saunders, 2002.

Pierson DJ, Kacmarek RM: *Foundations of Respiratory Care*. New York, Churchill Livingstone, 1993.

Shapiro BA, Cane RD, Harrison RA: Positive end-expiratory pressure in acute lung injury. *Chest* 83:558-563, 1983.

Shapiro BA, Cane RD, Harrison RA: Positive end-expiratory pressure therapy in adults with special reference to acute lung injury: a review of the literature and suggested clinical correlations. *Crit Care Med* 12:127-141, 1984.

The Acute Respiratory Distress Syndrome Network: Ventilation with lower tidal volumes as compared with traditional tidal volumes for acute lung injury and the acute respiratory distress syndrome. *N Engl J Med* 342:1301-1308, 2000.

Wilkins RL, Stoller JK, Scanlon CL: *Egan's Fundamentals of Respiratory Therapy*, ed 8. St. Louis, Mosby, 2003.

Chapter 41

Initiation, Maintenance, and Weaning from Mechanical Ventilation

I. **Physiologic Effects of Positive Pressure Ventilation**
   A. Increased mean airway pressure
      1. Normally mean airway pressure is slightly negative (below atmospheric) during inspiration (Figure 41-1, *A*).
      2. Because positive pressure ablates the normal mechanisms for gas movement, intrapulmonary pressures are usually supraatmospheric (see Figure 41-1, *B*).
      3. The extent that intrapulmonary pressure is increased depends on
         a. Tidal volume (V_T)
         b. Inspiratory time (T_I)
         c. Inspiratory:expiratory (I:E) ratio
         d. Respiratory rate (RR)
         e. Airway resistance (R_{AW})
         f. Pulmonary and thoracic compliance
   B. Increased mean intrathoracic pressure (see Figure 41-1, *B*)
      1. Transmission of intrapulmonary pressure to the intrathoracic space depends on pulmonary and thoracic compliance. The stiffer the lung, generally the lower the amount of pressure transmitted from the intrapulmonary to the intrathoracic space. In contrast, the stiffer the thorax, the greater the amount of pressure transmitted to the intrathoracic space.
      2. In most patients requiring mechanical ventilation, the mean intrathoracic pressure changes from negative to positive.
   C. Decreased venous return (see Figure 41-1, *B*)
      1. Because intrathoracic pressures become positive with the application of mechanical ventilation, the thoracic pump mechanism assisting venous return is eliminated.
      2. As a result the pressure gradient favoring venous flow to the right side of the heart is decreased and right ventricular filling is impaired.
      3. Positive pressure, especially positive end-expiratory pressure (PEEP), also increases pulmonary vascular resistance, which decreases right ventricular filling and cardiac output.
      4. Positive pressure also increases right ventricular afterload and can result in right ventricular hypertrophy with a shift in the ventricular septum and compromised left ventricular function.
      5. However, in patients with left ventricular dysfunction positive pressure may decrease left ventricular afterload, increasing cardiac output and left ventricular function.

737

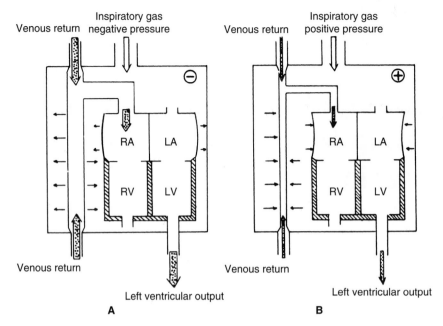

FIG. 41-1 A, Effect of spontaneous ventilation on intrathoracic pressure and cardiac output. **B,** Effect of positive pressure on intrathoracic pressure and cardiac output.

     6. Frequently the decreased transmural pressure across the vena cava is large enough to require fluid therapy to maintain appropriate right ventricular filling as mechanical ventilation is initially applied.

     7. Most patients are hypoxemic, acidotic, and hypercapnic before the institution of mechanical ventilation, which causes an increased sympathetic tone. The normalization of acid-base balance, the relief of hypoxemia, and the decrease in work of breathing (WOB) with mechanical ventilation result in a marked decrease in sympathetic tone. This may result in

        a. Decreased vascular tone and relative hypovolemia

        b. Decreased heart rate

        c. Decreased force of myocardial contraction

D. Decreased cardiac output

     1. Because venous return and sympathetic tone are decreased, there is some decrease in cardiac output.

     2. With appropriate fluid therapy and pharmacologic support, adequate cardiac output can be maintained.

E. Increased intracranial pressure (ICP)

     1. Because venous return is decreased, blood pools in the periphery and in the cranium.

     2. The increased volume of blood in the cranium increases ICP.

F. Decreased urinary output

     1. Decreased cardiac output results in decreased renal blood flow, which alters renal filtration pressures and decreases urine formation.

     2. Decreased venous return and decreased right atrial pressures are interpreted as a decrease in overall blood volume. As a result, antidiuretic hormone levels and natriuretic peptide levels are increased and urine formation is decreased (see Chapters 13 and 14).

G. Decreased WOB
1. Because the ventilator provides at least part of the force necessary to ventilate, the patient's WOB decreases.
2. The amount of work performed by the ventilator and the amount performed by the patient vary, depending on the approach used to ventilate and the actual setting of ventilating parameters.

H. Mechanical bronchodilation
1. Positive pressure causes a mechanical dilation of the conducting airways.
2. The transmural pressure gradients affecting the airways are always greater than during normal spontaneous ventilation.
3. However, intubation usually results in an increase in resistance to flow in the upper airway and puts the patient at risk for contamination of the lower respiratory tract.

I. Increased deadspace ventilation
1. Because positive pressure distends conducting airways and inhibits venous return, the portion of the V_T that is deadspace increases.
2. There also is an alteration in the normal distribution of ventilation. A greater percentage of ventilation goes to the apices and less to the bases than in spontaneous ventilation.
3. Normal deadspace/V_T ratios are 0.20 to 0.40; however, mechanical ventilation will cause these ratios to increase to 0.40 to 0.60 in the normal individual.
4. The level of ventilation required by a patient depends on the Pa_{CO_2}, alveolar ventilation, and tissue CO_2 production.

$$Pa_{CO_2} \propto \dot{V}_{CO_2}/\dot{V}_A \qquad (1)$$

or

$$Pa_{CO_2} = (\dot{V}_{CO_2} \times 0.863)\,(\dot{V}_E \times [1 - \frac{V_D}{V_T}]) \qquad (2)$$

where $\dot{V}_{CO_2}$ is CO_2 production, $\dot{V}_A$ is alveolar ventilation, $\dot{V}_E$ is minute ventilation, V_D is deadspace volume, and V_T is tidal volume.

J. Increased intrapulmonary shunt
1. With positive pressure ventilation, gas distribution and pulmonary perfusion are altered.
2. Ventilation to the most gravity-dependent aspects of the lung is decreased, whereas blood flow to these areas is increased.
3. Normal intrapulmonary shunts are approximately 2.0% to 5.0%; however, mechanical ventilation may increase the shunt fraction to approximately 10% in the normal individual.
4. Allowing some level of spontaneous ventilation (triggering the breath) minimizes the ventilation/perfusion mismatch.

K. The setting of ventilator parameters may induce hyperventilation or hypoventilation.

L. RR, V_T, T_I, and flow rate may all be manipulated.

M. Effect on gastrointestinal (GI) tract
1. The stress produced by positive pressure ventilation may lead to increased gastric secretion and gastric bleeding, resulting in the development of stress ulcers.
2. Agents that maintain gastric acidity may be useful to prevent ventilator-associated pneumonia (VAP).
3. Gastric distention does develop in some patients as a result of aerophagia (swallowing of air), requiring the use of a nasogastric tube.

N. Pneumonia
1. Many patients mechanically ventilated develop ventilator-associated pneumonia (VAP).
2. VAP is not a result of the ventilator circuit if appropriate precautions are taken (see Chapter 3).
3. VAP is a result of aspiration of contaminated oral and gastric secretions.

    4. The incidence of VAP can be reduced by
      a. Maintaining patients at a 30-degree head-up angle
      b. Maintaining a good seal with the airway cuff at peak inspiratory pressure. Cuff pressure should be 20 to 25 cm H_2O.
      c. Providing good oral hygiene on an every 2- to 4-hour basis
      d. Maintaining gastric acidity

O. Nutritional effects
    1. Appropriate nutritional support is difficult during mechanical ventilation.
    2. Respiratory muscle wasting and an increased risk of pneumonia and pulmonary edema develop if patients are underfed.
    3. Ventilatory requirements are increased because of increased CO_2 production if patients are overfed.

P. Sleep
    1. Mechanical ventilation disturbs normal sleep patterns.
    2. Sleep deprivation may produce delirium, patient-ventilatory dys-synchrony, and sedation-induced ventilator dependency.

Q. Effect on psychologic status: The continued stress associated with mechanical ventilation may result in
    1. Insomnia
    2. Anxiety
    3. Frustration
    4. Depression
    5. Apprehension
    6. Fear

II. Ventilator-induced Lung Injury
  A. The application of mechanical ventilation can cause lung injury, referred to as
    1. Oxygen toxicity
    2. Barotrauma
    3. Volutrauma
    4. Atelectrauma
    5. Biotrauma

  B. Oxygen toxicity
    1. High inhaled oxygen concentrations result in the formation of oxygen free radicals (e.g., superoxide, hydrogen peroxide, and hydroxyl ion).
    2. These free radicals cause ultrastructional changes in the lung similar to acute lung injury (ALI).
    3. In animal models inhalation of 100% oxygen causes death in 48 to 72 hours.
    4. Healthy volunteers breathing 100% oxygen develop inflammatory airway changes in 24 hours.
    5. However, concern regarding oxygen toxicity should never prevent the use of a high F_IO_2 in a patient who is hypoxemic.
    6. An F_IO_2 of 1.0 should always be used
      a. During suctioning
      b. During transport
      c. During periods of instability
      d. Whenever concern about an adequate Po_2 arises.
    7. But F_IO_2 should always be lowered as soon as possible to the lowest level maintaining the Pao_2 >60 mm Hg.
    8. Concerns about oxygen toxicity should not override concerns about tissue hypoxia.
    9. Ideally the F_IO_2 should be maintained ≤0.6 to minimize concerns regarding toxicity.
    10. There is some evidence that the presence of severe lung injury provides protection from oxygen toxicity.

C. Barotrauma
1. Barotrauma is the most acute and immediately severe form of ventilator-induced lung injury.
2. Barotrauma is literally air within a body space or compartment.
3. It is a result of disruption of the alveolar capillary membrane that allows air to dissect along fascial planes and accumulate within the pleural space or some other compartment (Figure 41-2).
4. The higher the peak alveolar (plateau) pressure and the greater the lung disease, the greater the likelihood of barotrauma.
5. Subcutaneous emphysema is air within the tissue.
6. The development of barotrauma can be minimized by limiting the peak alveolar pressure.
D. Volutrauma (Figure 41-3)
1. Volutrauma is lung parenchymal damage similar in presentation to acute respiratory distress syndrome (ARDS).

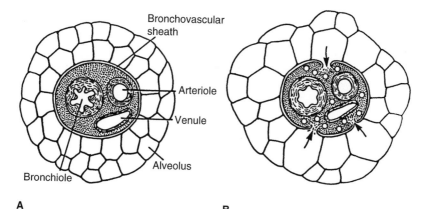

A   **B**

FIG. 41-2 Schematic of how air dissects across the lung parenchyma, resulting in barotrauma.

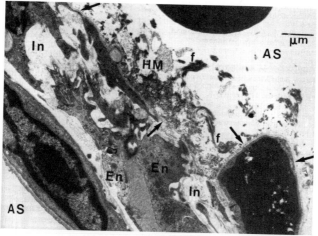

FIG. 41-3 Electron microscopic view of the cross-section of the alveolar-capillary complex of a rat ventilated with large tidal volumes at a peak pressure of 45 cm H_2O with zero positive end-expiratory pressure. Markedly altered alveolar septum with three capillaries. At the right side, the epithelial lining is destroyed, denuding the basement membrane *(arrows)*. Hyaline membrane (HM) composed of cell debris and fibrin (f) is present. Two endothelial cells (En) of another capillary are visible inside the interstitium (In). At the lower left side, a monocyte fills the lumen of a third capillary with a normal blood-air barrier.

2. Volutrauma is a result of localized overdistention of the lung.
3. It is manifested by an increase in the permeability of the alveolar capillary membrane, the development of pulmonary edema, the accumulation of neutrophils and protein, the disruption of surfactant production, the development of hyaline membranes, and a decrease in compliance of the lung.
4. Overdistending volume is best determined by assessing transpulmonary pressure (alveolar-pleural pressure).
   a. However, pleural pressure is generally not available in patients requiring mechanical ventilation.
   b. The end-inspiratory plateau pressure (P_{plat}) is clinically the best indicator of overdistention.
   c. P_{plat} in all patients should be maintained <30 cm H_2O unless the chest wall is stiff.
   d. A stiff chest wall results in a decreased transpulmonary pressure for any given P_{plat}.
   e. As a result patients with the following
      (1) Abdominal distention
      (2) Massive fluid overload
      (3) Marked obesity
      (4) Thoracic deformities
   May receive P_{plat} >30 cm H_2O without an increased likelihood of inducing lung injury.
5. Ideally to prevent volutrauma P_{plat} should be maintained <25 cm H_2O in all patients.
6. If the P_{plat} is <25 cm H_2O, VTs of 6 to 10 ml/kg ideal body weight (IBW) can be used.
7. IBW is determined by the following formulas.

$$\text{Male} = 50 + 2.3 \text{ [height (inches)} - 60)] \tag{3}$$

$$\text{Female} = 45.5 + 2.3 \text{ [height (inches)} - 60] \tag{4}$$

8. If the P_{plat} is 25 to 30 cm H_2O VTs should be maintained between 5 and 8 ml/kg IBW.
9. If the P_{plat} is ≥30 cm H_2O, VT should be ≤6 ml/kg IBW.

E. Atelectrauma
   1. Ventilator-induced lung injury is caused by the recruitment and derecruitment of unstable lung units during each ventilator cycle.
   2. Disruption of the alveolar capillary membrane is caused by the stress and strain exerted on the alveolar wall by lung recruitment.
   3. The application of 30 cm H_2O to an open lung unit can result in the development of approximately 140 cm H_2O stress on the wall of the collapsed alveoli adjacent to it.
   4. This repeated stress with each breath causes injury.
   5. To avoid this form of lung injury adequate PEEP must be applied to avoid the end-expiratory collapse of unstable lung (see Chapter 40) (Figure 41-4).
   6. As a general rule the following levels of PEEP should be applied to mechanically ventilated patients.
      a. 0 to 5 cm H_2O for patients without lung injury
      b. 8 to 12 cm H_2O for patients with ALI
      c. 12 to 16 cm H_2O for patients with ARDS

F. Biotrauma
   1. The activation of inflammatory mediators in the lung by the use of an overdistending VT and repetitive opening and closing of unstable lung units.
   2. This can cause inflammatory injury to the lung.
   3. There also are good animal data to indicate that cells and other substances can be translocated from the lung to systemic circulation by inappropriate ventilatory patterns, resulting in lung injury.
   4. The translocated inflammatory mediators can cause injury to other organs.
   5. Clinical studies clearly show that systemic inflammatory mediator levels are decreased by a ventilatory pattern that is lung protective.

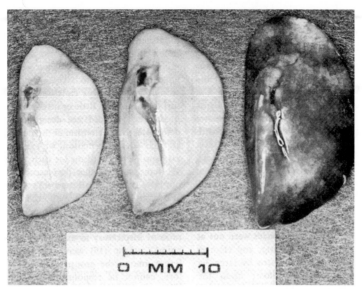

FIG. 41-4 Comparison of lungs excised from rats ventilated with peak pressure of 14 cm H_2O, zero positive end-expiratory pressure (PEEP), peak pressure of 45 cm H_2O, 10 cm H_2O PEEP, and peak pressure 45 cm H_2O, zero PEEP (left to right). The perivascular groove is distended with edema in the lungs from rats ventilated with peak pressures of 45 cm H_2O. The lung ventilated at 45 cm H_2O, zero PEEP is grossly hemorrhaged.

      6. Many believe that multisystem organ failure can be caused by the use of inappropriate ventilatory patterns.
  G. Lung protective ventilation
      1. This term refers to a ventilatory pattern that prevents the lung from the development of ventilator-induced lung injury.
      2. The key aspects of this pattern are
          a. Avoidance of overdistention: P_{plat} as low as possible, always <30 cm H_2O, and small VTs
          b. The application of sufficient PEEP to avoid collapse of lung at end expiration

III. **Indications for Mechanical Ventilation**
Numerous pathophysiologic conditions may necessitate mechanical ventilation. However, each may be categorized into one of the following general indications.
  A. Apnea: The cessation of breathing
  B. Acute ventilatory failure: A P_{CO_2} of >50 mm Hg and a pH <7.30.
  C. Impending acute ventilatory failure
      1. This is a clinical impression based on serial laboratory data and clinical findings indicating that the patient is progressing toward ventilatory failure.
      2. Clinical problems frequently resulting in impending acute ventilatory failure may be categorized as
          a. Primary pulmonary abnormalities, such as
             (1) ARDS
             (2) Pneumonia
             (3) Pulmonary emboli
          b. Secondary (nonpulmonary) abnormalities associated with the inability to effectively ventilate
             (1) Sepsis
             (2) Ventilatory muscle fatigue
             (3) Nutritional deficiencies

        (4)   Chest injury

        (5)   Thoracic abnormalities

        (6)   Pleural disease

        (7)   Myoneural disease

        (8)   Neurologic disease

3. Clinical evaluation of the patient in impending acute ventilatory failure

    a.   Vital signs: With increased cardiopulmonary stress, pulse and blood pressure typically increase. If bacterial infection is present, temperature also increases.

    b.   Ventilatory parameters: As WOB increases

        (1) V_T decreases

        (2)   RR increases

        (3)   Accessory muscle use increases

    c.   Paradoxical breathing may occur.

    d.   Retractions may be noted.

    e.   Ventilatory reserve is decreased: V_T becomes a greater percentage of vital capacity.

    f.   Development of impending acute ventilatory failure may demonstrate, for example

        (1)   Progressive muscle weakness in patients with neuromuscular or neurologic diseases

        (2)   Continued progress of pulmonary or pleural infections

        (3)   Increasing fatigue associated with any cardiorespiratory disease. Fatigue can be the primary factor precipitating impending acute ventilatory failure in any disease state.

        (4)   Serial blood gases demonstrating a trend toward acute ventilatory failure. For example

	9:00 AM	10:00 AM	11:00 AM	12:00 PM
pH	7.53	7.46	7.38	7.32
P_{CO_2} (mm Hg)	28	35	42	48
HCO_3^- (mEq/L)	22	23	24	25
P_{O_2} (mm Hg)	60	55	50	43

        Along with these results, the patient's RR, heart rate, and blood pressure continue to increase, whereas the V_T decreases.

        (5)   Without intervention to break this trend, a blood gas value measured at 1:00 PM may show a pH of 7.28 and a P_{CO_2} of 54 mm Hg, and at 2:00 PM the pH may be 7.24 and the P_{CO_2} 62 mm Hg.

        (6)   As a result the decision may be made at 12:00 to institute mechanical ventilation because the patient is in impending acute ventilatory failure.

  D. Inability to oxygenate

    1. An inability to oxygenate without failure to ventilate is an unlikely indication for mechanical ventilation.

    2. In most settings oxygenation problems can be managed with oxygen therapy, continuous positive pressure ventilation via mask, and cardiovascular stabilization.

    3. However, there are some patients in whom the increased WOB caused by a failure to oxygenate leads to ventilatory failure and the need for intubation and mechanical ventilation.

IV. Patient-Ventilatory Synchrony

  A. A critically important aspect of provision of ventilatory support is ensuring that the patient and ventilator are working in unison, not in opposition.

  B. The basic interaction between the patient and the ventilator can be described by the equation of motion.

$$P_T = P_E + P_R \tag{5}$$

Which states that the total pressure (P_T) needed to deliver a V_T is equal to the pressure to overcome the elastic properties of the respiratory system (P_E) and the resistive properties of the respiratory system (P_R).

C. P_E can be written as V_T divided by compliance (C) or

$$P_E = \frac{V_T}{C} \tag{6}$$

D. P_R can be written as flow ($\dot{V}$) multiplied by airway resistance (R).

$$P_R = \dot{V} \times R \tag{7}$$

E. As a result the equation of motion describes the pressure required to deliver a breath as the relationship between V_T, compliance, flow, and resistance.

$$P_T = \frac{V_T}{C} + (\dot{V} \times R) \tag{8}$$

F. P_T is generated by the ventilator (P airway), by the patient's muscular efforts (P muscle), or a combination of both.

$$P_T = P\ airway + P\ muscle \tag{9}$$

G. During spontaneous unassisted ventilation all of the effort (pressure) needed to deliver a V_T is provided by the patients' muscular effort, whereas during controlled ventilation (no patient effort), the ventilator provides all of the pressure needed to deliver a V_T.

H. During assisted ventilation the patient and the ventilator share the effort needed to deliver a breath.
  1. In this setting care must be taken to ensure that the ventilator provides a sufficient V_T and adequate peak flow rate is delivered in an appropriate time to meet the patient's ventilatory demand.
  2. During volume ventilation when patients are sedated and ventilation changes from assisted to controlled, peak airway pressure generally increases because the patient no longer is providing muscular effort assisting in gas delivery.
  3. During pressure ventilation V_T decreases when the transition is made from assisted to controlled ventilation for the same reason.

I. Patient-ventilator dys-synchrony occurs primarily when the following ventilator parameters do not meet the patient's ventilatory demand or are not set properly.
  1. Trigger sensitivity
  2. Initial flow rate
  3. Flow pattern
  4. T_I
  5. V_T

J. As discussed in detail in Chapter 40, auto-PEEP also contributes to dys-synchrony.

K. Trigger sensitivity (see Chapter 39) should always be set as sensitive as possible without causing auto-triggering. Flow triggering is usually more effective than pressure triggering.

L. Initial flow rate
  1. Figure 41-5 illustrates the effect of an inadequate peak inspiratory flow rate on patient effort.
  2. The ideal relationship between patient effort and ventilator response to a volume-targeted breath is depicted in Figure 41-5, *A*. The airway pressure versus time curve during assisted ventilation should be the same as that during controlled ventilation except for the pressure decrease to trigger the ventilator.
  3. The greater the difference between these two curves, the greater the WOB performed by the patient.

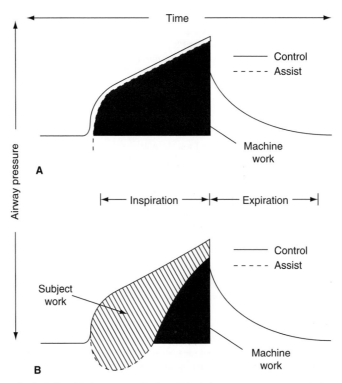

FIG. 41-5 A, Theoretical relationship between actual and ideal airway pressure curve during assisted mechanical breaths (assist/control or synchronized intermittent mandatory ventilation). No difference should exist between control breath and assisted breath. **B,** Actual airway pressure curve differences. The hatched area represents work performed by the patient during an assisted volume limited breath. If inspiratory flows and inspiratory times are inappropriate, patient work of breathing during assisted breathing may equal that during spontaneous breathing.

4. In Figure 41-5, *B,* the dotted line is the airway pressure curve during assisted ventilation, and the hatched area between the solid and dotted lines represents the work done by the patient. The greater the area, the greater the patient work.
5. Any time the airway pressure curve is concave or not matching the idealized curve, the patient is performing much of the WOB.
6. By increasing the peak inspiratory flow, patient work can be minimized.
   a. Figure 41-6 illustrates the impact of increasing peak flow and decreasing TI on the airway pressure curve and patient WOB.
   b. As you go from left to right in Figure 41-6, patient effort decreases because peak flow increases.
   c. In most adults receiving assisted volume-targeted ventilation, peak flows ≥80 L/min are needed to meet patient demand.
M. Flow waveform
   1. Essentially two waveforms are available during volume-targeted ventilation.
      a. Square
      b. Decelerating
   2. With square wave flow, gas flow is constant throughout inspiration.
   3. With decelerating flow, gas flow peaks at the onset of inspiration and decreases as inspiration continues.
   4. During assisted ventilation a decelerating flow pattern generally is most useful because it allows a high initial peak flow to meet patient demand but decelerates over time, ensuring that TI will be long enough to match patient demand.

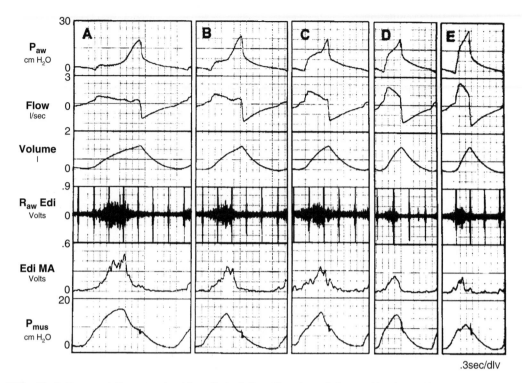

FIG. 41-6 Representative example of the effect of alternations in peak flow and inspiratory time on airway pressure (P_{aw}), the raw diaphragmatic electromyography (EMG) signal (R_{aw} Edi), the diaphragmatic EMG signal after removal of the electrocardiographic interference and rectification, and the calculated pressure output of the inspiratory muscles (P_{mus}). As flow increases note the reduction in EMG activity and muscle output.

    5. With a decelerating flow pattern compared with a square wave flow pattern
        a. Peak airway pressure is lower.
        b. End inspiratory P_{plat} is equal.
        c. If peak flows are the same, TI is longer.
    6. During controlled ventilation either a square or decelerating flow pattern can be used.
  N. TI should always match the patient's desired TI.
    1. In most patients a TI of ≤1.0 second is most appropriate.
    2. Some markedly stressed patients desire a TI as short as 0.6 second.
    3. Patients with chronic restrictive lung disease may desire a TI of 0.5 second.
    4. Regardless of the use of pressure or volume ventilation, TI during patient-triggered ventilation should always match the patient's desired TI.
  O. VT
    1. The average resting VT of all mammals is approximately 6.0 ml/kg IBW.
    2. As a result patients requiring ventilatory support *if not* stressed should also require an actual delivered VT of approximately 6.0 ml/kg IBW.
    3. However, the VT desired by many patients is greater because of an increased ventilatory demand.
    4. As discussed in Section II, Ventilator-Induced Lung Injury, the greater the VT, the greater the potential for end-inspiratory overdistention. As a result VT should be related to P_{plat}.
        a. If the P_{plat} is <25 cm H_2O, VT should be 6 to 10 ml/kg IBW.
        b. If P_{plat} is 25 to 30 cm H_2O, VT should be ≤8 ml/kg IBW.
        c. If P_{plat} is ≥30 cm H_2O, VT should be ≤6 ml/kg IBW.

P. Pressure ventilation
1. As discussed in Chapter 39, pressure ventilation is better able to meet the ventilatory demands of the stressed patient than volume ventilation.
2. Because flow delivery in pressure ventilation increases as demand increases, adequate flow is provided unless the pressure level is too low.
3. With pressure ventilation adjustments of the following may be needed to ensure synchrony.
    a. Pressure level
    b. Rise time
    c. Inspiratory termination criteria
    d. TI
4. Pressure level may be either too high or too low.
    a. In patients with a small VT and rapid rate, pressure may need to be increased; however, rise time and inspiratory termination criteria should also be evaluated.
    b. In some patients the pressure level may force too large a VT. Decreasing the VT may improve synchrony.
5. Rise time should be adjusted to allow a rapid increase in inspiratory pressure to the set level but no increase in pressure beyond the level set (see Chapter 39).
6. Inspiratory termination criteria (pressure support only) should be set to ensure the patient and ventilator end the breath at the same time (see Chapter 39).

Q. Auto-PEEP can cause marked dys-synchrony.
1. As noted in Figure 41-7 the greater the auto-PEEP level, the greater the likelihood that the patient will not trigger the ventilator with each of his or her inspiratory efforts.
2. In those with chronic obstructive pulmonary disease (COPD; dynamic airway obstruction) the application of PEEP can minimize triggering effort and improve patient-ventilator synchrony.
3. Refer to Chapter 40 for details.

V. **Gas Exchange Targets**
A. Ideally the blood gases of all patients mechanically ventilated should be equal to textbook normal values.
B. However, the cost in relationship to ventilator-induced lung injury may be excessive.
C. As a result, in many patients target blood gas values are different from textbook normal values.
D. As an overall guideline PaO_2 levels in critically ill patients should be maintained ≥60 to 70 mm Hg, and in some patients with severe ARDS a PaO_2 of >50 mm Hg may be acceptable.

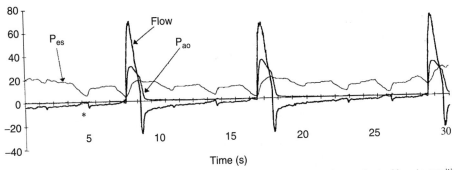

FIG. 41-7 Esophageal pressure (P_{es}), airway opening pressure (P_{ao}), and flow in a patient with auto-positive end-expiratory pressure (PEEP) and air trapping on volume assist/control mode. The units are cm H_2O for the pressure tracing and L/min for flow. The patient's inspiratory efforts are identified by the negative P_{es} swings. The PEEP is set at zero. P_{ao} appropriately decreases to zero during expiration, demonstrating little circuit or valve resistance. Auto-PEEP is evident, with one triggered breath every three to four efforts. Prolonged expiratory flow is caused by airflow limitation. P_{es} swings have little effect in retarding the expiratory flow and even less effect on P_{ao}, depending on the phase of ventilation.

E. In COPD patients $Paco_2$ should always be maintained at the patient's "baseline" level.
   1. This is the level defined by the patient's ability to spontaneously ventilate.
   2. If COPD patients are ventilated to normal $Paco_2$ levels (35 to 45 cm H_2O) they will not be able to wean from ventilatory support because they cannot generate the muscular effort without ventilator assistance needed to maintain arterial $Paco_2$ at normal levels.
   3. In many COPD patients $Paco_2$ is maintained between 50 and 80 mm Hg.
F. In patients with ARDS and especially in patients with asthma, permissive hypercapnia may be unavoidable.
   1. Permissive hypercapnia is the setting of the ventilator in a manner that allows the $Paco_2$ to increase above normal (50 to 100 mm Hg).
   2. Permissive hypercapnia is allowed because the cost from a ventilator-induced lung injury perspective is too high to maintain the normal $Paco_2$ (i.e., the P_{plat} has exceeded 30 cm H_2O, the V_T is > 6 ml/kg IBW, and the rate is increased to the level that auto-PEEP begins to develop).
   3. A number of physiologic effects are attributed to permissive hypercapnia.
      a. Shift in the oxyhemoglobin dissociation curve to the right
      b. Decreased alveolar Po_2
      c. Stimulation and depression of the cardiovascular system
         (1) An increase in $Paco_2$ results in a variety of hemodynamic effects (Figure 41-8).
         (2) Increased cardiac output is common in most patients.
      d. Central nervous system depression
      e. Stimulation of ventilation
      f. Dilation of vascular beds
      g. Increased ICP

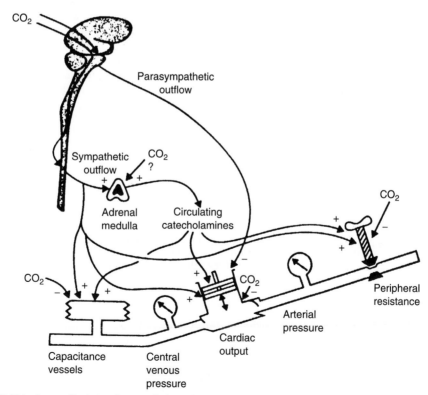

FIG. 41-8 This diagram illustrates the complexity of the mechanisms by which CO_2 influences the circulatory system.

       h.   Anesthesia (Pa_{CO_2} >200 mm Hg)
       i.   Decreased renal blood flow (Pa_{CO_2} >150 mm Hg)
       j.   Leakage of intracellular potassium (Pa_{CO_2} >150 mm Hg)
       k.   Alteration in the action of pharmacologic agents (a result of intracellular acidosis)

  4. Permissive hypercapnia is best tolerated in patients with
       a.   A healthy cardiovascular system
       b.   The absence of metabolic acidosis
       c.   Good peripheral perfusion
  5. The major limiting factor to permissive hypercapnia is acidosis.
  6. Patients can tolerate marked increases in Pa_{CO_2} if not associated with marked acidosis.
  7. Most young patients and those without cardiovascular disease can tolerate a pH of approximately 7.20 without cardiovascular problems.
  8. However, the more compromised the cardiovascular system, the less likely a patient will tolerate acidosis.
  9. Permissive hypercapnia is contraindicated in the patient with increased ICP.
 10. In some patients the systemic administration of buffers may be indicated to control the acidosis.

VI. Ventilator Commitment
  A. Ventilate with bag and mask, and then establish an artificial airway.
  B. Attach patient to the ventilator and adjust settings (see Section VII, Determination of Setting on the Ventilator).
  C. Stabilize the cardiovascular system.
     1. Before manual ventilation the patient's sympathetic tone is pronounced because of
       a.   Hypercarbia
       b.   Acidosis
       c.   Hypoxemia
       d.   Generalized increased stress
     2. Because manual ventilation and mechanical ventilation inhibit venous return and typically reverse hypercarbia, acidosis, and hypoxemia, a decreased sympathetic tone results. This may result in hypotension when manual or mechanical ventilation is instituted.
     3. The use of narcotics may also add to the hypotensive state.
     4. Fluid therapy may be essential during ventilator commitment (see Chapter 14).
     5. Some patients also may require the use of sympathomimetics for β_1 effects (see Chapter 17).
  D. Record baseline values for
     1. Vital signs
     2. Blood gases
  E. Institute appropriate cardiovascular and pulmonary monitors.
     1. Electrocardiogram
     2. Arterial line
     3. Central venous line
     4. Pulmonary artery line
  F. Sedate as indicated to improve synchrony.

VII. Determination of Settings on the Mechanical Ventilator
  A. In all patients mechanically ventilated the following issues are always of concern regardless of the reason for ventilatory support.
     1. Ventilator-induced lung injury (see Section II, Ventilator-Induced Lung Injury)
     2. Patient-ventilatory synchrony (see Section IV, Patient-Ventilator Synchrony)
     3. Target blood gases (see Section V, Target Blood Gases)
     4. Cardiovascular stability especially at the onset of invasive mechanical ventilation
  B. Ventilator management of COPD (see Chapter 21)
     1. Pathophysiologic concerns
       a.   The primary concern is *auto-PEEP* (see Chapter 40).
       b.   Secondary issues are gas delivery and insurance of patient-ventilator synchrony.

BOX 41-1
COPD: Initial Ventilator Settings

Noninvasive Ventilation: First-Line Therapy
- Mode: Assist/control (pressure) or pressure support
- Tidal volume: 6 to 8 ml/kg ideal body weight (IBW)
- Positive end-expiratory pressure: 3 to 8 cm H_2O
- Ventilating pressure: 8 to 12 cm H_2O
- Inspiratory time: <1.0 second
- F_1O_2: To maintain PaO_2 >60 mm Hg
- Back-up rate: 8 to 10, actual patient's rate determines baseline $PaCO_2$

Invasive Ventilation
- Mode assist/control (pressure preferred) or pressure support
- Tidal volume dependent on plateau pressure
  - 6 to 10 ml/kg IBW plateau pressure: <25 cm H_2O
  - ≤8 ml/kg IBW plateau pressure: 25 to 30 cm H_2O
  - ≤6 ml/kg IBW plateau pressure: >30 cm H_2O

- Peak flow (volume ventilation): ≥80 L/min to meet peak inspiratory demand
- Flow waveform (volume ventilation): Decelerating
- Inspiratory time: Equal to the patient's desired neuroinspiratory time normally 0.6 to 1.0 second.
- Rise time (pressure ventilation): Set to ensure initial flow meets patient demand.
- Inspiratory termination criteria (pressure support): Set to ensure synchronous termination of inspiratory, ≥25%
- PEEP: Usually 5 to 10 cm H_2O to offset auto-PEEP and allow triggering
- F_1O_2: Set to maintain PaO_2 >60 mm Hg
- Rate: 8 to 16/min set to minimize auto-PEEP, but rate normally controlled by patient inspiratory effort
- Sedate as necessary

    c. Target blood gases should be equal to the patient's normal values.

    d. Weaning: COPD patients are some of the most difficult patients to wean. Some require a long course of weaning/rehabilitation, whereas others become ventilator dependent.

  2. Initial ventilator settings (Box 41-1)

    a. Always consider noninvasive ventilation as the initial approach to ventilatory support (see Chapter 43).

    b. Select settings that minimize dys-synchrony.

    c. Pressure-targeted modes are preferred over volume-targeted modes.

    d. Use PEEP to offset auto-PEEP and ensure triggering with each spontaneous breath.

    e. Minimize auto-PEEP by maintaining the lowest minute ventilation required.

  3. Management of gas exchange

    a. PCO_2 greater than patient "baseline": Increase V_T if plateau <25 cm H_2O, and if P_{plat} ≥25 cm H_2O increase rate unless auto-PEEP develops. If auto-PEEP increases, focus attention on improving bronchial hygiene.

      (1) Bronchodilators

      (2) Decreased mucosal edema

      (3) Secretion removal

    b. PCO_2 below patient's baseline, decrease rate and then V_T unless P_{plat} is >25 cm H_2O, then decrease V_T first.

    c. Manage PaO_2 by altering F_1O_2 unless the acute exacerbation is compounded by ALI or ARDS.

  4. Ongoing management

    a. Key issue is rest for the first 24 to 72 hours.

    b. Patient should be able to trigger the ventilator, but ventilator settings should ensure work is performed by the ventilator.

    c. As patient recovers

      (1) Convert to pressure support

      (2) Decrease PEEP

      (3) Adjust F_1O_2

d.   Assess ability to spontaneously ventilate (see Section IX, Weaning and Ventilator Discontinuation).

e.   Some require rehabilitation and long-term ventilatory support.

f.   Patients physiologically appearing ready for ventilator discontinuation but repeatedly failing spontaneous breathing trials should be considered for extubation to noninvasive positive pressure ventilation (NPPV).

C.   Ventilator management of ARDS (see Chapter 23)

1.   Pathophysiologic concerns

a.   The primary concern is inducing greater lung injury by the process of mechanical ventilation. Ventilation should always be provided in a lung-protective manner.

b.   Recruitable lung should be opened and stabilized.

2.   Initial ventilator setting (Box 41-2)

a.   Use lung protective ventilator settings.

b.   After initial stabilization hemodynamically, recruit the lung.

c.   Set PEEP after recruitment at the level maintaining the benefit of lung recruitment (see Chapter 40).

d.   Appropriately sedate to ensure conformance with small V_T.

3.   Lung recruitment maneuvers

a.   These maneuvers are the short-term application of an increased airway pressure to open those parts of the lung that are collapsed.

b.   Clearly there is a potential for injury, and careful monitoring is required; however, the short-term application of pressure up to approximately 45 cm H_2O does not seem to cause lung injury.

c.   Recruitment maneuvers are applied because the collapsed lung

(1)   Requires increased P_{plat} to ventilate

(2)   Requires increased F_IO_2 to oxygenate

(3)   Decreases surfactant function

(4)   Increases the likelihood of the development of pneumonia

d.   The desired outcome of a recruitment maneuver is the movement of the lung from the inflation to the deflation limb of the pressure-volume curve of the lung. This results in a larger lung volume at any PEEP level (Figure 41-9).

e.   For recruitment maneuvers to be most effective they should be performed

(1)   On the first or second day of ventilatory support

(2)   Only after hemodynamic stability is established

BOX 41-2

ARDS/ALI: Initial Ventilator Settings

- Mode assist/control (pressure or volume) or pressure support
- Tidal volume dependent on plateau pressure
  - 6 to 10 ml/kg ideal body weight (IBW) plateau pressure: <25 cm H_2O
  - <8 ml/kg IBW plateau pressure: 25 to 30 cm H_2O
  - <6 ml/kg IBW plateau pressure: >30 cm H_2O
- Positive end-expiratory pressure (PEEP): 10 cm H_2O until stabilized
- F_IO_2: 1.0 until stabilized
- Inspiratory time: ≤1.0 second
- Peak flow: (volume ventilation) ≥80 L/min to meet patient demand
- Flow waveform: (volume ventilation) decelerating

- Once stabilized lung recruitment maneuver performed
- PEEP: Minimal level maintaining benefit of lung recruitment normally
  - 8 to 12 cm H_2O acute lung injury
  - 12 to 16 cm H_2O acute respiratory distress syndrome (ARDS)
- F_IO_2: Minimal level to maintain PaO_2 >60 mm Hg or in some severe ARDS >50 mm Hg
- Rate: ≤35/min, set to maintain $PaCO_2$ 35 to 50 mm Hg without causing auto-PEEP
- Permissive hypercapnia necessary in some patients
- Sedate as necessary

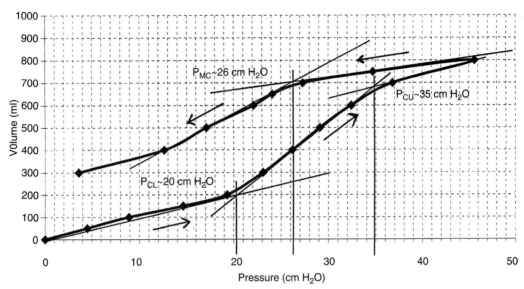

FIG. 41-9 Pressure-volume curve of the total respiratory system indicating the inflation and deflation limb. Arrows indicate direction of flow. P_{CL}, Lower inflection point-Pflex; P_{CU}, upper inflection point; P_{MC}, point of maximum compliance change.

        (3) They appear to be more successful in patients with secondary versus primary ARDS.
    f. The safest and most successful recruitment maneuvers use high continuous positive airway pressure (CPAP) levels for short periods.
        (1) CPAP of 30 to 45 cm H_2O
        (2) Applied for 30 to 40 seconds
        (3) Actual settings based on patient tolerance and response
    g. Before a recruitment maneuver is applied the patient should be
        (1) Sedated to near apnea, with no vigorous inspiratory effects
        (2) Stabilized hemodynamically
        (3) Oxygenated with an F_IO_2 of 1.0
    h. During the maneuver a respiratory therapist, nurse, and physician should carefully monitor the patient. Guidelines should be set defining when the maneuver should be terminated because of lack of tolerance. Typical guidelines could be
        (1) Mean arterial pressure (MAP): <60 mm Hg or a 20% decrease
        (2) Heart rate: >130 or <60 beats/min
        (3) Spo_2: <88%
        (4) New arrhythmias
    i. Change the ventilator mode to CPAP; no ventilation is provided during this recruitment maneuver.
        (1) A CPAP level of 30 cm H_2O for 30 to 40 seconds can be used first to determine patient tolerance.
        (2) If tolerated hemodynamically the CPAP level can be increased to 35 or 40 cm H_2O.
        (3) Maximum CPAP level recommended is 45 cm H_2O.
        (4) Some patients may require two or three recruitment maneuvers. However, between maneuvers patients should be ventilated and allowed to stabilize for 15 to 20 minutes before a second maneuver is performed.

    j. Lung recruitment maneuvers are generally contradicted if the patient is/has
        (1) Hemodynamically unstable
        (2) Preexisting pulmonary cysts
        (3) Preexisting bullous lung disease
        (4) Preexisting barotrauma
        (5) Unilateral lung disease
    k. After the lung recruitment maneuver, set PEEP at the lowest level maintaining the benefits of the maneuver.
    l. The best approach to achieve this is the use of a decremental PEEP trial (see Chapter 40).
    m. Regardless of approach used if the patient loses the benefit of the maneuver after a short time, the PEEP level was too low and needs to be increased.

4. Management of gas exchange
    a. $Paco_2$ should be managed by alteration in rate unless the P_{plat} is <25 cm H_2O, then VT may be increased.
    b. Pao_2 is managed by PEEP and F_IO_2.
        (1) Generally if the Pao_2 is low the first approach is to increase the PEEP level, followed by the F_IO_2.
        (2) If the Pao_2 is high the F_IO_2 should be decreased first until the F_IO_2 is <0.5, and then PEEP can be decreased.

5. Ongoing management
    a. Target $Paco_2$ levels are generally 35 to 50 mm Hg, but many patients require permissive hypercapnia because of high P_{plat}.
    b. In-line suction catheters should be used, and the ventilator should not be disconnected because collapse of lung units occurs in seconds in ARDS patients.
    c. If the ventilator is disconnected, the lung may need to be rerecruited.
    d. As the patient's status improves his or her mode can be changed to pressure support.
    e. Spontaneous breathing trials should be used to determine when mechanical ventilation should be discontinued.
    f. Patients with ALI generally require 8 to 12 cm H_2O PEEP, and those with ARDS require 12 to 16 cm H_2O PEEP.

D. Ventilator management of asthma (Box 41-3)
    1. Physiologic concerns
        a. As with COPD auto-PEEP is the primary concern.
        b. However, contrary to COPD, in patients with asthma airway obstruction is observed during inspiration and expiration.
        c. The increased airway resistance in patients with asthma is fixed compared with the dynamic obstruction observed only during exhalation in those with COPD.

BOX 41-3

Asthma: Initial Ventilator Settings

- Mode: Volume assist/control
- Peak airway pressure: May need pressure to 70 to 80 cm H_2O to deliver tidal volume (VT)
- Plateau pressure: <30 cm H_2O
- VT: 4 to 8 ml/kg ideal body weight
- Flow waveform: (volume ventilation) decelerating
- Peak flow: (volume ventilation) sufficient to deliver VT in defined inspiratory time
- Inspiratory time: 1.0 to 1.5 seconds to ensure distribution of inspiration
- Positive end-expiratory pressure (PEEP): 0 to 5 cm H_2O
- F_IO_2: To maintain Pao_2 >60 mm Hg
- Rate: 8 to 16/min, level that minimizes auto-PEEP
- Permissive hypercapnia required for first 12 to 48 hours or more
- Most patients require sedation to apnea

d. As a result it is as difficult to deliver a VT as it is for patients with asthma to exhale.

e. PEEP is not normally recommended to offset auto-PEEP in those with asthma. Applied PEEP in asthma patients is generally additive to auto-PEEP, increasing the total PEEP level.

f. Measurement of auto-PEEP is also a problem in those with asthma. As illustrated in Figure 41-10 some areas of the lung may be totally obstructed at end exhalation, preventing the pressures from being averaged when auto-PEEP is determined by an end-expiratory pause.

g. It is better to use P_{plat} to monitor auto-PEEP level in patients with asthma. If P_{plat} increases (provided VT is constant), auto-PEEP has increased, and if P_{plat} decreases, auto-PEEP level has decreased.

h. As with ARDS patients ventilator-induced lung injury is a major concern in those with asthma.

i. P_{plat} should always be kept as low as possible and always <30 cm H_2O.

j. However, peak pressures (volume ventilation) will need to be high (sometimes 70 to 80 cm H_2O) to provide the driving pressure to deliver a VT.

k. A high driving pressure is not desirable, but most of the pressure is dissipated in the endotracheal tube (ETT) and large airways and does not affect the lung parenchyma.

l. Without a high driving pressure, asthma patients cannot be ventilated.

m. Because of the difficulty in ventilating patients with severe asthma, permissive hypercapnia is unavoidable.

n. In many patients Pa_{CO_2} is 60 to 90 mm Hg or higher for the first 24 hours or longer.

o. For patients with asthma the cost to maintain a normal Pa_{CO_2} far exceeds the benefits.

p. Most asthma patients can tolerate a high Pa_{CO_2}, provided the pH is ≥7.20 and they have a normally functioning cardiovascular system.

End-expiratory airway occlusion

Measured AP = 5 cm H_2O

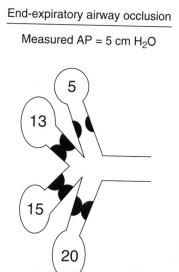

FIG. 41-10 A hypothetical model to explain underestimation of end-expiratory alveolar pressure by measured auto-positive end-expiratory pressure (auto-PEEP) in severe asthma. Alveolar pressure (cm H_2O) in four different lung units is shown. At end expiration, only the upper lung unit is in communication with the central airway, causing the airway occlusion pressure (measured auto-PEEP) to be much lower than end-expiratory alveolar pressure in the other hyperinflated but noncommunicating lung units. *AP*, Auto-PEEP.

2. Initial ventilator settings (see Box 41-3)
   a. In patients with asthma, volume assist/control is frequently the only mode that can effectively ventilate patients and still maintain a low P_{plat}.
   b. Because of the high inspiratory resistance TI may need to be approximately 1.0 to 1.5 seconds to ensure gas is able to distribute in the lung.
   c. RR should be set based on the development of auto-PEEP. A balance between minimum auto-PEEP and $PaCO_2$ must be established.
   d. Ideally a low rate with long expiratory time minimizes auto-PEEP.
   e. The factor most affecting auto-PEEP is minute ventilation. The lower the minute ventilation, the lower the auto-PEEP.

3. Management of gas exchange
   a. Little change in the level of mechanical ventilation is necessary because as pharmacology decreases the severity of the asthmatic attack and auto-PEEP decreases, $PaCO_2$ also decreases.
   b. As patients improve, the rate can be increased and the TI decreased to assist in normalizing the $PaCO_2$.
   c. F_IO_2 should be adjusted to maintain the PaO_2 >60 mm Hg and decreased as the patient's status improves.

4. Ongoing management
   a. The key issue is the use of bronchodilators and steroids to manage the severe asthma.
   b. As the patient improves he or she can be changed to pressure support.
   c. However, as patients improve and sedation is decreased, many poorly tolerate the ETT.
   d. Most asthma patients are simply extubated after their lung function has improved and sedation is decreased.

E. Ventilator management of cutaneous burns/inhalation injury
   1. Physiologic concerns
      a. Patients with burn/inhalation injury require ventilation because of:
         (1) Upper airway burns
         (2) Severe inhalation injury
         (3) Development of ARDS
         (4) Development of sepsis
         (5) Fluid overload
         (6) Pain management
         (7) High carboxyhemoglobin levels
         (8) Decreased chest wall compliance
      b. Inhalation injury patients may develop high levels of auto-PEEP because of inflammation, bronchospasm, and the inhibition of mucociliary transport.
      c. Many severe inhalation injury patients develop ARDS.
   2. Initial ventilatory settings (Box 41-4)
      a. If there are no inhalation injuries ventilation is fairly straightforward unless the patient has severe thoracic burns that decrease chest wall compliance as they heal. If this is the case
         (1) VT needs to be decreased; and
         (2) RR needs to be increased.
      b. Patients with inhalation injury frequently develop ARDS.
      c. However, management is complicated by the fact that air trapping and auto-PEEP also are common.
      d. Ventilator settings should be similar to ARDS, but care should be taken to ensure that air trapping is not increased by the application of PEEP.
   3. Management of gas exchange
      a. Permissive hypercapnia is a necessity for some patients because of the competing effects of auto-PEEP and ARDS.
      b. For those patients with stiff chest walls it is possible to allow P_{plat} to exceed 30 cm H_2O because of decreased chest wall compliance.

BOX 41-4

Burns/Inhalation Injury: Initial Ventilator Settings

If *no* Inhalation Injury
- Mode: Pressure assist/control
- Plateau pressure: <30 cm H_2O
- Tidal volume (VT): 6 to 10 ml/kg ideal body weight (IBW) dependent on plateau pressure
- Rate: 15 to 30/min based on chest wall compliance and metabolic rate
- Peak flow: (volume ventilation) sufficient to meet inspiratory time
- Flow waveform: (volume ventilation) decelerating
- F_1O_2: Sufficient to maintain PaO_2 >60 mm Hg
- Positive end-expiratory pressure (PEEP): 5 cm H_2O
- Inspiratory time: 1.0 second
- Sedation and pain control to apnea

If Inhalation Injury
- Mode: Pressure assist/control
- Plateau pressure: <30 cm H_2O
- VT: 5 to 8 ml/kg IBW
- Peak flow: (volume ventilation) sufficient to meet inspiratory time
- Flow waveform: (volume ventilation) decelerating
- PEEP: To manage oxygenation but may be additive to auto-PEEP
- F_1O_2: Maintain PaO_2 >60 mm Hg
- Inspiratory time: 0.8 to 1.2 seconds
- Rate: 10 to 25/min based on the balance between $PaCO_2$ and auto-PEEP level
- Permissive hypercapnia usually unavoidable
- Sedation and pain control to apnea

    c.   Oxygenation is managed by a combination of PEEP and F_1O_2.
    d.   PEEP level should be maximized if ARDS is present.
    e.   If carboxyhemoglobin >10%, maintain 100% oxygen.
    f.   If no ARDS is present, manage a decreased PO_2 with increasing F_1O_2.
  4. Ongoing management
    a.   Many patients have long ventilatory courses because of the need for multiple surgeries and decreased chest wall compliance.
    b.   Many patients are hypermetabolic and require high minute ventilation.
    c.   Weaning in some patients with inhalation and body surface burns is lengthy.
F. Ventilator management of chest trauma
  1. Pathophysiologic concerns
    a.   Blunt chest trauma can result in
       (1) Rib and sternum fractures resulting in a flail chest
       (2) Pulmonary contusion developing into ARDS
       (3) Tracheobronchial injury resulting in disruption of the airway (fistula formation)
       (4) Myocardial and vascular injury
       (5) Esophageal perforation
       (6) Diaphragmatic injury
    b.   Penetrating chest injuries frequently result in pneumothorax and extensive tissue damage.
  2. Initial ventilator settings (Box 41-5)
    a.   Most patients will not be capable of breathing spontaneously because of sedation and pain control; as a result the assist/control mode (pressure preferred) is indicated.
    b.   As with all patients P_{plat} should be <30 cm H_2O to avoid the development of additional lung injury.
    c.   PEEP level used varies considerably depending on level of lung injury.
    d.   In patients with ALI/ARDS apply PEEP as in ARDS patients.
    e.   In patients with large air leaks 0 to 5 cm H_2O PEEP should only be applied to avoid excessive air leak. However, if these patients develop ARDS higher PEEP levels are necessary.
  3. Management of gas exchange
    a.   In most patients $PaCO_2$ is easily managed by changes in RR.
    b.   However, in patients with ARDS and especially in those with large air leaks permissive hypercapnia may be necessary.

BOX 41-5

Chest Trauma: Initial Ventilator Settings

- Mode: Assist/control (pressure preferred)
- Tidal volume (VT) dependent on plateau pressure
  - 6 to 10 ml/kg ideal body weight (IBW) plateau pressure <25 cm H_2O
  - ≤8 ml/kg IBW plateau pressure 25 to 30 cm H_2O
  - ≤6 ml/kg IBW plateau pressure >30 cm H_2O
- Peak flow: (volume ventilation) dependent on VT and inspiratory time if controlled ventilation

- Flow waveform: (volume ventilation) decelerating
- Rate: Set to manage $PaCO_2$, normally 10 to 20/min
- Positive end-expiratory pressure: 5 to 10 cm H_2O depending on atelectasis; 0 to 5 if continuous severe air leak
- Inspiratory time: 1.0 second
- F_IO_2: To maintain PaO_2 > 60 mm Hg
- Sedate as necessary

    c. Oxygenation is managed usually by adjustment of F_IO_2.

    d. However, if ARDS develops PEEP should be adjusted as discussed in the management of ARDS.

  4. Ongoing management

    a. The chest wall generally stabilizes in 5 to 10 days, and most patients can be weaned after stabilization.

    b. Over time reduce ventilating pressure as the patient's status changes, and switch to pressure support as ventilatory capabilities stabilize.

    c. F_IO_2 can be decreased over time as PaO_2 improves.

G. Ventilatory management of head trauma

  1. Pathophysiologic concerns

    a. Head trauma results in an increase in ICP because of the fixed size of the skull.

    b. Increased ICP results in a decreased cerebral perfusion pressure (CPP).

    c. CPP is defined as the difference between MAP and ICP.

$$CPP = MAP - ICP \qquad (10)$$

    d. Normally

      (1) ICP: <10 mm Hg

      (2) MAP: approximately 90 mm Hg

      (3) CPP: >80 mm Hg

    e. CPP <60 mm Hg is associated with poor outcome in patients with acute head trauma.

    f. A normal response to an acute increase in ICP is hypertension and bradycardia; this is referred to as the Cushing response.

    g. An increase in ICP and a decrease in CPP may result in

      (1) Cheyne-Stokes breathing

      (2) Central neurogenic hyperventilation

      (3) Apnea

      (4) Neurogenic pulmonary edema that presents similarly to ARDS.

  2. Initial ventilator settings (Box 41-6)

    a. Most patients are treated with controlled ventilation because of the need for sedation to control ICP.

    b. If no lung injury is present it is easy to maintain ventilatory support with VT 6 to 10 ml/kg IBW and rates 15 to 20 breaths/min.

    c. Patients with lung injury should be treated as ARDS patients.

    d. PEEP is 0 to 5 cm H_2O if no lung injury.

    e. However, if head of the bed is elevated 30 degrees, patients tolerate up to 10 cm H_2O PEEP or higher without increasing ICP.

BOX 41-6

Head Trauma: Initial Ventilatory Settings

- Mode: Assist/control
- Tidal volume: 6 to 10 ml/kg ideal body weight
- Plateau pressure: ≤ 25 cm H_2O
- Peak flow: (volume ventilation) to maintain inspiratory time
- Flow waveform: (volume ventilation) decelerating

- Positive end-expiratory pressure: 5 cm H_2O but may need to be increased up to 10 cm H_2O if atelectasis
- F_IO_2: Set to maintain $PaO_2 > 80$ to 100 mm Hg
- Inspiratory time: 1.0 second
- Rate: 15 to 20/min set to maintain $PaCO_2$ at approximately 35 mm Hg
- Sedate to apnea

    f.   In patients with ARDS risks versus benefits of an elevated PEEP level on ICP must be balanced.

  3. Management of gas exchange

    a.   Patients should *not* be hyperventilated except for acute management of an increase in ICP. $PaCO_2$ of 25 to 35 mm Hg constricts cerebral vasculature and decreases ICP.

    b.   Sustaining hyperventilation results in renal compensation and a return of pH to normal, negating the effect of the decreased $PaCO_2$.

    c. $PaCO_2$ should be maintained at approximately 35 mm Hg.

    d.   Oxygenation is primarily managed by F_IO_2; ideally PaO_2 should be 80 to 100 mm Hg to ensure adequate cerebral oxygenation.

    e.   In patients with ARDS, PEEP and F_IO_2 are titrated to manage PaO_2.

  4. Ongoing management

    a.   Manage as discussed until ICP returns to normal.

    b.   If patients have an intact ventilatory drive they may be changed to pressure support.

    c.   Many patients require low-level ventilatory support for lengthy periods because of poor ventilatory drive even after ICP normalizes.

    d.   However, once ventilatory drive has normalized and stabilized, patients wean rapidly.

 H. Ventilatory management of postoperative respiratory failure

  1. Physiologic concerns

    a.   Surgeries that involve the thoracic or abdominal cavities result in impairment of ventilatory function

    b.   As a result lung volume can decrease 20% to 30% after thoracic or cardiac surgery and up to 60% with upper abdominal surgery.

  2. Initial ventilator setting (Box 41-7)

    a.   If previous COPD ventilate as COPD.

    b.   If the patient develops ARDS ventilate as ARDS.

    c.   If no previous pulmonary disease or complications ventilation is fairly straightforward.

BOX 41-7

Postoperative Ventilatory Failure: Initial Ventilator Settings

- Mode: Assist/control or pressure support
- Tidal volume: 8 to 10 ml/kg ideal body weight
- Plateau pressure: <25 cm H_2O
- Peak flow: (volume ventilation) to establish inspiratory time during control ventilation, >80 L/min during assisted ventilation
- Flow waveform: (volume ventilation) decelerating

- Inspiratory time: ≤ 1.0 second
- Positive end-expiratory pressure: 5 to 10 cm H_2O dependent on level of atelectasis
- F_IO_2: To maintain PaO_2 >70 mm Hg
- Rate: 10 to 20/min to maintain patient's baseline $PaCO_2$

3. Management of gas exchange
   a. Manage Pa_{CO_2} first by altering rate.
   b. If Pa_{CO_2} is elevated and P_{plat} is <25 cm H_2O, V_T may also be increased.
   c. Oxygenation is managed primarily by F_IO_2.
   d. However, if there is extensive atelectasis, PEEP up to approximately 10 cm H_2O may be needed.
4. Ongoing management
   a. Ventilatory management is usually short term, 4 to 48 hours.
   b. Weaning is rapid unless COPD or ARDS is present.

I. Ventilatory management of neuromuscular disease
   1. Physiologic concerns
      a. Respiratory failure is a result of muscular weakness.
      b. Recovery is frequently slow, requiring a lengthy ventilatory course.
      c. However, ventilation is straightforward because of the absence of lung disease.
   2. Initial ventilator settings (Box 41-8)
      a. Some patients desire large V_T (<12 ml/kg IBW).
      b. Oxygenation normally is not a problem.
   3. Management of gas exchange
      a. Because of the large V_T manage CO_2 by altering rate.
      b. Manage Pa_{O_2} by F_IO_2.
      c. Low PEEP is all that is required.
   4. Ongoing management
      a. Ventilatory course is usually lengthy.
      b. Weaning can be slow because of slow recovery of muscle weakness.

J. Ventilatory management of chronic restrictive pulmonary disease
   1. Physiologic concerns
      a. Primary concern is the decrease in respiratory system compliance.
      b. This requires a small V_T and a rapid rate.
      c. Patients generally also have a marked increase in ventilatory demand.
      d. Auto-PEEP is not a problem in these patients.
   2. Initial ventilatory settings (Box 41-9)
      a. In some patients noninvasive ventilation should be initially used.
      b. T_I is short: 0.5 to 0.8 second.
      c. RRs are rapid: 20 to 35 breaths/min.
      d. As with all patients with restrictive pulmonary disease concerns regarding P_{plat} exist.
      e. Only low level of PEEP is required.
   3. Management of gas exchange
      a. Permissive hypercapnia may be necessary in some patients.
      b. Pa_{CO_2} should be managed by rate.
      c. Pa_{O_2} is managed by adjustment of F_IO_2.
   4. Ongoing maintenance
      a. As with COPD ventilatory muscle rest is essential before weaning is successful.
      b. Many patients with pulmonary fibrosis are end stage and may become ventilator dependent.

BOX 41-8

Neuromuscular Disease: Initial Ventilator Setting

- Mode: Assist/control
- Tidal volume: <12 ml/kg ideal body weight
- Plateau pressure: <25 cm H_2O
- Inspiratory time: 1.0 to 1.2 seconds
- Peak flow: (volume ventilation) to ensure inspiratory time
- Flow waveform: (volume ventilation) decelerating
- Positive end-expiratory pressure: 5 cm H_2O
- F_IO_2: To maintain Pa_{O_2} >70 mm Hg
- Rate: 10 to 16/min to maintain patient's baseline Pa_{CO_2}

BOX 41-9

Chronic Restrictive Pulmonary Disease: Initial Ventilator Settings

Noninvasive Positive Pressure Ventilation: In Patients with Thoracic Deformities but no Intrinsic Lung Disease
- Mode: Assist/control (pressure) or pressure support
- Tidal volume (V_T): 4 to 6 ml/kg ideal body weight (IBW)
- Positive end-expiratory pressure: ≤5 cm H_2O
- Ventilating pressure: 10 to 15 cm H_2O
- F_1O_2: To maintain PaO_2 >60 mm Hg
- Inspiratory time: 0.5 to 0.8 second
- Rate: 20 to 35/min

Invasive Ventilation
- Mode: Assist/control (pressure preferred) or pressure support
- V_T: 4 to 8 ml/kg IBW
- Plateau pressure: Ideally <25 cm H_2O
- Peak flow: >80 L/min to meet peak inspiratory demand (volume ventilation)
- Flow waveform: (volume ventilation) decelerating
- Inspiratory time: 0.5 to 0.8 second equal to neuroinspiratory time
- Positive end-expiratory pressure: 0 to 5 cm H_2O
- F_1O_2: To maintain PaO_2 >60 mm Hg
- Rate: 20 to 35/min to maintain patient's baseline $PaCO_2$

    c. Patients with chest wall deformities frequently require nocturnal NPPV after extubation.

    d. Care should always be exercised to avoid excessive work during assisted ventilation.

K. Ventilator management of cardiac disease

    1. Physiologic concerns

        a. During unassisted breathing the negative intrathoracic pressure facilitates venous return.

        b. However, if the myocardium is compromised as in a recent myocardial infarction or congestive heart failure, the markedly negative intrathoracic pressure associated with vigorous breathing results in

            (1) Increased left ventricular preload

            (2) Development of pulmonary edema

            (3) Decreased cardiac output

            (4) Increasing hypoxemia

            (5) Even greater WOB

        c. Stressed ventilatory muscles consume up to approximately 40% of the cardiac output, limiting blood flow to other organs.

        d. As a result positive pressure, because it increases mean intrathoracic pressure, may have a beneficial effect on cardiac output since it

            (1) Decreases venous return

            (2) Decreases ventricular preload

            (3) Decreases ventricular afterload

        e. However, if the patient is hypovolemic positive pressure will further compromise hemodynamics unless hypovolemia is managed properly.

        f. Positive pressure has the greatest negative impact on the cardiovascular system when pulmonary compliance is normal but chest wall compliance is decreased because venous return is markedly decreased.

        g. The effects an increase in intrathoracic pressure has on hemodynamics are a result of the combined effects of

            (1) Vascular volume

            (2) Vascular tone

            (3) Pulmonary vascular resistance

            (4) Left and right ventricular function

2. Initial ventilator settings (Box 41-10)
   a. In patients with congestive heart failure with pulmonary edema noninvasive CPAP is first-line therapy.
   b. If congestive heart failure with pulmonary edema is associated with hypercapnia, NPPV is the initial treatment of choice.
   c. However, if the presentation of congestive heart failure is complicated by myocardial infarction, intubate and invasively ventilate.
   d. Sedation of intubated patients is necessary to establish hemodynamic stability. Marked ventilatory efforts add to hemodynamic instability.
3. Management of gas exchange
   a. Oxygenation should be managed by a combination of PEEP and F_IO_2 adjustment.
   b. If pulmonary edema persists with good vascular volume, increasing PEEP may improve oxygenation and myocardial function.
   c. PaO_2 should be maintained at approximately 80 to 100 mm Hg if possible.
   d. Ventilation can usually be managed by adjustment of rate.
3. Ongoing management
   a. Improvement in overall status and length of mechanical ventilation depend on improvement in cardiovascular function.
   b. Weaning may be slow because removal of positive pressure may result in low-grade pulmonary edema.
L. Ventilatory management of drug overdose
   1. Physiologic concerns
      a. The length of ventilatory support depends on the specific drug ingested.
      b. Major problems exist if patients have aspirated.
      c. In this setting ARDS may develop.
   2. Initial ventilatory settings (Box 41-11)

BOX 41-10

Cardiac Disease: Initial Ventilator Settings

Noninvasive Positive Pressure

Continuous positive airway pressure: If only hypoxemic respiratory failure 8 to 12 cm H_2O with F_IO_2 1.0

Noninvasive positive pressure ventilation: If hypercapnic ventilatory failure
- Positive end-expiratory pressure (PEEP): 5 to 8 cm H_2O
- Ventilatory pressure: 8 to 12 cm H_2O
- Tidal volume (VT): 6 to 8 ml/kg ideal body weight (IBW)
- F_IO_2: 1.0
- Inspiratory time: Equal to patient neuroinspiratory time, ≤ 1.0 second
- Rate: 15 to 25/min

If Intubated
- Mode: Assist/control
- VT: 8 to 10 ml/kg IBW
- Plateau pressure: <25 cm H_2O
- PEEP: 5 to 10 cm H_2O
- Inspiratory time: 1.0 second
- Peak flow: (volume ventilation) to ensure inspiratory time
- Flow waveform: (volume ventilation) decelerating
- F_IO_2: 1.0
- Rate: 15 to 25/min to maintain patient's baseline $PaCO_2$

BOX 41-11

Drug Overdose: Initial Ventilator Settings

- Mode: Assist/control
- Tidal volume: 8 to 10 ml/kg ideal body weight
- Plateau pressure: <25 cm H_2O
- PEEP: 5 cm H_2O
- Peak flow: (volume ventilation) to ensure inspiratory time
- Flow waveform: (volume ventilation) decelerating
- Inspiratory time: 1.0 second
- F_IO_2: To maintain PaO_2 >70 mm Hg
- Rate: 10 to 20/min to maintain patient's baseline $PaCO_2$

        a. Ventilator settings are relatively straightforward.

        b. If aspiration has occurred, management may need to be similar to that of ARDS.

    3. Management of gas exchange

        a. Maintain $Paco_2$ by adjusting rate.

        b. If P_{plat} is <25 mm Hg V_T can be increased to manage $Paco_2$.

        c. Manage Pao_2 with F_Io_2 unless aspiration, and then manage as ARDS.

    4. Ongoing management

        a. Normally ventilatory management is short term.

        b. Management is only prolonged when aspiration and ARDS are present.

VIII. **Monitoring the Patient/Ventilator System**

    A. Monitoring the patient and the functions of the ventilator should be performed as frequently as the clinical situation dictates. Most patient/ventilator systems should be evaluated every 4 hours. However, the highly unstable patient may require hourly or continuous evaluation.

    B. The patient's response to mechanical ventilation should be the primary focus of the evaluation.

        1. Determine spontaneous RR and heart rate.

        2. Measure blood pressure.

        3. If hemodynamic monitoring is used, evaluate all available parameters.

        4. Record peak pressure and P_{plat}.

        5. Assess patient/ventilator synchrony.

            a. Ensure all patient inspiratory efforts trigger a breath.

            b. Ensure patient T_I and ventilator T_I are equal.

            c. Ensure the patient and the ventilator end the breath at the same time.

            d. Ensure gas delivery meets patient inspiratory demand.

            e. Ensure Spo_2 (pulse oximetry saturation) is ≥90% to 92%.

            f. Evaluate patient compliance and resistance *when indicated,* usually in long-term ventilator-dependent patients (see Chapter 5).

            g. Arterial blood gases need to be evaluated once a day unless the patient is unstable.

               (1) Changes in PEEP and F_Io_2 can be evaluated by Spo_2.

               (2) Changes in level of ventilation may not require immediate blood gas evaluation, and changes in hemodynamics may be sufficient to evaluate response.

            h. Patients with airflow obstruction or rapid rates should have auto-PEEP levels evaluated with each assessment.

            i. Evaluate the patient's airway.

               (1) Position of the ETT

               (2) Obstruction of the tube

               (3) Pressure in the cuff should be 20 to 25 cm H_2O to avoid aspiration.

               (4) Kinking of the ETT

    C. Evaluate the ventilatory system

        1. Drain all tubing of condensate.

        2. Verify ventilator parameters are set as ordered.

            a. Volume ventilation: High and low pressure alarms are critical to set.

            b. Pressure ventilation: High and low volume alarms are critical to set.

            c. High and low F_Io_2 alarms should be set.

            d. Loss of PEEP alarm should be set.

IX. **Ventilator Discontinuation/Weaning**

The following issues ideally should be resolved before patients are considered for ventilatory discontinuation and are the issues that prevent patients failing weaning trials from successfully weaning.

    A. The disease process necessitating ventilatory support should be reversed.

    B. No active acute pulmonary disease process should be present.

    C. Vital signs should be stable.

1. Fever even if not of pulmonary origin
    a. Increases oxygen consumption
    b. Increases CO_2 production
2. Tachycardia and hypertension are indicative of increased level of stress.
3. Bradycardia and hypotension, possibly indicating a lack of myocardial reserves and poor peripheral perfusion

D. Nutritional status should be optimized (see Chapter 24)
    1. This is of particular concern if patients have been ventilated for a lengthy period and have a chronic underlying disease process.
    2. If a patient is receiving hyperalimentation, it may be preferable to delay ventilator discontinuance until hyperalimentation is complete.
        a. This is particularly true if all nonprotein calories are administered as carbohydrates.
        b. When lipids are not administered, the respiratory quotient for the conversion of carbohydrates to lipids is >8.0.
        c. As a result, the patient's CO_2 production is markedly increased.
        d. Patients with marginal cardiopulmonary reserves may not be able to meet the demands of ventilator discontinuance when coupled with an increased CO_2 load.

E. Adequate cardiovascular reserves
    1. Normal pulse and blood pressure
    2. No arrhythmias
    3. Good peripheral perfusion
    4. The pulmonary artery catheter should have been removed.

F. Normal renal function

G. Intact central nervous system

H. Normally functioning GI tract

I. Proper electrolyte and fluid balance (see Chapter 14)
    1. Electrolyte abnormalities may result in muscular weakness. Specifically the following electrolytes should be normal.
        a. K^+
        b. Cl^-
        c. Ca^{+2}
        d. PO_4^{-3}
        e. Mg^{+2}
        Note: Any electrolyte, fluid, or major organ system malfunction results in an increase in physiologic stress. This, coupled with the added stress of spontaneous ventilation, may be enough to cause a patient to fail a weaning trial and require ventilatory support.

J. Adequate gas exchange capabilities
    1. Acceptable arterial blood gas values
        a. $PaCO_2$ at patient's normal level
            (1) For most patients this is approximately 40 mm Hg.
            (2) For COPD patients, it may be at an elevated $PaCO_2$ level.
        b. Normal pH
        c. No indication of excessive deadspace or intrapulmonary shunt
        d. PaO_2 >60 mm Hg with F_IO_2 <0.5 and PEEP ≤5 mm Hg

K. Adequate ventilatory capabilities
    1. Numerous indexes have been proposed to identify ventilatory capabilities.
    2. However, none of these indexes is capable of accurately identifying *all* patients who will wean from ventilatory support.
    3. The following have been shown to indicate in *some* patients the ability to breathe spontaneously.
        a. Vital capacity: >10 ml/kg body weight
        b. Maximum inspiratory pressure (MIP)
            (1) <−30 cm H_2O
            (2) >−20 cm H_2O is a good indicator of the need for continued ventilatory support.

    c. Spontaneous RR: <35 breaths/min

    d. Rapid shallow breathing index (RSBI): <105 (RR divided by V_T in liters) is the best of these indexes but is still problematic.

    e. V_T: >3.5 ml/kg body weight

    f. Minute volume: <10 L/min

    g. Deadspace to V_T ratio (V_D/V_T): <0.5

    h. Percent intrapulmonary shunt: <15%

    i. WOB: <1.2 J/L

    j. Maximum voluntary ventilation (MVV): >2 times minute ventilation

L. Psychologic preparation

    1. The transition from mechanical ventilation to spontaneous ventilation produces a great deal of anxiety in some patients. This is particularly evident in patients ventilated for more than several days.

    2. To relieve some of the anxiety

        a. Carefully explain the procedure in detail.

        b. Attempt to develop the patient's confidence by reinforcing the improvement noted in their disease process.

        c. Assure patients that they will be continually monitored throughout the time they are ventilating spontaneously and that you will respond to their needs.

        d. Do not tell patients they will never need the ventilator again.

            (1) If this is done and ventilatory support must be reestablished, it is not uncommon for patients to lose confidence in themselves and the medical team caring for them.

            (2) It is more appropriate to inform patients that their capability of ventilating spontaneously is going to be evaluated. If they are ventilating adequately, they will be allowed to continue; however, if they deteriorate clinically, mechanical ventilation will be reinstituted.

M. Approaches to weaning

    1. Spontaneous breathing trials

        a. The patient is removed from ventilatory support placed on a T piece or left attached to the ventilator with no ventilatory support and CPAP set at zero.

        b. The patient's cardiorespiratory response is monitored for 30 to 120 minutes on unassisted breathing. If none of the following are observed for a sustained period, the patient is considered ready for ventilator discontinuation.

            (1) RR: >35/minute

            (2) SpO_2: <90%

            (3) Pulse: >140 beats/min or 20% increase

            (4) Arterial blood pressure: ≥20% change; systolic, >180; and diastolic, >90

            (5) Diaphoresis

            (6) Increased anxiety

        c. Note that $Paco_2$ is not part of the above assessment.

            (1) $Paco_2$ is a late indicator of failure.

            (2) Changes in ventilatory status and vital signs are more indicative of ability to withstand the stress of ventilation than $Paco_2$.

            (3) In many patients $Paco_2$ may be normal, but physiologic stress is marked.

        d. In patients who fail an initial spontaneous breathing trial and who have auto-PEEP because of airway obstruction, 5 cm H_2O CPAP may be applied during the trial.

        e. In patients with nasal intubation or small for their size ETTs, 5 to 7 cm H_2O pressure support may be applied during the spontaneous breathing trial.

        f. If a patient fails a spontaneous breathing trial, the patient should be placed on appropriate ventilatory support to rest.

        g. Spontaneous breathing trials generally need only be applied daily.

    2. Decreasing levels of pressure support

        a. With this approach pressure support is slowly decreased over time.

        b. When 2 to 4 hours of ventilatory support can be tolerated with a pressure support level of 5 to 7 cm H_2O, the patient is considered weaned.

      c. The same variables indicating failure of a spontaneous breathing trial are used to indicate failure of a pressure support wean.

    3. Decreasing synchronized intermittent mandatory ventilation (SIMV) rate

      a. The SIMV rate is decreased 2/min as tolerated every 2 to 4 hours.

      b. When the SIMV rate is equal to 4/min and can be tolerated for 2 to 4 hours the patient is considered ready for extubation.

      c. The same variables indicating failure of a spontaneous breathing trial are used to indicate failure of an SIMV weaning trial.

N. The most successful approach to weaning patients is the spontaneous breathing trial.

    1. Other approaches to weaning prolong the ventilatory course.

    2. Regardless of the indication for ventilatory support or the length of ventilatory support, a spontaneous breathing trial should be used to assess readiness for discontinuation of ventilatory support.

O. Protocolized weaning from ventilatory support

    1. This is a well-defined set of criteria that are followed in assessment of the patient's status, in the performance of a spontaneous breathing trial, and in the discontinuation of ventilatory support.

    2. All protocols should define a specific level of assessment daily.

    3. Patient's meeting the assessment criteria are placed on a daily spontaneous breathing trial.

    4. Those passing the trial are extubated unless there was a reason to *not* extubate.

      a. Upper airway obstruction

      b. Ongoing aspiration concern

      c. An inability to manage secretions

P. More than 80% of all ventilated patients can be rapidly discontinued from ventilatory support with the first spontaneous breathing trial.

Q. Approximately 18% to 19% of patients require a series of spontaneous breathing trials over a number of days before ventilator discontinuation.

R. Approximately 1% of all ventilated patients require a lengthy period of weaning from ventilatory support.

    1. Even these patients are weaned by spontaneous breathing trial.

    2. However, they require multiple days of successful 12 to 16 hours of unassisted spontaneous breathing before they are allowed to go 24 hours without ventilatory support.

    3. These patients also frequently require extensive rehabilitation to successfully wean.

    4. However, some of these patients will remain ventilator dependent.

    5. Patients remain ventilator dependent for a physiologic reason. One or more of the concerns outlined in Section IX. A to L are the reasons why patients fail to wean from ventilatory support.

BIBLIOGRAPHY

Amato MBP, Barbas CSV, Medeiros DM: Effect of a protective-ventilation strategy on mortality in the acute respiratory distress syndrome. *N Engl J Med* 338:347-354, 1998.

Burton GC, Hodgkin JF, Ward JJ: *Respiratory Care*, ed 4. Philadelphia, JB Lippincott, 1997.

Hess DJ, Kacmarek RM: *Essentials of Mechanical Ventilation*, ed 2. New York, McGraw Hill Publishing, 2002.

Hess DJ, MacIntyre NR, Mishoc SC, Galvin WF, Adams AB, Saposnick AB: *Respiratory Care Principles and Practice.* Philadelphia, WB Saunders, 2002.

Kacmarek RM, Hess DR, Stoller JK: *Monitoring in Respiratory Care.* St. Louis, Mosby, 1993.

Pierson DJ, Kacmarek K: *Foundations of Respiratory Care.* New York, Churchill Livingstone, 1992.

Shapiro BA, Cane RD, Harrison RA: Positive end-expiratory pressure in acute lung injury. *Chest* 83: 558-563, 1983.

Shapiro BA, Kacmarek RM, Cane RD, et al: *Clinical Application of Respiratory Care*, ed 4. St. Louis, Mosby, 1991.

The Acute Respiratory Distress Syndrome Network: Ventilation with lower tidal volumes as compared with traditional tidal volumes for acute lung injury and the acute respiratory distress syndrome. *N Engl J Med* 342:1301-1308, 2000.

Tobin MJ: *Principles and Practice of Mechanical Ventilation.* New York, McGraw Hill, 1994.

Wilkins RL, Stoller JK, Scanlon CL: *Egan's Fundamentals of Respiratory Care*, ed 8. St. Louis, Mosby, 2003.

Chapter 42

High Frequency Ventilation

I. **Definitions**
   A. High frequency ventilation (HFV) is a form of mechanical ventilation that uses small tidal volumes (VTs approaching deadspace volume or less) and high respiratory rates (>120 breaths/min).
   B. Basically four different types of high frequency approaches to ventilation have been used.
      1. High frequency positive-pressure ventilation (HFPPV): This approach uses conventional ventilators to provide HFV.
         a. Respiratory rate ranges from 120 to 240 breaths/min.
         b. VT is set at 3 to 5 ml/kg.
         c. Inspiratory-to-expiratory (I:E) ratios are set at approximately 1:2.
         d. Positive end-expiratory pressure (PEEP) can be set at any level.
         e. Technically HFPPV is applied via conventional ventilators or pneumatic valve systems.
         f. With all systems, exhalation is passive.
         g. No additional or secondary gas is entrained.
      2. High frequency jet ventilation (HFJV): This approach normally combines the use of a jet ventilator and a conventional ventilator.
         a. Respiratory frequency ranges from 120 to 1200 breaths/min or 2 Hz to 20 Hz. One hertz (Hz) equals 60 breaths/min.
         b. VT is estimated to be approximately 2 to 5 ml/kg.
         c. The I:E ratio is set at approximately 1:2.
         d. PEEP can be set at any level.
         e. All systems use a ventilator specifically designed for HFJV and a secondary gas source, commonly a conventional ventilator.
         f. Each ventilation system uses a 14- to 18-gauge small-bore injector in which gas is periodically introduced at high pressure (15 to 50 pounds per square inch) into a specially designed endotracheal tube adapter (Figure 42-1). However, the small-bore injector can also be inserted directly into the cricothyroid membrane.
         g. Gas is also entrained from a secondary source, mixing with the injector flow to establish VT (see Figure 42-1).
         h. Exhaled gas leaves via a separate route (see Figure 42-1).
         i. Gas flow through the injector is interrupted at clinician-set intervals by pneumatic, fluidic, or electronically controlled solenoid valves.
         j. With all systems exhalation is passive.
         k. The jet flow is humidified by water dripped in front of the injector. The entrained gas is normally humidified.

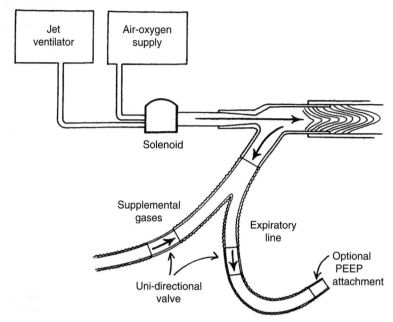

FIG. 42-1 Essential design features of a high frequency jet ventilator.

3. High frequency oscillation (HFO)
   a. The most common approach to HFV used today is HFO.
   b. Requires a unique self-contained system to provide ventilation
   c. Basically a bias flow of gas passes across the airway, exiting through a variable resistor.
   d. A mechanism to oscillate the flow is included perpendicular to the bias flow (Figure 42-2).
      (1) A piston
      (2) A high frequency speaker
      (3) A rotating valve
   e. The oscillation causes the inspiratory phase to be positive pressure and the expiratory phase to be negative pressure.
   f. The force of the oscillation is referred to as the delta pressure: The total pressure change from inspiration to expiration. If the delta pressure is 60 cm H_2O, +30 cm H_2O is developed during inspiration and −30 cm H_2O is developed during expiration. This is above and below the mean airway pressure.
   g. The resistance to the bias flow and the total bias flow controls the mean airway pressure.
   h. With some systems the I:E ratio can be adjusted from 1:1 to 1:2.
   i. Frequency can vary with most HFO systems from 3 Hz to 20 Hz.
   j. As with other ventilatory systems, F_IO_2 can be adjusted from 0.21 to 1.0.
   k. PEEP is not set during HFO. However, during HFO especially at high frequency settings, the mean airway pressure is essentially equal to the PEEP level because the delta pressure is markedly decreased by the time it reaches the alveolar level.
   l. High frequency flow interruption is a form of HFO that does not have a negative expiratory phase. The bias flow is simply interrupted to allow passive exhalation to occur.
4. High frequency percussive ventilation (HFPV)
   a. This approach to HFV is truly a combination of conventional ventilation and HFV.
   b. As noted in Figure 42-3 gas is delivered as a pressure-limited conventional breath with oscillations superimposed on the breath.

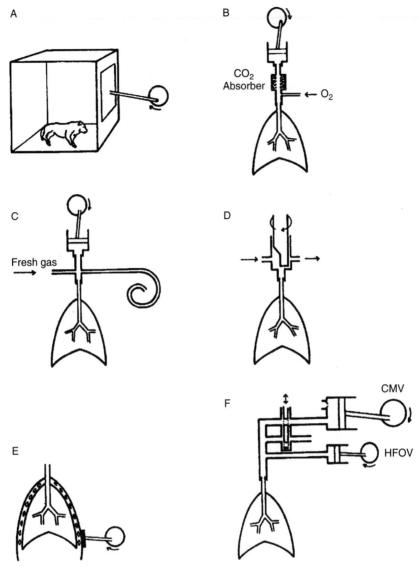

FIG. 42-2 Schematic representation of six different types of high frequency oscillation (HFO) systems. **A,** Whole body oscillation administered either in a dynamic pressure chamber or by whole body mechanical ventilation. **B,** A closed HFO system in which CO_2 is absorbed. **C,** Bias flow oscillator: Oscillations can be provided by many mechanisms: piston, a high frequency speaker, or other vibrating membrane. **D,** Rotating valve that interrupts a high pressure gas source. **E,** Oscillations coupled to the thorax. **F,** HFO ventilation combined with conventional ventilation similar to high frequency percussive ventilation.

    c. Oscillations can be delivered either during inspiration only or during inspiration and expiration. Throughout the ventilatory cycle patients may breathe spontaneously in association with the conventional and high frequency breaths.

    d. Thus the conventional gas delivery and high frequency approaches to ventilation can be adjusted.

    e. HFPV operates by using a high frequency injector that injects gas flow to operate a sliding Venturi valve used to entrain a secondary humidified flow of gas (Figure 42-4).

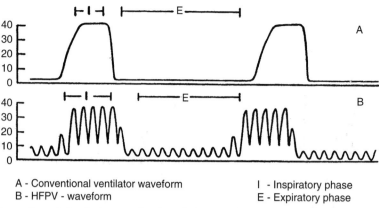

A - Conventional ventilator waveform
B - HFPV - waveform

I - Inspiratory phase
E - Expiratory phase

FIG. 42-3 Comparison of standard conventional ventilation waveform and high frequency percussive ventilation waveform with high frequency oscillations superimposed on a standard pressure targeted ventilation waveform.

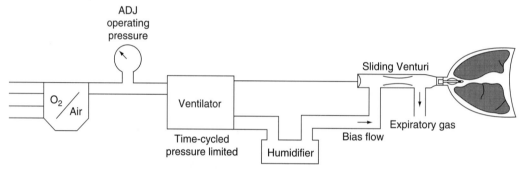

FIG. 42-4 Schematic of a high frequency percussive ventilation system. Gas from an air/oxygen blender is delivered to the ventilator. The ventilator is time cycled, pressure limited, and allows spontaneous breathing to occur throughout the respiratory cycle. The two gas sources originate from the ventilator. The first powers a nebulizer that provides humidified gases that are entrained by the sliding Venturi valve. The second carries pulsatile gas under pressure to power the sliding Venturi valve.

II. **Mechanism of Gas Exchange**
   A. During normal spontaneous breathing and conventional mechanical ventilation (CMV) the two factors responsible for gas exchange are
      1. Convection
      2. Diffusion
   B. Convection is primarily responsible for gas movement to the level of the terminal bronchioles and diffusion from the terminal bronchioles to the alveoli.
   C. During HFV many other factors come into play ensuring that CO_2 elimination can be maintained despite V_T being equal to or smaller than deadspace volume (Figure 42-5).
   D. The following have been proposed as possible mechanisms for gas movement during HFV.
      1. Pendelluft gas movement: Because neighboring gas units have varying compliance and resistance, filling of lung units is uneven (underventilation of some and overventilation of others); thus gas movement can occur from one lung unit to another that is convective movement within the lung.
      2. Convective dispersion by asymmetric velocity profiles: Gas in the center of a column moves faster than gas at the periphery. As a result gas can move to a greater depth in the lung than predicted by the V_T delivered. There is also coaxial or bidirectional gas

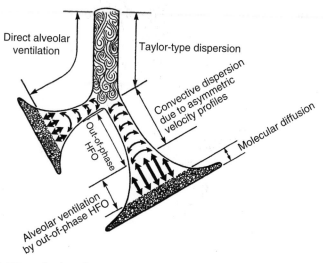

FIG. 42-5 More than one mechanism of gas movement may operate in various regions of the lung during high frequency ventilation. Moreover, mechanisms may act synergistically. Gas velocities decrease from the airway opening to the alveolus. See text for discussion.

movement. At the center of the airway, gas (O_2) moves into the lung, whereas at the periphery gas (CO_2) moves to the mouth.

3. Taylor dispersion (augmented dispersion): High-velocity gas movement enhances the development of turbulence in the conducting airways, causing eddies and swirling gas movement. This movement encourages dispersion of gas laterally and centrally.
4. Cardiogenic oscillation: The oscillations of the circulatory system assist gas movement especially at very high ventilatory frequencies.
5. Out-of-phase HFO: If the oscillation is out of phase with the normal resonance frequency of the lung, lateral and distal gas movement is enhanced.
6. Convection in larger airways: Most gas movement is still by gross movement of gas from one place to another.
7. At the alveolar level molecular diffusion accounts for gas movement.
8. The lung may be considered in three zones with reference to HFV (see Figure 42-5).
   a. Zone 1 is the large airways in which flow is turbulent. Here convection and Taylor dispersion are responsible primarily for gas movement.
   b. Zone 2 is the lower airways, where flow is laminar. Here gas movement is primarily by coaxial flow and asymmetric velocity profiles.
   c. Zone 3 is lung parenchyma, where no bulk movement occurs. Here gas movement is primarily by cardiac oscillations, pendelluft, and molecular diffusion.
9. Gas movement in the upper airway generally seems to be the major limiting factor in HFV.

III. **Ventilation and Oxygenation**
   A. With HFPPV, HFJV, and HFPV, ventilation and oxygenation are linked as in conventional ventilation. However, with HFO most consider the two processes uncoupled.
   B. Ventilation during HFO depends on
      1. Rate
      2. Delta pressure
      3. Bias flow
   C. CO_2 elimination is generally directly related to the delta pressure and the bias flow in HFO. Increasing both tends to increase V_T.

D. However, CO_2 elimination is *inversely* related to rate in HFO (i.e., as rate decreases, CO_2 elimination increases). The reason for this is that a decrease in rate in HFO results in an increase in VT.

1. A lower rate increases inspiratory time, allowing more time for VT delivery.
2. This also means that less of the delta pressure dissipates in the larger airways. More pressure extends into the lower respiratory tract.
3. At low rates (3 Hz) and high delta pressures (90 cm H_2O), as has been applied in adults, VT with HFO approaches that of normal breathing approximately 5 to 6 ml/kg of ideal body weight.
4. At rapid rates as seen in neonates (8 to 15 Hz) VT may be smaller than deadspace volume ($\leq$1 ml/kg ideal body weight).

E. Oxygenation in HFO depends on mean airway pressure.

1. The greater the mean airway pressure, the greater the functional residual capacity (FRC; or PEEP equivalent).
2. I:E affects mean airway pressure somewhat. The longer the inspiratory time, the greater the mean airway pressure.
3. Increasing the bias flow has a direct effect on mean airway pressure.

IV. **Respiratory and Cardiovascular Effects of HFV**

A. HFV when applied properly maintains the lung in a state of hyperinflation. This is more pronounced the greater the compliance of the lung. However, even with acute lung injury (acute respiratory distress syndrome [ARDS]), auto-PEEP develops with HFPPV, HFJV, and HFPV. Auto-PEEP is not developed during HFO.
B. HFV does not appear to alter surfactant production to the same extent as conventional ventilation. Compliance decreases over time with conventional ventilation but does not seem to be altered with HFV.
C. As long as PCO_2 is maintained at a normal or below normal level, apnea is common with the use of HFV. Although spontaneous breathing develops during rapid eye movement sleep, it is believed that inhibition of phrenic activity via the vagus nerve and activation of mechanoreceptors inhibit breathing at other times during HFV in some patients.
D. The frequency of barotrauma is equivalent to that of conventional ventilation.
E. Hemodynamic compromise is similar to that with conventional ventilation.
F. The other overall respiratory and cardiovascular effects of HFV are similar to conventional ventilation.

V. **Indications**

A. Upper airway surgery and bronchoscopy

1. HFPPV and HFJV are preferred over conventional ventilation in these clinical settings.
2. Both are capable of providing more efficient gas exchange than conventional ventilation with an open airway.

B. Bronchopulmonary fistula

1. Initially HFV was considered superior to conventional ventilation in the presence of a large air leak.
2. At least theoretically gas distribution with conventional ventilation depends primarily on compliance, whereas as rate increases, gas distribution depends more on airway resistance.
3. Recent data indicate conventional ventilation and HFV are equally capable of ventilating in the presence of a bronchopulmonary fistula if acute lung injury is also present.
4. With major air leaks without acute lung injury, HFV may ventilate more effectively.

C. Acute lung injury

1. In the adult population HFV provides no advantage over conventional ventilation. Based on currently available data they are equivalent.
2. In the neonatal population HFO has been used to treat any severely ill neonate and has been considered superior to conventional ventilation. However, the use of surfactant,

lung protective ventilatory strategies, and nitric oxide during ventilation has resulted in no demonstrable benefit in recent clinical trials from HFO over conventional ventilation.

VI. **Safety**
   A. Extreme care must be taken with the use of HFV systems because of the potential for tremendous increases in airway pressure in a short period.
   B. In addition to alarms, mechanisms to abort gas delivery must be included. This is of particular concern with HFJV.

VII. **Humidification**
   A. A major problem with HFJV is humidification. No efficient mechanism to appropriately humidify the 20 to 60 L of gas delivered per minute during HFJV is available.
   B. As a result of insufficient humidification, necrotizing tracheobronchitis and squamous metaplasia of the bronchial mucosa with submucosal inflammatory cell infiltration are common during HFJV.
   C. However, gas used during HFPPV, HFO, and HFPV can be easily humidified and causes no greater problems than conventional ventilation.

VIII. **The Use of HFO in Adult ARDS**
   A. Initial setting
      1. F_IO_2 at or greater than that used during CMV
      2. Rate: 3 to 8 Hz, generally started at 5 Hz
      3. Delta pressure: 40 to 90 cm H_2O, generally started at 60 cm H_2O
      4. I:E: 1:1 or 1:2, generally started at 1:1
      5. Bias flow: 40 L/min
      6. Mean airway pressure: between 20 and 35 cm H_2O initially
         a. 3 to 5 cm H_2O higher than that during CMV
         b. Set at 35 to 40 cm H_2O to recruit the lung then decrease to the lowest level maintaining oxygenation.
      7. When mean airway pressure can be decreased to 20 cm H_2O, patients are frequently converted to conventional ventilation at the same mean airway pressure then weaned as tolerated.

IX. **Sedation**
   A. It has been the rule that adults on HFO have been heavily sedated.
   B. However, neonates can frequently be maintained on HFO while still capable of spontaneous breathing.
   C. Sedation requirements should be adjusted to the patient's needs.

BIBLIOGRAPHY

Branson RD, Hess DR, Chatburn RL: *Respiratory Care Equipment*, ed 2. Philadelphia, Lippincott, Williams & Wilkins, 1999.

Carlon GC, Howland WS: High-frequency ventilation in intensive care and during surgery. *Lung Biology in Health and Disease Series*. New York, Marcel Dekker Inc., 1985.

Carlon GC, Howland WS, Ray C, et al: High-frequency jet ventilation. A prospective randomized evaluation. *Chest* 84:551-559, 1983.

Carlon GC, Miodownik S, Ray C Jr, et al: Technical aspects and clinical implications of high frequency jet ventilation with a solenoid valve. *Crit Care Med* 9:47-50, 1981.

Carlon GC, Ray C Jr, Klain M, et al: High-frequency positive pressure ventilation in management of a patient with bronchopleural fistula. *Anesthesiology* 52:160-162, 1980.

Chang HF: Mechanisms of gas-transport during ventilation by high frequency oscillation. *J Appl Physiol* 56:553-563, 1984.

Derdak S, Mehta S, Steard TE: High-frequency oscillatory ventilation for acute respiratory distress syndrome in adults. *Am J Respir Crit Care Med* 166:801-808, 2002.

Forese AB, Bryan AC: High frequency ventilation. *Am Rev Respir Dis* 135:1363-1374, 1987.

Fort P, Framer C, Westerman J: High-frequency oscilatory ventilation for adult respiratory distress syndrome—a pilot study. *Crit Care Med* 25: 937-947, 1997.

Hess DR, Kacmarek RM: *Essentials of Mechanical Ventilation*, ed 2. New York, McGraw-Hill Publishing, 2003.

Holzapfel L, Perrin RF, Gaussorgues P, et al: Comparison of high-frequency jet ventilation to conventional ventilation in adults with respiratory distress syndrome. *Intensive Care Med* 13:100-105, 1987.

Hurst JM, Branson RD, David K: High-frequency percussive ventilation in the management of elevated intracranial pressure. *J Trauma* 28:1363-1367, 1988.

Mehta S, Lapinsky SE, Hallett DC: Prospective trial of high-frequency oscillation in adults with acute respiratory distress syndrome. *Crit Care Med* 29:1360-1369, 2001.

Ray C, Miodownik S, Carlon G, et al: Pneumatic-to-electric analog for high frequency jet ventilation of disrupted airways. *Crit Care Med* 12:711-712, 1984.

Rossing TH, Slutsky AS, Lehr JL, et al: Tidal volume and frequency dependence of carbon dioxide elimination by high-frequency ventilation. *N Engl J Med* 305:1375-1379, 1981.

Slutsky AS: Mechanisms affecting gas transport during high frequency oscillation. *Crit Care Med* 12:713-717, 1984.

Slutsky AS, Drazen JM, Ingram RH Jr, et al: Effective pulmonary ventilation with small-volume oscillations at high frequency. *Science* 209:609-611, 1980.

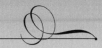
Noninvasive Positive Pressure Ventilation

I. **Noninvasive Positive Pressure Ventilation**

Noninvasive positive pressure ventilation (NPPV) is the application of positive pressure by non-invasive means to patients with acute or chronic respiratory failure.

A. Many have considered acute respiratory failure caused by the following as situations in which NPPV should be applied (Box 43-1).
1. Chronic obstructive pulmonary disease (COPD), acute exacerbation
2. Cardiogenic pulmonary edema
3. Asthma
4. Neurologic/neuromuscular disease
5. Weaning from ventilatory support
6. Extubation failure
7. Acute lung injury
8. Immunosuppressed patients
9. Patients awaiting lung transplantation
10. Do not intubate/do not resuscitate (DNI/DNR) status

B. COPD, acute exacerbation
1. Multiple randomized controlled trials of the use of NPPV in patients with COPD have indicated improved outcome.
2. Patients with a moderate to severe acute exacerbation of COPD and treated with NPPV
   a. Are less likely to be intubated
   b. Are less likely to develop nosocomial pneumonia
   c. Have a shorter mechanical ventilation time
   d. Have a shorter intensive care unit (ICU) stay
   e. Have a shorter hospital stay
   f. Have decreased hospital mortality
3. NPPV is a "standard of care" to manage an acute exacerbation of COPD.
4. NPPV for COPD should be the first-line therapy in all institutions caring for these patients.

C. Cardiogenic pulmonary edema
1. NPPV has been useful for patients with cardiogenic pulmonary edema who are unable to effectively ventilate (Paco$_2$, >45 cm H$_2$O).
2. Patients with only hypoxemic acute respiratory failure should be treated with 8 to 12 cm H$_2$O continuous positive airway pressure (CPAP).

BOX 43-1

Indications for NPPV in Acute Respiratory Failure

- Acute exacerbation of COPD, standard of care, should be considered for all patients.
- Cardiogenic pulmonary edema
  - Hypoxemic respiratory failure only: CPAP
  - Hypercapnic respiratory failure: NPPV
  - Myocardial infarction: Intubation
- Weaning failure: May be useful in some patients
- Immunosuppressed patients: NPPV should be used

- Lung transplant candidate: In many very useful
- Acute lung injury: May prevent timely intubation and place some patients at greater risk
- Asthma: Poorly tolerated by most asthma patients
- Neuromuscular/neurologic disease: Considered first-line therapy
- DNI/DNR patients: Useful but patients must understand that NPPV is life support

NPPV, Noninvasive positive pressure ventilation; *COPD*, chronic obstructive pulmonary disease; *CPAP*, continuous positive airway pressure; *DNI/DNR*, do not intubate/do not resuscitate.

3. Patients with a myocardial infarction or suspected myocardial infarction should not receive NPPV or CPAP; they should be intubated and invasively ventilated.
4. During NPPV 100% oxygen should initially be delivered when the indication is cardiogenic pulmonary edema.

D. Asthma
   1. Patients with severe asthma have a difficult time tolerating a tight-fitting mask.
   2. These patients tend to be claustrophobic.
   3. Case studies from a few centers have indicated success with NPPV for patients with asthma.
   4. However, most do not recommend NPPV or CPAP for acute severe asthma.
   5. Heliox does work well for many patients with acute severe asthma to reduce work of breathing (see Chapter 34).

E. Neurologic/neuromuscular disease
   1. NPPV works well for these patients when applied for short-term or long-term use for those with progressively deteriorating diseases.
   2. No randomized controlled trials have been performed, but dozens of case series demonstrate improved gas exchange and avoidance of intubation.
   3. NPPV should always be considered for patients with neurologic/neuromuscular disease before a decision to intubate is made.

F. Weaning from ventilatory support
   1. A series of randomized controlled trials have evaluated elective extubation to NPPV for patients who have failed to respond to weaning trials.
   2. However, other randomized controlled trials have shown no benefit from elective extubation.
   3. Extubation to NPPV should be considered for patients who have failed to respond to multiple attempts at weaning but all clinical signs indicate they should be weaned.
   4. Patients who are extubated after passing a weaning trial but subsequently develop respiratory failure should also be considered for NPPV; however, existing data seem to indicate NPPV does not prevent reintubation.

G. Acute lung injury (ALI)
   1. Mask CPAP has been used over the years to manage acute hypoxemic respiratory failure from ALI.
   2. A number of groups have used NPPV with varying success to manage hypoxemic respiratory failure.
   3. However, the NPPV failure rate has been high in these patients (>60%), and mortality of those failing NPPV has also been high (>60%).
   4. It is frequent that either CPAP or NPPV is maintained too long, delaying the decision to intubate.
   5. As a result during intubation an increased risk of cardiac arrest exists.

6. NPPV or CPAP should be cautiously applied to patients with ALI, and if a beneficial response is not observed in a few hours, intubation should not be delayed.

H. Immunosuppressed patients

1. These patients almost always develop nosocomial pneumonia if intubated and have a high mortality when intubated.

2. As a result NPPV should always be considered first-line therapy to manage ventilatory failure.

3. Randomized controlled trials indicate a decrease in intubation rate and mortality if NPPV is used.

I. Patients awaiting lung transplantation

1. Many of these patients benefit from the short-term and long-term use of NPPV.

2. Intubation in transplantation candidates, similar to immunosuppressed patients, frequently results in the development of nosocomial pneumonia.

J. DNI/DNR patients

1. NPPV has been used to provide relief of hypercarbic and hypoxemic respiratory failure and to provide palliative care for these patients.

2. Because NPPV is life support patients should fully understand what it is they are receiving before it is started.

3. NPPV is useful for these patients to

a. Prolong life until family members arrive

b. Allow patients to be transported home to die

c. Provide comfort during the last hours of life

4. The expected outcome of NPPV in this setting is different from that in any of the other settings in which NPPV is applied.

II. **Initiation of NPPV**

A. Successful application of NPPV requires different skills than the successful application of invasive ventilation.

B. The therapist must fully understand the indications, benefits, and limitations of NPPV.

C. Patients *must* be part of the process. They must fully understand what is to be done and *must* be cooperative if the application is to be successful.

D. The initial application period can be time consuming. Frequently 60 to 90 minutes of a therapist's time is required during initial application.

E. After appropriate patient instruction a mask is selected (see Section V, The Mask).

1. Initial application ideally is by the patient holding the mask to his or her face.

2. If the patient is incapable of holding the mask, the therapist should hold the mask.

3. Do not strap the mask to the patient's face until he or she is completely accepting of the mask and all questions of the patient have been answered.

F. Initial ventilator setting should be low (Box 43-2).

1. Positive end-expiratory pressure (PEEP): 0 to 4 cm H_2O

2. Ventilatory pressure (pressure support, <5 cm H_2O)

BOX 43-2
NPPV Ventilator Setting

Initial Settings	Final Setting
PEEP: 0 to 4 cm H_2O	PEEP: 4 to 8 cm H_2O improves trigger synchrony
Ventilating pressure: <5 cm H_2O	Ventilating pressure: 8 to 12 cm H_2O establishes V_T
Expected V_T: 100 to 300 ml	Peak pressure: ≤20 cm H_2O
F_IO_2: Maintain SpO_2 >90%	V_T: 400 to 600 ml
Rate: Patient determined	F_IO_2: Maintain SpO_2 >90%
	Rate: Patient determined

NPPV, Noninvasive positive pressure ventilation; *PEEP*, positive end-expiratory pressure; *V_T*, tidal volume.

      3. Expected tidal volume (VT): 100 to 300 ml
      4. Set F_IO_2 to ensure SpO_2 >90%

  G. Do not increase pressure setting until the patient is comfortable with the application of positive pressure.

  H. Remember the application of high pressure by mask is uncomfortable and needs to be applied gradually for maximum patient acceptance.

  I. Slowly adjust PEEP to improve inspiratory trigger capability (offset the effect of auto-PEEP). Normally maximum setting is 4 to 8 cm H_2O.

  J. Increase pressure support level until an effective VT is delivered (400 to 600 ml). In most cases 8 to 12 cm H_2O pressure support is all that is necessary.

  K. Peak airway pressure should be kept <20 cm H_2O if possible. This prevents gastric distention because the gastric opening pressure is approximately 20 to 25 cm H_2O.

  L. Rate should be patient determined; set back up rate at 8 to 12/min, depending on patient ventilatory rate.

  M. Throughout this process constant encouragement and reinforcement of the purpose of NPPV should be provided.

  N. Only after the patient is fully accepting and comfortable with NPPV should the therapist leave the room.

  O. Ideally patients receiving NPPV for acute respiratory failure should be located in the emergency room, the ICU, or a special care unit where near-constant observation is possible.

III. Assessment of NPPV

  A. If within 2 hours of applying NPPV the following changes in patient's status are observed, NPPV was successful.
    1. $PaCO_2$ decreases
    2. pH increases
    3. PO_2 improves
    4. Respiratory rate decreases
    5. Heart rate and blood pressure normalize
    6. Ventilatory pattern normalizes

  B. However, if none of the above occurs intubation should be considered because NPPV is not having a positive impact on the patient's clinical status.

  C. Many patients present between these two extremes.
    1. $PaCO_2$ is not improved.
    2. pH is not improved.
    3. However, the patient's clinical status appears improved.
      a. Respiratory rate is decreased.
      b. Heart rate and blood pressure normalize.
    4. The patient appears more comfortable and is not using accessory muscles to ventilate.

  D. In this setting NPPV has unloaded cardiopulmonary stress but has not yet altered gas exchange.
    1. The patient should be allowed to continue on NPPV but should be closely observed for additional signs of benefit or failure.
    2. Many patients may take a longer period before definitive blood gas data indicating success or failure are observed.

  E. Be careful not to prolong the unsuccessful application of NPPV to avoid marked difficulty in intubating the patients who fail to respond (i.e., cardiac arrest).

IV. Type of Ventilator Used to Provide NPPV (Box 43-3)

  A. Any ventilator ever manufactured can be used to provide NPPV.

  B. However, most in the United States use either BiLevel pressure ventilators (Figure 43-1) or ICU ventilators.

  C. Most home care and subacute care ventilators available in the United States are not designed to provide NPPV. However, this situation is rapidly changing.

  D. BiLevel pressure ventilators deliver pressure-targeted breaths with at least the same efficiency as ICU ventilators.

BOX 43-3

*Type of Ventilators for NPPV**

BiLevel Pressure Ventilators	ICU Ventilators
Advantages	*Advantages*
• Good gas delivery system	• Good gas delivery system
• Leak compensation	• Monitors, alarms, waveforms
• Automatic adjustment of:	• Accurate and precise F_IO_2 delivery
• Inspiratory trigger sensitivity	
• Expiratory cycling criteria	*Disadvantages*
	• No leak compensation
Disadvantages	• No automatic adjustment of:
• Lack of monitoring	• Inspiratory trigger sensitivity
• Lack of alarms	• Expiratory cycling criteria
• Lack of pressure and flow waveforms	
• Lack of precise and accurate F_IO_2	

*The ideal NPPV ventilator combines the advantages of both types of ventilators.
NPPV, Noninvasive positive pressure ventilation; *ICU,* intensive care unit.

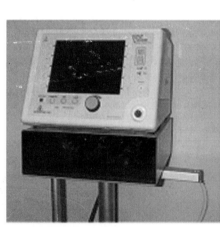
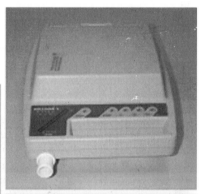
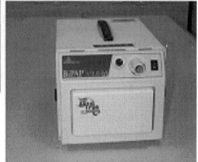

FIG. 43-1 Picture of various BiLevel pressure ventilators currently available.

    E. Many BiLevel pressure ventilators also
        1. Automatically adjust trigger sensitivity to changes in system leak
        2. Automatically adjust expiratory cycling criteria to changes in system leak
        3. Better ensure patient ventilator synchrony than noninvasively applied ICU ventilators
    F. However, *most* BiLevel pressure ventilators
        1. Can allow rebreathing of CO_2 (Figure 43-2)
            a. This is now avoided on newer models of BiLevel pressure ventilators by ensuring minimal PEEP is 4 cm H_2O.
            b. The inclusion of a secondary expiratory valve can avoid CO_2 breathing.

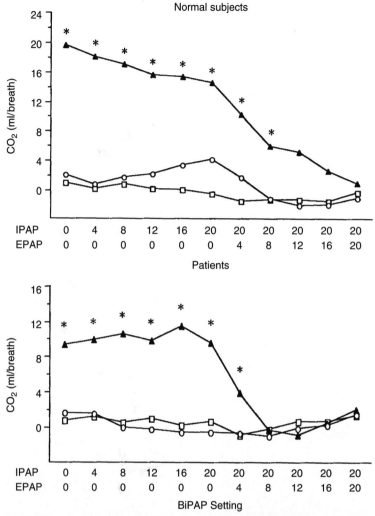

FIG. 43-2 Volume of CO_2 rebreathing in normal subjects and patients during noninvasive positive pressure ventilation with a BiLevel ventilator. ▲, Whisper swivel exhalation port; O, plateau pressure valve; □, non-breathing valve. CO_2 is rebreathed with the standard whisper swivel exhalation port unless approximately 4 cm H_2O positive end-expiratory pressure is applied. *$p < 0.05$.

    c. Rebreathing occurs when the flow from the ventilator is low during expiration (no or little PEEP) and the patient exhales completely into the circuit (oronasal mask).

    d. Because the ventilator has low internal resistance and only a small hole for exhalation (whisper swivel), exhaled gas can move into the single circuit gas delivery tubing all the way back to the ventilator.

    e. As a result on the next breath the exhaled CO_2 is rebreathed.

  2. Do not incorporate patient monitoring or alarms

  3. Do not allow visualization of airway pressure and flow waveforms, making it difficult to identify large leaks and patient-ventilator dysynchrony

  4. Do not allow for the delivery of high and precise F_1O_2

G. ICU ventilators can be used during NPPV; however, the disadvantages are

  1. No leak compensation

  2. Inability on most to adjust expiratory cycling criteria during pressure support

    a. As a result in some patients, pressure assist/control instead of pressure support is needed because pressure assist/control has a set inspiratory time (see Chapter 39).

    b. Simply set the inspiratory time equal to the patient actual inspiratory time.

    c. Gas delivery during pressure support and pressure assist/control is the same.

    d. The only difference other than the ability to set a backup rate is the mechanism that terminates inspiration.

       (1) With pressure support, a decrease in inspiratory flow to a set percentage

       (2) With pressure assist/control, a set time

  H. The ideal ventilator for NPPV is a BiLevel pressure ventilator designed for ICU use that includes

    1. Monitoring of the patient

    2. System alarms

    3. Pressure and flow waveforms

    4. The ability to deliver high and precise F_IO_2

V. The Mask (Figure 43-3)

  A. A large number of nasal and oronasal masks are currently available from multiple manufacturers.

  B. Differences in opinion regarding the use of nasal or oronasal masks during acute respiratory failure exist. Table 43-1 lists the pros and cons of each mask type.

  C. We prefer the use of an oronasal mask for acute respiratory failure because it is easier to ensure better ventilation with the oronasal mask than a nasal mask: fewer leaks.

  D. Other facial interphases can be used, but the majority of patients can be effectively treated with an oronasal or nasal mask.

  E. However, 24 to 48 hours after initial application, when the acute failure is resolved, many patients prefer a nasal mask.

  F. Proper mask fit is a critical factor affecting successful application of NPPV.

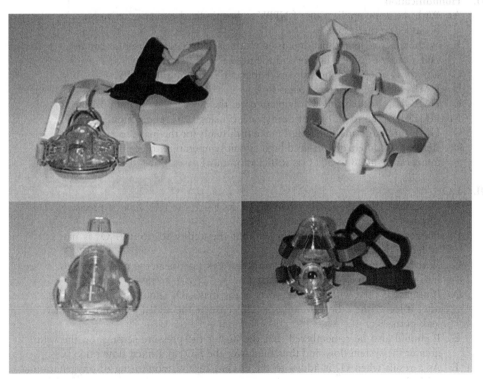

FIG. 43-3 Various nasal and oronasal masks used for noninvasive positive pressure ventilation.

TABLE **43-1**		
Nasal versus Oronasal Masks		
	Nasal	**Oronasal**
Ability to ventilate	Fair	Very good
Claustrophobia	Low	High
Ability to speak	Good	Poor
Ability to cough	Good	Limited
Air leak	Large	Small
Deadspace	Small	Large

    G. Regardless of mask type the top of the mask should rest about one fourth to one third of the way from top of the bridge of the nose.

       1. If the mask rests higher on the nose there is a greater likelihood of leaks around the nose into the eyes.

       2. The mask should conform to the lateral border of the nose.

    H. With nasal masks the bottom of the mask should rest above the upper lip.

    I. With oronasal masks they should either rest below the lower lip or at the chin, depending on mask design.

    J. If the mask is properly sized little force is necessary to maintain a good seal.

    K. When the mask is strapped to a patient's face, two fingers should be able to be comfortably placed between the strap and the patient's face.

    L. Too tight a strapped mask causes skin breakdown on the nose.

    M. It is always a good idea to bring a number of differently sized masks from a variety of manufacturers to ensure that the mask that best conforms to the patient's anatomy can be used.

VI. Humidification

    A. With the acute application of NPPV to hospitalized patients, active humidification should be added to the system.

    B. Without active humidification dried retained pharyngeal secretions can be a major problem and a cause of NPPV failure and the need to intubate.

    C. *Do not use* heat and moisture exchangers (HMEs) during NPPV.

    D. HMEs increase resistance to gas flow.

    E. HMEs require all exhaled volume to enter the device, usually not possible because of leaks.

    F. HMEs have up to 100 ml of deadspace, causing CO_2 rebreathing.

    G. HMEs are large and bulky and make it difficult for the mask to be secured.

    H. Active humidifiers do not need high circuit temperature to be effective. Maintaining circuit temperature at 28 to 30° C is sufficient in most cases.

VII. F_IO_2

    A. As stated earlier the ideal system is one in which the F_IO_2 can be precisely set and monitored.

    B. However, if a BiLevel ventilator without the ability to titrate F_IO_2 is used, O_2 must be added to the circuit.

    C. With the standard NPPV circuit with the leak port near the mask, O_2 should be titrated into the mask to ensure the highest F_IO_2.

    D. If a mask is used with the leak ports in the mask, O_2 should be added to the circuit right after it leaves the BiLevel ventilator. This ensures the added O_2 is not all lost via the mask leak ports.

    E. It should also be remembered that the higher the pressure settings on the ventilator, the greater the system flow and thus the lower the F_IO_2 at a fixed flow rate.

    F. As a result when O_2 is added to the circuit, careful monitoring of oxygenation status is critical.

VIII. **Aerosolized Pharmacologic Agents**
   A. Medications can be aerosolized during NPPV.
   B. However, because of the leaks and high flow, some of the drug will be lost to the environment; as a result higher doses may be necessary.
   C. To maximize drug delivery, the nebulizer or metered dose inhaler should be placed between the leak port and the mask.

IX. **Weaning**
   A. Contrary to invasive ventilation NPPV can easily be stopped for short periods and the patient evaluated.
   B. Most patients can ingest clear liquids during their short periods without NPPV.
   C. If patients can tolerated long periods without NPPV, solid food can be ingested.
   D. Weaning is accomplished by increasing the amount of time patients are without NPPV.
   E. Many patients decide by refusing to continue when NPPV is ready to be discontinued.

BIBLIOGRAPHY

Antonelli M, Conti G, Moro ML, et al: Predictors of failure on noninvasive positive pressure ventilation in patients with acute hypoxemic respiratory failure: a multi-center study. *Intensive Care Med* 27:1718-1728, 2001.

Bunburaphong T, Imanaka H, Nishimura M, Hess D, Kacmarek RM: Performance characteristics of Bilevel pressure ventilators: a lung model study. *Chest* 111:1050-1060, 1997.

Chu CM, Chan VL, Wong IWY, Leung WS, Lin AWN, Cheung KF: Noninvasive ventilation in patients with acute hypercapnic exacerbation of chronic obstructive pulmonary disease who refused endotracheal intubation. *Crit Care Med* 32:372-377, 2004.

Ferguson GT, Gilmartin M: CO_2 rebreathing during BiPAP® ventilatory assistance. *Am J Respir Crit Care Med* 151:1126-1135, 1995.

Ferrer M, Esquinas A, Arancibia F, et al: Noninvasive ventilation during persistent weaning failure: a randomized controlled trial. *Am J Respir Crit Care Med* 168:70-76, 2003.

Ferrer M, Esquinas A, Leon M, et al: Noninvasive ventilation in severe hypoxemic respiratory failure: a randomized clinical trial. *Am J Respir Crit Care Med* 168:1438-1444, 2003.

Girault C, Briel A, Hellot MF, et al: Noninvasive mechanical ventilation in clinical practice: a 2-year experience in a medical intensive care unit. *Crit Care Med* 31:552-559, 2003.

Kacmarek RM: Noninvasive positive-pressure ventilation: the little things do make the difference! *Respir Care* 48:919-921, 2003.

Keenan SP, Powers C, McCormack DG, Block G: Noninvasive positive-pressure ventilation for post-extubation respiratory distress. *JAMA* 287:3238-3244, 2002.

Kwok H, McCormack J, Cece R, Houtchens J, Hill N: Controlled trial of oronasal versus nasal mask ventilation in the treatment of acute respiratory failure. *Crit Care Med* 31:468-473, 2003.

Mehta S, Hill N: Noninvasive ventilation. *Am J Respir Crit Care Med* 163:540-577, 2001.

Nava S, Carbone G, DiBattista N, et al: Noninvasive ventilation in cardiogenic pulmonary edema: a multicenter randomized trial. *Am J Respir Crit Care Med* 168:1432-1437, 2003.

Schettino GPP, Chatmongkolchart S, Hess D, Kacmarek RM: Position of exhalation port and mask design affect CO_2 breathing during noninvasive positive pressure breathing. *Crit Care Med* 31:2178-2182, 2003.

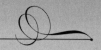

Chapter 44

Tracheal Gas Insufflation

I. **Tracheal Gas Insufflation**

Tracheal gas insufflation (TGI): The addition of a secondary gas flow during mechanical ventilation at the level of the carina to wash CO_2 from the deadspace of the large airways, endotracheal tube (ETT), and ventilator circuit (Figure 44-1).

   A. At end exhalation large airways, the ETT and the ventilator circuit deadspace contain a large amount of CO_2.

   B. Washing the CO_2 from these areas decreases the CO_2 of the gas moving to the alveoli during the next inhalation.

   C. As a result, over time the arterial PCO_2 decreases.

   D. Numerous case series in patients have demonstrated that TGI at flows of approximately 6 to 15 L/min decrease $PaCO_2$ (Figure 44-2).

   E. The greater the $PaCO_2$ at the time of initiating TGI, the greater the decrease in $PaCO_2$.

   F. The greater the TGI flow, the greater the effect on $PaCO_2$.

   G. The greater the volume of deadspace washed of CO_2, the greater the effect on arterial PCO_2.

II. **TGI Methodology**

   A. Figure 44-3 illustrates a typical TGI system.

   B. A small-gauge catheter is placed into or along side the ETT with its tip setting just past the tip of the ETT in the trachea.

   C. In most settings the tube is directed toward the carina (direct TGI).

   D. However, the flow through the catheter may also be directed up toward the ETT (e.g., indirect or reverse TGI).

   E. TGI can also be applied continuously or intermittently (during exhalation only).

   F. By simply attaching the TGI catheter to a flowmeter, continuous flow TGI can be performed.

   G. To accomplish expiratory phase-only TGI, the flow delivery must be coordinated with the ventilator (i.e., activation of TGI flow must begin and end during the expiratory phase).

   H. There are also some data to show that tracheal gas exsufflation (TGE; negative pressure applied to the catheter during expiration) also reduces PCO_2. However, TGE must be coordinated with the ventilator, only being applied during the expiratory phase.

III. **Concerns with TGI**

   A. Humidification: Clearly the TGI flow must be humidified to avoid the development of dried retained secretions.

   B. Airway injury: A high flow of gas from the TGI catheter can cause the tip of the catheter to wipe in the airway causing injury to the tracheal wall.

   C. With TGE, humidification and airway injury are not problems because the system only removes gas from the airway.

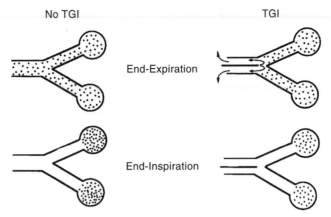

FIG. 44-1 With no tracheal gas insufflation (TGI) flow, CO_2 in the central airways, endotracheal tube, and circuit deadspace is delivered to the alveoli with each breath. With TGI the CO_2 in these areas is cleared by the TGI flow by end-expiration, decreasing CO_2 moved to the alveoli with each breath and thus decreasing $Paco_2$.

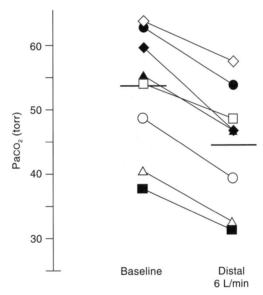

FIG. 44-2 Effect of 6 L/min continuous flow tracheal gas insufflation (TGI) in eight patients with acute respiratory distress syndrome. Before TGI, $Paco_2 = 53.1 \pm 3.1$ mm Hg; during TGI, $Paco_2 = 45.0 \pm 2.1$ mm Hg.

D. A major concern with TGI is the ability to shut down the system if there is an obstruction of the airway proximal to the tip of the catheter (i.e., between the ventilator circuit "wye" and the tip of the TGI catheter).

E. If the TGI flow is not stopped when this occurs, rapid overdistention of the airway and the potential for barotrauma rapidly develop.
1. To avoid these problems the TGI system must shut down whenever the ventilator senses obstruction.
2. This is necessary regardless whether the TGI flow is continuous or intermittent.

F. Direct TGI causes the total applied positive end-expiratory pressure (PEEP) to increase because the TGI flow is directed toward the lower airway at end expiration.

G. Indirect TGI causes the total PEEP to decrease because flow is directed toward the endotracheal tube and ventilator tubing, causing a Venturi effect and reducing PEEP.

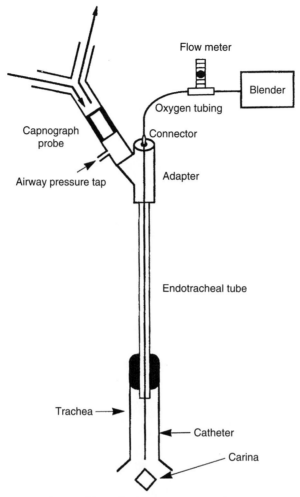

FIG. 44-3 A typical system used to provide tracheal gas insufflation (TGI), with the TGI catheter placed through the endotracheal tube into the trachea just above the carina.

    H. Monitoring of airway pressures and tidal volumes (VTs) is difficult during TGI.
        1. With continuous flow TGI it is impossible to measure VT, plateau pressure, and PEEP level.
        2. During expiratory TGI if the TGI flow is coordinated with the ventilator, plateau pressure and PEEP can be measured by flow interruption.
        3. Actual VT in volume ventilation delivered during continuous flow TGI can be estimated by subtracting the TGI volume (flow × inspiratory time) from the total exhaled volume.
        4. During expiratory TGI the inspiratory VT can be easily measured.

IV. Setting TGI
    A. During continuous TGI, VT and airway pressure are increased during volume ventilation (Figure 44-4) unless the VT is adjusted downward by a volume equal to the TGI flow added during inspiration.
        1. If 6 L/min of continuous TGI flow is delivered, 100 ml volume of gas is delivered each second by the TGI system.
        2. If inspiratory time is 1.0 second, decrease the delivered VT by 100 ml to keep the delivered VT and plateau pressure constant.

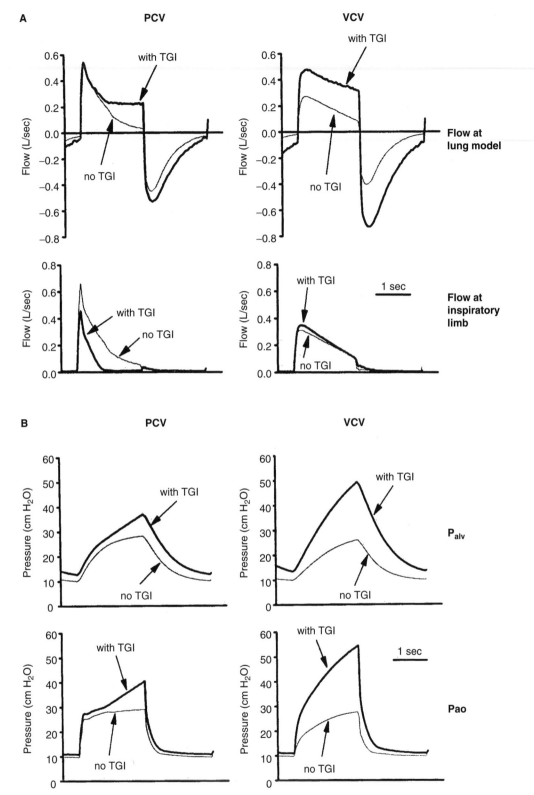

FIG. 44-4 A, Flow versus time tracings of delivered gas flow measured at airway opening and distal to the entrance of the tracheal gas insufflation (TGI) flow in pressure-controlled ventilation (PCV) and volume-controlled ventilation (VCV) with and without the addition of 12 L/min TGI flow in a lung model. **B,** Pressure versus time tracings of system pressure measured at airway opening (Pao) and distal to the entrance of the TGI flow (P_{alv}) in PCV and VCV, with and without the addition of 12 L/min TGI flow in a lung model.

B. In pressure control ventilation, continuous flow TGI will increase the V_T and plateau pressure if the ventilator-delivered flow decreases to zero before the end of the inspiratory phase (see Figure 44-4).
   1. When the ventilator flow returns to zero, the ventilator cannot maintain a constant plateau pressure if a secondary flow of gas (TGI) is maintained.
   2. Thus adding a continuous TGI flow has a high probability of increasing V_T and plateau pressure during pressure control ventilator.
C. Pressure relief and flow relief valves can be added to the ventilator circuit to avoid pressure and volume increases.
D. The use of expiratory phase-only TGI avoids the increase in volume and pressure during volume- and pressure-targeted ventilation.
E. However, to measure plateau pressure and end expiratory pressure during TGI (continuous and intermittent) the TGI flow must be coordinated with the ventilator.

V. **Indications**
   A. TGI is useful during permissive hypercapnia for patients with acute respiratory distress syndrome (ARDS) with an existent metabolic acidosis or a marked respiratory acidosis.
   B. It is useful for ARDS patients in whom it is desirable to decrease plateau pressure without necessarily changing $Paco_2$ (i.e., to maintain the same $Paco_2$ in patients with increased intracranial pressure who also have ARDS) and to maintain a normal $Paco_2$ without exposing the lungs to high peak alveolar pressure and V_Ts.

VI. **TGI Is Experimental.**
   A. Commercially designed systems that incorporate the safety features described previously are not available in the United States.
      1. TGI should be considered a *research tool* until commercially designed systems become available.

BIBLIOGRAPHY

Adams AB: Catheters for tracheal gas insufflation. *Respir Care* 46:177-184, 2001.

Adams AB: Tracheal gas insufflation (TGI). *Respir Care* 41:285-293, 1996.

Blanch LL: Clinical studies of tracheal gas insufflation. *Respir Care* 46:158-166, 2001.

DeRobertis E, Sigurdsson SE, Drefeldt B, Jonson B: Aspiration of airway dead space: a new model to enhance CO_2 elimination. *Am J Respir Crit Care Med* 159:728-733, 1999.

Hess DR, Gillette MA: Tracheal gas insufflation and related techniques to introduce gas flow into the trachea. *Respir Care* 46:119-129, 2001.

Kacmarek RM: Complications of tracheal gas insufflation. *Respir Care* 46:167-176, 2001.

Nahum A: Animal and lung model studies of tracheal gas insufflation. *Respir Care* 46:149-157, 2001.

Ravencraft SA: Tracheal gas insufflation: adjunct to conventional mechanical ventilation. *Respir Care* 41:105-111, 1996.

Takahashi T, Bugedo G, Adams AB, et al: Effects of tracheal gas insufflation and tracheal gas exsufflation on intrinsic PEEP and carbon dioxide elimination. *Respir Care* 44:918-924, 1999.

Chapter 45

Prone Positioning

I. **Indication (Box 45-1)**
   A. There is currently only one indication for prone positioning: Acute respiratory distress syndrome (ARDS).
   B. The specific level of oxygenation deficit indicating a need for prone positioning has not been precisely defined.
   C. However, many would agree that if the following is required and the Pa_{O_2} is still <70 mm Hg, prone positioning should be considered.
      1. F_IO_2: >0.60
      2. Lung recruitment maneuvers tried
      3. Positive end-expiratory pressure (PEEP): ≥ 15 cm H_2O
   D. Animal studies indicate that prone positioning is lung protective (i.e., ventilator-induced lung injuries are less severe in the prone position than in the supine position).

II. **Contraindications of Prone Positioning**
   A. Spinal cord injury
   B. Recent thoracic or abdominal surgery
   C. Hemodynamic instability
   D. Unstable airway
   E. Marked obesity
   F. However, correcting hemodynamic and airway instability eliminates the contraindication.

III. **Mechanism of Action**
   A. In the supine position, especially in ARDS because of the increased weight of the lung, there is a large transpulmonary pressure gradient between nondependent and dependent lung.
   B. The reasons for this gradient when supine are the following.
      1. Approximately 60% of the lung is in the dependent position. This is because the lung in the supine position is essentially triangular shaped with the base of the triangular most dependent.
      2. The heart and great vessels sit on top of the lungs.
      3. The posterior basilar segments of the lungs are under the diaphragm.
   C. In ARDS the force exerted by these factors pulls the lung from the anterior chest wall, creating a negative anterior transpulmonary pressure gradient and a positive posterior or dependent transpulmonary pressure gradient.
   D. This causes most of the functional residual capacity (FRC) to occupy the nondependent lung and most of the tidal volume (V_T) to go to the nondependent lung.
   E. A large $\dot{V}/\dot{Q}$ mismatch is created because most perfusion in the supine position goes to the dependent lung.

789

BOX 45-1

Prone Positioning

- Indication: ARDS
  - PaO_2: <70 mm Hg
  - F_IO_2: >0.60
  - PEEP: ≥15 cm H_2O
  - Failure to respond to recruitment maneuvers
- Positioning: Requires four people
  - One RT to manage airway
  - One RN to manage vascular lines
  - Two others turning
- Maintain in prone position ≥20 hours per day

- Move from prone position when
  - PaO_2: >60 mm Hg
  - F_IO_2: ≤0.40
  - PEEP: ≤8 cm H_2O
- Complications
  - Extubation
  - Loss of vascular line
  - Arrhythmias
  - Hemodynamic instability

ARDS, Acute respiratory distress syndrome; *PEEP*, positive end-expiratory pressure; *RT*, respiratory therapist; *RN*, registered nurse.

F. On positioning in the prone position many of these issues are reversed.
1. The majority of the lung is now nondependent.
2. The heart and great vessels are now dependent.
3. The impact of the abdomen on the posterior-basilar lung segments is eliminated.
4. Prone positioning also decreases chest wall compliance.
5. As a result, the transpulmonary pressure gradient is more evenly distributed from non-dependent to dependent lung.
6. Blood flow also is more evenly distributed from nondependent to dependent lung.
7. In the prone position a greater percentage of the FRC volume is dependent and VT is more evenly distributed.
8. All of this results in improved $\dot{V}/\dot{Q}$ matching and PaO_2 increases.

IV. **Response to Prone Positioning**
A. Numerous care series indicate that approximately 70% of ARDS patients when placed in the prone position experience a >20% increase in PaO_2 at the same ventilator settings.
B. Figure 45-1 depicts the possible responses of patients turned prone. Unfortunately no good explanation is available as to why some respond to prone positioning and others do not.
1. No response in approximately 20% to 30% of patients (nonresponders)
2. An increase in PaO_2 that is sustained when returned supine occurs in approximately 30% to 40% of patients (persistent responders).
3. An increase in PaO_2 when prone but a loss of the PaO_2 benefit when returned to the supine position occurs in approximately 30% to 40% of patients (nonpersistent responders).
C. Some patients mobilize a large amount of secretions when turned prone. This may account for the sustained increase in PaO_2.
D. In some patients the areas of atelectasis/consolidation seem to change when moved supine to prone to supine. Thus when turned supine the benefit of prone positioning is lost.

V. **The Process of Turning Prone**
A. At least four staff members are necessary to turn a patient prone.
1. One therapist to only pay attention to the airway
2. One nurse to only pay attention to vascular lines
3. Two other individuals to turn the patient
B. Before turning care should be taken to ensure
1. The endotracheal tube is properly placed and secured.
2. Vascular lines are properly placed and secured.
3. The airway is well suctioned.
4. The patient is hemodynamically stable.

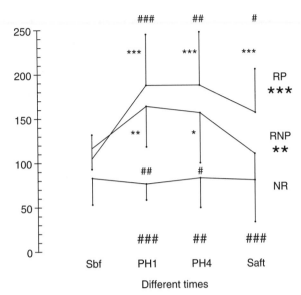

FIG. 45-1 Evolution of Pao_2/F_IO_2 before, during, and after the first 4 hours of the prone trial in the different groups. *Sbf,* 1 hour before prone; *PH1,* first hour during prone; *PH4,* fourth hour during prone; *Saft,* 1 hour after returning to supine; *NR,* nonresponders; *RNP,* responders nonpersistent; *RP,* responders persistent. $^*P < 0.05$; $^{**}P < 0.01$; $^{***}P < 0.001$. Results between the four times (analysis of variance [ANOVA]) are indicated with larger asterisk than results between PH1, PH4, and Saft to Sbf (t test). $\#P < 0.05$; $\#\#P < 0.01$; $\#\#\#P < 0.001$. Results between the three groups (ANOVA) are indicated with larger # than results between RNP and RP to NR. Nonsignificant results are not indicated.

C. The therapist maintaining the airway and the nurse maintaining the vascular lines should also carefully observe the response of the patient during prone placement: cardiac monitor, pulse oximeter, and function of the mechanical ventilator.

D. As the patient is turned the therapist at the airway should be ready to immediately suction the patient's airways.
1. In some patients a large amount of secretion is mobilized as soon as the patient is prone.
2. There are cases in which the volume is so large that the patient cannot be ventilated until the secretions are removed.

E. After stabilization in the prone position, ventilator settings may need to be adjusted.
1. F_IO_2 decreased
2. PEEP decreased but only after decreasing F_IO_2
3. Because of the lower chest wall compliance in the prone position, VT or ventilating pressure may need to be adjusted.

F. Two specific positions during prone placement have been advocated.
1. Figure 45-2 depicts complete prone positioning.
   a. In this position the head, chest, and hip need to be properly supported to prevent trauma and allow free movement of the abdomen.
   b. Free abdominal movement is especially critical if the patient is obese.

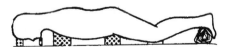

FIG. 45-2 When prone, patients ought to be supported by foam rubber pads under the upper thorax and pelvis. The head should be supported under the chin, cheeks, and forehead. It is essential that pressure on the eyes be avoided at all times.

2. The second position is the swimmer's position, which is the more commonly used prone position.
   a. The patient's head is turned to one side.
   b. The arm on that side is placed in front of the patient's face.
   c. The leg on the same side is bent at the knee and hip.
   d. The arm on the opposite side is left along the body and that leg is straight.
   e. A pillow is placed under the shoulder, chest, and hip on the side the patient is facing.

VI. **How Long to Leave Prone**
   A. All mammals sleep in the prone position.
   B. When placed supine and sedated, dependent atelectasis develops in all laboratory animals.
   C. After approximately 2 hours supine and sedated, these animals' PaO_2 decreases markedly.
   D. Patients undergoing surgery in the supine position rapidly develop atelectasis and require higher F_IO_2.
   E. As a result patients needing prone positioning should be kept prone indefinitely.
   F. From a practical perspective patients should be kept prone >20 hours per day if the oxygenation and lung protective effects of prone positioning are to be maximized.
   G. Patients only need to be placed supine for nursing care, ideally only once per day for as short a time as possible.
   H. The greater the percentage of the day patients are prone, the greater the benefit from prone positioning.

VII. **When to Move Patient from Prone Position**
   A. Patients should be moved from prone position before attempts to wean begin.
   B. Most patients can be moved from prone position when a PaO_2 >60 mm Hg can be sustained by an F_IO_2 ≤0.40 and a PEEP ≤8 cm H_2O.

VIII. **Complications of Prone Positioning (Box 45-2)**
   A. The most devastating complication of prone positioning is the loss of an artificial airway. This should be extremely infrequent if the aforementioned proper precautions are taken.
   B. Loss of vascular lines or urinary catheters; this can be avoided with proper care during positioning.
   C. From the perspective of the family, facial edema is a major concern.
      1. Family should be notified that disfiguring facial edema is common.
      2. Fortunately the edema resolves as quickly as it forms when patients are again placed supine.
   D. Development of transient cardiac arrhythmias or hyper/hypotension; it normally can be rapidly corrected with fluid or drug therapy.
   E. Apical atelectasis

BOX 45-2

Complications of Prone Positions

- In moving 294 patients to the prone position, the following complications were observed.
- Two cases of apical atelectasis
- One intravascular line loss
- One intravascular line compression
- One endotracheal tube extubation
- One transient supraventricular tachycardia

From Chatte G, et al: Prone position in mechanically ventilated patients with severe acute respiratory failure. *Am J Respir Crit Care Med* 155:473-488, 1997.

BIBLIOGRAPHY

Albert RK: Prone ventilation. *Clin Chest Med* 21:511-517, 2000.

Albert RK, Hubmayr RD: The prone position eliminates compression of the lungs by the heart. *Am J Respir Crit Care Med* 161:1660-1665, 2000.

Blanch L, Mancebo J, Perez M, et al: Short-term effects of prone position in critically ill patients with acute respiratory distress syndrome. *Intensive Care Med* 23:1033-1039, 1997.

Cakar N, Van der Kloot T, Youngblood M, et al: Oxygenation response to a recruitment maneuver during supine and prone positions in an oleic acid-induced lung injury model. *Am J Respir Crit Care Med* 16:11949-11956, 2000.

Chatte G, Sob J, Dubois J, et al: Prone position in mechanically ventilated patients with severe acute respiratory failure. *Am J Respir Crit Care Med* 155:473-478, 1997.

Colmenero-Ruiz M, Pola-Gallego de Guzman D, Jimenez-Quintant MM, et al: Abdomen release in prone position does not improve oxygenation in an experimental model of acute lung injury. *Intensive Care Med* 27:566-573, 2001.

Gattinoni L, Tognoni G, Pesenti A, et al: Effect of prone positioning on the survival of patients with acute respiratory failure. *N Engl J Med* 345:568-573, 2001.

Lamm WJE, Graham MM, Albert RK: Mechanism by which the prone position improves oxygenation in acute lung injury. *Am J Respir Crit Care Med* 150:184-193, 1994.

Messerole E, Peine P, Wittkopp S, et al: The pragmatics of prone positioning. *Am J Respir Crit Care Med* 165:1359-1363, 2002.

Mure M, Glenny RW, Domino KB, et al: Pulmonary gas exchange improves in the prone position with abdominal distension. *Am J Respir Crit Care Med* 157:1785-1790, 1998.

Mure M, Martling CR, Lindahl SGE: Dramatic effect on oxygenation in patients with severe acute lung insufficiency treated in the prone position. *Crit Care Med* 25:1539-1544, 1997.

Offner PJ, Haenel JB, Moore EE, et al: Complications of prone ventilation in patients with multisystem trauma with fulminant acute respiratory distress syndrome. *J Trauma* 48:224-228, 2000.

Pelosi P, Croci M, Calappi E, et al: Prone positioning improves pulmonary function in obese patients during general anesthesia. *Anesth Analg* 83:578-583, 1996.

Piedalue F, Albert RN: Prone positioning in acute respiratory distress syndrome. *Respir Care Clin* 9:495-509, 2003.

Stocker R, Neff T, Stein S, et al: Prone positioning and low-volume pressure-limited ventilation improve survival in patients with severe ARDS. *Chest* 111:1008-1017, 1997.

Chapter 46

Liquid Ventilation

I. **History of Liquid Ventilation**
   A. The first successful use of total liquid ventilation was in dogs in 1966.
   B. During this period liquid ventilation was researched in the hope that individuals would be able to remain under water for long periods with respiration supported by a fluid media.
   C. The first fluid used for liquid ventilation was saline.
   D. Fuhrman first described partial liquid ventilation in 1991.
   E. The first reported series of patients (neonates) maintained with partial liquid ventilation was in 1996.
   F. The last randomized controlled trial of partial liquid ventilation in adults was completed in 2001.

II. **Definitions and Descriptions**
   A. Total liquid ventilation
      1. The movement of a liquid into and out of the lungs with each breath.
      2. This is accomplished with a system similar to an extracorporeal membrane oxygenation system.
      3. A gas exchanger, heater, and pump are necessary.
      4. Total liquid ventilation systems have only been used on animal models; no patient has ever been maintained with a total liquid ventilation system.
   B. Partial liquid ventilation
      1. The lung is filled with a liquid to approximately 50% to 100% of functional residual capacity (FRC).
      2. On top of the liquid the patient is conventionally mechanically ventilated.
      3. Partial liquid ventilation is the only approach ever used in patients.
   C. Perfluorocarbons
      1. Carbon-based chemicals are used as the liquid media for all approaches to liquid ventilation.
      2. A number of different perfluorocarbons have been used in animal models, but only one, Perflubron (C_8F_{17} Br; Alliance Pharmaceuticals, San Diego, CA) has been used in patients.
      3. Box 46-1 lists the physical properties of Perflubron.
      4. Other perfluorocarbons used for liquid ventilation include
         a. FC-100: Has a lower surface tension than Perflubron and spreads more rapidly but carries less oxygen and carbon dioxide.
         b. FC-3280: Has a vapor pressure 10 times that of Perflubron.
         c. Perfluorodecalin: Has a lower spreading coefficient and lipid solubility than Perflubron.

BOX 46-1
Physical Properties of Perflubron

Colorless	Carbon dioxide solubility, 210 ml/100 ml
Odorless	Surface tension, 18 dynes/cm
Insoluble in water	Density, 1.92 g/ml
Biologically inert	Spreading coefficient, +2.7 dynes/cm
Chemically stable	Vapor pressure, 11 mm Hg
Oxygen solubility, 63 ml/100 ml	

III. **Mechanisms of Action of Perflubron**
   A. Alveolar tamponade
      1. Because Perflubron has a high density it prevents fluid and protein from moving across the alveolar capillary membrane into the lung.
      2. Thus Perflubron reduces the amount of fluid in the lung.
   B. Antiinflammatory effects
      1. Perflubron improves survival of pneumonia in animal models.
      2. In cell cultures it decreases the number of viable bacteria.
   C. Pulmonary lavage
      1. The high density and the insolubility of Perflubron move cellular debris from the lung periphery to the top of the Perflubron column for removal by suctioning.
      2. It is occasionally necessary to instill saline into the airway to remove thick secretions on the top of a Perflubron column.
      3. In some patients fiberoptic bronchoscopy is necessary.
   D. Redistribution of pulmonary blood flow
      1. Because Perflubron primarily distributes to gravity-dependent lung, its high density moves blood flow to the nondependent lung.
      2. Because most gas ventilation during partial liquid ventilation is in nondependent lung, $\dot{V}/\dot{Q}$ matching is improved.
   E. Lung recruitment
      1. The high density of the Perflubron recruits atelectatic lung units.
      2. This primarily occurs in the dependent lung.
      3. However, because of the low surface tension of Perflubron, it improves the stability of lung units throughout the lung.
   F. Prevention of alveolar collapse
      1. Partial liquid ventilation has been referred to as "liquid positive end-expiratory pressure (PEEP)."
      2. It provides a selective application of PEEP based on its density.
      3. The most gravity-dependent lung is affected most.

IV. **Filling of the Lung with a Perfluorocarbon**
   A. The only method to fill the lung with a perfluorocarbon is to slowly instill it into the lung (Figure 46-1).
   B. This instillation can be controlled by intravenous pump, but careful monitoring during instillation is critical.
   C. Adverse events have been frequently reported during dosing.
      1. Hypoxemia
      2. Hypertension
      3. Hypotension
      4. Bradycardia
      5. Tachycardia
      6. Pneumothorax

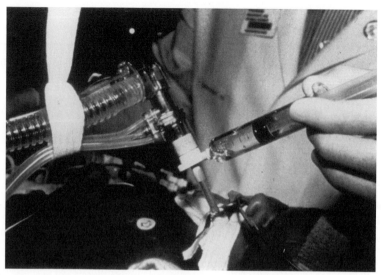

FIG. 46-1 The administration of Perflubron to a patient using a syringe. The dose is slowly instilled in the airway, filling the lung to between 50% and 100% of functional residual capacity.

    D. Because perfluorocarbons have a high vapor pressure, they rapidly evaporate, requiring regular refilling.

    E. The evaporation rate for adults is approximately 1 ml/kg/hr but depends on minute ventilation.

  V. **Conventional Ventilation During Partial Liquid Ventilation**

    A. A high level of PEEP ($\geq$13 cm H_2O) is required during partial liquid ventilation to move the Perflubron out of central airways.

    B. If inadequate PEEP is applied, high peak airway pressure is necessary.

    C. Tidal volume (VT) should be low during partial liquid ventilation.

    D. During most human trials in the 1990s, large VTs were used that resulted in a high pneumothorax rate.

    E. VTs should be maintained at approximately 6 ml/kg ideal body weight.

    F. Respiratory rate is limited by air trapping.

    G. The rate should not prevent normal exhalation.

    H. Spontaneous ventilation should be avoided during partial liquid ventilation because of increased work of breathing.

    I. Heavy sedation is required.

 VI. **Monitoring During Partial Liquid Ventilation**

    A. Figure 46-2 illustrates a lung filled with Perflubron to FRC.

    B. Because of the bromide atom on the end of the Perflubron chain, the Perflubron is easily identified on radiographs.

    C. Pneumothorax, consolidation, and the complete outline of the lung are easy to observe in the Perflubron-filled lung.

    D. Careful monitoring for the development of pneumothorax is critical. The incidence of pneumothorax during partial liquid ventilation is high.

    E. Plateau pressure should be kept <30 cm H_2O as in all forms of mechanical ventilation.

    F. Hemodynamic stability should be carefully monitored because of the high local mean airway pressure established.

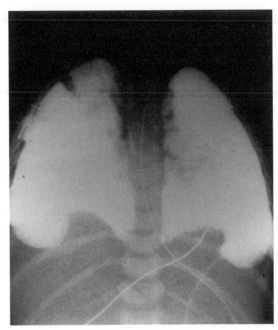

FIG. 46-2 Chest radiograph of a patient with lungs filled with Perflubron. Because of the bromide atom in the Perflubron molecule, Perflubron is easily identified on chest radiography. Pneumothorax and consolidation are easily observed in the Perflubron-filled lung.

VII. **Effect on Outcome**
   A. Partial liquid ventilation has not demonstrated an improvement in outcome in patients with acute respiratory distress syndrome (ARDS).
   B. As a result it is unlikely that it will become part of the normal clinical care of patients with ARDS in the near future.
   C. Experimentation using high frequency oscillation is ongoing in animal models.
   D. Many believe perfluorocarbons may be useful in single small doses to help recruit the lung.
   E. Animal trials using vaporized or aerosolized perfluorocarbons are currently ongoing.
   F. The entire concept of liquid ventilation must still be considered experimental.

BIBLIOGRAPHY

Arnold JH: High-frequency oscillatory ventilation and partial liquid ventilation: liquid breathing to a different beat (frequency). Editorial. *Crit Care Med* 28:2600-2602, 2000.

Doctor A, Mazzoni MC, DelBalzo U, DiCanzio J, Arnold JH: High-frequency oscillatory ventilation of the perfluorocarbon-filled lung: preliminary results in an animal model of acute lung injury. *Crit Care Med* 27:2500-2507, 1999.

Ferreyra G, Goddon S, Fujino Y, Kacmarek RM: The relationship between gas delivery patterns and the lower inflection point of the pressure-volume curve during partial liquid ventilation. *Chest* 117:191-198, 2000.

Fuhrman BP, Peczan PR, DeFrancisis M: Perfluorocarbon-associated gas exchange. *Crit Care Med* 19:712-718, 1991.

Fujino Y, Kirmse M, Hess D, Kacmarek RM: The effect of mode, inspiratory time, and positive end-expiratory pressure on partial liquid ventilation. *Am J Respir Crit Care Med* 159:1087-1095, 1999.

Hirschl RB, Croche M, Gore D: Prospective, randomized controlled pilot study of partial liquid ventilation in acute respiratory distress syndrome. *Am J Respir Crit Care Med* 165:781-787, 2002.

Kacmarek RM: Liquid ventilation. *Respir Care Clin* 8:187-200, 2002.

Kacmarek RM: Combination therapy. *Respir Care Clin* 7:663-681, 2001.

Kirmse M, Fujino Y, Hess D, Kacmarek RM: Positive end-expiratory pressure improves gas exchange and pulmonary mechanics during partial liquid ventilation. *Am J Respir Crit Care Med* 158:1550-1556, 1998.

Leach CL, Greenspan JS, Rubenstein SD, et al: Partial liquid ventilation with Perflubron in premature infants with severe respiratory distress syndrome. *N Engl J Med* 335:761-767, 1996.

Smith KM, Mrozek JD, Simonton SC, et al: Prolonged partial liquid ventilation using conventional and high-frequency ventilatory techniques: gas exchange and lung pathology in an animal model of respiratory distress syndrome. *Crit Care Med* 25: 1888-1897, 1997.

Thome UH, Schulze A, Schnabel R, Franz AR, Pohlandt F, Hummler HD: Partial liquid ventilation in severely surfactant-depleted, spontaneously breathing rabbits supported by proportional assist ventilation. *Crit Care Med* 29:1175-1180, 2001.

Chapter 1—*Figure 1-4,* from Pierson DJ, Kacmarek RM: *Foundations of Respiratory Care.* New York, Churchill Livingstone, 1992; *Figure 1-5,* from Pierson DJ, Kacmarek RM: *Foundations of Respiratory Care.* New York, Churchill Livingstone, 1992.

Chapter 2—*Figure 2-1,* from Wilkins RL, Stoller JK, Scanlan CL: *Egan's Fundamentals of Respiratory Care,* ed 8. St. Louis, Mosby, 2003; *Figure 2-2,* from Wilkins RL, Stoller JK, Scanlan CL: *Egan's Fundamentals of Respiratory Care,* ed 8. St. Louis, Mosby, 2003; *Figure 2-3,* from Kacmarek RM, et al: *Monitoring in Respiratory Care.* St. Louis, Mosby, 1993; *Figure 2-4,* from Wilkins RL, Stoller JK, Scanlan CL: *Egan's Fundamentals of Respiratory Care,* ed 8. St. Louis, Mosby, 2003; *Figure 2-5,* from Pierson DJ, Kacmarek RM: *Foundations of Respiratory Care.* New York, Churchill Livingstone, 1992; *Figure 2-6,* from Comroe JR: *The Lung,* ed 2. Chicago, Year Book Medical Publishers, 1962; *Figure 2-7,* from Comroe JR: *The Lung,* ed 2. Chicago, Year Book Medical Publishers, 1962; *Figure 2-8,* from Wilkins RL, Stoller JK, Scanlan CL: *Egan's Fundamentals of Respiratory Care,* ed 8. St. Louis, Mosby, 2003; *Figure 2-9,* from Pierson DJ, Kacmarek RM: *Foundations of Respiratory Care.* New York, Churchill Livingstone, 1992; *Figure 2-10,* from Kacmarek RM, et al: *Monitoring in Respiratory Care.* St. Louis, Mosby, 1993; *Figure 2-11,* from Kacmarek RM, et al: *Monitoring in Respiratory Care.* St. Louis, Mosby, 1993; *Figure 2-12,* modified from Moser KM, Spragg RG: *Respiratory Emergencies,* ed 2. St. Louis, Mosby, 1982; *Figure 2-13,* from Kacmarek RM, et al: *Monitoring in Respiratory Care.* St. Louis, Mosby, 1993; *Figure 2-14,* from Pierson DJ, Kacmarek RM: *Foundations of Respiratory Care.* New York, Churchill Livingstone, 1992; *Figure 2-15,* from Pierson DJ, Kacmarek RM: *Foundations of Respiratory Care.* New York, Churchill Livingstone, 1992; *Figure 2-16,* from Pierson DJ, Kacmarek RM: *Foundations of Respiratory Care.* New York, Churchill Livingstone, 1992.

Chapter 3—*Figure 3-1,* from Thibodeau GA, Patton KT: *Anatomy and Physiology,* ed 5. St. Louis, Mosby, 2003; *Figure 3-2,* from Hess DR, et al: *Respiratory Care: Principles and Practice.* Philadelphia, WB Saunders, 2002.

Chapter 4—*Figure 4-1,* from Hicks GH: *Cardiopulmonary Anatomy and Physiology.* Philadelphia, WB Saunders, 2000; *Figure 4-2,* from Beachey W: *Respiratory Care Anatomy and Physiology: Foundations for Clinical Practice.* St. Louis, Mosby, 1998; *Figure 4-3,* from Hicks GH: *Cardiopulmonary Anatomy and Physiology.* Philadelphia, WB Saunders, 2000; *Figure 4-4,* from Hess DR, et al: *Respiratory Care: Principles and Practice.* Philadelphia, WB Saunders, 2002; *Figure 4-5,* from Hicks GH: *Cardiopulmonary Anatomy and Physiology.* Philadelphia, WB Saunders, 2000; *Figure 4-6,* from Hicks GH: *Cardiopulmonary Anatomy and Physiology.* Philadelphia, WB Saunders, 2000; *Figure 4-7,* from Hicks GH: *Cardiopulmonary Anatomy and Physiology.* Philadelphia, WB Saunders, 2000; *Figure 4-8,* from Shapiro BA, Harrison RA, Kacmarek RM, et al: *Clinical Application of Respiratory Care,* ed 3. Chicago, Year Book Medical Publishers, 1985; *Figure 4-9,* from Shapiro BA, Harrison RA, Kacmarek RM, et al: *Clinical Application of Respiratory Care,* ed 3. Chicago, Year Book Medical Publishers, 1985; *Figure 4-10,* from Pierson DJ, Kacmarek RM: *Foundations of Respiratory Care.* New York, Churchill Livingstone, 1992; *Figure 4-11,* from Shapiro BA, Harrison RA, Kacmarek RM, et al: *Clinical Application of Respiratory Care,* ed 3. Chicago, Year Book Medical Publishers, 1985; *Figure 4-12,* from Wilkins RL, Stoller JK, Scanlan CL: *Egan's Fundamentals of Respiratory Care,* ed 8. St. Louis, Mosby, 2003; *Figure 4-13,* from Hess DR, et al: *Respiratory Care: Principles and Practice.* Philadelphia, WB Saunders, 2002; *Figure 4-14,* from Hicks GH: *Cardiopulmonary Anatomy and Physiology.* Philadelphia, WB Saunders, 2000; *Figure 4-15,* from Wilkins RL, Stoller JK, Scanlan CL: *Egan's Fundamentals of Respiratory Care,* ed 8, St. Louis, Mosby, 2003; *Figure 4-16,* from Seeley RR, Stephens TD, Tate P: *Anatomy and Physiology,* ed 3. New York, McGraw-Hill, 1995; *Figure 4-17,* from Wilkins RL, Stoller JK, Scanlan CL: *Egan's Fundamentals of Respiratory Care,* ed 8.

St. Louis, Mosby, 2003; *Figure 4-18,* from Osmond DG: Functional anatomy of the chest wall. In Roussos C, MacKlem PT, editors: *The Thorax, Part A, Lung Biology in Health and Disease,* ed 2. New York, Marcel Dekker, 1995.

Chapter 5—*Figure 5-1,* from Shapiro BA, Harrison RA, Kacmarek RM, et al: *Clinical Application of Respiratory Care,* ed 3. Chicago, Year Book Medical Publishers, 1985; *Figure 5-2,* from Spearman CB, Sheldon RL, Egan DL: *Egan's Fundamentals of Respiratory Therapy,* ed 4. St. Louis, Mosby, 1982; *Figure 5-6,* from Culver BH: Mechanics of ventilation. In Culver BH, editor: *The Respiratory System: Syllabus for Human Biology.* Seattle, University of Washington Health Science Academic Services, 1990; *Figure 5-7,* from Berne RM, Levy MN: *Principles of Physiology,* ed 2. St. Louis, Mosby, 1996; *Figure 5-8,* from Culver BH: Mechanics of ventilation. In Culver BH, editor: *The Respiratory System: Syllabus for Human Biology.* Seattle, University of Washington Health Science Academic Services, 1990; *Figure 5-9,* from Comroe JR: *Physiology of Respiration.* Chicago, Year Book Medical Publishers, 1965; *Figure 5-10,* from Shapiro BA: *Clinical Application of Respiratory Care,* ed 2. Chicago, Year Book Medical Publishers, 1979; *Figure 5-12,* from Shapiro BA, Harrison RA, Kacmarek RM, et al: *Clinical Application of Respiratory Care,* ed 3. Chicago, Year Book Medical Publishers, 1985; *Figure 5-13,* from Kacmarek RM: The role of pressure support ventilation in reducing work of breathing. *Respir Care* 33:99-120, 1988.

Chapter 6—*Figure 6-1,* from Spearman CB, Sheldon RL, Egan DF: *Egan's Fundamentals of Respiratory Therapy,* ed 4. St. Louis, Mosby, 1982; *Figure 6-2,* from Guyton AC, Hall JE: *Textbook of Medical Physiology,* ed 10. Philadelphia, WB Saunders, 2000; *Figure 6-3,* from Hicks GH: *Cardiopulmonary Anatomy and Physiology.* Philadelphia, WB Saunders, 2000; *Figure 6-4,* from Guyton AC, Hall JE: *Textbook of Medical Physiology,* ed 10. Philadelphia, WB Saunders, 2000; *Figure 6-5,* from Hicks GH: *Cardiopulmonary Anatomy and Physiology.* Philadelphia, WB Saunders, 2000; *Figure 6-6,* from Hicks GH: *Cardiopulmonary Anatomy and Physiology.* Philadelphia, WB Saunders, 2000.

Chapter 7—*Figure 7-1,* from Hicks GH: *Cardiopulmonary Anatomy and Physiology.* Philadelphia, WB Saunders, 2000; *Figure 7-2,* from Hicks GH: *Cardiopulmonary Anatomy and Physiology.* Philadelphia, WB Saunders, 2000; *Figure 7-3,* from Pierson DJ, Kacmarek RM: *Foundations of Respiratory Care.* New York, Churchill Livingstone, 1992; *Figure 7-4,* modified from Shapiro BA, Harrison RA, Walton JR: *Clinical Application of Blood Gases,* ed 3. Chicago, Year Book Medical Publishers, 1982; *Figure 7-5,* from Kacmarek RM, Mack CW, Dimas S: *The Essentials of Respiratory Care,* ed 3, redrawn in Pierson DJ, Kacmarek RM: *Foundations of Respiratory Care.* New York, Churchill Livingstone, 1992; *Figure 7-6,* from Kacmarek RM, Mack CW, Dimas S: *The Essentials of Respiratory Care,* ed 3, redrawn in Pierson DJ, Kacmarek RM: *Foundations of Respiratory Care.* New York, Churchill Livingstone, 1992.

Chapter 8—*Figure 8-1,* from Shapiro BA, Harrison RA, Walton JR: *Clinical Application of Arterial Blood Gases,* ed 4. Chicago, Year Book Medical Publishers, 1989; *Figure 8-2,* from Shapiro BA, Harrison RA, Walton JR: *Clinical Application of Arterial Blood Gases,* ed 4. Chicago, Year Book Medical Publishers, 1989; *Figure 8-3,* from Pierson DJ, Kacmarek RM: *Foundations of Respiratory Care.* New York, Churchill Livingstone, 1992; *Figure 8-4,* from Pierson DJ, Kacmarek RM: *Foundations of Respiratory Care.* New York, Churchill Livingstone, 1992; *Figure 8-5,* from Shapiro BA, Harrison RA, Walton JR: *Clinical Application of Blood Gases,* ed 4. Chicago, Year Book Medical Publishers, 1989; *Figure 8-6,* from Shapiro BA, Harrison RA, Walton JR: *Clinical Application of Blood Gases,* ed 4. Chicago, Year Book Medical Publishers, 1989; *Figure 8-7,* from Shapiro BA, Harrison RA, Walton JR: *Clinical Application of Blood Gases,* ed 4. Chicago, Year Book Medical Publishers, 1989; *Figure 8-8,* from Pierson DJ, Kacmarek RM: *Foundations of Respiratory Care.* New York, Churchill Livingstone, 1992.

Chapter 9—*Figure 9-1,* from Waugh A, Grant A: *Ross and Wilson Anatomy and Physiology in Health and Illness,* ed 9. London, Churchill Livingstone, 2001; *Figure 9-2,* from Thibodeau GA, Patton KT: *Anatomy and Physiology,* ed 5. St. Louis, Mosby, 2003; *Figure 9-3,* from Shapiro BA,

Harrison RA, Kacmarek RM, et al: *Clinical Applications of Respiratory Care,* ed 3. Chicago, Year Book Medical Publishers, 1985; *Figure 9-4,* from Guyton AC, Hall JE: *Textbook of Medical Physiology,* ed 10. Philadelphia, WB Saunders, 2000; *Figure 9-5,* from Shapiro BA, Harrison RA, Kacmarek RM, et al: *Clinical Applications of Respiratory Care,* ed 3. Chicago, Year Book Medical Publishers, 1985; *Figure 9-6,* from Thibodeau GA, Patton KT: *Anatomy and Physiology,* ed 5. St. Louis, Mosby, 2003; *Figure 9-7,* from Waugh A, Grant A: *Ross and Wilson Anatomy and Physiology in Health and Illness,* ed 9. London, Churchill Livingstone, 2001; *Figure 9-8,* from Wilson KJW, Waugh A: *Ross and Wilson Anatomy and Physiology in Health and Illness,* ed 8. London, Churchill Livingstone, 1996; *Figure 9-9,* from Wilson SF, Giddens JF: *Health Assessment for Nursing Practice,* ed 2. St. Louis, Mosby, 2001 [as appears in Thibodeau GA, Patton KT: *Anatomy and Physiology,* ed 5. St. Louis, Mosby, 2003]; *Figure 9-10,* from Thibodeau GA, Patton KT: *Anatomy and Physiology,* ed 5. St. Louis, Mosby, 2003; *Figure 9-11,* from Jacob SW, Francone CA, et al: *Structure and Function in Man,* ed 4. Philadelphia, WB Saunders, 1978; *Figure 9-12,* from Waugh A, Grant A: *Ross and Wilson Anatomy and Physiology in Health and Illness,* ed 9. London, Churchill Livingstone, 2001; *Figure 9-13,* from Rushmer RF: *Cardiac Diagnosis: A Physiologic Approach,* ed 3. Philadelphia, WB Saunders, 1970; *Figure 9-14,* from Thibodeau GA, Patton KT: *Anatomy and Physiology,* ed 5. St. Louis, Mosby, 2003; *Figure 9-15,* from Rushmer RF: *Cardiac Diagnosis: A Physiologic Approach,* ed 3. Philadelphia, WB Saunders, 1970; *Figure 9-16,* from Thibodeau GA, Patton KT: *Anatomy and Physiology,* ed 5. St. Louis, Mosby, 2003.

Chapter 10—*Figure 10-1,* from Ross G: *Essentials of Human Physiology,* ed 2. Chicago, Year Book Medical Publishers, 1982; *Figure 10-2,* from Ross G: *Essentials of Human Physiology,* ed 2. Chicago, Year Book Medical Publishers, 1982; *Figure 10-3,* from Thibodeau GA, Patton KT: *Anatomy and Physiology,* ed 5. St. Louis, Mosby, 2003; *Figure 10-4,* from Shapiro BA, Harrison RA, Kacmarek RM, et al: *Clinical Applications of Respiratory Care,* ed 3. Chicago, Year Book Medical Publishers, 1985; *Figure 10-5,* from Thibodeau GA, Patton KT: *Anatomy and Physiology,* ed 5. St. Louis, Mosby, 2003; *Figure 10-6,* from Mountcastle VB: *Medical Physiology,* ed 14. St. Louis, Mosby, 1980; *Figure 10-7,* from Thibodeau GA, Patton KT: *Anatomy and Physiology,* ed 5. St. Louis, Mosby, 2003; *Figure 10-8,* from Thibodeau GA, Patton KT: *Anatomy and Physiology,* ed 5. St. Louis, Mosby, 2003; *Figure 10-9,* from Shapiro BA, Harrison RA, Kacmarek RM, et al: *Clinical Applications of Respiratory Care,* ed 3. Chicago, Year Book Medical Publishers, 1985; *Figure 10-10,* from Ruch TC, Patton HD: *Physiology and Biophysics,* ed 20. Philadelphia, WB Saunders, 1974; *Figure 10-11,* from Thibodeau GA, Patton KT: *Anatomy and Physiology,* ed 5. St. Louis, Mosby, 2003.

Chapter 11—*Figure 11-1,* from Spearman CB, Sheldon RL, Egan DF: *Egan's Fundamentals of Respiratory Therapy,* ed 4. St. Louis, Mosby, 1982; *Figure 11-2,* from Rushmer RF: *Cardiac Diagnosis: A Physiologic Approach,* ed 3. Philadelphia, WB Saunders, 1970; *Figure 11-3,* from Shapiro BA, Harrison RA, Kacmarek RM, et al: *Clinical Applications of Respiratory Care,* ed 3. Chicago, Year Book Medical Publishers, 1985; *Figure 11-4,* from Spearman CB, Sheldon RL, Egan DF: *Egan's Fundamentals of Respiratory Therapy,* ed 4. St. Louis, Mosby, 1982; *Figure 11-5,* from Shapiro BA, Harrison RA, Kacmarek RM, et al: *Clinical Applications of Respiratory Care,* ed 3. Chicago, Year Book Medical Publishers, 1985; *Figure 11-6,* from Hicks GH: *Cardiopulmonary Anatomy and Physiology.* Philadelphia, WB Saunders, 2000; *Figure 11-7,* from Mountcastle VB: *Medical Physiology,* ed 14. St. Louis, Mosby, 1980.

Chapter 12—*Figure 12-1,* from Little RC: *Physiology of the Heart and Circulation,* ed 2. Chicago, Year Book Medical Publishers, 1981; *Figure 12-2,* redrawn from Rushmer RF: *Structure and Functions of the Cardiovascular System,* ed 2. Philadelphia, WB Saunders, 1976 [as appears in Wilkins RL, Stoller JK, Scanlan CL: *Egan's Fundamentals of Respiratory Care,* ed 8. St. Louis, Mosby, 2003]; *Figure 12-3,* from Wilkins RL, Krider SJ, Sheldon RL: *Clinical Assessment in Respiratory Care,* ed 4. St. Louis, Mosby, 2000; *Figure 12-4,* from Wilkins RL, Krider SJ, Sheldon RL: *Clinical Assessment in Respiratory Care,* ed 4. St. Louis, Mosby, 2000; *Figure 12-5,* from Spearman CB, Sheldon RL, Egan DF: *Egan's Fundamentals of Respiratory Therapy,* ed 4. St. Louis, Mosby, 1982; *Figure 12-6,* from Shapiro BA, Harrison RA, Kacmarek RM, et al: *Clinical Applications of Respiratory Care,* ed 3. Chicago, Year Book Medical Publishers, 1985; *Figure 12-7,* from Mountcastle VB: *Medical*

Physiology, ed 14. St. Louis, Mosby, 1980; *Figure 12-8*, from Hess DR, et al: *Respiratory Care: Principles and Practice*, Philadelphia, WB Saunders, 2002; *Figure 12-9*, from Daily EK, Schroeder JS: *Techniques in Bedside Hemodynamic Monitoring*, ed 2. St. Louis, Mosby, 1981.

Chapter 13—*Figure 13-1*, from Guyton AC, Hall JE: *Textbook of Medical Physiology*, ed 10. Philadelphia, WB Saunders, 2000; *Figure 13-2*, from Guyton AC, Hall JE: *Textbook of Medical Physiology*, ed 10. Philadelphia, WB Saunders, 2000; *Figure 13-3*, from Brundage DJ: *Renal Disorders*. St. Louis, Mosby, 1992; *Figure 13-4*, from Guyton AC, Hall JE: *Textbook of Medical Physiology*, ed 10. Philadelphia, WB Saunders, 2000; *Figure 13-5*, from Vander AJ: *Renal Physiology*, ed 2. New York, McGraw-Hill, 1980; *Figure 13-6*, from Vander AJ: *Renal Physiology*, ed 2. New York, McGraw-Hill, 1980; *Figure 13-7*, from Vander AJ: *Renal Physiology*, ed 2. New York, McGraw-Hill, 1980; *Figure 13-8*, from Vander AJ: *Renal Physiology*, ed 2, New York, McGraw-Hill, 1980.

Chapter 14—*Figure 14-1*, from Hicks GH: *Cardiopulmonary Anatomy and Physiology*. Philadelphia, WB Saunders, 2000; *Figure 14-6*, from Shapiro BA, Harrison RA, Kacmarek RM, et al: *Clinical Application of Respiratory Care*, ed 3. Chicago, Year Book Medical Publishers, 1985.

Chapter 15—*Figure 15-1*, from Pierson DJ, Kacmarek RM: *Foundations of Respiratory Care*. New York, Churchill Livingstone, 1992.

Chapter 16—*Figure 16-1*, from Guyton AC, Hall JE: *Textbook of Medical Physiology*, ed 10. Philadelphia, WB Saunders, 2000; *Figure 16-2*, from Guyton AC, Hall JE: *Textbook of Medical Physiology*, ed 10. Philadelphia, WB Saunders, 2000; *Figure 16-3*, from Guyton AC, Hall JE: *Textbook of Medical Physiology*, ed 10. Philadelphia, WB Saunders, 2000; *Figure 16-4*, from Rau JL: *Respiratory Care Pharmacology*, ed 6. St. Louis, Mosby, 2002; *Figure 16-5*, from Rau JL: *Respiratory Care Pharmacology*, ed 6. St. Louis, Mosby, 2002; *Figure 16-6*, from Rau JL: *Respiratory Care Pharmacology*, ed 6. St. Louis, Mosby, 2002; *Figure 16-7*, from Rau JL: *Respiratory Care Pharmacology*, ed 6. St. Louis, Mosby, 2002; *Figure 16-8*, from Guyton AC, Hall JE: *Textbook of Medical Physiology*, ed 10. Philadelphia, WB Saunders, 2000; *Figure 16-9*, from Guyton AC, Hall JE: *Textbook of Medical Physiology*, ed 10. Philadelphia, WB Saunders, 2000.

Chapter 17—*Figure 17-2*, from Hess DR, et al: *Respiratory Care: Principles and Practice*. Philadelphia, WB Saunders, 2002; *Figure 17-5*, from Rau JL: *Respiratory Care Pharmacology*, ed 6. St. Louis, Mosby, 2002; *Figure 17-6*, from Rau RL: *Respiratory Care Pharmacology*, ed 6. St. Louis, Mosby, 2002; *Figure 17-7*, from Rau JL: *Respiratory Care Pharmacology*, ed 6. St. Louis, Mosby, 2002; *Figure 17-8*, from Rau JL: *Respiratory Care Pharmacology*, ed 6. St. Louis, Mosby, 2002; *Figure 17-9*, from Rau JL: *Respiratory Care Pharmacology*, ed 6. St. Louis, Mosby, 2002; *Figure 17-10*, from Rau JL: *Respiratory Care Pharmacology*, ed 6. St. Louis, Mosby, 2002; *Figure 17-11*, from Rau JL: *Respiratory Care Pharmacology*, ed 6. St. Louis, Mosby, 2002.

Chapter 18—*Figure 18-1*, from DesJardins T, Burton GG: *Clinical Manifestations and Assessment of Respiratory Diseases*, ed 4. St. Louis, Mosby, 2002; *Figure 18-2*, modified from Wilkins RL, Dexter JR, editors: *Respiratory Diseases: A Case Study Approach to Patient Care*. Philadelphia, FA Davis, 1998; *Figure 18-3*, from Wilkins RL, Sheldon RL, Krider SJ: *Clinical Assessment in Respiratory Disease*. St. Louis, Mosby, 1985; *Figure 18-4*, from Shapiro BA, Harrison RA, Kacmarek RM, et al: *Clinical Application of Respiratory Care*, ed 3. Chicago, Year Book Medical Publishers, 1985; *Figure 18-5*, from Shapiro BA, Harrison RA, Walton JR: *Clinical Application of Blood Gases*, ed 3. Chicago, Year Book Medical Publishers, 1982; *Figure 18-6*, from Kacmarek RM, Cycyk-Chapman MC, Young-Palazzi PJ, Romagnoli DM: Determination of maximal inspiratory pressure: a clinical study and literature review. *Respir Care* 34:868-878, 1989.

Chapter 19—*Figure 19-1*, from Ruppel G: *Manual of Pulmonary Function Testing*, ed 8. St. Louis, Mosby, 2003; *Figure 19-3*, from Wilkins RL, Stoller JK, Scanlan CL: *Egan's Fundamentals of Respiratory Care*, ed 8. St. Louis, Mosby, 2003; *Figure 19-5*, from Ruppel G: *Manual of Pulmonary Function Testing*, ed 8. St. Louis, Mosby, 2003; *Figure 19-6*, from Ruppel G: *Manual* *of Pulmonary Function Testing,* ed 8. St. Louis, Mosby, 2003; *Figure 19-7,* from Ruppel G: *Manual of Pulmonary Function Testing,* ed 8. St. Louis, Mosby, 2003; *Figure 19-8,* from Ruppel G: *Manual of Pulmonary Function Testing,* ed 8. St. Louis, Mosby, 2003; *Figure 19-9,* from Ruppel G: *Manual of Pulmonary Function Testing,* ed 8. St. Louis, Mosby, 2003; *Figure 19-10,* from Ruppel G: *Manual of Pulmonary Function Testing,* ed 8. St. Louis, Mosby, 2003; *Figure 19-11,* from Ruppel G: *Manual of Pulmonary Function Testing,* ed 8. St. Louis, Mosby, 2003; *Figure 19-12,* from Ruppel G: *Manual of Pulmonary Function Testing,* ed 8. St. Louis, Mosby, 2003; *Figure 19-13,* from Ruppel G: *Manual of Pulmonary Function Testing,* ed 8. St. Louis, Mosby, 2003.

Chapter 20—*Figure 20-1,* from Albert RK, Spiro SG, Jett JR: *Comprehensive Respiratory Medicine.* London, Mosby, 1999; *Figure 20-2,* from Albert RK, Spiro SG, Jett JR: *Comprehensive Respiratory Medicine.* London, Mosby, 1999; *Figure 20-3,* from Albert RK, Spiro SG, Jett JR: *Comprehensive Respiratory Medicine.* London, Mosby, 1999; *Figure 20-4,* from Albert RK, Spiro SG, Jett JR: *Comprehensive Respiratory Medicine.* London, Mosby, 1999; *Figure 20-5,* from Albert RK, Spiro SG, Jett JR: *Comprehensive Respiratory Medicine.* London, Mosby, 1999; *Figure 20-6,* from Farzan S: *A Concise Handbook of Respiratory Diseases,* ed 3. Norwalk, CT, Appleton and Lange, 1992; *Figure 20-7,* from Ruppel G: *Manual of Pulmonary Function Testing,* ed 8. St. Louis, Mosby, 2003.

Chapter 21—*Figure 21-1,* from Pepe PE, Marini JJ: Occult positive end-expiratory pressure in mechanically ventilated patients with airflow obstruction. The auto-PEEP effect. *Am Rev Respir Dis* 126:166-170, 1982; *Figure 21-2,* from Chao DC, Acheinhorn DJ, Stearn-Hassenpflug M: Patient-ventilator trigger asynchrony in prolonged mechanical ventilation. *Chest* 112:1592-1599, 1997; *Figure 21-3,* from Leatherman JW, Ravenscroft SA: Low measured auto-positive end-expiratory pressure during mechanical ventilation of patients with severe asthma: hidden auto-positive end-expiratory pressure. *Crit Care Med* 24:541-546, 1996; *Figure 21-4,* from Ranson RD, Campbell RS, Davis K, et al: Altering flowrate during maximum pressure support ventilation (PSV$_{max}$): Effects on cardiorespiratory function. *Respir Care* 35:1056-1064, 1990; *Figure 21-5,* from MacIntyre NR, Ho L: Effects of initial flow rate and breath termination criteria on pressure support ventilation. *Chest* 99:134-138, 1991; *Figure 21-6,* from Branson RD, Campbell RS: Pressure support ventilation, patient-ventilator synchrony, and ventilator algorithms. *Respir Care* 43:1045-1047, 1998.

Chapter 22—*Figure 22-1,* from Albert RK, Spiro SG, Jett JR: *Comprehensive Respiratory Medicine.* London, Mosby, 1999; *Figure 22-2,* from Albert RK, Spiro SG, Jett JR: *Comprehensive Respiratory Medicine.* London, Mosby, 1999; *Figure 22-3,* from Albert RK, Spiro SG, Jett JR: *Comprehensive Respiratory Medicine.* London, Mosby, 1999; *Figure 22-4,* from Albert RK, Spiro SG, Jett JR: *Comprehensive Respiratory Medicine.* London, Mosby, 1999; *Figure 22-5,* from Albert RK, Spiro SG, Jett JR: *Comprehensive Respiratory Medicine.* London, Mosby, 1999.

Chapter 23—*Figure 23-1,* from Ware LB, Matthay MA: The acute respiratory distress syndrome. *N Engl J Med* 342:1339, 2000; *Figure 23-2,* from Ware LB, Mattbay MA: The acute respiratory distress syndrome. *N Engl J Med* 342:1339, 2000; *Figure 23-3,* from Webb HH, Tierney DF: Experimental pulmonary edema due to intermittent positive pressure ventilation with high inflation pressures: protection by positive end-expiratory pressure. *Am Rev Respir Dis* 110:556-565, 1974; *Figure 23-4,* from Maunder RJ, Pierson DJ, Hudson LD: Subcutaneous and mediastinal emphysema. Pathophysiology, diagnosis, and management. *Arch Intern Med* 144:1447-1453, 1984; *Figure 23-5,* courtesy of John Marini, MD, Pulmonary Medicine and Critical Care, Regions Hospital, St. Paul, MN; *Figure 23-6,* from ACCP/SCCM Consensus Conference: Definitions for Sepsis and Organ Failure and Guidelines for the Use of Innovative Therapy in Sepsis. *Chest* 101:1644-1655, 1992; *Figure 23-7,* from Wiedemann H: Systemic pharmacologic therapy of ARDS. *Respir Care Clin* 4:741, 1998.

Chapter 24—*Figure 24-2,* from Respironics, Wallingford, CT.

Chapter 25—*Figure 25-1,* from Eubanks DH, Bone RC: *Comprehensive Respiratory Care.* St. Louis, Mosby, 1985; *Figure 25-3,* from Eubanks DH, Bone RC: *Comprehensive Respiratory Care.* St. Louis, Mosby, 1985.

Chapter 26—*Figure 26-1,* from Dubowitz LMS, Dubowitz V, Goldberg C: Clinical assessment of gestational age in the newborn infant. *J Pediatr* 77:1-10, 1970; *Figure 26-2,* modified from Ballard JL, Novak KK, Drive M: A simplified score for assessment of fetal maturation of newly born infants. *J Pediatr* 95:769-774, 1979 [as appears in Wilkins RL, Stoller JK, Scanlan CL: *Egan's Fundamentals of Respiratory Care,* ed 8. St. Louis, Mosby, 2003]; *Figure 26-3,* from Eubanks DH, Bone RC: *Comprehensive Respiratory Care.* St. Louis, Mosby, 1985.

Chapter 27—*Figure 27-2,* from Pierog SH, Ferrara A: *Medical Care of the Sick Newborn,* ed 2. St. Louis, Mosby, 1976; *Figure 27-5,* from An international classification of retinopathy of prematurity. The Committee for the Classification of Retinopathy of Prematurity. *Arch Ophthalmol* 102:1130-1134, 1984; *Figure 27-6,* from Ross Laboratories, Clinical Education Aid no. 7 [G163], Columbus, OH, 1978; *Figure 27-7,* from Ross Laboratories, Clinical Education Aid no. 7 [G163], Columbus, OH, 1978; *Figure 27-8,* from Ross Laboratories, Clinical Education Aid no. 7 [G163], Columbus, OH, 1978; *Figure 27-9,* from Merenstein G, Gardner SL: *Handbook of Neonatal Intensive Care,* ed 5. St. Louis, Mosby, 2002; *Figure 27-10,* from Merenstein G, Gardner SL: *Handbook of Neonatal Intensive Care,* ed 5. St. Louis, Mosby, 2002; *Figure 27-11,* from Ross Laboratories, Clinical Education Aid no. 7 [G163], Columbus, OH, 1978; *Figure 27-12,* from Ross Laboratories, Clinical Education Aid no. 7 [G163], Columbus, OH, 1978; *Figure 27-13,* from Ross Laboratories, Clinical Education Aid no. 7 [G163], Columbus, OH, 1978; *Figure 27-14,* from Ross Laboratories, Clinical Education Aid no. 7 [G163], Columbus, OH, 1978; *Figure 27-15,* from Ross Laboratories, Clinical Education Aid no. 7 [G163], Columbus, OH, 1978; *Figure 27-16,* from Ross Laboratories, Clinical Education Aid no. 7 [G163], Columbus, OH, 1978; *Figure 27-17,* from Wong DL, Hockenberry-Eaton M, Wilson D, et al: *Nursing Care of Infants and Children,* ed 6. St. Louis, Mosby, 1999.

Chapter 28—*Figure 28-6,* from *Respiratory Care Procedure Manual.* Boston, Massachusetts General Hospital, 2003; *Figure 28-7,* from Chapman RA, Toomasian JM, Bartlett RH: *ECMO Extracorporeal Membrane Oxygenation Technical Specialist Manual,* Department of Surgery, University of Michigan, Ann Arbor, Michigan, 1988.

Chapter 32—*Figure 32-1,* from Carlin BW, Clauser JL, Ries AL: *Chest* 94:239-241, 1988; *Figure 32-2,* from Kacmarek RM, Stanek KS, McMahon KM, et al: Imposed work of breathing during synchronized intermittent mandatory ventilation via home care ventilators. *Respir Care* 35:405-414, 1990; *Figure 32-3,* from Kacmarek RM, Stanek KS, McMahon KM, et al: Imposed work of breathing during synchronized intermittent mandatory ventilation via home care ventilators. *Respir Care* 35:405-414, 1990; *Figure 32-4,* from Kacmarek RM, Stanek KS, McMahon KM, et al: Imposed work of breathing during synchronized intermittent mandatory ventilation via home care ventilators. *Respir Care* 35:405-414, 1990; *Figure 32-5,* from Hill NS: Clinical applications of body ventilators. *Chest* 90:897-905, 1986; *Figure 32-6,* courtesy of Emerson Company, Boston, MA.

Chapter 33—*Figure 33-1,* from Spearman CB, Sheldon RL, Egan DF: *Egan's Fundamentals of Respiratory Therapy,* ed 4. St. Louis, Mosby, 1982; *Figure 33-2,* from Spearman CB, Sheldon RL, Egan DF: *Egan's Fundamentals of Respiratory Therapy,* ed 4. St. Louis, Mosby, 1982; *Figure 33-3,* from Spearman CB, Sheldon RL, Egan DF: *Egan's Fundamentals of Respiratory Therapy,* ed 4. St. Louis, Mosby, 1982; *Figure 33-4,* from Spearman CB, Sheldon RL, Egan DF: *Egan's Fundamentals of Respiratory Therapy,* ed 4. St. Louis, Mosby, 1982; *Figure 33-5,* from Wilkins RL, Stoller JK, Scanlan CL: *Egan's Fundamentals of Respiratory Care,* ed 8. St. Louis, Mosby, 2003; *Figure 33-6,* from Spearman CB, Sheldon RL, Egan DF: *Egan's Fundamentals of Respiratory Therapy,* ed 4. St. Louis, Mosby, 1982; *Figure 33-7,* from Spearman CB, Sheldon RL, Egan DF: *Egan's Fundamentals of Respiratory Therapy,* ed 4. St. Louis, Mosby, 1982; *Figure 33-8,* from Wilkins RL, Stoller JK, Scanlan CL: *Egan's Fundamentals of Respiratory Care,* ed 8. St. Louis, Mosby, 2003; *Figure 33-9,* from Spearman CB, Sheldon RL, Egan DF: *Egan's Fundamentals of Respiratory Therapy,* ed 4. St. Louis, Mosby, 1982; *Figure 33-10,* from Spearman CB, Sheldon RL, Egan DF: *Egan's Fundamentals of Respiratory Therapy,* ed 4. St. Louis, Mosby, 1982; *Figure 33-11,* reprinted with permission from NFPA 99-2002, Health Care Facilities, Copyright 1999, National Fire Protection Association, Quincy,

MA 02269. This reprinted material is not the complete and official position of the NFPA on the referenced subject, which is referenced only by the standard in its entirety; *Figure 33-12,* from McPherson SP, Spearman CB: *Respiratory Care Equipment,* ed 3. St. Louis, Mosby, 1985; *Figure 33-13,* modified from McPherson SP, Spearman CB: *Respiratory Therapy Equipment,* ed 5. St. Louis, Mosby, 1995 [as appears in Wilkins RL, Stoller JK, Scanlan CL: *Egan's Fundamentals of Respiratory Care,* ed 8. St. Louis, Mosby, 2003].

Chapter 34—*Figure 34-1,* from Wilkins RL: *Egan's Fundamentals of Respiratory Care,* ed 8. St. Louis, Mosby, 2003; *Figure 34-2,* from Shapiro BA, Harrison RA, Walton JR: *Clinical Application of Blood Gas,* ed 3. Chicago, Year Book Medical Publishers, 1982; *Figure 34-3,* from Kacmarek RM: Oxygen therapy techniques. In Kacmarek RM, Stoller JK, editors: *Current Respiratory Care.* Toronto, BC Decker, 1988 (with permission from Elsevier); *Figure 34-4,* from Kacmarek RM: Oxygen therapy techniques. In Kacmarek RM, Stoller JK, editors: *Current Respiratory Care.* Toronto, BC Decker, 1988 (with permission from Elsevier); *Figure 34-5,* from *Respiratory Care Procedure Manual.* Boston, Massachusetts General Hospital, 2003; *Figure 34-6,* from Kacmarek RM: In-hospital administration of oxygen. In Kacmarek RM, Stoller JK , editors: *Current Respiratory Care.* Toronto, BC Decker, 1988 (with permission from Elsevier); *Figure 34-7,* from Kacmarek RM: In-hospital administration of oxygen. In Kacmarek RM, Stoller JK, editors: *Current Respiratory Care.* Toronto, BC Decker, 1988 (with permission from Elsevier); *Figure 34-8,* from Kacmarek RM: In-hospital administration of oxygen. In Kacmarek RM, Stoller JK, editors: *Current Respiratory Care.* Toronto, BC Decker, 1988 (with permission from Elsevier); *Figure 34-9,* courtesy of VIASYS Healthcare, Yorba Linda, CA; *Figure 34-10,* courtesy of Vapotherm, Annapolis, MD; *Figure 34-11,* from Tiep PB, Nicotra B, Carter R, et al: Evaluation of a low-flow oxygen conserving nasal cannula. *Am Rev Respir Dis* 130:500-502, 1984; *Figure 34-12,* from Gonzales SC, Huntington D, Romo R, et al: Efficiency of the oxymizer pendant in reducing oxygen requirements of hypoxemic patients. *Respir Care* 31:681-688, 1986; *Figure 34-13,* from Spofford B, Christopher K, McCarty D, et al: Transtracheal oxygen therapy: a guide for the respiratory therapist. *Respir Care* 32:345-352, 1987; *Figure 34-16,* courtesy of Datex-Ohmeda, Inc., a General Electric Company, Madison, WI; *Figure 34-17,* from Hess DR, et al: *Respiratory Care: Principles and Practice.* Philadelphia, WB Saunders, 2002.

Chapter 35—*Figure 35-1,* from Wilkins RL, Stoller JK, Scanlan CL: *Egan's Fundamentals of Respiratory Care,* ed 8. St. Louis, Mosby, 2003; *Figure 35-2,* from Hess DR, et al: *Respiratory Care: Principles and Practice.* Philadelphia, WB Saunders, 2002; *Figure 35-3,* modified from Rau JL Jr: *Respiratory Care Pharmacology,* ed 5. St. Louis, Mosby, 1998; *Figure 35-4,* modified from Spiro S, MacCochran G: Delivery of medication to the lungs. In Albert R, Spiro S, Jett J, editors: *Comprehensive Respiratory Medicine.* St. Louis, Mosby, 1999; *Figure 35-5,* A-D, modified from Peterson BD: Heated humidifiers. *Respir Care Clin North Am* 4:243-260, 1998; *Figure 35-5, E,* courtesy of Hudson RCI, Temecula, CA; *Figure 35-6,* modified from Barnes TA: *Core Textbook for Respiratory Care Practice,* ed 2. St. Louis, Mosby, 1994 [as appears in Wilkins RL, Stoller JK, Scanlan CL: *Egan's Fundamentals of Respiratory Care,* ed 8. St. Louis, Mosby, 2003]; *Figure 35-7,* from Wilkins RL, Stoller JK, Scanlan CL: *Egan's Fundamentals of Respiratory Care,* ed 8. St. Louis, Mosby, 2003; *Figure 35-8,* from Wilkins RL, Stoller JK, Scanlan CL: *Egan's Fundamentals of Respiratory Care,* ed 8. St. Louis, Mosby, 2003.

Chapter 36—*Figure 36-1,* from Hess DR, et al: *Respiratory Care: Principles and Practice.* St. Louis, Mosby, 2002; *Figure 36-13,* from Wilkins RL, Stoller JK, Scanlan CL: *Egan's Fundamentals of Respiratory Care,* ed 8. St. Louis, Mosby, 2003; *Figure 36-15,* from Eubanks DH, Bone RC: *Comprehensive Respiratory Care.* St. Louis, Mosby, 1985; *Figure 36-17,* from Wilkins RL, Stoller JK, Scanlan CL: *Egan's Fundamentals of Respiratory Care,* ed 8. St. Louis, Mosby, 2003; *Figure 36-19,* from Hess DR, et al: *Respiratory Care: Principles and Practice.* Philadelphia, WB Saunders, 2002.

Chapter 37—*Figure 37-1,* from Shapiro BA, Harrison RA, Walton JR: *Clinical Application of Arterial Blood Gases,* ed 3. Chicago, Year Book Medical Publishers, 1982; *Figure 37-2,* from Shapiro BA, Harrison RA, Walton JR: *Clinical Application of Arterial Blood Gases,* ed 3. Chicago, Year Book Medical Publishers, 1982; *Figure 37-3,* from Shapiro BA, Peruzzi WT, Kozlowski-Templin R: *Clinical*

Application of Blood Gases, ed 5. Chicago, Mosby, 1994; *Figure 37-4,* from Shapiro BA, Peruzzi WT, Kozlowski-Templin R: *Clinical Application of Blood Gases,* ed 5. Chicago, Mosby, 1994; *Figure 37-5,* from Shapiro BA, Peruzzi WT, Kozlowski-Templin R: *Clinical Application of Blood Gases,* ed 5. Chicago, Mosby, 1994; *Figure 37-6,* courtesy of SenDx Medical, Inc., a Radiometer Company, Carlsbad, CA; *Figure 37-7,* courtesy of i-STAT Corporation, East Windsor, NJ; *Figure 37-8,* from Wilkins RL, Stoller JK, Scanlan CL: *Egan's Fundamentals of Respiratory Care,* ed 8. St. Louis, Mosby, 2003; *Figure 37-9,* from Wilkins RL, Stoller JK, Scanlan CL: *Egan's Fundamentals of Respiratory Care,* ed 8. St. Louis, Mosby, 2003; *Figure 37-10,* modified from Gardner RM: *J Cardiovasc Nurs* 1:79, 1987 [as appears in Wilkins RL, Stoller JK, Scanlan CL: *Egan's Fundamentals of Respiratory Care,* ed 8. St. Louis, Mosby, 2003]; *Figure 37-11,* from Wilkins RL, Stoller JK, Scanlan CL: *Egan's Fundamentals of Respiratory Care,* ed 8. St. Louis, Mosby, 2003; *Figure 37-12,* from Swedlow DB: Capnometry and capnography: the anesthesia disaster early warning system. *Semin Anesth* 5:194-202, 1986; *Figure 37-13,* from Swedlow DB: Capnometry and capnography: the anesthesia disaster early warning system. *Semin Anesth* 5:194-202, 1986; *Figure 37-14,* from Body S, Hartigan P, Sherman S, et al: Nitric oxide: delivery, measurement, and clinical application. *J Cardiothoracic Vasc Anesth* 9:748-763, 1995; *Figure 37-15,* from Wilkins RL, Stoller JK, Scanlan CL: *Egan's Fundamentals of Respiratory Care,* ed 8. St. Louis, Mosby, 2003.

Chapter 38—*Figure 38-1,* from Hess DR, et al: *Respiratory Care: Principles and Practice.* Philadelphia, WB Saunders, 2002; *Figure 38-2,* from Hess DR, et al: *Respiratory Care: Principles and Practice.* Philadelphia, WB Saunders, 2002; *Figure 38-3,* from Hess DR, et al: *Respiratory Care: Principles and Practice.* Philadelphia, WB Saunders, 2002; *Figure 38-5,* from Passy-Muir, Irvine, CA; *Figure 38-7,* from Wilson D: Airway appliances and management. In Kacmarek RM, Stoller JK, editors: *Current Respiratory Care.* Toronto, BC Decker, 1988 (with permission from Elsevier); *Figure 38-8,* modified from McPherson SP: *Respiratory Therapy Equipment,* ed 4. St. Louis, Mosby, 1989 [as appears in Wilkins RL, Stoller JK, Scanlan CL: *Egan's Fundamentals of Respiratory Care,* ed 8. St. Louis, Mosby, 2003; *Figure 38-9,* from Bortner PL, May RA: Artificial airways and tubes. In Eubanks DH, Bone RC, editors: *Principles and Applications of Cardiorespiratory Care Equipment.* St. Louis, Mosby, 1994; *Figure 38-10,* from Hess DR: Managing the artificial airway. *Respir Care* 44:759-772, 1999.

Chapter 39—*Figure 39-1,* modified from Wilkins RL, Stoller JK, Scanlan CL: *Egan's Fundamentals of Respiratory Care,* ed 8. St. Louis, Mosby, 2003. *Figure 39-2,* from Hess DR, et al: *Respiratory Care: Principles and Practice.* Philadelphia, WB Saunders, 2002; *Figure 39-3,* from Hess DR, et al: *Respiratory Care: Principles and Practice.* Philadelphia, WB Saunders, 2002; *Figure 39-4,* from Hess DR, et al: *Respiratory Care: Principles and Practice.* Philadelphia, WB Saunders, 2002; *Figure 39-5,* from Hess DR, et al: *Respiratory Care: Principles and Practice.* Philadelphia, WB Saunders, 2002; *Figure 39-6,* from Hess DR, et al: *Respiratory Care: Principles and Practice.* Philadelphia, WB Saunders, 2002; *Figure 39-7,* from Marini JJ, Rodriguez RM, Lamb VJ: The inspiratory workload of patient-initiated mechanical ventilation. *Am Rev Respir Dis* 134:902-909, 1986; *Figure 39-8,* from Kacmarek RM et al: *Monitoring in Respiratory Care.* St. Louis, Mosby, 1993; *Figure 39-9,* from Hess DR, et al: *Respiratory Care: Principles and Practice.* Philadelphia, WB Saunders, 2002; *Figure 39-10,* from Hess DR, et al: *Respiratory Care: Principles and Practice.* Philadelphia, WB Saunders, 2002; *Figure 39-11,* from Wilkins RL, Stoller JK, Scanlan CL: *Egan's Fundamentals of Respiratory Care,* ed 8. St. Louis, Mosby, 2003; *Figure 39-12,* from Marini JJ, Smith TC, Lamb VJ: External work output and force generation during SIMV. *Am Rev Respir Dis* 138:1169-1179, 1988; *Figure 39-13,* from Imsand C, Feihl F, Perret C, Fitting JW: Regulation of inspiratory neuromuscular output during SIMV. *Anesthesiology* 80:13-22, 1994; *Figure 39-14,* from Hess DR, et al: *Respiratory Care: Principles and Practice.* Philadelphia, WB Saunders, 2002; *Figure 39-15,* from MacIntyre N, Nishimura M, Usada Y, et al: The Nagoya Conference on System Design and Patient-Ventilator Interaction During Pressure Support Ventilation. *Chest* 97:1463-1466, 1990; *Figure 39-16,* from Branson RD, Campbell RS, Davis K, et al: Altering flow rate during maximum pressure support ventilation (PSV max): effects on cardiorespiratory function. *Respir Care* 35:1056-1063, 1990; *Figure 39-17,* from Branson RD, Campbell RS: Pressure support ventilation, patient-ventilator synchrony, and ventilator algorithms. *Respir Care* 43:1043-1047, 1998; *Figure 39-18,* from Tokioka H, Tanaka T, Ishizu T, et al: The effect of breath termination criteria on breathing patterns and the work of breathing during pressure support ventilation. *Anesth Analg* 92:161-165, 2001; *Figure 39-19,* from Guttman J, Eng LE, Fabry B, et al: Continuous calculation of intratracheal pressure in tracheally, intubated patients. *Anesthesiology* 79:503-509, 1993; *Figure 39-20,* from Fabry B, Haberthun C, Zappe D et al: Breathing pattern and additional work of breathing in spontaneously breathing patients with different ventilatory demands during inspiratory pressure support and automatic tube compensation. *Intensive Care Med* 23:545-551, 1997; *Figure 39-21,* from Branson P, Davis K: Dual control modes: combining volume and pressure breaths. *Respir Care Clin North Am* 7:397-408, 2001; *Figure 39-22,* from Younes M: Proportional assist ventilation, a new approach to ventilatory support. *Am Rev Respir Dis* 145:114-120, 1992; *Figure 39-23,* from Younes M: Proportional assist ventilation, a new approach to ventilatory support. *Am Rev Respir Dis* 145:114-120, 1992; *Figure 39-25,* from Neuman P, Golisch W, Strohmeyer A, et al: Influence of different release times on spontaneous breathing pattern during airway pressure release ventilation. *Intensive Care Med* 28:1742, 2002.

Chapter 40—*Figure 40-1,* from Shapiro BA, Harrison RA, Kacmarek RM, et al: *Clinical Application of Respiratory Care,* ed 3. Chicago, Year Book Medical Publishers, 1985; *Figure 40-3,* from Pierson DJ, Kacmarek RM: *Foundations of Respiratory Care.* New York, Churchill Livingstone, 1992; *Figure 40-4,* modified from Goddon S, Fujino Y, Hromi JM, Kacmarek RM: Optimal mean airway pressure during high frequency oscillation. *Anesthesiology* 94:862-868, 2001; *Figure 40-5,* from Pepe PE, Marini JJ: Occult positive end-expiratory pressure in mechanically ventilated patients with airflow obstruction: the auto-PEEP effect. *Am Rev Respir Dis* 126:166-170, 1982; *Figure 40-6,* from Shapiro BA, Harrison RA, Kacmarek RM, et al: *Clinical Application of Respiratory Care,* ed 3. Chicago, Year Book Medical Publishers, 1985; *Figure 40-7,* From Kacmarek RM, et al: *Monitoring in Respiratory Care.* Chicago, Year Book Medical Publishers, 1993; *Figure 40-8,* from Smith TC, Marini JJ: Impact of PEEP on lung mechanics and work of breathing in severe airflow obstruction. *J Appl Physiol* 65:1488-1499, 1988; *Figure 40-9,* from Pierson DJ, Kacmarek RM: *Foundations of Respiratory Care.* New York, Churchill Livingstone, 1992; *Figure 40-10,* From Kacmarek RM, et al: *Monitoring in Respiratory Care.* Chicago, Year Book Medical Publishers, 1993; *Figure 40-11,* from Chao DC, et al: Patient-ventilator trigger asynchrony in prolonged mechanical ventilation. *Chest* 112:1592-1599, 1997.

Chapter 41—*Figure 41-1,* from Spearman CB, Sheldon RL, Egan DF: *Egan's Fundamentals of Respiratory Therapy,* ed 4. St. Louis, Mosby, 1982; *Figure 41-2,* from Maunder RJ, Pierson DJ, Hudson LD: Subcutaneous and mediastinal emphysema: pathophysiology, diagnosis, and management. *Arch Intern Med* 144:1447-1453, 1984; *Figure 41-3,* from Dreyfuss D, Basset G, Solar P, Saumon G: Intermittent positive pressure hyperventilation with high inflation pressures produces pulmonary microvascular injury in rats. *Am Rev Respir Dis* 132:880-884, 1985; *Figure 41-4,* from Webb HH, Tierney D: Experimental pulmonary edema due to intermittent positive pressure ventilation with high inflation pressure, protection by positive end expiratory pressure. *Am Rev Respir Dis* 110:556-565, 1974; *Figure 41-5,* from Marini JJ, Rodriguez RM, Lamb V: The inspiratory workload of patient-initiated mechanical ventilation. *Am Rev Respir Dis* 134:902-909, 1986; *Figure 41-6,* from Fernandez R, Mendez M, Younes M: Effect of ventilatory flow rates on respiratory timing in normal humans. *Am J Respir Crit Care Med* 159:710-719, 1999; *Figure 41-7,* from Chao DC, et al: Patient-ventilator trigger asynchrony in prolonged mechanical ventilation. *Chest* 112:1592-1599, 1997; *Figure 41-8,* from Nunn JF: Carbon dioxide. In Nunn JF, editor: *Applied Respiratory Physiology,* ed 2. London, Butterworth and Co., 1977; *Figure 41-9,* from Goddon S, Fujino Y, Hromi JM, Kacmarek RM: Optimal mean airway pressure during high frequency ventilation. *Anesthesiology* 94:862-868, 2001; *Figure 41-10,* from Leatterman JW, Ravenscraft SA: Low measured auto-PEEP end-expiratory pressure during mechanical ventilation of patients with severe asthma. Hidden auto-positive end expiratory pressure. *Crit Care Med* 24:541-546, 1996.

Chapter 42—*Figure 42-1,* from Carlon CC: High frequency jet ventilation: a prospective randomized evaluation. *Chest* 84:551, 1983; *Figure 42-2,* from Carlon GC, Howland WS: *High Frequency Ventilation in Intensive Care and During Surgery, Lung Biology in Health and Disease Series.* New York, Marcel Dekker, 1985; *Figure 42-3,* from Hurst JM, Branson RD, Davis K Jr: High frequency percussive ventilation in the management of elevated intracranial pressure. *J Trauma* 28:1363-1367,

1988; *Figure 42-4,* from Hurst JM, Branson RD, Davis K Jr: High frequency percussive ventilation in the management of elevated intracranial pressure. *J Trauma* 28:1363-1367, 1988; *Figure 42-5,* from Chang HK: Mechanisms of gas transport during ventilation by high-frequency oscillation. *J Applied Physiol* 56:553-563, 1984.

Chapter 43—*Figure 43-2,* from Ferguson GI, Gilmartin M: CO_2 rebreathing during B_iPAP ventilatory assistance. *Am J Respir Crit Care Med* 151:1126-1135, 1995.

Chapter 44—*Figure 44-1,* from Ravenscraft SA: Tracheal gas insufflation: adjunct to conventional mechanical ventilation. *Respir Care* 41:105-111, 1996; *Figure 44-2,* from Ravenscraft SA, et al: Tracheal gas insufflation augments CO_2 clearance during mechanical ventilation. *Am J Respir Crit Care Med* 148:345-351, 1993; *Figure 44-3,* from Adams AB: Tracheal gas insufflation [TGI]. *Respir Care* 41:285-293, 1996; *Figure 44-4,* from Imanaka H, Kacmarek RM, Ritz R, et al: Tracheal gas insufflation-pressure control versus volume control ventilation: a lung model study. *Am J Respir Crit Care Med* 153:1019-1029, 1996.

Chapter 45—*Figure 45-1,* from Chatte G, et al: Prone position in mechanically ventilated patients with severe acute respiratory failure. *Am J Respir Crit Care Med* 155:473-488, 1997; *Figure 45-2,* from Mure M, et al: Dramatic effects on oxygenation of inpatients with severe acute lung insufficiency treated in the prone position. *Crit Care Med* 25:1539-1544, 1997.

Page references followed by "f" indicate figures, by "t" indicate tables, and by "b" indicate boxes.